STUDY GUIDE

to

DSM-5®

STUDY GUIDE

to

DSM-5®

Edited by

Laura Weiss Roberts, M.D., M.A.
Alan K. Louie, M.D.

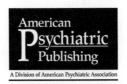

American Psychiatric Publishing
A Division of American Psychiatric Association

Washington, DC
London, England

To buy 25–99 copies of this or any other APP title at a 20% discount, please contact Customer Service at appi@psych.org or 800–368–5777. If you wish to buy 100 or more copies of the same title, please e-mail us at bulksales@psych.org for a price quote.

Copyright © 2015 American Psychiatric Association
ALL RIGHTS RESERVED

Manufactured in the United States of America on acid-free paper
18 17 16 15 14   5 4 3 2 1
First Edition

Typeset in Adobe's AGaramond and Formata.

American Psychiatric Publishing
A Division of American Psychiatric Association
1000 Wilson Boulevard
Arlington, VA 22209-3901
www.appi.org

Library of Congress Cataloging-in-Publication Data
Study guide to DSM-5 / edited by Laura Weiss Roberts, Alan K. Louie.—First edition.
     p. ; cm.
   Includes bibliographical references and index.
   ISBN 978-1-58562-464-5 (alk. paper)
   I. Roberts, Laura Weiss, 1960– , editor. II. Louie, Alan K., 1955– , editor. III. American Psychiatric Publishing, publisher.
   [DNLM: 1. Diagnostic and statistical manual of mental disorders. 5th ed. 2. Mental Disorders—classification—Case Reports. 3. Mental Disorders—classification—Problems and Exercises. 4. Mental Disorders—diagnosis—Case Reports. 5. Mental Disorders—diagnosis—Problems and Exercises. 6. Diagnosis, Differential—Case Reports. 7. Diagnosis, Differential—Problems and Exercises. WM 18.2]
   RC457
   616.890076—dc23

                                                                                    2014030042

British Library Cataloguing in Publication Data
A CIP record is available from the British Library.

Contents

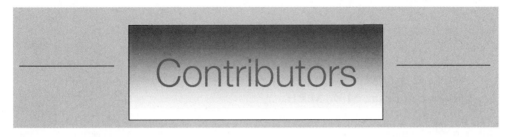
Contributors

Elias Aboujaoude, M.D., M.A.
Clinical Professor of Psychiatry and Behavioral Sciences, Stanford University School of Medicine, Stanford, California

Bruce A. Arnow, Ph.D.
Professor and Associate Chair, Department of Psychiatry and Behavioral Sciences, Stanford University School of Medicine, and Director, Psychosocial Treatment Clinic, Stanford University Medical Center, Stanford, California

Sepideh N. Bajestan, M.D., Ph.D.
Neuropsychiatry Fellow, Department of Psychiatry and Behavioral Sciences, Stanford University School of Medicine, Stanford, California

Richard Balon, M.D.
Professor, Departments of Psychiatry and Behavioral Neurosciences and Anesthesiology; Program Director, Adult Psychiatry Residency Program, Wayne State University School of Medicine, Detroit, Michigan

Cara Bohon, Ph.D.
Assistant Professor of Psychiatry and Behavioral Sciences, Stanford University School of Medicine, Stanford, California

Kimberly L. Brodsky, Ph.D.
Clinical Assistant Professor (Affiliated) of Psychiatry and Behavioral Sciences, Stanford University School of Medicine, Stanford, California; Attending Psychologist, VA Palo Alto Health Care System, Palo Alto, California

John H. Coverdale, M.D., M.Ed.
Professor of Psychiatry, Behavioral Sciences, and Medical Ethics, Baylor College of Medicine, Houston, Texas

Whitney Daniels, M.D.
Clinical Instructor of Psychiatry and Behavioral Sciences, Division of Child and Adolescent Psychiatry, Stanford University School of Medicine; Staff Psychiatrist, Lucile Salter Packard Children's Hospital, Stanford, California

Jennifer Derenne, M.D.
Clinical Associate Professor of Psychiatry and Behavioral Sciences, Stanford University School of Medicine, Stanford, California

Kathleen Kara Fitzpatrick, Ph.D.
Clinical Assistant Professor of Psychiatry and Behavioral Sciences, Stanford University School of Medicine, Stanford, California

M. Rameen Ghorieshi, M.D., M.P.H.
Adjunct Clinical Instructor of Psychiatry and Behavioral Sciences, Stanford University School of Medicine, Stanford, California; Psychiatrist, Palo Alto Center for Mind Body Health, Palo Alto, California

Cheryl Gore-Felton, Ph.D.
Associate Dean for Academic Affairs, Stanford University School of Medicine; Professor and Associate Chairman of Psychiatry and Behavioral Sciences, Stanford University School of Medicine, Stanford, California

Carlos C. Greaves, M.D.
Associate Clinical Professor of Psychiatry and Behavioral Sciences, Adjunct Faculty, Stanford University School of Medicine, Stanford, California

Thomas W. Heinrich, M.D.
Professor of Psychiatry and Behavioral Medicine, Professor of Family and Community Medicine, Director of the Division of Consultation-Liaison Psychiatry, Medical College of Wisconsin, Milwaukee, Wisconsin

Robert M. Holaway, Ph.D.
Clinical Assistant Professor of Psychiatry and Behavioral Sciences, Stanford University School of Medicine, Stanford, California

David S. Hong, M.D.
Assistant Professor of Psychiatry and Behavioral Sciences, Stanford University School of Medicine, Stanford, California

Honor Hsin, M.D., Ph.D.
Resident in Psychiatry and Behavioral Sciences, Stanford University School of Medicine, Stanford, California

Terence A. Ketter, M.D.
Professor of Psychiatry and Behavioral Sciences and Chief, Bipolar Disorders Clinic, Stanford University School of Medicine, Stanford, California

Cheryl Koopman, Ph.D.
Professor of Psychiatry and Behavioral Sciences, Stanford University School of Medicine, Stanford, California

John Lauriello, M.D.
Professor and Chairman of Psychiatry, University of Missouri School of Medicine, Columbia, Missouri

Alan K. Louie, M.D.
Professor, Associate Chair, and Director of Education, Department of Psychiatry and Behavioral Sciences, Stanford University School of Medicine, Stanford, California

Daniel Mason, M.D.
Resident in Psychiatry and Behavioral Sciences, Stanford University School of Medicine, Stanford, California

Shefali Miller, M.D.
Clinical Assistant Professor of Psychiatry and Behavioral Sciences, Stanford University School of Medicine, Stanford, California

Ruth O'Hara, Ph.D.
Associate Professor of Psychiatry and Behavioral Sciences, Stanford University School of Medicine, Stanford, California

Maurice M. Ohayon, M.D., D.Sc., Ph.D.
Professor of Psychiatry and Behavioral Sciences; Chief of the Division of Public Mental Health and Population Sciences, Stanford University School of Medicine, Stanford, California

Michael J. Ostacher, M.D., M.P.H., M.M.Sc.
Associate Professor of Psychiatry and Behavioral Sciences, Stanford University School of Medicine, Stanford, California; Staff Psychiatrist, VA Palo Alto Health Care System, Palo Alto, California

Yasmin Owusu, M.D.
Child and Adolescent Psychiatry Fellow, Department of Psychiatry and Behavioral Sciences, Stanford University School of Medicine, Stanford, California

Michelle Primeau, M.D.
Clinical Instructor of Psychiatry and Behavioral Sciences, Division of Sleep Medicine, Stanford University School of Medicine, Stanford, California

Tahir Rahman, M.D.
Assistant Professor of Psychiatry, University of Missouri School of Medicine, Columbia, Missouri

Daryn Reicherter, M.D.
Clinical Associate Professor, Department of Psychiatry and Behavioral Sciences, Stanford University School of Medicine, Stanford, California

Margaret Reynolds-May, M.D.
Resident in Psychiatry and Behavioral Sciences, Stanford University School of Medicine, Stanford, California

Laura Weiss Roberts, M.D., M.A.
Chairman and Katharine Dexter McCormick and Stanley McCormick Memorial Professor, Department of Psychiatry and Behavioral Sciences, Stanford University School of Medicine, and Chief, Psychiatry Service, Stanford Hospital and Clinics, Stanford, California; and Editor-in-Chief, Academic Psychiatry

Allyson C. Rosen, Ph.D.
Clinical Associate Professor (Affiliated) of Psychiatry and Behavioral Sciences, Stanford University School of Medicine, Stanford, California; Clinical Neuropsychologist, VA Palo Alto Health Care System, Palo Alto, California

Ann C. Schwartz, M.D.
Associate Professor, Department of Psychiatry and Behavioral Sciences, and Residency Training Director, Emory University, Atlanta, Georgia

Yelizaveta I. Sher, M.D.
Instructor of Psychiatry and Behavioral Sciences, Stanford University School of Medicine, Stanford, California

Daphne Simeon, M.D.
Associate Professor of Psychiatry, Mount Sinai School of Medicine, New York, New York

David Spiegel, M.D.
Willson Professor in the School of Medicine and Associate Chair of Psychiatry and Behavioral Sciences, Stanford University School of Medicine; Medical Director, Stanford Center for Integrative Medicine, Stanford University Medical Center, Stanford, California

Hans Steiner, M.D.
Professor of Psychiatry and Behavioral Sciences at the Lucile Salter Packard Children's Hospital, Emeritus, Stanford University School of Medicine, Stanford, California

Mickey Trockel, M.D., Ph.D.
Assistant Clinical Professor of Psychiatry and Behavioral Sciences, Stanford University School of Medicine, Stanford, California

Tonita E. Wroolie, Ph.D.
Clinical Assistant Professor of Psychiatry and Behavioral Sciences, Stanford University School of Medicine, Stanford, California

Jerome Yesavage, M.D.
Professor of Psychiatry and Behavioral Sciences and, by courtesy, of Neurology and Neurological Sciences, Stanford University School of Medicine, Stanford, California; Associate Chief of Staff for Mental Health, VA Palo Alto Health Care System, Palo Alto, California

Brian Yochim, Ph.D.
Clinical Assistant Professor (Affiliated) of Psychiatry and Behavioral Sciences, Stanford University School of Medicine, Stanford, California; Clinical Neuropsychologist, VA Palo Alto Health Care System, Palo Alto, California

Maya Yutsis, Ph.D.
Clinical Neuropsychologist, VA Palo Alto Health Care System, Palo Alto, California

Sanno E. Zack, Ph.D.
Clinical Assistant Professor of Psychiatry and Behavioral Sciences, Stanford University School of Medicine, Stanford, California

Disclosures of Interest

The contributors have declared all forms of support received within the 12 months prior to manuscript submission that may represent a competing interest in relation to their work published in this volume, as follows:

Elias Aboujaoude, M.D., M.A. *Research support:* Roche
Terence A. Ketter, M.D. *Grant/research support:* AstraZeneca, Cephalon, Eli Lilly and Company, Pfizer, and Sunovion; *Consultant fees:* Allergan, Avanir Pharmaceuticals, Bristol-Myers Squibb, Cephalon, Forest Pharmaceuticals, Janssen, Merck, Sunovion, and Teva; *Lecture honoraria:* Abbott Laboratories, AstraZeneca, GlaxoSmithKline, and Otsuka; *Publication royalties:* American Psychiatric Publishing. *Dr. Ketter's spouse is an employee of and holds stock in Janssen.*
John Lauriello, M.D. *Research support:* Sunovion (clinical trial), Janssen (event monitoring board), Shire (data safety monitoring board), Eli Lilly (paper, no remuneration); *Advisory panel:* Otsuka; *Pharmaceutical CME activity:* Otsuka, Sunovion
Shefali Miller, M.D. *Funds to travel to attend Investigators Meeting:* Elan Pharmaceuticals

The following contributors have no competing interests to disclose:
Bruce A. Arnow, Ph.D.; Sepideh N. Bajestan, M.D., Ph.D.; Richard Balon, M.D.; Cara Bohon, Ph.D.; Kimberly L. Brodsky, Ph.D.; John H. Coverdale, M.D., M.Ed.; Whitney Daniels, M.D.; Jennifer Derenne, M.D.; Kathleen Kara Fitzpatrick, Ph.D.; M. Rameen Ghorieshi, M.D., M.P.H.; Cheryl Gore-Felton, Ph.D.; Carlos C. Greaves, M.D.; Thomas W. Heinrich, M.D.; Robert M. Holaway, Ph.D.; David S. Hong, M.D.; Honor Hsin, M.D., Ph.D.; Cheryl Koopman, Ph.D.; Alan K. Louie, M.D.; Daniel Mason, M.D.; Ruth O'Hara, Ph.D.; Maurice M. Ohayon, M.D., D.Sc., Ph.D.; Michael J. Ostacher, M.D., M.P.H., M.M.Sc.; Yasmin Owusu, M.D.; Michelle Primeau, M.D.; Tahir Rahman, M.D.; Daryn Reicherter, M.D.; Margaret Reynolds-May, M.D.; Laura Weiss Roberts, M.D., M.A.; Allyson C. Rosen, Ph.D.; Ann C. Schwartz, M.D.; Yelizaveta I. Sher, M.D.; Daphne Simeon, M.D.; David Spiegel, M.D.; Hans Steiner, M.D.; Mickey Trockel, M.D., Ph.D.; Tonita E. Wroolie, Ph.D.; Jerome Yesavage, M.D.; Brian Yochim, Ph.D.; Maya Yutsis, Ph.D.; Sanno E. Zack, Ph.D.

Introduction

The *Diagnostic and Statistical Manual of Mental Disorders* (DSM) is the most widely used manual for the diagnosis of mental disorders. As such, it has tremendous influence over the clinical care and research of these disorders and the understanding of patients, families, and the public regarding mental disorders. Knowledge of and facility with DSM is a necessity for clinicians and other professionals who work with people living with or affected by mental disorders. DSM-5, the fifth full edition of this manual, is an essential resource for those training in all fields of physical and mental health.

DSM-5 represents years of investigation and debate about how to describe and organize mental illness processes and conditions. DSM-5 embodies the tensions between what to keep of the old and what to change with the new—tensions that are natural and expected for all rapidly evolving fields such as psychiatry. Until the next edition, DSM-5 will be a key reference point in this evolution for further hypothesis testing and for comparison with other formal schemata with compatible but not identical aims, such as the Research Domain Criteria of the National Institute of Mental Health (see www.nimh.nih.gov/research-priorities/rdoc/index.shtml) and the sequential iterations of the World Health Organization's *International Statistical Classification of Diseases and Related Health Problems* (ICD).

DSM-5 includes a chapter for each diagnostic class, each with a number of disorders that may be viewed along a spectrum. Each disorder is fully described, including epidemiological "statistical" information and evidence-informed criteria that must be met for a diagnosis of that disorder. This architecture for the text has been the traditional organization of the manual—that is, one that is essentially focused on psychopathology and is disorder centered. The overarching structure of DSM-5 differs from previous DSM versions in that diagnostic classes of disorders with overlapping or similar features have been placed, wherever possible, in an intentional sequence.

Left to the reader is learning how these disorders are expressed and manifest in individuals in one's clinical practice. The human experience of a condition—from the perspective of the affected individual and from the perspective of the clinician—cannot be captured in "criteria" and "statistics." What does a person say when he or she experiences one, or more, of these disorders? How does the clinician talk with a patient about these experiences? Clinicians may assign a diagnosis to a patient, but most certainly the person cannot be reduced to a set of criteria, a diagnosis, or a list of diagnoses. The biological, psychological, and sociological particulars of each individual color how an illness, a "diagnosis," is expressed. The *Study Guide to DSM-5* aims to help translate the printed diagnostic criteria of DSM-5 into the lived experiences of patients.

The *Study Guide to DSM-5* should be used side-by-side with the full text of DSM-5. In this *Study Guide,* we take a patient-centered approach, complementing the more disorder-centered organization of DSM-5. We introduce consistent features in the diagnostic chapters to help make the concepts of DSM-5 come to life. For example, each of the chapters in Part II offers case vignettes that illustrate patterns of illness, including expected and, at times, unexpected elements, and demonstrate how age, gender, and several other cultural factors influence the cases. Other vignettes highlight patient-clinician interactions in the process of an interview and provide sample questions asked by the clinician to better appreciate the patient's unique experience of a disorder. The diagnosis-oriented chapters in Part II also provide "diagnostic pearls" and points of importance to daily clinical practice. The *Study Guide* provides a context for all of the diagnoses in DSM-5, but instead of covering every diagnosis superficially, we chose to dive into greater detail ("in depth") for certain very interesting or very prevalent diagnoses that illustrate each diagnostic class.

Because this book is a study guide, we have tried to make it "learner friendly" to facilitate the processes of registering new information from DSM-5, recalling it, and then considering how it will apply in the reader's work. Part I puts DSM-5 in context, in terms of explaining diagnostic frameworks and indicating how these might shape work with patients. Part II focuses on the diagnostic classes in DSM-5. To stimulate learning about the disorders, each of these chapters has a self-assessment section, including key concepts, questions to discuss with colleagues and mentors, complicated cases, and short-answer questions and answers (the answers are generally based on information in either the *Study Guide* or DSM-5). Part III ("Test Yourself") is replete with more than 100 questions, including brief vignettes covering a wide range of diagnoses and patient circumstances to aid the application of DSM-5 to clinical work and training.

DSM-5 contains some sections that are not reviewed in this *Study Guide* due to space limitations. Examples include "Other Mental Disorders," "Medication-Induced Movement Disorders and Other Adverse Effects of Medication," "Other Conditions That May Be a Focus of Clinical Attention," "Conditions for Further Study," "Highlights of Changes From DSM-IV to DSM-5," and "Glossary of Technical Terms." The reader is encouraged to refer directly to DSM-5 in order to become familiar with these important elements. For instance, the DSM-5 section "Other Conditions That May Be a Focus of Clinical Attention" includes psychosocial stressors that may influence the presentation of a diagnosis. "Conditions for Future Study" describes conditions that are being studied to determine if they should or should not be considered as diagnoses in subsequent iterations of DSM. The learner will also find the section "Highlights of Changes From DSM-IV to DSM-5" and the "Glossary of Technical Terms" quite handy.

Because this *Study Guide* is a companion book to DSM-5, its content intentionally parallels that of DSM-5. At times, the terminology and even phraseology in the *Study Guide* may be the same as in DSM-5 to provide a bridge between specific text in the *Study Guide* and DSM-5. The authors of the *Study Guide to DSM-5* have permission from American Psychiatric Publishing to use material from DSM-5.

The descriptions of people throughout the *Study Guide*—for example, in case vignettes and questions and answers—are hypothetical. Any resemblance to actual people is completely by chance, and names have been chosen randomly. Some of these descriptions of people include interactions with a clinician and questions that a clinician might ask. These described interactions are only meant to be illustrative, and the clinician questions are only sample questions. The descriptions are not of complete clinical interviews or analyses of cases, and many essential details have been omitted due to space limitations.

The authors of this *Study Guide* have attempted to ensure that all information in the *Study Guide* is accurate at the time of writing and consistent with general psychiatric and medical standards. As medical research and practice continue to advance, however, information and standards may change. Specific situations may require a specific response not included in this *Study Guide*. The editors and authors cannot assume any legal liability for any mistakes of commission or omission in this study guide.

Because this is a study guide for a diagnostic and statistical manual, it is not about therapies and interventions, and no information in this *Study Guide* should be construed as providing treatment recommendations. For the above reasons and because human and mechanical errors sometimes occur, we recommend that readers follow the advice of physicians directly involved in their care or the care of a member of their family.

We thank the many authors of the chapters and question-and-answer sections in this *Study Guide,* who have been immensely generous with their expertise and responsiveness in preparing this book. We offer our unending appreciation to Ann Tennier and Melinda Hantke at Stanford University School of Medicine, and Ann Eng, Senior Developmental Editor at American Psychiatric Publishing, for their outstanding support in preparing the *Study Guide*. We acknowledge with gratitude American Psychiatric Publishing, Robert E. Hales, M.D., Editor-in-Chief, and John McDuffie, Associate Publisher, for making this project possible and advising us along the way. Laura Roberts wishes to thank her colleagues who have contributed to this book and to express her loving appreciation to her family. Alan Louie wishes to thank his wife, children, and parents for their loving support in the past and present.

We wish, most importantly, to thank *you,* Dear Reader—no matter what your discipline, profession, time of life, or walk of life—for your engagement with this *Study Guide*. We hope that our work will help in your learning and in your efforts to improve the lives of people who turn to you for understanding and for their care.

Laura Weiss Roberts, M.D., M.A.
Alan K. Louie, M.D.
Stanford, California

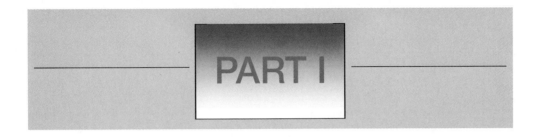

PART I

Foundations

Learning Objectives

- Describe the role, value, and limitations of DSM diagnostic criteria.
- Describe the role of the clinical interview in arriving at a psychiatric diagnosis conforming to DSM-5 criteria.
- Explain the biopsychosocial model and its relevance to the approach of DSM-5.
- Describe the role of psychiatric diagnoses in clinical communication.
- List patient benefits and burdens associated with receiving a psychiatric diagnosis.
- Characterize different approaches to diagnostic classification.

1

Diagnosis and DSM-5

Laura Weiss Roberts, M.D., M.A.
Mickey Trockel, M.D., Ph.D.

Clinicians see patterns. They see patterns in the experiences, behaviors, and physical findings of their patients. Clinicians seek to understand these aspects of patients' lives—the nature, timing, and sequence of experiences, findings, attributes, and behaviors—and in so doing, clinicians diagnose.

The diagnosis is an interpretation or judgment made with more or less certainty regarding how the pattern recognized in one patient's life compares with that of others seen throughout clinical medicine. It is through this comparative framework that a diagnosis can help guide the search for other distinguishing features of an illness process, may reveal an underlying cause, may inform the therapeutic approach to be undertaken, and may tell much about what the future holds for the patient and all who love and care for him or her. DSM-5 provides the current comparative framework for psychiatric illness.

DSM-5 is the fifth full version of the *Diagnostic and Statistical Manual of Mental Disorders*—a guidebook for characterizing significant mental health conditions that affect people throughout the world. DSM-5 has evolved to become more rigorous and comprehensive, as described in Chapter 3, "Understanding Different Approaches to Diagnostic Classification," and this manual represents the current thinking of master clinicians and scientists in psychiatry, a specialty of medicine; in clinical psychology; and in related health professions. Where convincing evidence is available, DSM-5 diagnoses are informed by evidence from the basic and clinical neurosciences and behavioral sciences. The diagnosis of mental health conditions, like physical health conditions, often relies on data that are descriptive or subjective in nature—at times with little empirical verification and often lacking clear biological explanation. (See Chapter 3 for greater detail on diagnostic classification systems and underlying ques-

3

tions of validity.) Because of these challenges, wherever possible DSM-5 includes the use of formal assessments or measures to bring greater consistency and precision to the diagnostic process. Taken together, the DSM-5 diagnoses represent a useful system for characterizing highly diverse phenomena across highly diverse settings.

Perhaps most importantly, DSM-5 diagnostic criteria offer a valuable framework for clinicians as they work to help their patients and also offer a common language between different specialties. The DSM diagnostic criteria may be used in communicating and generating ideas that will allow for a greater understanding of a patient's condition as well as its possible origins and likely future path. Diagnostic hypotheses may guide additional data gathering—obtaining more detailed information regarding the patient's history, for example, or new laboratory results—that in turn will allow some ideas to be eliminated and others to be supported. This iterative process of hypothesis generation and empirical testing is paramount to arrive at a well-reasoned and carefully substantiated diagnosis, the basis for therapeutic decision-making and for the best outcome for the patient.

Arriving at an accurate diagnosis is important to sound clinical care, yet being given a diagnosis brings burdens and risks, as well as benefits, to patients. The authority to render the diagnosis is the power to wield both the gift of understanding and relief on the one hand and the problem of labeling and possible stigmatization on the other. Lessening the weight of psychiatric disease burden while also seeking to "do no harm" can be a difficult balance to attain, especially given the prejudices and misunderstandings that exist throughout society related to neuropsychiatric diseases and related conditions. The hallmark of an excellent clinician is therefore not simply the capacity to diagnose an illness correctly. An excellent clinician possesses the professional judgment to diagnose an illness with rigor and also with an appreciation for the experience of the illness and the full meaning of having it "named" in the context of the patient's life.

Careful study of DSM-5 diagnostic criteria, coupled with clinical experience and informed by study of relevant basic and applied sciences, fosters the development of professional judgment. For both clinicians in training and experienced clinicians engaged in lifelong learning, the *Study Guide to DSM-5* helps in this goal.

DSM-5 and the Roles and Attributes of Diagnosis

There is a story about a man looking for his lost car keys one dark evening. He looks under the nearest lamppost, although he likely dropped the keys a block away. When asked why he was looking in that spot, he responded that he was looking in the only place he could—where he had enough light to see. Discerning the fundamental basis or underpinning of a patient's mental health complaint often requires looking where the light is dim at best. Indeed, in spite of increasing effort to bridge the gap between neuroscience discovery and clinical practice, few findings have as yet been able to shed much light on the exact causes of psychiatric diseases (Insel 2009). Although discouraging to some, the mystery of the functions and pathology of the human brain represents an extraordinary frontier. The observation that there are many unanswered questions in neuroscience is for many individuals a "call" to explore matters of importance to humankind.

Without definitive neuroscience to provide causal explanations of human health and disease, DSM-5 necessarily relies on descriptions—things patients experience and say about their experiences ("symptoms") and things observed by clinicians and others ("signs") and, to a lesser extent, laboratory findings and neuroimaging results. DSM-5, with its descriptive, or "phenomenological," rather than a causal, or "etiological," approach, has an alloy of scientific evidence and expert consensus opinion as its foundation. As such, with anticipated advances in science and deepening expertise, DSM-5 is an intentional "work in progress." DSM-5 is best understood as a systematic framework, informed by experience and evidence, that reflects maturation beyond prior diagnostic systems and yet, because it is a "living" document, is certain to change with time.

DSM-5 is an evolving and phenomenologically oriented diagnostic framework and has importance beyond clinical care, health science, and education in the health professions. This framework also has myriad applications in society and is used each day by teachers, attorneys, judges, policy makers, hospital administrators, insurers, and interested members of the public. For all who use DSM-5, it is wise to recall that biomedical science is a human endeavor and that the history of medicine is rich with examples in which incremental, systematic, and evidence-driven approaches focusing on observable phenomena yielded remarkable improvements in health outcomes, for example, even when underlying causes were unknown. Just as John Snow was able to identify the utility of avoiding consumption of contaminated water to prevent spread of cholera *before* the identification of its bacterial cause (Paneth 2004), the use of empirically derived, descriptive criteria-based diagnostic approaches can—and often does—yield relief of psychiatric morbidity. Unlike the cause of cholera—the bacterium *Vibrio cholerae*—the causes of psychiatric morbidity involve many biological pathways and complicated environmental interactions that will be elucidated gradually in the coming decades (Frances and Widiger 2012). Nevertheless, exciting basic and clinical neuroscience holds great promise at this time and its implications are revealed each day. While waiting for new and more clearly definitive scientific answers regarding the causes and prevention of mental illness, clinicians will use the increasingly rigorous and careful descriptive approach of DSM-5 to help in applying this work in all settings, whether clinical, community, classroom, or court.

For the clinician and for the patient, the DSM-5 diagnosis serves many functions and has many attributes. The diagnosis may be understood as a hypothesis, as a way of communicating, as a source of distress, as a risk, and as a therapeutic "gift." Each of these aspects of the diagnosis is important, with bearing on the approach of the clinician and the health of patients.

Diagnosis as a Hypothesis

The DSM-5 diagnostic criteria allow clinicians to form hypotheses about their patients' mental health difficulties that imply commonality with other patients who present with similar symptom clusters and patterns. When the hypothesis is well founded, a knowledge base derived from the clinical history of other patients with the same diagnosis is available as a basis of understanding to build on in the process of evaluating data gathered through further diagnostic inquiry and in making treatment decisions.

When clinicians apply systematic reasoning to the clinical evaluation process, they use clinical data to formulate and test diagnostic hypotheses. Early conceptualization of diagnostic reasoning posited that establishing a clinical diagnosis involves hypothesis testing, in which a limited set of hypotheses formulated early in the process guides further data gathering (Elstein et al. 1978). Health education methods often focus on this process, teaching clinicians to use initial presenting clinical data to create what is called a *differential diagnosis*—a short list of plausible diagnosis hypotheses. Clinicians are taught to use the differential diagnosis to focus additional data gathering and to use evolving clinical information to narrow and refine the diagnostic possibilities that may be at work in the situation. More recent application of evidence-based medicine adds precision to the process by employing decision theory, in which new data are used to adjust estimated probability of diagnoses (Elstein and Schwartz 2002).

For routine medical cases, careful hypothesis testing may progress to more efficient pattern recognition. More advanced clinicians will find it necessary to engage in deductive reasoning–driven hypothesis testing only when confronted with the most complex cases (Elstein and Schwartz 2002; Moayyeri et al. 2011). Although expert psychiatric clinicians are likely to become more efficient at DSM-5–based pattern recognition with time, there is unique utility of careful hypothesis testing during the process of psychiatric diagnosis, even for experienced clinicians. DSM-5 criteria are based almost entirely on latent (unobservable) variables. The necessary reliance on latent variables reduces reliability and validity in any diagnostic process and is the bane of current psychiatric clinical practice. Perhaps to a higher degree than in most other medical fields, the adage "knowing is the enemy of learning" rings true in psychiatric diagnosis. Overreliance on pattern recognition to establish an efficient diagnosis dismisses the opportunity to discover an alternative and more accurate explanation of a patient's problem.

Consider a 30-year-old woman with depressed mood, poor concentration, low energy, weight gain, and psychomotor slowing over the last 2 months. Her pattern "looks" like a major depressive episode, and this diagnosis may, in the end, be accurate. However, if the clinician looks no further, he may miss an underlying, and correctable, hypothyroid problem responsible for the patient's symptoms. The correct diagnosis would be readily discoverable through careful deductive reasoning to evaluate a limited set of plausible diagnoses. This example serves as a reminder of the importance of professional judgment in the use of DSM-5 criteria. The DSM-5 diagnostic system—which, of necessity, is oriented toward patterns of observations, findings, and symptoms rather than causal explanations—if applied without care will give rise to superficial, premature, and incorrect diagnostic conclusions. To fulfill professional responsibilities with patients, clinicians must engage in careful consideration of reasonable alternative diagnoses and must rigorously test diagnostic hypotheses against available data, even in apparently simple and straightforward cases.

Case Example: Importance of Refining a Diagnostic Hypothesis

Ms. Evans, age 27, was awaiting honorable discharge from her service in Iraq with the U.S. Navy when her colleagues noticed she looked increasingly fearful and was talking about hearing voices telling her the world was going to be destroyed in 2020. With Ms.

Evans's permission, the evaluating psychiatrist interviewed one of her closest colleagues, who indicated that Ms. Evans had not been taking good care of her personal hygiene for several months. Ms. Evans said she was depressed. The psychiatrist also learned that Ms. Evans's performance of her military job duties had declined during this time and that her commanding officer had recommended she be evaluated by a psychiatrist approximately 2 weeks earlier, for possible depression.

On interview, Ms. Evans endorsed believing the world was going to end soon and indicated that several times she has heard an audible voice that repeated this information. She has a maternal uncle with schizophrenia, and her mother has a diagnosis of bipolar I disorder. Ms. Evans's toxicology screen is positive for tetrahydrocannabinol (THC). The evaluating psychiatrist informed Ms. Evans that she had made a tentative diagnosis of schizophrenia.

Questions to Consider

- In thinking about this case, what are your thoughts regarding the tentative diagnosis of schizophrenia that the psychiatrist shared with Ms. Evans?
- Should the psychiatrist have made a tentative diagnosis?
- Should the psychiatrist have shared this information with Ms. Evans at this time?
- Will Ms. Evans's future situation, such as clinical care, military status, employment, and family and personal life, be affected significantly by this diagnostic hypothesis?
- What substantiation may be possible with additional clinical data?
- What are the benefits and burdens that go with this diagnostic hypothesis?

The time invested in refining a diagnostic hypothesis pays dividends in the process of formulating, implementing, and evaluating a treatment plan. An accurate psychiatric diagnosis opens the door to a growing body of evidence-based treatments and slowly emerging adaptive treatment algorithms (Lavori and Dawson 2008) that will help mental health clinicians tailor treatment to the presentation and initial treatment response of individual patients. A hypothesized diagnosis will also help clinicians evaluate observed treatment response against expected treatment response characterized in available literature on the basis of other patients with the same diagnosis. This comparison may also provide additional data that help clinicians to further refine the dynamic diagnostic hypothesis-making process. At several points during the course of clinical care, open discussion of the working diagnostic hypothesis with the patient can facilitate collaborative, ethically sound, treatment decision-making. When the clinician and the patient are collaboratively working together to make treatment decisions, the likelihood that treatment plans will be successfully implemented increases.

Diagnosis as a Way of Communicating

To the degree that the DSM-5 criteria are reliable, deriving a diagnosis facilitates precision and parsimony in clinical communication. A working diagnosis facilitates communication between individual patients and their clinicians, between members of a treatment team, between clinicians and researchers, and in conversations with families and stakeholders such as insurers, employers, and teachers. In one or a few short words, a diagnosis summarizes a wealth of descriptive information in all of these contexts.

Patients are increasingly aware of mental health diagnostic criteria, because of the explosion of Internet-based health education. Although Internet-based information varies in accuracy, a large number of patients now recognize symptoms of common diagnoses such as major depressive disorder. Some patients can and do present for mental health evaluation with an opening statement such as "I'm worried I have post-traumatic stress disorder." Other patients are likely to accurately report a diagnosis they received previously from another clinician. Some patients may not present with a preconceived notion of their own diagnosis but will recognize some of the symptoms associated with their hypothesized diagnosis, because of experience with a friend or family member who had the same diagnosis. In all of these scenarios, the short words making up the diagnostic title convey, to varying degrees, a large amount of shared understanding that facilitates communication between the patient and clinician.

Information sharing with a treatment team and in clinical consultation ideally will be efficient and accurate. A diagnosis rapidly provides a wealth of information regarding clinical signs, symptoms, and probable course of illness from volumes of relevant research and immense clinical experience. Consider the following beginning to a case presentation:

> Mr. Samuels, a 25-year-old man, was brought to the emergency department by his father for assessment after he was found wandering in the park, muttering under his breath that he needed to get away from the FBI. He had left his house 2 days earlier after appearing increasingly anxious and withdrawn.

Now, consider the amount of additional information included in this initial case description by including a short statement regarding a clearly determined diagnosis:

> Mr. Samuels, a 25-year-old man *with a previously well-established diagnosis of schizophrenia*, was brought to the emergency department by his father for assessment after he was found wandering in the park, muttering under his breath that he needed to get away from the FBI. He had left his house 2 days earlier after appearing increasingly anxious and withdrawn.

The short description "a 25-year-old man with a previously well-established diagnosis of schizophrenia" immediately evokes a common understanding based on study of professional literature and experience with other patients with the same diagnosis. Although an astute listener will always be mindful of less likely possible explanations, a listener is more likely, when hearing the second presentation, to focus on a narrowed set of highly relevant concerns. An accurate diagnosis facilitates effective and efficient "dense" communication in clinical teaching, consultation, and all forms of treatment team collaboration.

Clinical diagnoses also convey salient information that when coupled with associated epidemiology, helps guide public policy for funding of research and clinical services. Expert groups of clinicians determine diagnostic criteria. Epidemiologists then use diagnostic criteria to estimate incidence, prevalence, and other parameters that indicate public health burden associated with the disease. One example is the measure of years of life lost due to disability (YLD). For example, depressive disorders are the leading cause of YLD throughout the world, for both men and women, across higher- and lower-income countries (World Health Organization 2008). Alcohol use disorders, schizophrenia, and bipolar disorder are also on the "top 10" list. Average disability-adjusted life years lost (DALY) is another measure in which mental disorders are prominent. The DALY measure characterizes years of life lost both to premature mortality and to living with disability associated with having a specific diagnosis. In middle-income and high-income countries throughout the world, depressive disorders represent the diagnosis with the highest DALY estimates, and in low-income countries, these disorders are the eighth leading cause of years lost from premature death and disability. By 2030, depressive disorders are anticipated to be the greatest source of disease burden throughout the world, moving ahead of the current leading causes—causes that are infectious and communicable in nature. These indicators of public health burden assist policy makers in deciding how to allocate funding for research leading to prevention and treatment of specific diagnostic criteria–defined diseases and for funding population-based preventive services and clinical treatment services.

Diagnosis as a Source of Distress

Diagnoses with poor prognoses, such as schizophrenia, may bring distress and only partial hope. It is widely understood that among individuals who receive a diagnosis of schizophrenia, those with the greatest capacity to understand the nature of their illness are at greatest risk for subsequent depression and suicide (Crumlish et al. 2005; Kao and Liu 2011). In these cases, clinicians may appropriately wonder whether disclosing a diagnosis is likely to do more harm than good. The distress of living with severe symptoms that are only partially amenable to treatment is made even more severe by societal stigmatization. Patients suffering from mental illness, because of the intrinsic character of their diseases, may have more difficulty establishing and maintaining meaningful interpersonal relationships. Because of how mental disorders are viewed, people living with these conditions are likely to fear discrimination at work, in seeking housing, and in purchasing life and health insurance policies.

Although some psychiatric diagnoses may carry less burden of stigma now than in the past, some data suggest that patients with psychotic illness were more commonly stigmatized as violent and dangerous at the end of the twentieth century than they were half a century earlier (Phelan et al. 2000). A thought-provoking qualitative analysis of narrative interviews of 46 people with mental illness suggested that almost all people with mental illness worry about stigma (Dinos et al. 2004). Those with substance dependence or psychotic disorders are most affected by stigma, as poignantly illustrated in the remarks of an African Caribbean woman with schizophrenia: "Schizophrenic is the worst diagnosis because I've heard it in the newspapers and on TV, that they are really mad schizophrenic people, they are very dangerous to society, they've got no control. So obviously I came under that category" (Dinos et al. 2004, p. 177). In speaking with people who have received psychiatric diagnoses, the clinician needs to consider the distress of living with an illness process, as well as the psychosocial impact of how the diagnosis is perceived.

In most clinical encounters, there are both significant benefits and detriments associated with rendering a diagnosis. Diagnostic decisions are necessary to formulate treatment plans and to foster understanding and insight of the patient who must navigate the experience of illness and a system of care. Families and societal stakeholders (e.g., employers, insurers) may become involved, often introducing concerns and perhaps prejudices and greater sources of distress to the ill individual. In many cases, the understanding, legitimacy, and hope a diagnosis offers patients are true gifts. However, juxtaposed against these benefits are real risks of societal stigma and internal loss of self-esteem and self-efficacy (Corrigan and Watson 2002). Patients may benefit greatly from clinician willingness to weigh carefully the benefits and risks associated with rendering a diagnosis, the balance of which will vary across diagnostic categories and across individual patients within diagnostic categories.

Case Example: Diagnosis-Related Stigma

During Matthew's senior year in high school, his girlfriend of 2 years broke up with him and he felt devastated. His parents were worried because he was feeling "nervous" and "upset," skipped several meals, and stayed in his room for most of the day on weekends for about 2 weeks in a row. His sleep pattern and energy remained the same. His parents brought him to a physician, who diagnosed Matthew with major depressive disorder and provided Matthew with a prescription for antidepressant medication. He took the medication for about 6 weeks and then stopped.

Seven years later, Matthew was completing a medical screen for a job as a pilot for a major passenger airline. When asked about mental health history, he honestly reported the previous diagnosis of major depressive disorder. He also accurately reported that he had not experienced these symptoms before or since the one episode he experienced during his senior year of high school. The interview had gone very well, but he was not offered the job. The company representative who informed him that he had not been selected for the job simply reported that there were a very large number of highly qualified applicants and that the decision was difficult but that in the end another candidate was deemed the best fit for the position. Matthew was left wondering whether his past diagnosis hurt his chances when seeking this very competitive job.

Questions to Consider

- Did Matthew's physician do him a disservice in issuing a diagnosis of major depressive disorder?
- What confidence do you have in the diagnosis that Matthew was given?
- How likely is it that Matthew's diagnosis will hurt his chances for competitive employment that requires a baseline health screening?
- If you were hiring someone to care for your child or your elderly parents and you had access to all the applicants' mental health history, all other things being equal, would a diagnosis of major depressive disorder influence your hiring decision?

Diagnosis as a Risk

In addition to the balance of psychosocial benefits and risks of psychiatric diagnoses, most diagnoses lead to a treatment plan that conveys probable benefits and risks. An appropriate view of benefits and risks inherent in the diagnostic process is further complicated by the reality that psychiatric diagnosis is not a process with perfect precision. Even when the brightest clinicians have the best training and the best intentions, their diagnostic conclusions will not be perfectly accurate. As summarized in Table 1–1, evaluation of the balance of benefits and risks associated with receiving a psychiatric diagnosis (and associated treatment where indicated) requires consideration of diagnoses that are accurate (true positive and true negative) and inaccurate (false positive and false negative).

TABLE 1–1. **Summary considerations to keep in mind when rendering a psychiatric diagnosis**

Diagnosed with the disorder

Has the disorder	**Does not have the disorder**
True positive cases: A. Most likely to benefit from research and clinical experience related to the diagnosis B. Likely to be subjected to typical side-effect burden and economic cost of treatment, as well as psychosocial effects of the diagnostic label	False positive cases: A. Less likely to benefit from research and clinical experience related to the diagnosis B. Likely to be subjected to typical side-effect burden and economic cost of treatment, as well as psychosocial effects of the diagnostic label *More detrimental when side-effect burden or economic cost of treatment is high, and when psychosocial effects of the diagnosis label are high*

Diagnosed as not having the disorder

Has the disorder	**Does not have the disorder**
False negative cases: A. Subject to consequences of delayed treatment B. Potentially spared some exposure to typical side-effect burden and cost of treatment, as well as psychosocial effects of the diagnostic label *More detrimental when severity of illness is high and when benefit-to-risk ratio of treatment is high*	True negative cases: A. Spared consequences and cost of unnecessary treatment B. Spared psychosocial effects of the diagnostic label

TRUE POSITIVE DIAGNOSES

Many individuals who present for evaluation to a trained mental health clinician will have a DSM-5–defined diagnosis and will receive a diagnosis from their clinician that accurately categorizes the problem they present with. This is the category most readers probably have had in mind as we have alluded to benefits and risks associated with psychiatric diagnoses. These are the patients who are most likely to benefit from the growing body of research defining effective treatment strategies for the problem they are experiencing. There are at least two reasons for this:

1. These patients are more likely than patients without their diagnosis to be similar to the people who participated in clinical trials targeting individuals who have the same diagnosis.
2. The clinician caring for these patients may be more effective in deriving treatment solutions on the basis of his or her own clinical experience of what has worked with previous patients who had the same diagnosis.

A clinician who has derived a highly effective method for helping patients with bipolar I disorder stay on their medication will be of more benefit to a patient whom the clinician has accurately diagnosed with bipolar I disorder than to a patient with major depressive disorder whom the clinician has inaccurately diagnosed with bipolar I disorder.

FALSE POSITIVE DIAGNOSES

Patients who are inaccurately labeled with a diagnosis they do not have suffer burdens associated with the hypothesized characterization without the benefit of an evidence-based treatment plan derived from the clinician's previous experience and research focused on a population with equivalent signs and symptoms. The error is particularly unfortunate when the diagnosis indicates a lifetime of medication use that renders significant metabolic, cognitive, or other serious side effects. In some cases the diagnostic error may not be the fault of the clinician. Consider the case of an adolescent who had a single manic episode while taking his friend's psychostimulant prescribed for attention-deficit/hyperactivity disorder. The clinician faces a difficult diagnostic puzzle if sufficient time has elapsed between the episode and a warranted toxicology screen and the patient denies use of substances because he fears punishment if his parents find out that he illicitly used his friend's medication. The history of a single manic episode in this context may suggest a diagnosis of bipolar disorder to even the most careful and experienced clinician.

In many cases, however, an errant diagnosis can be avoided through appropriate assessment and understanding of diagnostic criteria. For example, consider the case of a young woman who has a history of a manic episode while taking two antidepressant medications for treatment of a major depressive episode. An inappropriate diagnosis of bipolar disorder in this case can—and in similar actual cases does—lead to significant unnecessary exposure to the ill effects of mood-stabilizing and/or atypical antipsychotic medications, as well as the psychosocial burden associated with the errant diagnosis.

The likelihood of inappropriately receiving a psychiatric diagnosis may be increasing with each DSM version due to the increased number of officially canonized diagnoses. The original DSM, published in the middle of the twentieth century, listed 6 disorders, whereas DSM-5 lists 157. The iterations of the *International Statistical Classification of Diseases and Related Health Problems* (ICD) present an even greater concern in this respect, because the number of codes listed in the ICD-10 has grown to 16,000 and the number of codes in the companion inpatient procedure coding system for the United States (ICD-10 PCS) has increased to more than 76,000. Clinicians who are socialized by their training to be wary of missing a diagnosis (i.e., who are focused on preventing false negative diagnoses) may be less cognizant of the potential harm associated with false positive diagnoses. Nevertheless, the imperfect process of psychiatric diagnosis will also miss some diagnoses that should be rendered.

FALSE NEGATIVE DIAGNOSES

Failure to make a diagnosis that should have been made can also lead to unintended, unnecessary harm. A person who is looking for help for an underlying psychiatric illness that is not detected by a clinician will probably not benefit from optimal treatment—treatment that in some cases can be lifesaving. In the most extreme cases, this risk is most alarmingly apparent. A substance-related disorder that leads to reckless driving and a traffic fatality could have been averted by timely diagnosis and treatment. A case of treatable postpartum depression inappropriately assumed to be a minor adjustment disorder may lead to detriments in mother-child interactions, later associated with increased mental illness burden and decreased quality of life for years to come in the life of the mother's newborn child.

Alternatively, some patients present with temporary anxiety, stress, or loss that is circumstantially bounded and may not warrant a psychiatric diagnosis. For these individuals the greatest diagnostic gift a clinician may offer is reassurance that the experience does not convey a psychiatric diagnosis, along with appropriate support and assistance where warranted and desired.

TRUE NEGATIVE DIAGNOSES

Although some individuals stand to lose benefits associated with a hoped-for diagnosis when seeking psychiatric evaluation, most will be relieved to know they do not have a significant mental health disorder. News that what ails the patient is not a suspected DSM diagnosis may indeed be reassuring to a bereaved individual, for example, and to most others suffering from difficult but "normal" human experience. For a small minority of individuals, not receiving a certain diagnosis may mean lack of insurance coverage for desired help or lack of perceived legitimacy sought via a clinical explanation of real suffering. For example, a military veteran who suffered significant trauma during armed conflict but does not meet criteria for posttraumatic stress disorder could interpret the accurate diagnostic message as meaning his suffering is not as legitimate as is the suffering of others who do have posttraumatic stress disorder. Still, for the vast majority of patients, an accurate declaration of the absence of a significant mental health disorder will be welcome news.

In almost all circumstances, an accurate (true positive or true negative) diagnosis yields a more optimal benefit-to-risk ratio than an inaccurate (false positive or false negative) diagnosis. An accurate diagnosis maximizes the clinical benefit-to-risk ratio, in spite of potential legal, economic, social, and other complicating variables.

Diagnosis as a Gift

Most patients would like their clinicians' help with two things: 1) an understanding of the symptoms they are experiencing (Salmon et al. 2004) and 2) a solution to alleviate these symptoms. A diagnosis can be a gift that helps meet both of these needs.

An accurately rendered diagnosis clearly explored with a patient can help the patient feel that the clinician understands the patient's suffering and that the clinician can draw from a clinical knowledge base derived from working with other patients who have suffered the same problem and from the experience of colleagues working with similar patients. Receiving a medical diagnosis can begin to give patients a sense of clarity, affirmation, or legitimacy in the experience of their suffering. A clinical interview conducted with empathy and kindness—even by a novice or a learner in a clinical situation—is sufficient to help a patient feel that the clinician understands what suffering the patient is experiencing. Hearing a professional diagnosis helps a patient feel that the clinician understands *why* the patient is suffering. This beneficial psychological effect may exist even though the DSM-based diagnoses are based much more on useful descriptive constructs than on validated biological models of pathology. The experience of receiving a diagnosis may be particularly validating to psychiatric patients with emotional suffering that is mostly unobservable to or misunderstood by others. A diagnostic explanation can help a patient feel more understood and less harshly judged. A patient who suffered severe child abuse and has regular disturbing nightmares and a paralyzing fear of intimacy is likely to feel more understood and less judged after learning that many other people who have been exposed to similar traumatic experiences have reacted in the same way. The same patient may benefit from knowing that this reaction is officially termed posttraumatic stress disorder and is well recognized and studied. For this patient, the gift of diagnosis also extends hope of recovery and the restoration of a better life. For many individuals, a diagnosis may bring some, if somewhat paradoxical, comfort. These include the person with an eating disorder who has previously been told to "just *eat* something"; the person with social phobia who has been told to "just get out of the house"; or the profoundly depressed person who is unable to muster enough energy and motivation to get out of bed—and who has been told to "just snap out of it."

A good clinician will convey the gift of a diagnosis wrapped in optimism and founded in a growing body of literature describing treatment strategies proven successful for patients with the same diagnosis. For example, a severely depressed patient and her clinician will then have the option of selecting a best-fit treatment strategy that includes evidence-based psychotherapy, an antidepressant medication, or both. A patient with posttraumatic stress disorder and his clinician can also begin to map out an evidence-based treatment plan that, although challenging to implement when appropriately including a strategy such as cognitive processing therapy (Resick and Schnicke 1992) or prolonged exposure therapy (Foa et al. 1999), offers evidence-based fuel for optimistic hope of significant—even life-trajectory-changing—recovery. Patients with some anxiety disorders, including debilitating panic disorder, may be overjoyed to learn that their symptoms can be alleviated, in many cases, with only 4–8 weeks of appropriate treatment (Gould et al. 1995). There are, however, many patients who present with dire need for relief from mental health problems for which decades of research have rendered less optimal solutions.

The Compassionate, Astute Diagnostician

The task of the modern clinician is to use the wisdom and proven practices of the past while learning continuously about emerging evidence and, all the while, working tirelessly to improve approaches to health care. Alleviating the suffering and enabling greater well-being of patients—rather than unthoughtful adherence to tradition or unquestioning "uptake" of tentative new information—are, and should be, the aims that guide clinical practice in the DSM-5 era.

Diagnostic accuracy depends to a large extent on content mastery (Elstein and Schwartz 2002). Experts are more accurate than novices. Clinicians can accelerate their progress from novice to expert through study coupled with clinical experience.

Most training programs insist that budding clinicians study a significant amount of material before engaging in direct patient care. The reason for this is obvious. Although both study and clinical experience facilitate clinical content mastery, only one of these is accomplished without any burden to patients who may not benefit much from care rendered by a complete novice. This principle holds some truth for all clinicians. Study accelerates and supplements learning derived from clinical experience and will help clinicians optimize the benefit-to-risk ratio of care they provide to their patients (Box 1–1). Careful study of DSM-defined diagnoses will help clinicians maximize diagnostic accuracy.

Box 1–1. Summing up: psychosocial considerations in arriving at an accurate psychiatric diagnosis

Andrea is a 16-year-old with a police record for possession of cocaine. She presents 2 weeks following delivery of her baby with depressed mood and loss of interest in playing with her new baby girl. She indicates that these symptoms began 1 week earlier, after she left her home in New Orleans to live in a small town with her aunt. Andrea indicates that she gets along well with her aunt but misses her friends and that it is hard for her to stay awake during the day because her baby daughter wakes up every hour at night. Andrea finds it hard to focus on her home-school coursework and feels tired all the time. She is feeling guilty about not being able to get much done. When asked about suicidal thoughts, Andrea states that she would never consider doing anything to hurt herself because her baby "needs a mother." She has been abstinent from all illicit drug use, alcohol, and tobacco since learning she was pregnant. The father of the baby is now in jail. Andrea has elected to keep the baby, and her aunt supports her decision. However, during an initial welfare visit, social services informed Andrea and her aunt that they will be periodically evaluating Andrea's fitness to care for her child. The initial welfare visit was initiated after a neighbor reported to child protective services that he had knocked on the door to see why the baby had been crying for 2 hours and saw through the window that Andrea was sleeping on the couch while the crying baby lay on the floor on a blanket. Andrea indicates that she wants help but is worried that social services may not look favorably on a mental health diagnosis in their evaluation of her capacity to care for her baby.

Questions to Consider

- What are your thoughts about the diagnostic considerations that Andrea's psychiatrist should keep in mind?
- How will an accurate diagnosis bring benefit to Andrea?
- What psychosocial issues are of importance in this situation, and how do they influence the process of arriving at a diagnosis?

DSM-5 and the antecedent DSM versions are similar to other classification systems, such as the ICD, in that each edition has arisen through a sequential process of review of the emerging evidence and thoughtful consensus building. Some components of DSM-5 are identical to prior versions—for instance, the diagnostic scheme for personality disorders presented in Section II, "Diagnostic Criteria and Codes."

Many components represent novel or more refined approaches, moving beyond the prior versions of DSM quite substantially. DSM-5 is not assumed to be perfect or "final"—indeed, the manual is certain to be replaced as the understanding of diseases and dysfunction of the brain evolves—and the learner who uses the *Study Guide to DSM-5* will be wise to understand the evolving nature of the DSM process.

This *Study Guide* is designed to help clinicians at all levels of experience master the new DSM-5 diagnostic system. With the emergence of DSM-5, in a sense we are all novices to the newly revised diagnostic system and will benefit from systematic study together. Happy studying!

Self-Assessment

Questions to Discuss With Colleagues and Mentors

1. Have you ever made a diagnosis with unexpected results?
2. Have you ever delayed a diagnosis you wish you had made more rapidly?
3. When is rendering a psychiatric diagnosis most worrisome in your experience? Why?
4. Are there clinical circumstances in which you have found it better not to share your diagnostic hypothesis with your patient? If yes, when?

Short-Answer Questions

1. To what degree is the DSM-5 diagnostic system based on neuroscience discovery?
2. How do psychiatric diagnoses facilitate clinical communication?
3. What are some significant benefits to patients associated with an accurate psychiatric diagnosis?

Answers

1. The DSM-5 diagnostic system sought to incorporate recent best-evidence and, where possible and appropriate, neuroscientific findings. The DSM-5 is a phenomenologically oriented diagnostic system rather than an etiologically governed diagnostic approach.
2. In developing and refining a diagnostic hypothesis, the clinician must engage in a careful dialogue with the patient. The astute clinician will seek to clarify the patient's personal history, the symptoms experienced, the impact of living with an illness process, relevant background, and the concerns of the patient. The dialogue may further allow the clinician to reconcile any incongruities in the patient's presentation and narrative, prior documentation, and collateral medical and psychosocial information.
3. Placing the experience of the patient into a diagnostic framework can help the patient to understand features of the illness process and anticipated outcomes. Receiving a diagnosis paradoxically can be reassuring and provide validation for patients who may feel that their symptoms are poorly understood by others.

Recommended Readings

Corrigan PW (ed): On the Stigma of Mental Illness: Practical Strategies for Research and Social Change. Washington, DC, American Psychological Association, 2005

Frances AJ, Widiger T: Psychiatric diagnosis: lessons from the DSM-IV past and cautions for the DSM-5 future. Annu Rev Clin Psychol 8:109–130, 2012

Kraemer HC: Validity and psychiatric diagnoses. JAMA Psychiatry 70:138–139, 2013

Regier DA, Narrow WE, Clarke DE, et al: DSM-5 field trials in the United States and Canada, part II: test-retest reliability of selected categorical diagnoses. Am J Psychiatry 170:59–70, 2013

References

Corrigan PW, Watson AC: The paradox of self-stigma and mental illness. Clin Psychol 9:35–53, 2002

Crumlish N, Whitty P, Kamali M, et al: Early insight predicts depression and attempted suicide after 4 years in first-episode schizophrenia and schizophreniform disorder. Acta Psychiatr Scand 112:449–455, 2005

Dinos S, Stevens S, Serfaty M, et al: Stigma: the feelings and experiences of 46 people with mental illness. Qualitative study. Br J Psychiatry 184:176–181, 2004

Elstein AS, Schwartz A: Clinical problem solving and diagnostic decision making: selective review of the cognitive literature. BMJ 324:729–732, 2002

Elstein AS, Shulman LS, Sprafka SA: Medical Problem Solving: An Analysis of Clinical Reasoning. Cambridge, MA, Harvard University Press, 1978

Foa EB, Dancu CV, Hembree EA, et al: A comparison of exposure therapy, stress inoculation training, and their combination for reducing posttraumatic stress disorder in female assault victims. J Consult Clin Psychol 67:194–200, 1999

Frances AJ, Widiger T: Psychiatric diagnosis: lessons from the DSM-IV past and cautions for the DSM-5 future. Annu Rev Clin Psychol 8:109–130, 2012

Gould RA, Ott MW, Pollack MH: A meta-analysis of treatment outcome for panic disorder. Clin Psychol Rev 15:819–844, 1995

Insel TR: Translating scientific opportunity into public health impact: a strategic plan for research on mental illness. Arch Gen Psychiatry 66:128–133, 2009

Kao YC, Liu YP: Suicidal behavior and insight into illness among patients with schizophrenia spectrum disorders. Psychiatr Q 82:207–220, 2011

Lavori PW, Dawson R: Adaptive treatment strategies in chronic disease. Annu Rev Med 59:443–453, 2008

Moayyeri A, Soltani A, Moosapour H, et al: Evidence-based history taking under "time constraint." J Res Med Sci 16:559–564, 2011

Paneth N: Assessing the contributions of John Snow to epidemiology: 150 years after removal of the broad street pump handle. Epidemiology 15:514–516, 2004

Phelan JC, Link BG, Stueve A, et al: Public conceptions of mental illness in 1950 and 1996: what is mental illness and is it to be feared? J Health Soc Behav 41:188–207, 2000

Resick PA, Schnicke MK: Cognitive processing therapy for sexual assault victims. J Consult Clin Psychol 60:748–756, 1992

Salmon P, Dowrick CF, Ring A, et al: Voiced but unheard agendas: qualitative analysis of the psychosocial cues that patients with unexplained symptoms present to general practitioners. Br J Gen Pract 54:171–176, 2004

World Health Organization: The Global Burden of Disease: 2004 Update. Geneva, World Health Organization, 2008. Available at: http://www.who.int/healthinfo/global_burden_disease/2004_report_update/en. Accessed September 22, 2013.

Arriving at a Diagnosis

The Role of the Clinical Interview

John H. Coverdale, M.D., M.Ed.
Alan K. Louie, M.D.
Laura Weiss Roberts, M.D., M.A.

DSM-5 provides information, language, and formal criteria that together serve as tools that the diagnostician brings to an interaction with another person to ascertain whether a psychiatric disorder is present. The art of diagnosis relates to how these tools are applied in situ—in real people, real situations, and real settings. The clinical interview occurs in this specific context, and it is the central process for arriving at a sound psychiatric diagnosis.

Making a Diagnosis in Context

A clinical interview is shaped by its context. Context may be broken down by asking who, what, when, where, and why questions. Each of these questions should be considered explicitly for each clinical interview. For instance, who is the diagnostician conducting the interview, where is the interview situated, and when is the interview taking place? Is the person to be interviewed a student being seen by a social worker in a college health center just before final exams, an individual meeting with a clinical psychologist to see if he meets criteria to volunteer for a research protocol, or an inmate being evaluated by a forensic psychiatrist in a jail? The student, volunteer, and inmate might all have the same diagnosis, but the context of each interview will influence the nature of the interaction and how each person looks, reacts to questions, offers information, and so on. Taken one step further, people of different cultural and ethnic backgrounds, primary languages, genders, and ages will respond differently when seeking services for routine mental health needs in a familiar clinic in comparison with needs that are acute and life-threatening in an unfamiliar emergency facility. Many other scenarios may be imagined, covering people with varying attributes, diverse locations, and different time frames—each context will influence the presentation of a particular diagnosis.

Why does context matter? Attention to context matters because a formulaic or mechanical approach to making diagnoses in these highly varied scenarios may lead to poorly executed interviews and possibly even incorrect diagnoses.

As a consequence, before starting the interview, the diagnostician should focus on the "why" and the "what" questions. Why is the interview being conducted? Why is this interview, at this time, important? The answer to the "why" questions thus informs "what" type of interview should be performed, including the prioritization and framing of queries and topics to be covered in the interaction. Review of the three scenarios presented in the previous paragraph will illustrate the salience of these questions and how their answers influence the effectiveness of the interview on a very practical level:

- The first scenario involved a social worker meeting with a student at a college health center. This student was seeking help for psychological symptoms being experienced before final exams. The social worker wanted the student to speak freely about these symptoms, and to encourage this openness, she had assured the student that their discussions would be confidential, unless the student divulged information that the social worker was mandated to report (e.g., actively intending to harm another person). Notably, the social worker said she would not share information with the student's professors or dean. The interview questions clarified mental health issues and led to development of a supportive treatment plan with the student.
- In the second scenario, the volunteer was undergoing a screening interview to determine whether he met the inclusion and exclusion criteria set by the research protocol. The questions were not aimed at developing a treatment plan for the volunteer; indeed, he had been informed that he should not expect the research study to bring benefit for his mental health issues. This interview included an informed consent procedure that described the protocol and key safeguards, such as the approval and oversight by an institutional review board and a process for avoiding identification of the research volunteer in any subsequent publication.
- In the third scenario, the court set up the interview by the forensic psychiatrist. The forensic psychiatrist informed the inmate at the beginning of the interview that she had been appointed by the court and could not serve in a clinical, caregiving role and that any responses would not remain confidential. In fact, any disclosures made by the inmate were likely to appear in a psychiatric report for the court. (The use of DSM-5 in a forensic setting is complicated, and the reader should refer to the "Cautionary Statement for Forensic Use of DSM-5" in DSM-5 Section I.)

These scenarios illustrate practical aspects of context that shape a clinical interview, but a more abstract notion of context also exists and has relevance when arriving at a diagnosis.

The Biopsychosocial Model

The biopsychosocial model is a view of context that appreciates, and is open-minded to, the range of biological, psychological, and social factors that interact with and contribute to a patient's presentation and concerns. This more abstract notion has been generally referred to as the biopsychosocial paradigm, proposed and developed by George Engel in 1977, which posits that biological, psychological, and social domains together play a role in the development of disease or illness (Engel 1977). The biopsychosocial model is a paradigm intended to encompass the full set of factors that pertain to human experience and suffering, including, by extension, cultural and spiritual factors. The biopsychosocial model is antithetical to a reductionist approach. Patients should be assisted to talk about what is important to them within each domain. The following text describes the model first in the social context and then in the psychological and biological contexts.

SOCIAL CONTEXT

The practical questions of who, what, when, where, and why often address much of the social context. The social perspective is a natural starting place as the interview commences and as each party might wonder, "Why are we here and what are we doing here?" Usually, each party is taking on a role described in the society—for example, a role as a therapist, researcher, patient, research volunteer, and inmate. Very important to the success of the interview is whether the parties are in agreement about what these roles are and whether each willingly accepts his or her role. These issues are best understood, made transparent, and, if necessary, negotiated at the outset of the interview. If the social context is not agreed upon, then the rest of the interview is essentially going to be out of context.

PSYCHOLOGICAL CONTEXT

The social context, important as it may be, especially as a starting point, is not the only context to consider when making diagnoses. Individual psychology, encompassing the personal experience and background of the individual being interviewed, greatly affects the success of the interview. The most overt individual characteristic involves language. The interviewee may not fluently speak the language of the interviewer or may not be able to fully communicate in any language. Even with the assistance of a medical translator, the interviewer may not be sure if criteria are truly met. For instance, the DSM-5 criteria for major depressive disorder in the English language inquire if "depressed mood" is present. Some languages do not have words that are clearly equivalent to these English words. Additionally, individuals raised in divergent cultures may actually experience and manifest a symptom, such as depressed mood, variably. In one culture, an individual may experience depressed mood as a thought (e.g., "I think about depressing things"), whereas someone in another culture may experience it as a bodily sensation (e.g., "I am so fatigued"). The diagnostician has to make a judgment about how to weigh such factors when making a diagnosis. Even when no language or cultural differences exist, the individual context may still cause ambiguity, because everyone has dissimilar worldviews and values. For example, many DSM-5 criteria assess whether the individual reports being distressed by symptoms. This assessment, however, is mitigated by what level of distress an individual views as part of normal life, is not embarrassed to disclose, or has become aware of in his or her life.

BIOLOGICAL CONTEXT

Now that we have touched on the social and psychological contexts, the biological context remains. Psychiatry is a medical specialty that is concerned, in the main, with cognitive, emotional, and behavioral disorders and processes or conditions that are mediated by the brain. Although the "nurture" factors—that is, the social and psychological components—are strong determinants of a psychiatric diagnosis, the "nature" factors are also significant, especially for certain conditions. Indeed, a diagnosis may be understood to be a direct and inevitable result of an individual's fundamental biology (e.g., genetic makeup). With the realities of scientific neglect of psychiatric disorders historically, the challenges associated with advancing scientific understanding of multidetermined complex genetic disorders, and the observation that the sequencing of the human genome occurred only recently, this biological domain remains, for the most part, unexplored.

Currently, measures of biological markers that may correlate with or substantiate diagnoses are unavailable. Thus, we look to the future, when such markers, perhaps involving brain imaging or genetic findings, may be included in DSM criteria. For now, weak proxies of these measures are elicited during an interview. For instance, an interviewer wants to know if an interviewee has a family history of a psychiatric disorder, especially if the disorder is thought to be highly heritable on the basis of epidemiological data. Also, the interviewer searches for evidence of any medical disorder or of substance or medication use that may be directly inducing symptoms of a diagnosis.

Summary

In sum, psychiatric diagnoses occur in social, psychological, and biological contexts, and a goal of the psychiatric interviewer is to become informed of these contexts and to weigh them in applying diagnostic criteria and arriving at diagnoses. As discussed earlier, the interviewer should start with answering the questions of who, what, when, where, and why as they relate to the interview. The balance of this chapter addresses the details of "how" to conduct the interview and the psychiatric assessment in general. Interested readers may also wish to refer to excellent resources on interviewing that informed this narrative, listed in the "Recommended Readings" section at the end of this chapter.

Approach to the Psychiatric Interview and Assessment

The clinical interview and assessment in psychiatry are intended to identify whether or not a patient has a mental health problem, the nature of any problem(s), and the specific diagnoses. The assessment process is aimed at developing a comprehensive, valid, and reliable database for the purpose of ameliorating the problems with which the patient presented by identifying and treating specific medical and psychiatric diagnoses. The components of such a comprehensive approach include obtaining a history, conducting a mental status examination, investigating possible medical problems, pursuing collateral records and other informants (not covered in this book), administering relevant and validated assessment tools, and physical and laboratory examinations. The psychiatric interview, which is a critical component of a comprehensive assessment, serves to identify all of the factors (i.e., biological/medical, psychological, social/cultural) that influence the presenting problems and that pertain to the provision of safe and beneficial preventions and treatments.

Despite the clear objectives of the psychiatric interview and assessment, patients should be encouraged to talk about what is important to them during assessment processes. This approach is complementary to a narrower elicitation of symptoms and details in arriving at a specific diagnosis. Thus, in patient-centered interviewing, clinicians should help the patient to lead the conversation to aspects of his or her life (i.e., psychosocial factors) that might be important in understanding the determinants of the problems and diagnoses. For example, homeless individuals who seek mental health care constitute a biopsychosocially vulnerable population with potential unmet needs. These needs could include undertreated medical, dietary, and psychiatric conditions complicated by victimization from crimes, violence, sexual exploitation, and alcohol and substance abuse. A reductionist "checklist" approach to diagnosis alone is ineffective in identifying and managing the complex biopsychosocial problems with which these patients might present. Indeed, such a necessarily broad approach to assessments and interviewing is fundamentally humanizing.

We begin with a note about professionalism in clinical interviewing. Respect for persons is, indeed, the principle that is first and foremost in the clinical professions. This text is written with the purpose of identifying, in very general terms, how to sensitively acquire clinical data that each practitioner should consider in accordance with his or her respective professional responsibilities and privileges. Practitioners of all types of clinical licensure are urged to keep in mind the professional virtues that are the ethical basis of clinical practice. In particular, they should consider the four fundamental professional virtues of integrity, compassion, self-effacement, and self-sacrifice: *Integrity* is the lifelong commitment to the practice of medicine in accordance with the standards of intellectual and moral excellence. *Compassion* in medicine is the deep regard for the experience of the patient and, as a corollary, the commitment to serve the well-being of the patient, including relief of the patient's pain and suffering, through identification with the patient's distress. *Self-effacement* refers to the notion of humility. *Self-sacrifice* and self-effacement in medicine are apparent when the clinician sets aside personal concerns and interpersonal differences so that the patient's interests are best served. These virtues were introduced into the history of medical ethics by John Gregory (1724–1773) and, as described by Laurence McCullough (1998), provide the basis for the concept of fiduciary and constitute the starting point to the clinical professional approach to psychiatric interviewing and assessment.

Psychiatric Interview

Psychiatric history taking necessitates a thoughtful, systematic, and disciplined inquiry. Although psychiatric interviews are dynamic and interactive processes, a general interview structure is required to promote efficiency and to facilitate the recognition of diagnostic patterns and symptoms. This structure should be sufficiently flexible that the interviewer allows patients to talk about what is important to them, follows their cues and leads, and is sensitive to their mental state, comfort level, and personality style.

The interview of a new patient should begin with introductions, including a statement of purpose and degree of confidentiality. An early focus should be on developing rapport and a working alliance. Patients should be given an opportunity to talk about what is important to them. The early phases of the interview are necessarily open-ended in identifying the history of the presenting problem(s) and symptoms, including the events that led up to those problems. Listening and empathically responding, deepening rapport, and seeking clarification should be priorities, especially for this beginning stage of the interview. Such an open-ended approach should be followed by screening for symptoms across diagnostic categories.

Some essential elements of the psychiatric interview include, but are not limited to, identifying information (e.g., age, gender, marital status), presenting problem, history of the presenting problem, past psychiatric history, suicidal and/or homicidal history, substance use history (including alcohol), medical history, family history, and personal and social histories. In Part II of this *Study Guide,* more details on how to obtain the psychiatric history are provided in relation to specific diagnostic categories.

Interviewing Techniques

Getting valid information from patients enhances the comprehensiveness of information concerning clinical risks and consequences and thus enriches clinical judgment. Eliciting accurate information from patients can be challenging, especially when patients are reluctant to divulge sensitive information for whatever reason. Interviewers may also be reluctant to enter into areas that are uncomfortable for themselves, perhaps in anticipation of discomfort in the patient. Feelings of discomfort in the interviewer can unhinge judgment and impede further inquiry or alternatively might lead to questions that invite a negative versus affirmative response by the patient. A key strategy for validly obtaining information on sensitive issues is for the interviewer to recognize any feelings of discomfort or distress during the interview, in either the patient or the interviewer, and to prevent those feelings from becoming negatively influential.

Sensitive areas of inquiry include the patient's sexual history, alcohol and drug history, history of possible victimization or violence, and suicidal or homicidal ideation. Inquiry into the possibility of a history of sexual abuse, for example, should be routinely conducted.

A number of strategies can be used for obtaining valid information (Shea 1998). One is to wait to ask questions of a potentially sensitive nature later in the interview, after rapport is established. A second strategy is to provide the patient with a rationale for sensitive questions. For example, the interviewer might tell the patient that questions about sexual history are important for understanding risk for unwanted pregnancies and sexually transmitted infections. A third strategy is for the interviewer to respond to leads that the patient provides and that open the gate into sensitive areas, while using language that facilitates and normalizes the expression of true responses.

In one approach to the last strategy, the interviewer asks questions that assume that the patient has experienced a particular event or feeling. The patient's willingness to affirm such an experience might become further enhanced by the interviewer's telling the patient how such an experience or feeling is common, even expectable, given certain circumstances. For example, when asking what suicidal thoughts a depressed patient is experiencing, the interviewer might tell the patient that depression is almost always associated with suicidal thoughts. Initial negative responses by the patient, especially when these are counterintuitive, should invite clarification and additional inquiry. Moreover, specific incidences and details of behavior (e.g., sexual, abusive, suicidal, violent) should be obtained. For example, a patient might be asked whether arguing with a family member ever leads to physical blows.

Interviewing People From Special Groups

CHILDREN

When assessing children, clinicians should obtain information from a variety of sources, including family members, schools, and medical records. Because children are sensitive to stress in families, the family is an especially important source of information. Furthermore, because very young children are less verbal and less able to sit still for a formal interview, their feelings can be assessed by how they play and what they draw, as well as by what is attributed to objects such as dolls and stuffed animals. As in any vulnerable population, clinicians should be vigilant to identify possible neglect or abuse.

OLDER ADULT PATIENTS

Because new medical problems commonly arise in older age, and because patients with preexisting mental disorders commonly have unidentified or unmet medical needs, clinicians should be especially assiduous to thoroughly assess possible biological contributions to a psychiatric presentation. Older age, rapidity of symptom onset, concomitant medical illnesses, and alcohol or substance abuse are examples of factors that should heighten a suspicion of biological etiologies. Thus, the medical history, physical examination, laboratory tests, and ancillary investigations are routinely important in assessing geriatric patients with psychiatric problems. These patients are also vulnerable to adverse social circumstances, and a comprehensive assessment should determine functional capacity and ability to maintain safety in the home. Self-neglect will become more prevalent in an aging population. In addition, being careful to ensure that the older patient is physically comfortable and can hear the interviewer is essential for a successful interview.

CULTURALLY DISTINCT GROUPS

Culture constitutes a wide developmental, social, and interpersonal matrix relevant to all psychiatric assessments and presentations. Culture should be considered broadly and not be narrowly interpreted as a matter of ethnicity or race. Everyone has a distinctive personal culture that may be determined by a number of individual characteristics as diverse as age, immigration history, religion, occupation, sexual orientation, school affiliation, club or sports membership, veteran status, linguistic capabilities, and so on. Given that people identify with a conglomerate of cultures and given the wide diversity of beliefs even within a given culture, the clinician should approach each patient as unique and respect cultural differences. Clinicians should learn with enthusiasm about cultural factors that can contribute to individual psychiatric presentations and integrate relevant protective or exacerbating factors into an understanding of why the patient presented. For example, immigrant or minority population status may be associated with challenges in accessing care, and any such barriers should be identified and addressed. Also of note, both clinicians and patients will be influenced by values related to their own cultures, and these may significantly affect the interaction between them as clinician and patient. For instance, cultures differ with regard to expectations about how authoritarian the clinician will be toward the patient and how questioning the patient will be toward the clinician.

DSM-5 provides a Cultural Formulation Interview in Section III, "Emerging Measures and Models." This interview is a structured approach to evaluating the interaction of culture and psychiatric and substance use disorders in a patient. Two versions are provided: one to administer to the patient and one for interviewing an informant about the patient. This structured interview guides a clinician through specific questions in a stepwise fashion, helping to define cultural factors and their possible influence on treatment. DSM-5 also includes a Glossary of Cultural Concepts of Distress in its Appendix.

Mental Status Examination

The mental status examination (MSE) assesses specific details of the patient's appearance, mental experiences, and behaviors. This structured assessment uses a relatively consistent terminology. The general components of the MSE often include appearance and behavior, motor activities, speech, affect and mood, form and content of thought, perception, and cognition. Table 2–1 lists a limited number of examples of details that might be found in each component of an MSE report. The table is not a universal or fully inclusive list; readers are directed to references on the MSE (e.g., Strub and Black 1999).

TABLE 2–1. Components of the mental status examination, with examples[a]

Appearance and behavior: level of consciousness, attentiveness or distractibility, attitude toward the examiner, eye contact, clothing, grooming

Motor behavior: agitation or retardation, mannerisms, abnormal movements, gait

Speech: rate, volume, quantity, prosody

Affect and mood: *affect* is the feeling state of the patient as observed by the examiner (e.g., hostile, sad, happy, fearful, blunted, flat); *mood* is the patient's self-described feeling state (e.g., anxious, depressed, angry)

Form of thought (thought process): connectivity between ideas; perseveration; coherence; looseness of associations

Thought content: suicidal and/or homicidal ideas, intentions, or plans; delusions; obsessions

Perception: illusions, hallucinations, derealization, depersonalization

Cognition: orientation, attention, memory (different types), spatial abilities, abstract thinking, judgment, insight

[a]Examples are not all-inclusive.

Assessment

The psychiatric interview and MSE may be supplemented by administration of validated and reliable assessment tools. These tools reduce subjectivity in assessments and enable a formal evaluation of outcomes of treatment. There are many such validated tools, both self-administered and clinician-administered. Some tools provide information across a range of diagnostic areas, whereas others focus on narrow areas, such as patients' emotional or cognitive abilities. Some tools seek to determine the nature, severity, and duration of certain features of illness. Clinicians should learn about the strengths and weaknesses of diagnostic tools, including their validity, sensitivity, and specificity, and learn how to apply them to individual patients in conjunction with the psychiatric interview.

DSM-5 includes a chapter, "Assessment Measures," in Section III, "Emerging Measures and Methods," that features the following measures:

- DSM-5 Self-Rated Level 1 Cross-Cutting Symptom Measure—Adult
- Parent/Guardian-Rated DSM-5 Level 1 Cross-Cutting Symptom Measure—Child Age 6–17
- Clinician-Rated Dimensions of Psychosis Symptom Severity
- World Health Organization Disability Assessment Schedule 2.0 (WHODAS 2.0)

Of note, each of these measures assesses symptoms in a dimensional manner—that is, the symptoms are rated according to points along a continuum (e.g., from mild to severe). This rating system is in contrast to systems that merely indicate if a symptom is present or absent, in a categorical manner. Most of the criteria in DSM-5 are categorical; in other words, the person is rated as either having a symptom or not having it. The dimensional ratings allow a more graduated and nuanced characterization of symptoms (see Chapter 3, "Understanding Different Approaches to Diagnostic Classification").

The DSM-5 Cross-Cutting Symptom Measure, with separate versions for adults and children, is used to rate symptoms in a variety of domains along a continuum. Of note, the symptoms are not necessarily aligned with one diagnosis, and the endorsement of one symptom does not connote a specific diagnosis because several diagnoses may manifest this symptom. For instance, the symptoms of sleep disturbance may apply to several possible diagnoses. Thus, the term *cross-cutting* is used, because these symptoms cross diagnostic lines and provide a picture of the patient's presentation without assigning a diagnosis. This depiction of the patient's symptoms is holistic, and it complements and adds information to the categorical system of the diagnostic criteria in DSM-5.

In addition to the two cross-cutting measures, DSM-5 includes two other dimensional measures. The Clinician-Rated Dimensions of Psychosis Symptom Severity is a rating scale for the severity of eight symptoms of psychosis. The WHODAS 2.0 is used to measure the degree of disability, secondary to a health or mental health condition, experienced in everyday life during the last 30 days. The WHODAS 2.0 has a dimensional scale with a 5-point rating system ranging from having no problem doing a chore to not being able to do it at all. The 36 listed chores include daily functions, such as moving about physically, grooming oneself, and interacting with people. This scale measures functioning without regard to diagnosis; disability may be secondary to any health or mental health condition, although knowledge of the specific condition(s) is not required.

The three types of scales in the DSM-5 "Assessment Measures" chapter may be considered along with the diagnostic interview. All three scales are dimensional in construction and are not designed to make diagnoses. The diagnostic interview seeks to determine DSM-5 diagnoses; the assessment measures add value and nuance by attempting to quantify and track symptom severity and disabilities associated with the diagnoses made through the interview.

There is a potentially complex interplay between psychiatric and medical conditions. Medical conditions can cause psychiatric disorders, including mood, anxiety, psychotic, and cognitive disorders. Medical conditions can also adversely impact preexisting mental disorders. Also, patients with medical conditions might experience psychological problems that occur in connection with having been diagnosed with those conditions. In turn, preexisting psychiatric conditions can cause, underlie, or be associated with medical problems. Clinicians should be vigilant in identifying these interactions.

Physical examination and laboratory tests, in conjunction with the medical history and medical review of symptoms, serve to better identify salient medical issues. Identification of medical problems is an essential part of a comprehensive biopsychosocial prevention and treatment plan. The physical examination, when appropriate, should be thorough and adhere to examination standards. Laboratory tests and other diagnostic tests should be prudently ordered and justified in light of their relevance and costs.

Summary

The clinical interview plays an essential role in arriving at an accurate diagnosis. How an interview is conducted is an expression of the professionalism of the interviewer, and it serves as the cornerstone of the relationship between the clinician and patient. As described in this chapter, the clinical interview is grounded in a nonreductionist biopsychosocial model that gives importance to the whole person in context (Box 2–1). Oftentimes patients may be in distress or have significant impairments that become evident in a clinical interview, and sensitive information is, and should be, elicited in an indepth psychiatric interview. For these reasons, special care to address the comfort of the patient and to demonstrate respect toward the patient is warranted in psychiatry. The psychiatric interview, in particular, relies on a rigorous MSE and systematic inclusion of information from medical records and other informants, assessment (including formal measures), physical examination, and laboratory testing.

Box 2–1. Thoroughness of the clinical interview as essential in clarifying the diagnosis

Mr. Ortiz, an 18-year-old Hispanic man, was brought to the emergency room by his parents, desperately concerned about their son, who had gone without food or water for 2 days. The patient reported, "There is no point to it." Mr. Ortiz had for several months experienced a pervasive feeling of being "not-alive-not-not-alive" and feeling as if he recognized his family but "without knowing or feeling anything" about them. His mother said that he kept repeating that "everything is unreal" and that he felt "like a robot—but one that is alive." She said he was frightened and sad "all of the time." This experience of detachment had occurred suddenly and had not relented, although it seemed worse at night. Mr. Ortiz had been able to function at first, but as graduation from his senior year of high school approached, he had greater difficulty and refused to leave the house. His mother said, "Sometimes he just lies there in his bed and cries and shakes."

Mr. Ortiz had been hospitalized in another city and only recently discharged. The patient had not told the doctors about his internal experiences of detachment and derealization but would only acknowledge that he "felt different" and endorsed being "depressed." The doctors relied on the family reports of the sudden change in the patient's behavior. The father reported that "the doctors did every possible test—brain scans, tests for seizures, tests for drugs, tests for infections and metals and rare diseases—and found nothing wrong. How can there be nothing wrong?" There were no neurodevelopmental or medical issues in the patient's past, no relevant family history, and no current or previous substance use. Other than the symptoms described, the patient did not endorse hallucinations or unusual beliefs. The discharge diagnosis, according to the father, was "depression."

Mr. Ortiz had a reported history of depression, and he fully met criteria for depersonalization/derealization disorder at the time of the assessment in the emergency room. Over the next 2 years, however, he developed many more symptoms, including the belief that demons were responsible for his detachment, and he began to hear "whispers." Dark, threatening, and religious themes entered his artwork, which became much more chaotic and disorganized. His speech pattern changed—"now he just talks in circles and we can't understand his point," according to his mother. Mr. Ortiz said that he did not "have the energy of life because other people need it." His earlier diagnosis of depersonalization/derealization disorder was replaced with schizophrenia.

Questions to Consider

- How is a thorough clinical interview, informed by the biopsychosocial model, helpful in clarifying the diagnostic issues present in this clinical case?
- What special efforts must a clinical interviewer take in order to conduct a successful interview with this patient?
- What additional information is needed to clarify the diagnosis or diagnoses present in this case?

Self-Assessment

Questions to Discuss With Colleagues and Mentors

1. How does the clinician apply the biopsychosocial model for the practice of psychiatry and related fields?
2. How do the professional virtues of integrity, compassion, self-effacement, and self-sacrifice apply to the routine practice of psychiatry and related fields?
3. What methods, including wording of questions, are used to facilitate patients' disclosure of sensitive information and to screen for selected disorders?
4. What areas of the comprehensive psychiatric interview are challenging or discomforting for the reader, and what steps can be taken to increase comfort and skills in those areas?
5. How does the clinician incorporate a physical and laboratory examination into the assessment of psychiatric patients?

Short-Answer Questions

1. What is the virtue of self-effacement, and what are the implications of self-effacement for managing patients from different cultures?
2. How should a clinician begin a psychiatric interview with a new patient?
3. What techniques can be used for eliciting accurate information from patients on sensitive topic areas?

Answers

1. The virtue of self-effacement requires the clinician's humility. This virtue enables clinicians to put aside differences when these should not count as important in the clinical relationship. Clinicians should therefore strive to learn about the cultures of each of their patients and to respect cultural differences.
2. A new interview should begin with a general introduction and statement of purpose. Providing patients with an early opportunity to talk about what is important to them by using open-ended questions and by responding empathically should help to develop rapport and a working alliance with patients.
3. The interviewer should identify levels of discomfort in the interviewer and/or patient when asking questions that might impede a sensitive and accurate inquiry. Factors that enhance patients' willingness to answer honestly include developing rapport before asking questions of a sensitive nature, explaining the rationale for the questions, gently following leads, using facilitative or normalizing language, getting behavioral details, and being flexible to patients' personality style.

Recommended Readings

Poole R, Higgo R: Psychiatric Interviewing and Assessment. New York, Cambridge Press, 2006

Shea SC: Psychiatric Interviewing: The Art of Understanding: A Practical Manual for Psychiatrists, Psychologists, Counselors, Social Workers, Nurses and Other Mental Health Professionals, 2nd Edition. Philadelphia, PA, WB Saunders, 1998

Sommers-Flanagan J, Sommers-Flanagan R: Clinical Interviewing, 4th Edition. New York, Wiley, 2012

Strub RL, Black FW: The Mental Status Examination in Neurology. Philadelphia, PA, FA Davis, 1999

Trzepacz PT, Baker RW: The Psychiatric Mental Status Examination. London, Oxford Press, 1993

References

Engel GL: The need for a new medical model: a challenge for biomedicine. Science 196:129–136, 1977

McCullough LB: John Gregory and the Invention of Professional Medical Ethics and the Profession of Medicine. Dordrecht, The Netherlands, Kluwer Academic, 1998

Shea SC: Psychiatric Interviewing: The Art of Understanding: A Practical Manual for Psychiatrists, Psychologists, Counselors, Social Workers, Nurses and Other Mental Health Professionals, 2nd Edition. Philadelphia, PA, WB Saunders, 1998

Strub RL, Black FW: The Mental Status Examination in Neurology. Philadelphia, PA, FA Davis, 1999

3

Understanding Different Approaches to Diagnostic Classification

Maurice M. Ohayon, M.D., D.Sc., Ph.D.

Laura Weiss Roberts, M.D., M.A.

Giving a name, a diagnosis, to an illness that is due to a specific and known cause is intuitively clear. Pneumococcal pneumonia, for example, is an illness in which the lung is infected with the bacterium *Streptococcus pneumoniae*. Typically affecting young children, elders, or the immunocompromised, this infection may cause individuals to experience high fever, cough, shortness of breath, rapid breathing, and chest pain. Untreated, this infection can lead to death or enduring disability. A person who has high blood sugar due to a lack of insulin because the insulin-producing beta cells of the pancreas are destroyed by an autoimmune process has type 1 diabetes. And a person who has broken a leg in a bicycle accident will have, well, a broken leg, which might be characterized as being a compound, complete, comminuted, or compression bone fracture.

When the causes of an illness are not certain, the ways of sorting and classifying the dysfunction and disruption in health—assigning names or "diagnoses" to the problems—are less intuitive. In the context of mental illness, the origins of most psychiatric disorders are unknown, and definitive biomarkers for various disorders have yet to be discovered. Years ago, psychiatric diagnoses were based on assumptions—primarily untestable assertions of causality. Without clear etiology, pathogenesis, or discernible biomarkers, psychiatric diagnoses have thus become defined phenomenologically—that is, by attaching the name of an illness to the specific set of symptoms and signs that together represent a psychiatric "syndrome."

The identification of clear boundaries between different syndromes is essential for the validity of diagnoses. However, drawing such boundaries has proven difficult with major depression, anorexia nervosa, schizophrenia, posttraumatic stress disorder, and alcohol dependence, among other illnesses. Because a clear diagnosis is useful in the extent that it provides information on etiology, treatment, and prognosis, the aim of differentiating such illness processes remains valuable. Endeavoring to improve diagnostic classification is the intent of DSM-5, which uses insights from clinical and epidemiological studies. In clinical studies, the diagnosis is based primarily on diagnostic investigation of complaints reported by the patient and/or the physician's observation of the patient. In epidemiology, symptoms are mostly findings that emerge through the process of systematic inquiry. For example, individuals are asked a series of questions about different core psychiatric symptoms; positive answers to core symptoms will trigger the investigation of additional symptoms in order to achieve a diagnosis. DSM-5 thus uses an approach that aligns with the manner a general practitioner uses in reaching diagnostic conclusions: with each answer, the diagnosis becomes more refined.

Case Example: Refining a Diagnosis

Mr. Ramos, a 48-year-old man with a long-standing diagnosis of schizoaffective disorder, lost his daughter 1 year ago in an accident in which she was struck by a car. He is Hispanic, and throughout his life he has had very traditional religious values and beliefs. He tells his psychiatrist that he is "in despair" but feels comforted by "visits" from his daughter each night. He "sees" her in the flutter of his window curtain each night as he is falling asleep. Her visits started just a couple of months ago. He discussed his daughter's visits with his priest, who according to the patient, "at first" thought that the visits were "nice" but recently told the patient that he was "concerned" and thought the patient ought to "tell his doctor" about the visits.

Mr. Ramos has never used alcohol or other substances. He endorses feeling sad "nearly" every day, particularly in the mornings, and has lost 15 pounds. He says that the weight loss has been unintended and states that it is because his daughter is no longer there to cook his favorite enchiladas and beans for him. He has been adherent to his medication regimen, which includes medication for psychotic and mood symptoms. He has worked for more than 30 years on his family's ranch.

Questions to Consider

- What "facts" does the psychiatrist have to help understand this clinical story?
- Mr. Ramos describes feeling "despair"—is this a symptom, and what is the differential diagnosis that goes with this finding?
- Mr. Ramos does not feel distressed by his daughter's "visits," yet they have become a cause for others' concern. How does this experience relate to the normative experience in the patient's religious community?
- What should be of greatest concern to the psychiatrist? For instance, what serious physical health problems occur as an individual falls asleep (e.g., hypnagogic hallucinations) at night? What additional clinical data are needed to refine the diagnostic picture?

When a diagnostic framework is created, clinical phenomena must be understood within, and may be organized into, different hierarchical levels and components:

- When creating a diagnosis, the framework represents the most basic level. Examples of items that may be included in such a list are results of laboratory tests, scores on assessment scales, or the endorsement of symptoms or complaints on a checklist.

   In this context, a *fact* is a characteristic for which it is possible to define a normative value and its boundaries (e.g., a mean value with its standard deviation). For example, members of the general population sleep, on average, 6 hours and 45 minutes (Ohayon et al. 2004). This amount—6.75 hours—is a statistical norm. Different patterns of sleep represent variations or deviations from this norm and establish the range of variations in sleep behavior. Research may be performed to explore the extreme variations to this norm (e.g., two standard deviations from the norm, or the 5th and 95th percentiles) and can examine the health-related consequences for individuals whose sleep patterns are at the extremes. This process of identifying norms and identifying the extremes from normative values (in this case, sleep behavior) is an evidence-driven way of distinguishing highly specific clinical features that by definition, signal the presence of specific diagnoses.

   A list of facts does not assign relevance or importance to the individual items. Nevertheless, it has value in that it can be used in research, such as in identifying norms in a given population. An example is the experience of hearing one's name spoken when no one is present. This "finding" could be seen as a symptom of a psychotic illness, but norm-based data reveal that this experience occurs commonly among individuals who are not in any sense "ill."

   In another illustration, parkinsonism has many causes and is not always indicative of Parkinson's disease. By contrast, however, are features referred to as "pathognomonic." For example, in psychiatry, "chipmunk facies" due to parotid gland swelling is tightly associated with the presence of bulimia nervosa; this appearance has very few, very rare other causes. In pediatrics, Koplik spots are mucosal lesions demonstrating the presence of prodromal measles infection; in neurology, Negri bodies are lesions in the brain demonstrating the presence of rabies infection; and in general medicine, Aschoff bodies are highly distinct inflammatory nodules in the heart, demonstrating the presence of rheumatic fever. The presence of pathognomonic findings becomes a fact that signals a diagnosis, but still making the diagnosis is a judgment rendered by the clinician.

- Complaints represent the second most basic level. Diagnostic classification schemes also may be oriented toward categorizing patient *complaints*—that is, concerns reported by a patient. The complaint matters in that it reveals what is perceived as being a health problem for the individual. For health researchers, studying patient complaints can help in understanding what the motives are for help seeking and how help seeking relates to symptom burden. Patient complaints, moreover, are reflective of perceived need for care across larger groups and populations, and in turn, may be used to evaluate the efficiency of health care providers in recognizing and meeting these perceived needs.

- *Symptoms* are facts and complaints or concerns of patients that relate to pathology and then may be interpreted by the clinician. The clinician's medical knowledge and degree of specialization influence how well symptoms are discerned and ascribed meaning. Symptoms may then be the fundamental element in a diagnostic framework, although they may have a subjective component.
- *Diagnostic criteria* are collections of symptoms and clinical observations grouped to define clinical entities easily so that health care providers reliably recognize them and are able to communicate about them. These collections of symptoms and clinical observations can be assembled into syndromes, which allow for more refined efforts at validation of more specific diagnostic entities. Criterion-level investigation also presents the opportunity to explore manifestations of illness for which affected individuals may ignore or not understand the relationship between the symptomatology and pathology or impairment. Thus, a *syndrome* is a collection of criteria or symptoms necessary for a diagnosis. However, other possible diagnoses (the differential diagnosis) may not have been ruled out yet.
- *Disorders* are based on the previous elements—facts, complaints, symptoms, criteria, and syndromes (Box 3–1). Disorders represent a well-defined collection of pathological elements grouped into a pattern recognized as necessary for a diagnosis to be made. Accuracy in defining diagnostic categories in this way matters for precise communication among clinicians, researchers, and teachers; and diagnoses are valuable for people living with these conditions so that appropriate interventions may be identified, introduced, and evaluated for their effectiveness.

Insights for Epidemiology

Several methods can be used to improve the diagnosis-making process through the field of epidemiology; these include the study of the origins, development, and effects of the disease across groups of individuals. These include binary, probabilistic, and fuzzy logic models. These models shed light on the strengths and weaknesses of different approaches, including categorical models—the approach of DSM.

Traditionally, *binary models* are used to mark the existence of a diagnosis; that is, they indicate the presence or absence of symptoms and diagnoses. This approach is rather artificial in the sense that there is little room to accommodate the perceptions and experiences of the individuals, which is particularly salient in psychiatry. Symptoms associated with mental illness are rarely black or white—they come in all shades of gray. For example, if a person endorses feeling "very" depressed or "somewhat" depressed, there is a sense that these reports are truly different for that individual. But when asked to choose either "yes" or "no," a person experiencing even a "little bit" of depression is more likely to answer "yes." Using different and subtler or more graduated ways of eliciting symptoms may improve the accuracy of diagnoses and reduce uncertainty at both the symptomatology and diagnosis levels.

In epidemiology, probabilistic and fuzzy models are two ways that can be applied to capture subtler, more nuanced findings regarding the presence of a disease process. The *probabilistic model* is shaped by Bayesian theory, and it attributes certainty degrees

Box 3–1. The difference between the "complaint" and the diagnosis

Ms. Rush is a 26-year-old single woman completing her Ph.D. in biosciences. She is referred to a psychiatrist at the university mental health center because she has requested sleeping pills. "I just can't sleep," she says.

Ms. Rush reports that she has had trouble sleeping since she was a teenager. She states that she wakes up several times each night and that this occurs three to four times per week ("it seems like every other night"). She sleeps, on average, 5 hours per night. She feels sleepy during the day and "has" to take a 1-hour nap almost every afternoon.

In the course of the initial visit, the psychiatrist learns that Ms. Rush has been experiencing difficulty with her doctoral studies and she feels that her life has been "extremely stressful" for about 1 year. She has lost 14 pounds in the past year. ("I didn't try to lose the weight—it just happened from the stress.") Her body mass index (BMI) is 23 kg/m^2. Eight months ago she and her boyfriend of 3 years broke up.

Ms. Rush acknowledges that she wakes up every morning feeling extremely depressed and down; the feeling decreases in the day but is always present, every day. She says she cannot find any pleasure in her life. She feels that everything is taking an enormous effort. She is always tired and lacks energy even when she is not doing anything. As a result, concentrating on her studies has become increasingly difficult. She feels like she is letting everybody down. She states that she doesn't think her decision to get the Ph.D. in biosciences was a good idea and that she will not get a job in the future, but now "there is no turning back." Ms. Rush says some days are so difficult that she thinks she should "finish it"—ending her life so that she will not be such a disappointment to her family and her mentor.

Ms. Rush denies previous psychiatric or medical history. She had "a difficult time" when she was in high school and says that this was about the same time that she started having difficulty sleeping. She does not drink coffee or caffeinated sodas, and she has never smoked cigarettes or used any drugs. She "almost never" drinks alcohol. She feels she should exercise more ("I try to take walks once or twice a week with my roommate"). She says that she has not had interest in sex for "more than a year."

On mental status examination, Ms. Rush was cooperative, thin, dressed in athletic sweats and worn tennis shoes, and wore no jewelry or makeup. She sat very quietly, with little movement, and she answered most questions with few words, often by only a "yes" or "no." Her speech was clear and normal in pitch, tone, and rhythm. She denied hallucinations but said that she sometimes heard someone calling to her as she fell asleep at night—"like someone is in my bedroom, but I call for my roommate and she isn't there." She denies unusual thoughts or fears but "once in a while" she feels like she is being punished, as though there was a plan for everything to go wrong in her life.

Questions to Consider

- Difficulty sleeping is Ms. Rush's complaint and is the reason she is referred for psychiatric care at the university health center, but what are Ms. Rush's symptoms?
- How does the concept of "the funnel" apply to this case?
- How might the presenting complaint lead a clinician to give an incorrect diagnosis of a sleep disorder?

on the symptoms and/or the diagnosis. This approach allows for the creation of a nat-ural framework that retains the characteristics of the diagnostic classification and can still be interpreted in the usual way in practice. The *fuzzy logic model* (Zadeh 1979) is based on the concept of reasoning in degrees and linguistic variables, as opposed to the numerical/quantitative "degree" techniques of probabilistic models. For example, one can feel "slightly" or "a lot" depressed during the day and experience feeling depressed "daily" or "nearly every day." The same can be said about continuous variables. For ex-ample, an individual is obese when his or her body mass index (BMI) is 30 kg/m^2 or greater. What can be said about an individual whose BMI is 29.8 kg/m^2? Is the conclu-sion that this individual is not obese? A pure Boolean reasoning would conclude so, whereas a physician would not. In fuzzy logic, one can determine the degree of mem-bership of "BMI" to the category "obese." Consequently, the fuzzy logic model has the advantage of accommodating the imprecision of the human language. Using fuzzy logic, diagnoses are given with different levels of certainty (Ohayon 1999).

The prevalence of major depressive disorder according to the three models is shown in Figure 3–1. The binary model tends to provide higher prevalence than the probabilistic and fuzzy models. The fuzzy model can provide different levels of cer-tainty—a richer approach that has considerable impact on how scientists determine prevalence. The probabilistic model falls in between the binary and the "certain" or stricter fuzzy model in the example of major depressive disorder in Figure 3–1. Com-pared to the binary model, the probabilistic model provides lower prevalence in younger and older segments of the population.

Thus, the models used to describe psychopathology are imperfect. Mainly, the va-lidity of psychopathological models is verified through the models' ability to repre-sent real phenomena by an identification mechanism between what is symbolic and what is real. Nevertheless, this mechanism is only and always a process of general-ization because the model remains an unverified representation of the real phenom-ena. Is the representation true to the underlying realities? The "trap" in this thinking is that a model may slide from its position of analogy to that of the mechanism it is supposed to represent, and then it risks becoming an *autoreferential model,* in which the inclusion or exclusion of phenomena are no longer determined by the real uni-verse but instead by the model itself.

This autoreferential tendency can be seen in explanatory psychiatric models in which only demonstrable elements are true. As classification systems evolve, this prob-lem of autoreference cannot be eliminated. The risk of autoreference does not emanate from either the classification itself, because it is only a tool, or its creators, who under-stand the imperfections of diagnostic classification. Instead, the risk may come from us-ers of diagnostic schemata who are "true believers" in the classification, who do not understand the intrinsic limitations that exist, and who do not understand the impor-tance of both skepticism and judgment in the use of diagnostic classification approaches. If users do not actively question the validity of the scheme or ask for further verification, the symbolic representation is misunderstood as "the real world," and false conclusions may result. However, this risk does not mean that psychiatrists should stop creating or using models. On the contrary, the development and refinement of models is necessary to open discussion and to allow the advancement of knowledge.

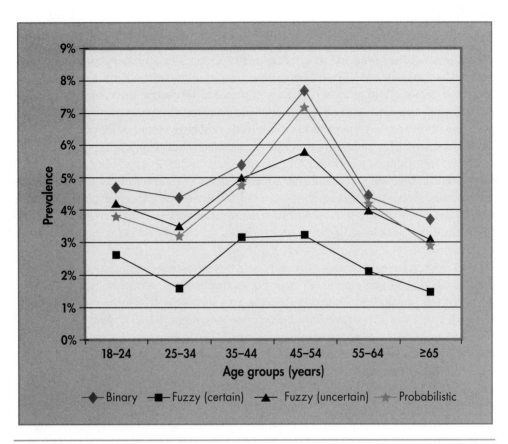

FIGURE 3–1. Prevalence of major depressive disorder according to binary, fuzzy, and probabilistic methods.

Source. M.M. Ohayon, personal data, July 2013.

Currently, categorical models—rather than binary, probabilistic, or fuzzy models—are the most widely used in the world. The *International Statistical Classification of Diseases and Related Health Problems* (ICD) by the World Health Organization and the *Diagnostic and Statistical Manual of Mental Disorders* (DSM) are two examples. With the progress in psychiatry, new classification entities are created; the objective is to achieve a better description of mental disorders while allowing a common language between researchers, clinicians, and mental health professionals. Nevertheless, these categorical models raise several concerns—mostly about their validity, because they are still anchored in phenomenology such as "facts" and "complaints." Some patients do not fit into any specific diagnostic category, while others fall into several. Despite an increase in the number of diagnoses, many disorders are not represented at all. This increase in the number of categories renders its use more difficult by clinicians. Further, the strong co-occurrence between some diagnostic classes suggests to some an inadequacy in the newly created categories. Finally, the absence of correlations between proposed classification entities and the efficacy of the different pharmacological treatments raises further concerns about their validity.

DSM Approach

DSM was originally valued as a research tool to provide common guidelines for investigators—rather than for its clinical utility. Over time, it has become firmly ingrained as the standard in psychiatric diagnosis among mental health professionals. However, making a diagnosis is not a mathematical problem: the sum of diagnostic criteria does not necessarily provide the best answer. The concept of diagnosis implies the ability to sort uncertainties and to decide between equally plausible solutions. Progressively, the distinction between concomitant (nonexclusive) diagnoses and concurrent diagnoses (those that exclude each other) is vanishing. This distinction is crucial because it bears important consequences in epidemiology and in clinical practice. Nonexclusive categorization essentially inflates the prevalence of some mental disorders. In the selection of treatment interventions, furthermore, the ambiguity and overlap of diagnostic categories increases the likelihood of nonresponse to treatment.

A classification system works, ideally, as a funnel, increasing the specificity in discerning or determining a given disease. For example, at the symptomatological level, 28.7% of the population endorses depressive symptoms. The prevalence progressively decreases to 5.2% of the population once the differential diagnosis is completed (Figure 3–2; M.M. Ohayon, personal data, July 2013). Consequently, by itself the presence of any depressive symptoms is helpful, but not in any way sufficient for planning treatment. Careful reflection on the differential diagnosis (i.e., engaging in the process of excluding other diagnoses) can help clinicians in this imprecise work. Consider the example of posttraumatic stress disorder. Although many people of the general population reported having been exposed to a traumatic event (15.5%), the prevalence progressively decreased with the addition of other diagnostic criteria, and only 3.9% met all the criteria for a diagnosis (M.M. Ohayon, personal data, July 2013). A third example relates to social anxiety disorder. Of the general population, 10.8% of people report experiencing discomfort in various social situations. However, only 3.4% of the population meet all the necessary symptoms and criteria for diagnosis of social anxiety disorder (M.M. Ohayon, personal data, July 2013).

DSM-5 preserves and advances the diagnostic classification scheme of DSM-IV. DSM-5 developers sought to capture emerging scientific evidence to more clearly separate or at times align diagnostic categories and to provide a clearer rationale for elevating and refining specific diagnoses. The overarching metastructure of DSM-5 was very intentional, creating a spectrum in which similar diagnostic categories were placed nearer to one another where possible. In DSM-5, there are 157 separate disorders, whereas there were 172 separate disorders in DSM-IV. Interestingly, with the decrease in total disorders in DSM-5, 15 new disorders were introduced (Table 3–1), 2 were eliminated (sexual aversion disorder and polysubstance-related disorder), and 22 were combined or consolidated with others (Table 3–2). Overall, classification of disorders emerging in childhood, sleep disorders, and substance-related disorders changed perhaps the most in DSM-5, whereas the personality disorders were preserved in their near-exact formulation from DSM-IV. As discussed in detail throughout this *Study Guide,* DSM-5 has changed the diagnostic criteria in highly utilized, important, and

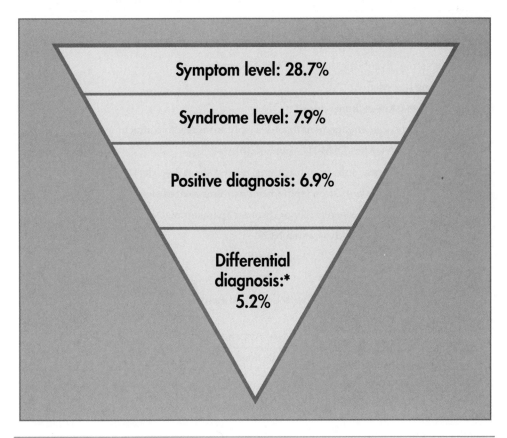

FIGURE 3–2.   Prevalence of depressive symptoms and diagnosis in the general population.

*Differential diagnosis refers to the positive diagnosis of a disorder excluding alternative, possible diagnoses.

Source.   M.M. Ohayon, personal data, July 2013.

long-standing disorders such as schizophrenia, bipolar disorder, major depression, posttraumatic stress disorder, and attention-deficit/hyperactivity disorder. DSM-5 also has moved away from "primary" and "secondary" attributions and eliminated the "not otherwise specified" language. Instead, it employs "other specified" and "unspecified" conditions, bringing DSM-5 closer to the language of the ICD system.

Diagnostic schemes evolve and are adaptive tools. The reader should seek to understand the value, application, and limitations of these tools—for DSM-5 as well as other diagnostic classification approaches. For learners, DSM-5 will prove to be helpful scaffolding for knowledge and will serve to inform clinical and scientific judgment, an expression of expertise and professionalism.

TABLE 3–1.   Disorders newly introduced in DSM-5 as compared with DSM-IV

1.   Social (pragmatic) communication disorder

2.   Disruptive mood dysregulation disorder

3.   Premenstrual dysphoric disorder (DSM-IV Appendix B)

4.   Hoarding disorder

5.   Excoriation (skin-picking) disorder

6.   Disinhibited social engagement disorder (split from reactive attachment disorder)

7.   Binge-eating disorder (DSM-IV Appendix B)

8.   Central sleep apnea (split from breathing-related sleep disorder)

9.   Sleep-related hypoventilation (split from breathing-related sleep disorder)

10.   Rapid eye movement sleep behavior disorder (parasomnia NOS)

11.   Restless legs syndrome (dyssomnia NOS)

12.   Caffeine withdrawal (DSM-IV Appendix B)

13.   Cannabis withdrawal

14.   Major neurocognitive disorder with Lewy bodies (dementia due to other medical conditions)

15.   Mild neurocognitive disorder (DSM-IV Appendix B)

Note.   DSM-IV Appendix B=diagnosis previously listed in "Criteria Sets and Axes Provided for Further Study"; NOS=not otherwise specified.

Self-Assessment

Questions to Discuss With Colleagues and Mentors

1.   What are the differences between a syndrome and a disorder? Why does this differentiation matter to a learner in the health professions?

2.   What are the advantages to a diagnostic classification system that uses descriptive phenomenological criteria as opposed to etiological or causal-based criteria?

3.   How does a clinician handle overlapping diagnostic criteria for different disorders?

4.   What does it mean to use binary, probabilistic, and fuzzy logic models in clinical care? How do these different approaches help in understanding the prevalence and impact of different illnesses?

TABLE 3–2. **Specific disorders newly combined in DSM-5 as compared with DSM-IV**

1. Language disorder (expressive language disorder and mixed receptive-expressive language disorder)

2. Autism spectrum disorder (autistic disorder, Asperger's disorder, childhood disintegrative disorder, Rett's disorder, and pervasive developmental disorder not otherwise specified)

3. Specific learning disorder (reading disorder, mathematics disorder, disorder of written expression, and learning disorder not otherwise specified)

4. Delusional disorder (shared psychotic disorder and delusional disorder)

5. Panic disorder (panic disorder without agoraphobia and panic disorder with agoraphobia)

6. Dissociative amnesia (dissociative fugue and dissociative amnesia)

7. Somatic symptom disorder (somatization disorder, hypochondriasis, undifferentiated somatoform disorder, and pain disorder)

8. Insomnia disorder (primary insomnia and insomnia related to another mental disorder)

9. Hypersomnolence disorder (primary hypersomnia and hypersomnia related to another mental disorder)

10. Non–rapid eye movement sleep arousal disorders (sleepwalking disorder and sleep terror disorder)

11. Genito-pelvic pain/penetration disorder (vaginismus and dyspareunia)

12. Alcohol use disorder (alcohol abuse and alcohol dependence)

13. Cannabis use disorder (cannabis abuse and cannabis dependence)

14. Phencyclidine use disorder (phencyclidine abuse and phencyclidine dependence)

15. Other hallucinogen use disorder (hallucinogen abuse and hallucinogen dependence)

16. Inhalant use disorder (inhalant abuse and inhalant dependence)

17. Opioid use disorder (opioid abuse and opioid dependence)

18. Sedative, hypnotic, or anxiolytic use disorder (sedative, hypnotic, or anxiolytic abuse and sedative, hypnotic, or anxiolytic dependence)

19. Stimulant use disorder (amphetamine abuse, amphetamine dependence, cocaine abuse, and cocaine dependence)

20. Stimulant intoxication (amphetamine intoxication and cocaine intoxication)

21. Stimulant withdrawal (amphetamine withdrawal and cocaine withdrawal)

22. Substance/medication-induced disorders (aggregate of mood, anxiety, and neurocognitive)

Short-Answer Questions

1. Which of the following diagnostic classification approaches is the most common throughout the world?

    A. Binary.
    B. Categorical.
    C. Etiological.
    D. Fuzzy.
    E. Probabilistic.

2. Which of the following lists is correctly ordered in terms of greatest prevalence to least prevalence?

    A. Disorder, symptom, syndrome.
    B. Disorder, syndrome, symptom.
    C. Symptom, disorder, syndrome.
    D. Symptom, syndrome, disorder.
    E. Syndrome, symptom, disorder.

3. Which of the following is a correct pair of a pathognomonic sign and the clearly related diagnosis?

    A. Chipmunk facies, bulimia nervosa.
    B. Compulsive behaviors, obsessive-compulsive personality disorder.
    C. Elevated heart rate, generalized anxiety disorder.
    D. Intrusive thoughts, posttraumatic stress disorder.
    E. Panic attacks, panic disorder.

Answers

1. B.   Categorical.
    The categorical approach is the most commonly used (e.g., *International Statistical Classification of Diseases and Related Health Problems* [ICD]).
2. D.   Symptom, syndrome, disorder.
    The list that is correctly ordered in terms of the greatest prevalence to least prevalence is symptom, syndrome, disorder. A diagnostic classification scheme narrows from widely experienced phenomena (such as a symptom of feeling sad or helpless) to a disorder (such as major depressive disorder).
3. A.   Chipmunk facies, bulimia nervosa.
    Elevated heart rate, panic attacks, compulsive behaviors, and intrusive thoughts occur in the context of many different disorders. Chipmunk facies due to parotid gland swelling is tightly associated with the presence of bulimia nervosa and has very rare other causes. For this reason, it may be considered pathognomonic of this disorder.

Recommended Reading

Regier DA, Narrow WE, Kuhl EA, Kupfer DJ: The Conceptual Evolution of DSM-5. Arlington, VA, American Psychiatric Publishing, 2011

References

Ohayon MM: Improving decision making processes with the fuzzy logic approach in the epidemiology of sleep disorders. J Psychosom Res 47:297–311, 1999

Ohayon MM, Carskadon MA, Guilleminault C, Vitiello MV: Meta-analysis of quantitative sleep parameters from childhood to old age in healthy individuals: developing normative sleep values across the human lifespan. Sleep 27: 1255–1273, 2004

Zadeh LA: A theory of approximate reasoning. Machine Intelligence 9:149–194, 1979

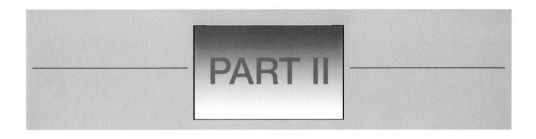

DSM-5 Diagnostic Classes

Learning Objectives

- Describe how the history may be used to differentiate among the disorders within and outside each respective diagnostic class.
- List interview questions that allow determination of which disorders within the diagnostic class the patient is manifesting, including disorders relating to substances and another medical disorder.
- Describe typical age at onset, risk factors, natural course, and complications of disorders in each diagnostic class.
- Outline the influences of gender and culture on disorders in each diagnostic class.
- Assess your practice for adequate screening and diagnosing of disorders in each diagnostic class.

Neurodevelopmental Disorders

David S. Hong, M.D.

"My son is too much to handle sometimes."

"I can tell my baby is different."

Development of the central nervous system is extremely intricate and complex, having implications for the multitude of functions that it innervates. Thus, neurodevelopmental disorders encompass impairments across a broad range of functions. Although phenomenology and affected domains in this diagnostic class are heterogeneous, they are unified within a developmental framework—symptoms are acquired or inherited early in development and are characterized by a divergence from an expected trajectory for gaining skills. Individuals are not, however, always diagnosed with these disorders in childhood. Often, diagnoses may not be made until adulthood, or clinical history may reveal that symptoms that started in childhood continue to exist in an attenuated form later in life. As a general rule, however, symptoms in this diagnostic class demonstrate early onset, are highly influenced by genetic and familial risk factors, and have a fairly pervasive course across several stages of development. Also, as with other diagnostic classes, impairments in this group of disorders must demonstrate significant impact on adaptive functioning, typically manifesting in learning or work environments.

Included in this class is a broad range of disorders, but diagnoses can be subgrouped generally according to the target cognitive or motor skill that demonstrates a disparity from typical development. Impairments in global domains such as intelligence would be diagnosed as intellectual disability (intellectual developmental disorder) or, when impairments do not meet full criteria, as global developmental delay. When specific speech and communication domains are affected, symptoms would be characterized under communication disorders (i.e., language disorder, speech sound disorder, childhood-onset fluency disorder [stuttering], social [pragmatic] communication disorder, unspecified communication disorder) or specific learning disorder. Disordered social communication is categorized under autism spectrum disorder or social (pragmatic) communication disorder.

Some disorders show overlap and impairment across several domains, such as attention-deficit/hyperactivity disorder (ADHD), in which both executive function and motor inhibition are affected, whereas others may be restricted to motor dysfunction, such as developmental coordination disorder, stereotypic movement disorder, and persistent (chronic) motor or vocal tic disorder. More complex syndromes, such as Tourette's disorder, encompass several motor domains, but are also commonly associated with executive function deficits and obsessive-compulsive symptoms. As a group, neurodevelopmental disorders are fairly complicated and heterogeneous both in etiology and clinical manifestations, but they also share significant similarities in onset, course, and susceptibility to genetic and familial factors.

Other disorders within this diagnostic class include unspecified intellectual disability (intellectual developmental disorder), other specified attention-deficit/hyperactivity disorder, unspecified attention-deficit/hyperactivity disorder, provisional tic disorder, other specified tic disorder, unspecified tic disorder, other specified neurodevelopmental disorder, and unspecified neurodevelopmental disorder.

The approach to diagnosing a child with a neurodevelopmental disorder can be challenging. First, the nature of symptoms and the typical age at presentation (i.e., during early development) often make it difficult to obtain all of the necessary information from a one-on-one clinical interview. Therefore, practitioners often need to be thoughtful and creative in their acquisition of information and may need to rely on other informants, such as family members, caregivers, and teachers, for additional clinical history. Standardized instruments that are designed to accommodate varying levels of developmental ability may also be of particular utility for this group. Second, the early age at presentation often means that receiving a diagnosis of a neurodevelopmental disorder is the first interaction a family will have with the mental health system. Therefore, clinicians need to be sensitive to the needs of the family throughout the process, especially because many disorders in this category are pervasive and symptoms will affect functioning over several stages of development, or in some cases, will be lifelong. Along a similar vein, practitioners have the opportunity to make a significant impact helping families obtain an accurate diagnosis and navigate the challenges of acquiring comprehensive interventions. In fact, successful diagnosis and treatment planning often require close interdisciplinary collaboration among mental health practitioners, medical specialists, educational staff, and agencies that provide specialized ancillary services.

A number of broad changes from DSM-IV occur in this diagnostic class. Most notably, DSM-5 diagnoses are consolidated around centralized domains of developmental delay, and diagnostic specifiers are introduced to characterize variations in symptom presentation. Changes include consolidation of social cognitive disorders under autism spectrum disorder and grouping of disorders in acquisition of academic skills under the specific learning disorder diagnosis. Strict age criteria are broadened to accommodate clinical variability in diagnostic presentations during the developmental period for intellectual disability, autism spectrum disorder, and ADHD. Readers will also note that several diagnoses that appeared in the DSM-IV chapter "Disorders Usually First Diagnosed in Infancy, Childhood, or Adolescence" have been relocated to other diagnostic classes in DSM-5; these include conduct disorder, oppositional defiant disorder, feeding and elimination disorders, separation anxiety disorder, selective mutism, and reactive attachment disorder. The DSM-5 neurodevelopmental disorders also include new diagnoses, such as global developmental delay and social (pragmatic) communication disorder. Careful review of DSM-5 will also reveal a number of minor changes, including, among others, the renaming of intellectual disability (intellectual developmental disorder), previously called "mental retardation"; utilizing adaptive functioning rather than IQ scores to define severity in intellectual disability; and using different symptom cutoffs in ADHD for older adolescents and adults.

───── IN-DEPTH DIAGNOSIS ─────

Intellectual Disability
(Intellectual Developmental Disorder)

The parents of a 6-year-old boy named Bryan have brought him to the clinic after being told by his school that Bryan is not ready to advance to first grade and will need to repeat a year. School reports indicate that he has not learned the alphabet and cannot count to 20 or recognize simple words by sight. He is also having difficulty engaging with peers and teachers, and demonstrates disruptive behaviors such as hand flapping and inability to sit still or pay attention during circle time. The school psychologist has just completed testing and found that Bryan has a full-scale IQ of 65 and is below expected grade level across several areas of academic achievement. Bryan was also noted to have "autistic traits" on a screening questionnaire.

Bryan's mother states that although she had difficulty getting pregnant, the pregnancy was otherwise uneventful and Bryan was born full term. She reports he was a "colicky" baby, was difficult to soothe and feed, and was late to start walking and talking (almost 2 years old), but she disregarded these issues because she felt that "boys are usually late with this kind of thing." On examination Bryan has prominent ears and a high forehead, appears anxious, avoids eye contact, and has poor enunciation of speech. Although his mother has a history of anxiety, there is no family history of intellectual disability. Bryan is an only child.

In this case, Bryan's IQ falls just below two standard deviations from the mean (<70), suggesting significant deficits in general mental abilities. Furthermore, Bryan presents with a constellation of symptoms that are consistent with fragile X syndrome, which is the most commonly inherited form of intellectual disability. Fragile X includes findings of characteristic facial features, stereotypic motor activity, and possible autistic symptoms. Although there is no clear evidence for family history of intellectual impairment, Bryan's mother has a history of anxiety and infertility issues, which may indicate that she carries a premutation. Fragile X syndrome is one of several genetic disorders with a relatively high prevalence rate; therefore, providers making an initial diagnosis of intellectual disability should be thoughtful about establishing an etiology when specific physical or medical features are present, because this diagnosis may have significant impact on clinical management and family planning. Furthermore, Bryan likely presents with features of ADHD and possibly autism spectrum disorder.

Approach to the Diagnosis

Individuals with intellectual disability are typically diagnosed at an early age. In severe cases, evidence for delayed cognitive development will be evident in the first few years of life. With subtler presentations, referrals may not be made until evidence is detected in the school setting. However, the diagnosis should reflect the presence of symptoms during the developmental period (Criterion C). Given that clinical presentation and associated symptoms will vary significantly with etiology, it is important to assess for signs of syndromic disorders even after establishing that criteria for intellectual disability are met. This entails a thorough assessment of behavioral symptoms, developmental history, family history, and physical traits. Because the majority of causes are linked to the period around birth, it is essential to obtain a thorough medical and developmental history for this time period. Further acquisition of collateral information from school systems and referrals to genetic and pediatric specialists may also be helpful for assessment and ongoing interdisciplinary management, if indicated.

Standardized intelligence testing establishes evidence of deficits in general mental abilities (Criterion A). Commonly, a score two standard deviations from the mean is considered evidence of cognitive impairment (e.g., a score $<70\pm5$ when the mean score is 100 and standard deviation is 15). It is important to remember that full-scale IQ scores may not accurately represent intellectual ability; therefore, clinical judgment should be used to interpret whether attention, cultural or language biases, motivation, or uneven intellectual abilities are affecting overall testing performance.

Also, impaired cognition is necessary but not sufficient to make a diagnosis of intellectual disability. It is important to demonstrate evidence of impaired adaptive functioning, which indicates how well an individual is able to adapt to everyday life across academic/intellectual, social, and practical domains, and to demonstrate social norms of personal independence (Criterion B). Adaptive behavior will necessarily reflect factors of age and sociocultural influences; therefore, these aspects should always be considered carefully when making a diagnosis. Particularly for individuals with more severe impairments, it is helpful to obtain information regarding adaptive functioning from other reliable informants or from evaluations or standardized testing specifically geared toward assessment of adaptive behavior. Notably, DSM-5 categorizes severity of intellectual disability on the basis of an individual's level of functioning relative to unaffected peers rather than IQ scores. Lastly, it is important to recognize that there are no exclusion criteria for this disorder; if the criteria for intellectual disability are met, a diagnosis should be made regardless of comorbid disorders.

As stated in DSM-5, "Individuals with a diagnosis of intellectual disability with co-occurring mental disorders are at risk for suicide…. Thus, screening for suicidal thoughts is essential in the assessment process. Because of a lack of awareness of risk and danger, accidental injury rates may be increased" (p. 38).

Getting the History

Parents bring their 9-year-old daughter to the clinic because of her cognitive delays. The interviewer determines whether the child lags behind expected age-appropriate development in general mental abilities, through assessment of overall acquisition of intellectual milestones and academic achievement. The interviewer asks the parents, "When did you first notice that your daughter might be having delays in her development?" and establishes that onset of deficits was before adolescence. Evaluation of impairments should assess reasoning, problem solving, abstract thinking, judgment, or learning. The interviewer asks, "Has your daughter ever had psychological testing or an IQ test?" and also determines whether any standardized assessment on adaptive scales has been done. If results are available, the interviewer should interpret them with careful clinical judgment to establish that global mental performance deviates significantly from the population mean and that other conditions may not better explain performance deficits. The interviewer then asks the parents to review the child's physical, medical, and family history, as well as any environmental exposures. The interviewer should maintain a high degree of suspicion for any factors that may explain the underlying cause of intellectual impairment. The interviewer then asks the child and her parents, "How do these symptoms present challenges for day-to-day function? School or work performance? Relationships with others?" The interviewer further determines the severity of function in academic, social, and practical domains.

As is typical with intellectual disability, this child is referred because of concerns by caregivers that she is having problems with cognitive development. The interviewer characterizes the nature of these deficits through the clinical interview and neuropsychological testing and ascertains that these impairments represent global difficulties with general mental abilities. The interviewer determines whether any factors may indicate a specific etiology or cause. In addition to a thorough clinical history, the interviewer will want to conduct a physical exam, with particular sensitivity to neurological signs or dysmorphic features. The interviewer may also consider the utility of referring this child to colleagues in other specialties if there is a high index of suspicion for a specific cluster of diagnoses. The interviewer will also want to ascertain how intellectual impairments are affecting specific domains of function. Collateral information from other providers, colleagues, and caregivers would be useful to determine adaptive function across a variety of contexts.

Tips for Clarifying the Diagnosis

- Establish level of general cognitive abilities by reviewing the patient's scores on standardized testing.
- Consider whether there are mitigating factors regarding the patient's performance on intelligence testing and whether mental abilities are affected across domains.
- Obtain collateral information on how intellectual impairments are affecting function in academic, social, and practical domains.

- Clarify when problems with intellectual function were first diagnosed; determine if onset occurred before adolescence.
- Consider whether intellectual impairment is accompanied by other developmental or physical impairments or by medical or family history that would suggest a specific etiology.

Consider the Case

> Mr. Mendez, a 26-year-old Hispanic man, is currently hospitalized for alcohol intoxication and withdrawal symptoms on the medical unit. Referral was made to the consultation-liaison psychiatry service to assess the patient and provide input on alcohol dependence and psychosocial issues. The internal medicine service is frustrated that Mr. Mendez is a "frequent flyer" with numerous similar hospitalizations over the past several years. He lives with his mother and has had significant difficulty independently managing activities of daily living since being hit by a car while riding his bike at age 11. Mr. Mendez sustained significant head trauma at that time and never returned to baseline function. His mother and close-knit family have since cared for him closely; however, they have had an increasingly difficult time managing him over the past several years. Maladaptive behaviors consist of poor insight; impaired cognitive abilities to reason, organize, and attend to basic self-care; and extreme impulsivity (they note that despite his small stature and some physical limitations, Mr. Mendez often gets into fights in the neighborhood). Mr. Mendez receives financial assistance for moderate intellectual disability and works part-time for his brother, stocking shelves; however, his family reports that after receiving any pay, Mr. Mendez immediately spends it on alcohol, leading to frequent inebriation and increased use of emergency services.

Mr. Mendez has an acquired etiology for intellectual disability, evidenced by a dramatically altered trajectory of cognitive development after sustaining serious head trauma during the developmental period. Because his intellectual disability likely results from traumatic brain injury, it would be appropriate to additionally give a diagnosis of major neurocognitive disorder. Further information regarding psychological testing is needed; however, clinical assessment suggests that he falls within the moderate range of impairment in the conceptual domain, given that he retains some verbal ability and possesses skills allowing him to work for his brother. The degree of impairment in the practical domain—impulsivity, excessive alcohol intake, inability to demonstrate progress toward independence—suggests an overall level of adaptive functioning that falls under the severe subtype. Providers should also consider to what extent Mr. Mendez's cultural identification may influence his family's perceptions of, or expectations for, his overall adaptive functioning. It is also clear in Mr. Mendez's case that his intellectual disability is a lifelong pervasive condition and demonstrates some of the challenges that occur during transition from childhood to adulthood for individuals with these impairments. Although a number of services are in place for children with intellectual disability through the school system and federal and state agencies, services available for adults with this condition are typically limited. In conjunction with varying levels in independence, insight, and judgment, the ability for adults with intellectual disability to navigate the medical system can be challenging. In Mr. Mendez's case, these issues have resulted in high utilization of emergency medical services and difficulty establishing appropriate care for comorbid disorders, such as likely alcohol dependence.

Differential Diagnosis

The differential diagnosis of intellectual disability is relatively limited because there are no exclusion criteria for this disorder. The diagnosis should be made when criteria are met, regardless of whether other diagnostic criteria are also fulfilled. Nevertheless, other psychiatric diagnoses should certainly be ruled out, including neurocognitive disorder with onset in childhood. Furthermore, it should be established that intelligence is globally affected; if deficits are narrowly limited to specific cognitive domains, diagnoses of specific learning disorder or communication disorder may be preferred. It is also important to take into consideration that impairments in these domains may make it difficult to assess global intellectual function, whether due to inability to participate in psychological testing or due to variable engagement or motivation in the assessment environment.

Given that diagnosis of intellectual disability does not have exclusion criteria, mastery of diagnostic criteria is relatively straightforward. The primary points regarding diagnosis are to assess whether impairments in general mental ability are not better explained by deficits in specific, restricted domains that may be falsely skewing testing of general mental abilities. A number of other diagnoses will also significantly influence aspects of cognitive function, including ADHD, autism spectrum disorder, mood disturbances, psychosis, and certain medical conditions. However, establishing the diagnosis may be facilitated by attention to age at onset; determination of episodic versus pervasive course; and a clear establishment of the developmental trajectory. As discussed in DSM-5, emphasis should also be placed on determining an underlying etiology, especially because the clinical manifestation of symptoms may vary significantly within this heterogeneous diagnostic category.

See DSM-5 for additional disorders to consider in the differential diagnosis. Also refer to the discussions of comorbidity and differential diagnosis in their respective sections of DSM-5.

Summary

- Intellectual disability represents global impairment of mental ability across cognitive domains.
- Psychological testing can confirm Criterion A for deficits in general mental abilities but may not reflect severity of functioning.
- Diagnosis of intellectual disability must always reflect impairment in adaptive functioning (Criterion B); cognitive impairment alone is not sufficient for diagnosis.
- Clinical approach to children with intellectual disability should include thorough developmental, family, and clinical histories to increase sensitivity for detecting syndromic manifestations.
- There are no exclusion criteria for diagnosis—intellectual disability should be diagnosed whenever criteria are met, regardless of occurrence with other comorbid diagnoses.

IN-DEPTH DIAGNOSIS

Autism Spectrum Disorder

The parents of a 2.5-year-old boy named Colin have presented to the outpatient child and adolescent psychiatry clinic with concerns that he speaks only three words ("mama," "dada," and "baby") and has not established a relationship with his parents or 5-year-old sister. The parents report that in retrospect, Colin did not seem "responsive" as an infant. They recall less cooing and decreased eye contact and copying of facial expressions in comparison to his older sister's behavior at the same age. However, they really started being concerned when he still had not acquired words by age 2 years. They note that over the past year, he has made only minimal gains in language skills—he speaks three words and appears to follow some simple commands, although neither of these behaviors is generally consistent or in context. Colin's parents note that he does not point or use gestures effectively; if he wants something, he will take them by the hand to an area and grunt, often getting frustrated and having a temper tantrum if they are unable to figure out what he wants. Colin also does not engage with peers and will completely ignore his sister, at times crawling over her to get where he wants. He primarily plays alone and obsessively with toys, lining up blocks by color or spinning wheels on trucks rather than rolling trucks on the floor. Colin is also somewhat clumsy for his age and frequently makes odd stretching postures with his fingers, but his medical history is otherwise unremarkable and his hearing has tested within normal limits. Family history is significant only for a paternal uncle who is "a bit odd" and "the black sheep of the family."

Colin's case demonstrates significant impairments in social reciprocity, structural language, and interactive play. These signs were evident early in childhood, although initial signs were likely already detectable in infancy. The solitary and restricted nature of Colin's play significantly diverges from what would be expected from age-matched peers. Similarly, his odd finger postures likely demonstrate restricted and stereotyped motor behaviors, which are also consistent with the diagnosis. Colin has significant delays in both expressive and receptive language; however, more notably in this case, he does not demonstrate other means of social communication, whether through nonverbal means, coordinated gestures, or expressions. It would be important to assess Colin's intellectual ability, although it will likely be challenging to obtain an accurate portrayal given that his social deficits may interfere with engagement in psychological testing and thereby affect performance. Although not presented in Colin's case description, it would also be important to screen for mood and anxiety symptoms, as well as problems with inattention, to assess whether other neuropsychiatric syndromes are contributing to his social deficits or are comorbid with an autism spectrum disorder diagnosis. Furthermore, additional clarity on initial age of concern, determination of whether Colin had demonstrated any sustained period of a typical developmental trajectory, and assessment for signs of any genetic predisposition or associated syndrome would be warranted. In this particular case, given a presumptive diagnosis of autism spectrum disorder, Colin likely exhibits impairments in social communication of level 3 severity. Further information regarding rigidity (including whether he demonstrates self-injurious behaviors) would be helpful in determining the degree of severity for restricted behaviors; however, his symptoms likely fall at least within level 2 severity.

Approach to the Diagnosis

The autism spectrum disorder diagnosis encompasses impairments in social cognitive abilities. Previously, distinct deficits in social interaction and social communication were required in Criterion A for this diagnosis; in DSM-5, Criterion A impairments now fall under three required categories: 1) social-emotional reciprocity, 2) nonverbal communicative behaviors, and 3) social interaction. To meet Criterion A, an individual must demonstrate persistent deficits in all three domains. Although a number of psychiatric disorders of childhood will adversely affect social functioning, either generally or in specific contexts, it is important to note that the core features of Criterion A for autism spectrum disorder indicate a pervasive impairment across social cognitive abilities that are integral for appropriate interpersonal relatedness. As an example, rather than impairment in language ability causing problems with social communication, the hallmark of this disorder is the inability to effectively understand or use the social aspects of language. The same holds true for nonverbal communication or maintenance of relationships. At times, discriminating the exact nature of these symptoms may be challenging, in which case structured social cognitive assessments may be useful in providing additional information.

Patients must also demonstrate at least two characteristics of restricted or repetitive behaviors (Criterion B), which can encompass repetitive speech; motor mannerisms; and use of objects, specific interests, rituals, or rigidity around routines. In DSM-5, restrictive or repetitive sensory behaviors also fall within this category, including sensitivity to textures, excessive touching or smelling of objects, and obsession with specific sights or sounds. Symptoms consistent with autism spectrum disorder must also be present in early childhood (Criterion C) and cause significant impairment in adaptive functioning (Criterion D).

Previously a number of additional subtypes were used to describe social impairments, including Asperger's disorder, childhood disintegrative disorder, and pervasive developmental disorder not otherwise specified. DSM-5 largely consolidates these diagnoses within the autism spectrum disorder diagnosis under the rubric of shared social cognitive deficits representing the core feature of impairment. Specifiers are now used to denote additional deficits in intelligence or language ability. Additionally, association with a genetic, medical, or environmental condition or a neurodevelopmental, mental, or behavioral disorder is defined using a specifier. There is also a specifier for associated catatonia. DSM-5 further defines level of severity for symptoms falling under the domains of social communication and restricted behaviors.

Getting the History

A pediatrician refers a 5-year-old child to the child psychiatry clinic due to concerns around delayed language and limited interaction with family members. The parents report their concerns that the child's development has differed significantly from that of his siblings. The interviewer asks them, "Can you tell me about his interactions with you and other family members?" The child's mother becomes tearful, stating that she always knew something was "wrong" and should have come to the doctor earlier but appears to have difficulty describing symptoms in detail. The interviewer asks, "How does he respond when you play with him?" leading the parents to respond that he has never engaged in games such as peekaboo, appears relatively uninterested in looking at their faces or eyes, and is generally oblivious to the presence of others. The interviewer queries whether the child has circumscribed stereotyped behaviors or interests that include at least two of the four symptom clusters for restricted and repetitive behaviors. The parents report extremely unusual sensory reactivity and cognitive rigidity. The interviewer asks about verbal and motor development, with specific attention to the child's delays in language. The interviewer also asks, "When did you first notice problems with language and social behaviors?" The interviewer establishes whether the child had acquired skills in the first years of life that were subsequently lost. The interviewer asks, "How are his symptoms affecting his day-to-day function at home and at preschool?" The interviewer asks about formal testing, including intelligence assessments, and questions whether any medical or genetic workup has been completed.

The symptoms in this case likely meet criteria for autism spectrum disorder. The child demonstrates pervasive developmental deficits in social-emotional reciprocity, nonverbal communication, and maintenance of relationships. It may be challenging to evaluate children with autism spectrum disorder, particularly when structural language impairments are present. Therefore, it is often important to obtain history from the family and other collateral sources to develop a comprehensive picture of a child's skills in a variety of contexts. Additionally, social cognitive ability is often difficult for individuals or family members to characterize. The psychiatrist is able to prompt the family by asking broad questions, which may be followed by more specific inquiries to establish that symptoms meet criteria for the condition. The interviewer also screens for other psychiatric disorders; however, further assessment of general mental abilities should be tested to determine whether social deficits are in line with or exceed other mental abilities, which would help to determine if the child meets criteria for the diagnosis. After establishing that social cognitive impairments exist, the psychiatrist also carefully ascertains how symptoms fall under specifiers defined in DSM-5.

Tips for Clarifying the Diagnosis

- Consider whether the child has difficulty understanding the perspective of others, and if so, how this difficulty manifests in the child's use of language, gestures, or play.
- Contemplate whether social interaction can be better explained by anxiety or specific social contexts, or whether symptoms are fairly pervasive across contexts and individuals.
- Question whether the child's interests and activities are narrower than would be expected given the child's age and cultural/socioeconomic background.
- Clarify the developmental history regarding onset of symptoms. Note whether the child has accompanying deficits in language or general intelligence.
- Determine whether social impairments exceed what would be expected, given the child's level of intelligence.
- Consider the impact of social communication deficits and restrictive/repetitive behaviors on overall functioning.

Consider the Case

A 17-year-old boy named Jon has been referred by his parents to the clinic for "having trouble getting along with people." Jon is a bright teenager who excels at academics, particularly in his stated interests of math and history, and when prompted he can expound at length on dates and events of colonial American history. He describes himself as being "socially awkward" and reports increasing feelings of isolation. Jon has a supportive family and has one or two friends at school who share his interest in computers and video games. He watches public programming on television but never watches sitcoms because he does not understand "why people find them funny." Jon has never had a girlfriend and rarely socializes with peers after school or on weekends, although he admits that he would like to do so. He is not able to recollect details from his childhood clearly but states that he always felt different from other kids and never had "best friends" growing up. He states that his parents never told him that he was behind developmentally and otherwise reports no notable psychiatric or medical history. During the interview, Jon presents as fairly robotic, with a flattened tone and stilted, adult-like language, which almost sounds like he is quoting text. When spoken to, Jon appears uncomfortable, avoiding eye contact and instead appearing to stare intently at the interviewer's mouth. Upon review of depressive symptoms, Jon states that "maybe" he feels down at times, and he goes on to express that people who commit suicide are "stupid" because there is always a logical reason to stay alive.

The case involving Jon demonstrates pervasive social deficits across contexts that are affecting his adaptive functioning, particularly in contrast to his desired level of social interaction. It is important to note that Jon's impairments are largely isolated to social functioning rather than general developmental delays. In fact, a cursory overview may suggest that Jon is generally functioning at a high level, particularly given the apparent absence of any intellectual impairment or language deficits. This may also explain why he is presenting for diagnostic assessment at a much later age than is typical for this disorder. However, despite his relative strengths, Jon recognizes significant social difficulties in engaging with others, and certain aspects of his clinical history, such as his limited peer interactions and narrow interests, may represent characteristic features of autism spectrum disorder. It would be important for the interviewer to get an understanding of the depth of Jon's interactions with his friends and his ability to develop and maintain those relationships, as well as to consider whether cultural differences affect the nature of his social interactions. Jon's stated inability to reciprocally understand others' perspectives may also be reflected in his lack of enjoyment or understanding of sitcoms, as well as in observed signs of nonverbal communication, such as impaired eye contact during the interview. He also demonstrates stereotyped speech and restricted interests in specific areas, although the extent to which these interests are excessively perseverative or circumscribed should be further assessed. In individuals who present in late adolescence or adulthood, determining the onset of symptoms is more challenging. In Jon's case it would be useful to obtain collateral information from family or friends to establish the developmental course of his symptoms. Also, how symptoms are affecting his function should be carefully assessed, especially because Jon's older age at diagnosis suggests that he may have already developed compensatory strategies for social deficits. In previous DSM categorizations, he may have fallen under the diagnosis of Asperger's disorder or high-functioning autism; however, using the DSM-5 schema, a diagnosis of autism spectrum disorder with specifiers denoting absence of accompanying intellectual or language impairments would be indicated. Furthermore, other comorbid disorders should be screened for, particularly depressive symptoms in Jon's case, because mood, anxiety, and attention disorders may either contribute to or result from core deficits in social functioning.

Differential Diagnosis

Many psychiatric disorders will have accompanying impairments in social functioning, but autism spectrum disorder is distinguished by social cognitive deficits representing the primary reason for symptoms. As an example, intellectual disability may be difficult to differentiate from autism spectrum disorder, because global impairments in mental functioning generally affect all cognitive domains, including social processing. However, a diagnosis of autism spectrum disorder should be made in an individual with intellectual disability when impairments in social communication and interaction exceed what would be expected for the individual's developmental level. Similarly, impairments in language, particularly receptive language, may also lead to secondary impairments in social functioning, requiring careful sensitivity on the part of an interviewer in defining the nature of core symptoms. In other instances, core social deficits may be present but are not accompanied by restricted or repetitive behaviors, as is the case in selective mutism and social communication disorder. In contrast, unusual motor stereotypies or repetitive behaviors in the absence of core deficits in social communication would be better categorized under stereotypic movement disorder, obsessive-compulsive disorder, or obsessive-compulsive personality disorder. The ubiquitous nature of social deficits and restrictive behaviors means there is a high degree of overlap of symptoms with other psychiatric disorders. It is also quite common for autism spectrum disorder to coexist with other conditions, if and when criteria are specifically met for comorbid disorders.

Evaluation of autism spectrum disorder may be complicated by the fact that impairment in communication is a primary feature of this condition, which may lead to misinformation in the diagnostic process. As an example, screening questions for psychotic symptoms, such as the item "hears voices when alone," may be interpreted literally, and a positive response may mean that the patient is listening to the radio rather than experiencing primary psychotic symptoms. Therefore, communication with individuals affected by autism spectrum disorder requires thoughtfulness about how information is perceived and understood. In cases where further diagnostic clarification is needed due to limited history or communication difficulties, standardized social cognitive assessments should also be considered.

Lastly, it should be noted that DSM-5 has centralized diagnoses characterized by impaired social communication and restrictive behavior with the goal of consolidating shared features across these diagnoses. Therefore, practitioners should pay particular attention to clarifying aspects of the diagnosis that may help distinguish variations in clinical presentation by careful screening for specifiers included under this diagnosis.

See DSM-5 for additional disorders to consider in the differential diagnosis. Also refer to the discussions of comorbidity and differential diagnosis in their respective sections of DSM-5.

Summary

- Specific attention should focus on social impairments and whether these arise from problems innately resulting from social cognitive abilities rather than from problems in other domains affecting social functioning.
- Restrictive and repetitive criteria may encompass a range of motor, interest, or behavioral aspects.
- Impairments will be pervasive and sustained, although manifestations will vary according to intellectual and language ability, as well as factors such as age.
- Compensatory strategies may influence presentation and time of diagnosis.
- Criteria for autism spectrum disorder define core features of social dysfunction; additional specifiers may be used to establish modifying factors, including severity, accompanying intellectual or language impairment, and presence of other related conditions.

——————— **IN-DEPTH DIAGNOSIS** ———————

Attention-Deficit/Hyperactivity Disorder

The mother of a 7-year-old boy named Shawn has brought him to the clinic because Shawn is experiencing problems in school and his mother is concerned that "he never sits still for a second." She reports that she has had multiple complaints over the past 2 years from Shawn's teachers, who state that his behavior is extremely disruptive—he is often getting out of his seat, talking with other classmates, and getting into arguments with peers during recess. His mother also has concerns about his behavior at home, although to a lesser degree than the concerns from school staff. She notes that he has always been an active child. She says that although he seems to be able to focus intently on an activity for hours at a time (e.g., playing video games), he also frequently gets out of his chair during meals, can never sit through a whole service at church, and tends to be more oppositional with boundaries than his siblings. She also observes that he is frequently losing his jackets and gloves and often forgets to complete or turn in homework assignments. She further describes Shawn as being very impulsive: "He is always saying the first thing on his mind"—which has caused problems with friends and family members on several occasions. Furthermore, when his attention is captured by a particular idea, he acts on it immediately, to the extent that he has walked out of a store or restaurant into the street by himself, causing his family to be extremely concerned about his personal safety. Upon observation during the interview, Shawn demonstrates a high degree of motor activity, jittering his legs constantly for the 5 minutes he is sitting in his chair, and then is noted to wander around the room, handling objects on the clinician's desk and frequently interrupting the conversation between the clinician and parent.

This case demonstrates a typical presentation of ADHD during an initial evaluation. There is evidence that Shawn has difficulty with both inattention and hyperactivity-impulsivity symptoms and would likely fall under the descriptive specifier for the combined inattentive and hyperactive-impulsive subtype. Although this presentation is fairly common in boys with this disorder, care should also be taken to ensure that Shawn's level of activity exceeds high-normal motor activity for boys of his age. Given that identification rates and symptom ratings of ADHD vary across cultural groups, his mother's interpretation of his behaviors should also be considered using a culturally competent approach. Further consideration regarding the variability of Shawn's symptoms should also be considered; although there is some evidence that he is able to maintain attention with activities that he finds interesting, predominant symptoms over the past several months indicate significant difficulty engaging in tasks with sustained mental effort, resulting in impaired functioning at school and at home. Additional collateral information, including parent and teacher rating scales, teacher interviews, and/or classroom observation, may be helpful in providing a more comprehensive picture of Shawn's symptoms across contexts. On the basis of the clinical interview, the severity of Shawn's symptoms likely would fall within the moderate to severe range. Additionally, it should be clarified whether Shawn's difficulties in school are due solely to ADHD, because these symptoms may mask specific learning disorders or other neurocognitive impairment. A thorough screening for other psychiatric conditions that are frequently comorbid with ADHD would be helpful, including an assessment of mood and anxiety symptoms and evaluation of disruptive or oppositional behavior.

Approach to the Diagnosis

Diagnosis of ADHD is challenging given the heterogeneous clinical nature of the disorder. Because ADHD symptoms may vary significantly over time and context, a high degree of suspicion and careful screening and assessment practices are required. The core features for ADHD in DSM-5 fall along two axes: inattention and hyperactivity-impulsivity. Impairments in either of these domains can manifest with a relatively broad range of symptoms; therefore, clinicians should take care to ensure that individuals meet required criteria before making a diagnosis. This care includes taking a thorough history to identify age at onset and placing symptoms in the context of where the individual is in his or her development. Furthermore, it is important to obtain family and medical histories, because certain risk factors may provide additional clues about the diagnosis, including low birth weight; toxin exposure; in utero exposure to smoking, substances, and/or alcohol; first-degree relatives with ADHD; and environmental stressors such as abuse and neglect. As listed in the DSM-5 differential diagnosis, a number of psychiatric and medical etiologies may also affect an individual's overall ability to maintain attention, motor activity, or impulse control; therefore, careful screening is needed to rule out alternative etiologies. However, because individuals with ADHD often will meet criteria for other comorbid diagnoses—particularly disruptive behaviors—criteria for these diagnoses should be carefully reviewed. Collateral information is also particularly useful in establishing both the diagnosis and the degree of functional impairment due to symptoms. This information may include standardized assessments from family members and teachers and neuropsychological testing.

Given that the clinical presentation for ADHD is temporally and contextually variable, care should be taken with DSM-5 specifiers in defining subtypes. Coding specifiers should take into account the predominant symptom presentation for the previous 6 months and include characterizations of severity from mild to severe. DSM-5 includes three classifications of symptoms—combined, predominantly inattentive, and predominantly hyperactive/impulsive—in addition to a course specifier indicating partial remission of symptoms.

As stated in DSM-5, "By early adulthood ADHD is associated with an increased risk of suicide attempts, primarily when comorbid with mood, conduct, or substance use disorders" (p. 61).

Getting the History

A 9-year-old child is brought into the pediatrician's office for a well-child check. Upon review of symptoms, his parents reveal that he has been having difficulty at school due to disruptive behaviors. The clinician asks the family, "What reports have you been receiving from school that have caused you to be concerned?" The parents respond that at a recent teacher conference, they were told that their son had difficulty paying attention, sitting still during class, and following instructions, but they feel that this may be due largely to teacher-student fit because his teacher in the previous year seemed better equipped to deal with these issues. The clinician follows up by asking the parents, "Can you tell me more about your son's development?" and asking for specific cognitive and motor milestones and other environmental, academic, or social factors that they feel might be influencing his current behavior in the classroom. The pediatrician asks, "Have you noticed similar behaviors at home?" and pays careful attention to determine if more than six symptoms are met under criteria for either inattention and/or hyperactivity-impulsivity. The parents describe symptoms of increased motor activity, although they feel that this activity may be normative because "all boys are active." They also report significant disorganization, impulsivity, and intrusiveness when he plays with siblings. The clinician then gently asks, "Do you feel as if these issues might be affecting your son's ability to thrive at school or in his relationships with his peers?" She asks the child how he feels things are going in school and at home, providing specific prompts as needed, such as whether he forgets what his teacher is saying in class, feels as if he cannot sit still, or forgets his things at school or home. She also reviews his medical, developmental, and family history to screen for risk factors that may provide additional diagnostic clues and assesses carefully for other medical or psychiatric conditions that may be contributing to the diagnosis. With the parents' consent, the clinician provides standardized assessment forms for the parents and their son's teachers to fill out before the next appointment.

The pediatrician in this case uses open-ended questions to contextualize the child's difficulties in school, carefully reviewing if his symptoms are consistent with an atypical developmental trajectory in core features of inattention and hyperactivity-impulsivity. She also systematically assesses whether other disorders might better explain the diagnosis or be comorbid with the patient's ADHD symptoms. Further investigation of mood and anxiety symptoms, as well as learning disorders, would be useful. The pediatrician demonstrates sensitivity to the parents' apparent concern about pathologizing their son's behavior by assessing whether they feel that symptoms exceed normative variation and are significantly affecting the patient's adaptive functioning. Additionally, she makes sure to obtain history from the patient regarding symptom presentation and effect on day-to-day function, while also arranging to gather further information from collateral sources through the use of standardized screening measures, which may provide further information in establishing a diagnosis.

Tips for Clarifying the Diagnosis

- Question when symptoms first appeared and whether symptoms exceed behavior that would be appropriate for an individual's stage of development.
- Understand how the symptoms manifest in different contexts and what others' impressions are regarding the individual's behavior in varied environments.
- Rule out other diagnoses, including medical etiologies that may better explain the clinical presentation.
- Question which symptom clusters have been predominant over the past 6 months along dimensions of inattention and/or hyperactivity-impulsivity.

Consider the Case

Ms. Jain, a 36-year-old professional woman, presents to the clinic for an "ADD evaluation." She reports lifelong problems with attention and organization, stating that she remembers always "daydreaming" in class. Although she managed to do fairly well in school, getting mostly high grades, she really started to struggle after beginning college. Ms. Jain remembers having significant problems managing her time, forgetting to turn in assignments, and often being described as forgetful and "dreamy" by her parents and teachers. Although she was able to manage a full course load, she always felt she had to work "three times as hard" as her peers to achieve the same results. After college, these problems crossed over into her professional work, where she is having significant difficulty organizing her office ("my desk is a chaotic mess"), has been missing important meetings, and has received negative feedback from managers regarding her organizational style. At home, she frequently misplaces her keys and mobile phone, and her lack of organization and impulsivity have caused frustration for her and her spouse. Ms. Jain particularly feels that symptoms have worsened since she gave birth to her two children; she needed to cut back from work after feeling overwhelmed with balancing full-time work and raising a family. Her 6-year-old son was recently diagnosed with ADHD, which prompted her to consider whether she also had the diagnosis. Medical history is otherwise significant for a remote history of an eating disorder during adolescence and infrequent migraines for which the patient takes opiate medications.

As demonstrated in this case, diagnosis of ADHD in adults may be challenging, particularly determining whether the person demonstrated symptoms before age 12 years. Obtaining historical records and collateral information from family and school sources may be of use in establishing this diagnostic criterion. Currently, Ms. Jain likely meets criteria for at least five symptoms of ADHD, with particularly prominent inattention symptoms. This symptom presentation is fairly typical for females with ADHD and is also more common in adults with the disorder because hyperactivity-impulsivity symptoms are more likely to attenuate over the course of development. Given that females with ADHD demonstrate fewer hyperactivity-impulsivity symptoms, they are also less likely to present with disruptive behaviors and may therefore escape detection of symptoms in childhood. This difference in symptom presentation may partly explain why Ms. Jain's impairments were not detected earlier in life even though symptoms were likely evident at that time. As an adult, Ms. Jain may face an additional challenge in obtaining an appropriate diagnosis for ADHD, particularly because she appears to be relatively high functioning. This challenge may in part be due to the difficulty in assessing the pervasiveness of symptoms over development but may also reflect her clinician's concerns that comorbid diagnoses are influencing her attention and cognitive function, as well as reservations about the high potential for misuse or abuse of first-line ADHD medications. However, careful clinical assessment should still allow an appropriate diagnosis to be established. In Ms. Jain's case, this assessment should include comprehensive screening for anxiety, depression, and eating disorder symptoms; assessment of interpersonal issues and adaptive functioning at home and at work; screening for abuse or misuse of pain medications; and a general medical workup.

Differential Diagnosis

ADHD may be difficult to discriminate from a number of other psychiatric disorders that affect higher cognitive functions of attention, motor, and impulse control. ADHD may be particularly difficult to discriminate from normative behaviors in early childhood. Oppositional defiant disorder and intermittent explosive disorder are also characterized by impaired impulse control, but specific features of hostility, aggression, and negativity are absent in individuals with ADHD alone. Hyperactivity is also seen in children with normative, high motor activity in the absence of other symptoms but should be distinguished from stereotypic movement disorder, autism spectrum disorder, and Tourette's disorder, in which motor behaviors are usually fixed and repetitive rather than generalized. Overall difficulties with attention, particularly in the school environment, may also be affected by mild intellectual disability and specific learning disorders, which can lead to frustration or disinterest in academic activities, although comorbid diagnoses can also be made when inattention persists in nonacademic tasks. Similarly, depressive, bipolar, anxiety, and psychotic disorders will affect attention and/or hyperactivity-impulsivity, although such effects are often clearly tied to specific mood or anxiety states and are more episodic in nature. External etiologies such as substance use disorders and side effects from prescribed medications (e.g., bronchodilators, thyroid hormone) may also closely mimic symptoms of ADHD and require thorough history and workup during assessment. Lastly, reactive attachment disorder and personality disorders share a number of nonspecific traits regarding emotional dysregulation and disorganization problems with inattention that require ongoing observation and assessment to distinguish these disorders from ADHD.

See DSM-5 for additional disorders to consider in the differential diagnosis. Also refer to the discussions of comorbidity and differential diagnosis in their respective sections of DSM-5.

Summary

- ADHD symptoms may vary significantly across contexts and developmental stage.
- Obtaining collateral information may be very helpful in establishing a comprehensive picture of symptoms and adaptive functioning in different environments.
- Impairments will broadly span clusters of inattention and hyperactivity-impulsivity, and predominant symptoms in these domains over the most recent 6 months will assist in establishing subtype.
- Difficulties with attention and hyperactivity can either mimic or be comorbid with a broad range of other etiologies, necessitating a thorough diagnostic evaluation and workup.

SUMMARY

Neurodevelopmental Disorders

Neurodevelopment is a dynamic process by which individuals acquire capacities in cognitive, physical, language, and social-emotional domains. This process is influenced by a number of factors, and there are many shared characteristics in the general framework and timeline by which these skills are acquired. Divergence from the expected sequence of events may reflect a derailment of the developmental process, and attention should be paid to how biological, psychological, or environmental factors may be affecting an individual's progress. The diagnostic class of neurodevelopmental disorders is designed to capture the presence of abnormal developmental processes, as well as to identify clinical symptoms that indicate an underlying pathological process. The domains that are affected may be heterogeneous, but the pervasive nature of symptoms over early developmental stages is shared in this group of disorders. Furthermore, symptoms for these groups may have a significant effect on an individual's functioning, with potentially severe consequences.

■ ■ ■

Diagnostic Pearls

- Concrete knowledge of developmental milestones is important for making accurate diagnoses.

- Comprehensive family histories may provide significant information in establishing a diagnosis, because many of these disorders are believed to have a strong genetic predisposition.

- With some exceptions, neurodevelopmental impairments tend to show a predominance in males.

- Disorders in this diagnostic class often share common features across cultural groups, but compensatory strategies used by families in dealing with symptoms may demonstrate sociocultural influences.

- Thorough medical histories will be useful in defining syndromes associated with neurodevelopmental disorders; physical exam findings and neurological signs may be particularly helpful.

- Increased access to and affordability of comprehensive genetic testing may make such testing a useful clinical modality for disorders in this class, particularly for intellectual disability and autism spectrum disorder.

- Collateral sources of information and standardized assessments are useful for diagnosis, particularly for individuals who are not able to participate fully in the diagnostic process.

Self-Assessment

Key Concepts: Double-Check Your Knowledge

What is the relevance of the following concepts to the various neurodevelopmental disorders?

- Developmental milestones
- General intelligence
- Cognitive subdomains
- Social cognition
- Attention
- Hyperactivity
- Motor ability

Questions to Discuss With Colleagues and Mentors

1. What distinguishes normative from atypical development? What defines early stages of development? How is adolescence defined?
2. What defines ability? How does ability differ among social, cognitive, executive functioning, and motor control domains?
3. How do impairments in neuropsychological domains interact with temperament, motivation, mood, or environment to define diagnoses?
4. What is the best way to screen for alternative etiologies for presenting symptoms? At what point is it best to make a referral or involve other team members? How much workup is appropriate for less commonly seen etiologies?
5. How much does making the appropriate diagnoses affect treatment and clinical outcome?
6. How does the clinician approach the treatment of patients with more than one disorder in this diagnostic class?

Case-Based Questions

PART A

> Gregory is a 13-year-old boy who was diagnosed prenatally with Down syndrome. His parents report a history of mild to moderate developmental delays: Gregory spoke his first words at age 1.5 years, and he started walking at age 2 years. Medical history is significant for surgical repair of a septal defect in infancy; short stature; vision impairment requiring glasses; and mild hearing loss bilaterally. His parents have brought him in for evaluation because of a recent increase in maladaptive behaviors at his middle school. Reports indicate that he is increasingly distracted and has trouble maintaining attention in his special day classroom and that he is more irritable and aggressive with his peers and staff than in the past.

What might be some contributing factors for Gregory's difficulties at school? Several issues are relevant in this case, most of which revolve around Gregory's diagnosis of Down syndrome. It would be important to determine the extent of his cognitive abilities and to assess for other conditions, such as specific learning disorder, ADHD, mood disorders, and/or difficulties arising from related medical conditions.

PART B

> Gregory's parents have brought his Individualized Education Program report, which includes results for psychological testing over the past several years. His full-scale IQ is in the 60 65 range, and academic achievement testing reveals lower scores across all domains. Teacher feedback suggests that Gregory appears withdrawn and less interested in class over the past several months, despite the absence of significant changes in his curriculum or classroom environment. He has also had a recent medical evaluation, including a hearing assessment, which showed no changes from his exam 1 year earlier.

How do you determine whether symptoms represent natural variation in the course of intellectual disability or emergence of a distinct disorder?   Psychological testing suggests that Gregory has general cognitive deficits, which is common for individuals with Down syndrome. However, intellectual impairments in this condition follow a relatively steady course. Although increasing cognitive demands may make existing deficits more pronounced as individuals progress through school, this change does not fully explain the relatively recent difficulties that Gregory has been experiencing. Similarly, sensory impairments may also result in academic and behavioral changes, but Gregory's medical issues appear to be addressed in the current case. Taken together, further evaluation for evidence of other psychiatric diagnoses would be warranted.

PART C

> More detailed history reveals that Gregory had problems with sustaining attention with difficult tasks when he was younger, although his parents did not feel it significantly affected his adaptive functioning at the time, particularly because he had a very supportive home and school environment. They also do not recollect that he was particularly fidgety or impulsive. When asked, Gregory focuses less on symptoms of attention or distractibility and instead endorses symptoms of depressed mood. He states that he increasingly feels alone and "different" from his peers and has many days when he feels too "sad" to go to school.

Does Gregory have ADHD and/or a depressive disorder?   Comorbid disorders are commonly seen with intellectual disability, which is not surprising given that impairments in general intellectual functioning may also contribute to difficulties in other cognitive domains, such as attention. Gregory's history suggests that he may have had at least some symptoms of ADHD in childhood, although his symptoms likely did not meet full criteria at that time. Furthermore, it is evident that he has difficulties with depressive symptoms. Depressive disorders are not uncommon in individuals with Down syndrome and can also be seen in people with intellectual disability. Cognitive impairments often contribute to significant difficulties in navigating school and home environments, thereby creating stressors that may exacerbate or contribute to depressive symptomatology. In turn, severe depressive symptoms may affect domains of attention and concentration. Gregory's case illustrates the interrelatedness of cognitive and social-emotional functions, as well as means by which cognitive difficulties can affect behavior and adaptive functioning. Further evaluation is warranted in his case, because he may in fact have symptoms consistent with both ADHD and a depressive disorder.

Short-Answer Questions

1. List three causes for intellectual disability.
2. Which of the following symptoms fall under the diagnostic criteria for autism spectrum disorder: limited facial expressions, echolalia, inaccurate word reading, clumsiness, lack of interest in peers, decreased sensitivity to temperature, self-injurious behavior?
3. Describe sex differences in the presentation of autism spectrum disorder.
4. How might the clinician differentiate between symptoms of bipolar disorder and ADHD?
5. List four medical conditions that may mimic symptoms of ADHD.
6. What is a difference in presentation for adults in comparison to children with ADHD?
7. How might intellectual disability be differentiated from specific learning disorder? Can these diagnoses coexist?
8. Which motor skills are affected in developmental coordination disorder?
9. Name at least two conditions to screen for when evaluating an individual for stereotypic movement disorder.
10. What is the distinguishing characteristic of Tourette's disorder from other tic disorders?

Answers

1. Down syndrome (trisomy 21) is the most common cause of intellectual disability; fragile X syndrome represents the most common *inherited* cause; and phenylketonuria is a metabolic disorder that leads to impairments in intellectual ability if left untreated.
2. Limited facial expressions and lack of interest in peers are characteristic deficits in social communication and interaction in autism spectrum disorder, and echolalia and decreased sensitivity to temperature represent typical restricted and repetitive behaviors associated with the disorder. Although subtle motor deficits may be observed in children with autism spectrum disorder, clumsiness is not a specific diagnostic feature. Likewise, self-injurious behavior may be observed in autistic children with severe features but is not part of the diagnostic criteria. Inaccurate word reading may suggest a diagnosis of language disorder or specific learning disorder.
3. Males are diagnosed with autism spectrum disorder four times more often than females, and there is some evidence to suggest that autistic girls are more likely to have accompanying intellectual disability.
4. Young children with bipolar disorder may also present with increased motor activity, impulsivity, and problems with attention and irritability, particularly

during hypomanic and manic episodes. However, these symptom presentations tend to be more episodic in nature and correlate with changes in mood state. The nature of motor activity is also usually more goal directed.

5. A wide range of conditions may also result in problems with attention, hyperactivity, and impulsivity; some medical etiologies include medication side effects (bronchodilators, neuroleptics, thyroid medications), thyroid disease, lead poisoning, obstructive sleep apnea, substance abuse, and sensory impairments such as hearing loss.

6. Adults with ADHD may be less likely to have overt symptoms of increased motor activity, but they may still experience an increased internal sense of restlessness or difficulty participating in sedentary activities. Also, for older adolescents and adults (ages ≥17 years) with ADHD, only five symptoms from the inattention or hyperactivity-impulsivity domains are required for diagnosis.

7. Intellectual disability involves impairment in general mental ability, whereas specific learning disorder involves an individual's ability to acquire skills in one or more academic domains, including reading, writing, or arithmetic. General intelligence will affect performance in specific academic skills, and individuals with specific learning disorder should also be evaluated for intellectual disability. Both diagnoses may be appropriate if difficulties in an academic skill exceed what would be expected given an individual's general intelligence.

8. Developmental coordination disorder covers a broad range of fine and gross motor skills, including general clumsiness, catching objects, handwriting, and riding a bike.

9. Trichotillomania and obsessive-compulsive disorder should be considered when assessing repetitive motor activity, because there may be instances where these disorders will be the more appropriate diagnosis.

10. Tourette's disorder can be distinguished from persistent motor or vocal tic disorder by virtue of having *both* motor and vocal features, and from provisional tic disorder based on duration of symptoms (>1 year).

5

Schizophrenia Spectrum and Other Psychotic Disorders

John Lauriello, M.D.
Tahir Rahman, M.D.

"I can't get my brother to eat; he thinks the food is poisoned."

*"I need to have a brain scan to find the transmitter
and get it out of there."*

Schizophrenia and the other psychotic disorders in this diagnostic class all share the common manifestation of psychosis. Psychotic thinking is a symptom, not a diagnosis by itself, and can be a presenting symptom of other disorders not in this class. *Psychosis* can be defined as a break in reality testing either by having sensory experiences that are not usual in a person (e.g., hallucinations) or by holding a belief or set of beliefs that is not accepted by most people (e.g., a delusion). Schizophrenia is a disease affecting thinking, communication, and behavior. Ever-growing research supports genetic, biochemical, and anatomical markers of schizophrenia. Less is known and researched on the other psychotic disorders.

The DSM-5 chapter on schizophrenia and other psychotic disorders includes abnormalities in one or more of the following domains: delusions, hallucinations, disorganized thinking (speech), grossly disorganized or abnormal motor behavior (including catatonia), and negative symptoms. The innovators of DSM-5 listed the disorders in this class as follows: schizotypal (personality) disorder, delusional disorder, brief psychotic disorder, schizophreniform disorder, schizophrenia, schizoaffective disorder, substance/medication-induced psychotic disorder, psychotic disorder due to another medical condition, and catatonia.

Overall, schizophrenia and its related psychotic disorders in DSM-5 have undergone moderate changes from the DSM-IV disorders. For schizophrenia, the five symptoms of Criterion A are the same (delusions, hallucinations, disorganized speech, grossly disorganized or catatonic behavior, and negative symptoms). Two or more of these symptoms are still required. However, in DSM-5, at least one of these must be a delusion, hallucination, or disorganized speech. This change eliminates the rare case under DSM-IV of an individual diagnosed with schizophrenia despite having only grossly disorganized or catatonic behavior and negative symptoms and no active psychotic symptoms. Another change in DSM-5 is that a clinician can no longer diagnose schizophrenia with only one Criterion A symptom if the patient is experiencing either a bizarre delusion or commenting voices. The final substantive change in the diagnosis of schizophrenia is the exclusion of subtypes, except for a specifier for catatonia. Thus, persons with schizophrenia no longer will be identified as paranoid, disorganized, and so on. The diagnosis continues to require markedly low levels of functioning in one or more major areas, such as work, interpersonal relations, or self-care. Continuous signs of the disturbance must persist for at least 6 months. Symptoms in Criterion A must be present for at least 1 month and may include periods of prodromal or residual symptoms. If there is a diagnosis of autism spectrum disorder or communication disorder of childhood onset, the diagnosis of schizophrenia requires the presence of prominent delusions or hallucinations.

These changes in the schizophrenia diagnosis also affect the other psychotic disorder diagnoses that require meeting the schizophrenia criteria but have shorter time durations of illness (i.e., schizophreniform disorder and brief psychotic disorder). If the length of time meeting the criteria is greater than 1 month but less than 6 months, the diagnosis of schizophreniform disorder should be used. If the symptoms are present for at least 1 day but less than 1 month, the diagnosis of brief psychotic disorder should be considered. Brief psychotic disorder can be further characterized depending on whether it occurs with or without a marked stressor or with peripartum onset (including within 4 weeks postpartum). Because these diagnoses depend on duration of illness, the diagnosis could change with greater time and continued symptoms.

An important consideration for the diagnosis of schizophrenia is whether the symptoms of Criterion A are due to a mood disorder. In other words, major depressive disorder and bipolar disorder must be ruled out. If the psychosis is only present when there is an identifiable mood disorder, then the psychosis is part of a mood disorder. A useful analogy is that the mood disorder is the fuel for the psychosis: put out the fuel (i.e., control the mood disturbance), and the psychosis is snuffed out. In contrast, if the symptoms of a psychotic disorder remain for at least 2 weeks after a diagnosed mood disorder is no longer clinically present, the fuel for the psychosis is independent of the mood disorder. In those situations, the diagnosis of schizoaffective disorder should be entertained. In DSM-5, the mood disorder, even if treated, must be present for the majority (>50%) of the duration of the illness. Another significant consideration before the diagnosis of schizophrenia can be made is whether a patient has a substance/medication-induced psychotic disorder or a psychotic disorder due to another medical condition. In both of these diagnoses, another explanation for the psychosis is suspected.

If Criterion A for schizophrenia is not met, several other diagnoses in this class can be considered. For example, if an individual manifests delusions alone for at least 1 month and the delusions do not markedly affect functioning, a delusional disorder should be considered. Subtypes of delusional disorder include erotomanic, grandiose, jealous, persecutory, somatic, and mixed. Some individuals manifest pervasive social and interpersonal difficulties that are "psychotic like" but do not meet the full symptom picture. Such individuals are often odd or eccentric and detached from others by lack of empathy or intimacy. In these cases, the diagnosis of schizotypal personality disorder may apply. In other cases, subclinical forms of delusions, hallucinations, and disorganized speech come to attention. A new diagnosis is attenuated psychosis syndrome (included in DSM-5 Section III as a condition for future study), which can be used to identify those persons who need immediate treatment and observation for potential progression to an established psychotic disorder. In some instances, the only disturbance is a pattern of abnormal movements and behavior that are identified as part of a catatonia (three or more abnormal psychomotor features). In DSM-5, catatonia is not treated independently, but it can occur in several disorders, including the following: catatonia associated with another mental disorder, catatonic disorder due to another medical condition, and unspecified catatonia. Finally, if there is psychosis that cannot be definitively placed in a specific disorder, a diagnosis of unspecified schizophrenia spectrum and other psychotic disorder may be appropriate.

In addition, other modifications affect the diagnoses of the other psychotic disorders. In schizoaffective disorder, the change of the word *substantial* to *majority* in Criterion C helps clarify the diagnosis significantly. Previously, the field debated what constituted a "substantial" duration of a mood disorder, and percentages varied from 15% to 50% of the illness length. The DSM-5 criteria specify that the mood disorder period must be present for the majority (>50%) of the time. This change should help standardize the diagnostic use of the category in both clinical and research practices. For delusional disorder, DSM-IV stipulated that the delusion must be nonbizarre; in DSM-5 any delusion may be present, but even a bizarre delusion must not markedly impair function or lead to obviously bizarre or odd behavior. Shared psychotic disorder is no longer a separate diagnosis in DSM-5. In circumstances of two persons sharing delusional and psychotic thinking, each person must meet the full criteria to receive the diagnosis of delusional disorder. In cases when the nondominant partner does not meet full criteria for any psychotic disorder, that person should be diagnosed using "other specified schizophrenia spectrum and other psychotic disorder" with the specifier "delusional symptoms in partner of individual with delusional disorder."

Diagnosing and treating persons with schizophrenia and the other psychotic disorders pose unique challenges. Many clinicians and family members have personal experiences with the symptoms of other mental illnesses. For example, feeling depressed, anxious, or overly preoccupied are common experiences, which may or may not progress to a diagnosis of a mental illness. In contrast, hallucinations and delusions are singular experiences. A clinician may merely be able to say, "I can only imagine what you are going through." Without a personal frame of reference for understanding the psychotic illnesses, a clinician can only wonder how hard it is for the person who manifests these symptoms initially and then chronically. The clinician may not be able to truly understand the symptoms but can understand and empathize with the distress and feeling of alienation resulting from these illnesses.

Often patients and families would like to know what the prognosis is with these disorders. Much will depend on the stage of the illness. If the symptoms are less than 6 months in duration and either schizophreniform disorder or brief psychotic disorder is diagnosed, the clinician must communicate a wait-and-see perspective. If the diagnostic criteria exceed the 6-month time limit, then a discussion of how to live with a potentially chronic disorder must ensue. In either case, the clinician's experience with the psychotic disorders is critical. An experienced clinician who has worked with a large number of patients with psychosis is usually aware of the highly variable outcomes, which depend on patients' insight into their illness, their premorbid level of functioning, and family and social supports. Clinicians should align themselves with their patients' goals and accentuate their patients' strengths and resilience in dealing with the illness.

IN-DEPTH DIAGNOSIS
Schizophrenia

> Mr. Kennedy is a 19-year-old sophomore in college who did well his freshman year but has had significant worsening of his grades recently. His parents are concerned because he calls them rarely, and when he does call, he seems distant and distracted. His parents note that they started to see changes when he came home after his first year, when he was working at a fantasy card store and often came home smelling of cannabis. They persuaded him to see a psychiatrist, although he declined at first. During the initial evaluation, while his parents were present, Mr. Kennedy was withdrawn and reluctant to talk. The psychiatrist asked to see him alone, and the parents left. When the psychiatrist asked if he enjoyed playing a particular fantasy game, Mr. Kennedy seemed to brighten and related how, although most people think it is just a game, he knew better. He related that he hears the voice of the "Grand Sorcerer," who told him the secrets to how people around him are pawns in a larger game of good versus evil. The psychiatrist asked how long he had been able to communicate with the Grand Sorcerer, and Mr. Kennedy said he had since the sorcerer came to him the previous summer (7 months before this evaluation). When asked if he communicated with the Grand Sorcerer after smoking cannabis, Mr. Kennedy said that he initially began to hear the voice after smoking cannabis but that he had not smoked for more than 3 months. A urine toxicology performed that day was negative for any illicit substances.

This case highlights several hallmark characteristics of a person with presumed schizophrenia. Age at onset is typically in the late teens and the mid-20s and is slightly younger in men than in women (mid-20s vs. late 20s). Mr. Kennedy is a male in his late teens who has demonstrated a disturbance in his expected level of functioning. In this case, a good student is now nearly failing his classes. The change in his behavior has concerned his family, and they are seeking some explanation from the psychiatrist. As in many cases, the strong suspicion that Mr. Kennedy has been smoking marijuana clouds the picture. The fact that he has not used marijuana for months but is still having difficulties tends to lead away from a purely substance-induced psychotic disorder. However, the use of illicit drugs can precipitate the onset of psychotic symptoms. The psychiatrist is able to engage Mr. Kennedy in an open conversation about fantasy games. This informal dialogue allows the young man to discuss his hallucinations and beliefs: he hears the Grand Sorcerer's voice, talks to that voice, and has an elaborate belief system centered on the game. The psychiatrist formulates a preliminary diagnosis of schizophrenia on the basis of the presence of psychosis, disturbance of functioning, and duration of symptoms for longer than 6 months. A cannabis-induced psychotic disorder may still be possible, but at this point that diagnosis is less likely because Mr. Kennedy has stopped marijuana use for a length of time.

Approach to the Diagnosis

Although the identification of hallucinations and delusions would seem to be the starting point for diagnosing schizophrenia, a change in level of functioning is most often the beginning of the diagnostic journey. The teenager whose grades are suffering or the new army recruit not doing well in boot camp either seeks help or has others seek it for him or her. The clinician is usually given a "chief complaint" or presenting problem. Discovering what is causing the problem is the clinician's first order of business. Clear indications of delusions and hallucinations direct the clinician toward schizophrenia and the related psychotic disorders. However, the presenting symptoms are often not clear-cut and may include misrepresentations, misattributions, and misperceptions, rather than frank delusions or hallucinations. The clinician begins to explore the symptoms, eliciting specific examples of each one. Understanding, in detail, what the person believes is a voice in his or her head is critical. Is it his or her own voice on a continuous ruminative loop or a distinct voice or voices alien to his or her own train of thought? Is the individual's avoidance of others a product of a delusion, a result of extreme shyness, or simply a way to deal with living in a well-documented dangerous neighborhood?

Listening to how the individual speaks and puts together thoughts is critical in understanding his or her information processing. Lack of education can have some effect on this process but cannot excuse all disorganization or poverty of speech. The clinician needs to talk to the person's family and friends and listen to what they say about the person's thought process, especially if it has changed.

Understanding the role of mood in diagnosing schizophrenia is critical. Individuals with schizophrenia have feelings, whether they readily show them or not. They are often susceptible to depression and rarely to mania. Determining whether the person's psychosis exists only under the umbrella of a mood disorder is critical and may take many months of observation and treatment response. Once the mood is stable, clearly identifying a remaining psychosis leads the clinician's diagnostic algorithm to either schizophrenia or schizoaffective disorder. Distinguishing these latter two diagnoses relies on a careful timeline of months and years and consideration of whether the mood disorder is active or in remission with treatment. If the mood disorder occupies the majority of the illness history, the diagnosis of schizoaffective disorder is more appropriate.

A clinician must avoid jumping to a diagnosis of schizophrenia without a comprehensive review of all other causations. Substance use, both prescribed and illicit, has become commonplace for many people. Possible nonpsychiatric diagnoses include autoimmune disorders, infections, and malignancies.

However, the clinician should not jump away from the diagnosis of schizophrenia if all evidence points to it. There is an understandable but countertherapeutic reluctance to tell patients and their families that the diagnosis is schizophrenia. Sometimes the diagnosis feels premature, despite the patient's clearly meeting the minimum duration of 6 months; sometimes the diagnosis can be too demoralizing for a clinician who recalls his or her chronic and disabled patients with schizophrenia.

The lifetime prevalence of schizophrenia is estimated to be approximately 0.3%–0.7%. Risk factors have been proposed for schizophrenia—including family history, late winter/early spring births, older paternal age, and birth complications—but no single risk factor has been clinically useful. Candidate genes have been identified, but they alone are not yet a definitive "test" for schizophrenia.

Morbidity data for persons with schizophrenia are often difficult to capture, but it is widely accepted that those with schizophrenia suffer from a greater burden of weight gain, diabetes, metabolic syndrome, cigarette smoking, cardiovascular and pulmonary disease, and substance abuse. A shared vulnerability for psychosis and medical disorders may explain some of these comorbidities. Psychotic symptoms tend to diminish over the life course, perhaps in association with normal age-related declines in dopamine activity. Negative symptoms are more common in males, tend to be the most persistent, and are associated with worse prognosis. Individuals with schizophrenia have a decrease in their life expectancy.

As stated in DSM-5, "Approximately 5%–6% of individuals with schizophrenia die by suicide, about 20% attempt suicide on one or more occasions, and many more have significant suicidal ideation. Suicidal behavior is sometimes in response to command hallucinations to harm oneself or others. Suicide risk remains high over the whole lifespan for males and females, although it may be especially high for younger males with comorbid substance use. Other risk factors include having depressive symptoms or feelings of hopelessness and being unemployed, and the risk is higher, also, in the period after a psychotic episode or hospital discharge" (p. 104).

Getting the History

Mr. Rivera, a 28-year-old man, presents to the clinic after a referral from his primary care doctor. His doctor is concerned that Mr. Rivera is overly occupied with a cough that does not appear to be due to any infection. In the doctor's office, Mr. Rivera seems distant and appears at times to look away and talk to himself.

The psychiatrist should be open-minded that Mr. Rivera may have a psychiatric condition but that it is also possible the cough is due to a biological cause yet to be determined. The clinician begins with questions about why Mr. Rivera is there and whether he understands his primary care provider's concern. Mr. Rivera says, "I am here because the doctor says it is all in my head." The clinician responds, "I am not sure whether that is true, so tell me about the cough." The psychiatrist goes beyond eliciting the symptoms of the cough (e.g., frequency, productive or not, other physical symptoms) and asks about Mr. Rivera's concerns about the cough: "What do you think is causing the cough? What are you afraid might happen if the cough continues?" In the interview, Mr. Rivera seems to look away and talk to himself. The psychiatrist asks, "I can't help noticing that you seem to be talking to someone besides me in the room. Are you comfortable telling me about that?" Mr. Rivera responds that he is hearing his mother talk to him, even though she died 3 years ago. The psychiatrist asks what he and his mother talk about. Though initially guarded, the man eventually says that his mother tells him that germs are everywhere and he needs to be afraid of them. The psychiatrist asks how long he has been able to communicate with his mother and if this communication is something that he finds helpful. Mr. Rivera says he has for the last year, and of course, it is a great help to talk to her. As he speaks, he talks with little emotion. To delve further, the clinician asks if the patient was upset about his mother's death. Mr. Rivera says with little expressed feeling that at first he was, but now he understands that she is still able to talk to him as if she were still alive. The psychiatrist asks if the cough has affected his work and learns that Mr. Rivera does not work now because there are too many germs "out there." The psychiatrist asks if he takes any prescribed medicine, home remedies, or even street drugs to help with the cough and germs. Mr. Rivera firmly states that he took prescribed antibiotics for a while but no longer does. He has consulted a healer in his neighborhood, who told him to breathe hot steamed water infused with garlic, which he occasionally does. He denies using any illicit substances.

The statement "once a clinician sees one case of schizophrenia, the clinician has seen one case of schizophrenia" is partially true. Specific details are unique to each patient, and it is often fascinating to hear the varied accounts patients present. The psychosis always comes in the context of the patient's life, family, stressors, and past events. Mr. Rivera presents with a physical symptom, which is a common entry into treatment. The facts about the physical symptom and the meaning of it to him are critical. Other patients might present after an identifiable breakdown in their functioning, a failed semester, or a new job they could not handle. Still others have had psychological difficulties from childhood and are diagnosed with a variety of other illnesses that either coexisted with or were harbingers of a fully manifested psychosis. The psychiatrist needs to be open-minded to the individual details but understand that central themes tend to emerge after working with many patients. These themes include preoccupations with beliefs that negatively affect functioning and odd thinking and behaviors that point to schizophrenia. Certain ways of expressing thoughts, often disconnected from the full range of emotions, are indicators of schizophrenia. The experienced clinician understands that schizophrenia is not a "one-visit" diagnosis but requires multiple assessments over time to confirm.

Tips for Clarifying the Diagnosis

- Determine if there is a psychosis. Ask the person about hearing voices or seeing things; delve into the details of these experiences. Is the voice separate from the person's own train of thought?
- Understand the person's cultural beliefs. A potentially helpful tip is to ask the individual's family members how they feel about the issues the person has reported. For example, if the family believes that dead relatives can speak to them, this experience may not be a delusion.
- Similarly, in evaluating level of functioning, ask what the person's parents and siblings do. If the individual engages in manual labor but everyone else in the family is a successful professional, this situation may signal a drop in the potential functioning of the person.
- Sometimes illicit substances cause many of the symptoms; however, do not be surprised if an individual ascribes his or her problem to substances even though little or no evidence supports that.

- When a person describes being paranoid, asking why someone is out to get the person specifically may be helpful; often this question brings out significant grandiose thinking.

Consider the Case

Ms. Smythe is a 42-year-old recent immigrant to the United States. She cites political and economic reasons for leaving her parents and extended family. Unable to find work in her professional field, she supports herself by working as a maid in a hotel. Generally friendly, she has made some acquaintances at work and at church. She misses her old life, especially her family, but hopes to bring her parents to the United States. In church, she enrolled in a vocational program that helps members find higher-paying work. While Ms. Smythe was in the program, the minister noticed that she was becoming increasingly disheveled and distracted. When asked about this, she became tearful and upset. She said everything was going so well until a man began to follow her home from work. At first she thought nothing of it, but now she was sure that he was from the secret police from her native country. Somehow he had been able to put listening devices in her apartment and had slipped a micro-tracking device in her food, which she can taste when she eats. When asked why anyone would go to such lengths to follow her, she whispered that she was the rightful heir to the throne and the man needed to stop her from taking power. The minister suggested she speak to someone at the community clinic and arranged for an appointment with a psychiatrist. On interview, the psychiatrist noted that Ms. Smythe seemed preoccupied and repeatedly looked out the window. When the psychiatrist asked what she was looking at, she stated nonchalantly that city buses with a certain advertisement were sending her codes from loyalists in her homeland. The psychiatrist noted that she spoke slowly and calmly and did not appear agitated. Ms. Smythe reported sleeping well and going to work as scheduled. Of note, she has no history of substance use and had been diagnosed 5 years earlier with hyperthyroidism, which is under good control.

Ms. Smythe presents with both usual and atypical features of schizophrenia. At age 42, she seems a bit "old" for the diagnosis, but it is not rare for a patient to present in the third or fourth decade. Her move to the United States is a significant stressor, compounded by having to leave her family. It is also not known whether she might have had previous or subclinical episodes in her native country. The minister noticed a change in her, but Ms. Smythe is still able to work and take care of herself. Her belief that she is being followed, the messages from the city buses (ideas of reference), and the possible gustatory hallucinations point to a psychotic manifestation. However, it is important to determine whether some of her experiences may be related to the culture and climate of her native country. It is possible that she may have to be much more independent in the United States than she was accustomed to in her homeland. This change might lead to a sense of insecurity that might seem paranoid. She may also have had traumatic events in her past that make her wary of others, so her psychotic symptoms may be intertwined with posttraumatic symptoms. As with all diagnoses, collecting information from family and friends may shed some light on many of these issues.

Studies have found that being a first- or second-generation immigrant is a risk factor for developing schizophrenia. A large study in the United Kingdom found increased rates in African and Afro-Caribbean immigrants. The adversities of people who migrate mirror those of native persons who experience racial discrimination, poverty, and disrupted families. Strong intact family and community support are postulated to be positive mitigating influences.

Determining whether Ms. Smythe's psychotic symptoms are secondary to a mood disorder is critical to making an accurate diagnosis. She believes herself to be the heir to the throne, an apparently grandiose belief. However, when asked, she says that she is neither depressed nor excessively happy. She is sleeping well, and no external observation of mania, including pressured speech, is described. Although thyroid abnormalities can lead to psychosis, there is no evidence so far of that, but a full thyroid panel should be obtained, as well as a toxicology screen, despite her report of not using substances. Depending on how long these symptoms have been occurring and how much they have affected her functioning, the presumptive diagnosis of schizophrenia could be confirmed.

Differential Diagnosis

The differential diagnosis of schizophrenia is a process of eliciting the cardinal symptoms represented in Criterion A and then determining whether these symptoms might be indicative of another disorder. Functional impairment is usually a main reason for the person to come to the attention of health care providers. The degree of functional impairment might help differentiate between more circumscribed disorders, such as delusional disorder or mood disorders. If the person has a noticeable presentation of depression or mania, mood disorders and schizoaffective disorder need to be immediately considered. The number of episodes and the recovery from psychosis with control of mood help differentiate mood disorders from schizophrenia. The continued manifestation of psychosis with control of mood (including treated time segments) directs the differential to either schizoaffective disorder or schizophrenia. Distinguishing these two can be difficult and requires a careful retrospective bookkeeping of the percentage of mood disorder versus the overall length of the psychotic illness.

Other important differentiators include length of illness and possible other external explanations for the symptoms. Along a time continuum, brief psychotic disorder is of less than 1 month in duration; schizophreniform disorder, less than 6 months in duration; and schizophrenia and schizoaffective disorder, greater than 6 months. If either an underlying medical condition or use of illicit substances is a possible source of the schizophrenic symptoms, it must be eliminated as the potential cause. The treatment of underlying medical conditions and the assurance of abstinence from substance use, when applicable, may lead to complete resolution of the schizophrenic symptoms and confirm a diagnosis of psychotic disorder due to another medical condition or substance/medication-induced psychotic disorder. Personality disorders (e.g., schizotypal personality disorder), communication disorders, and autism spectrum disorder must also be considered and usually include a long-standing pattern of behavior without the full-blown presentation of psychosis seen in schizophrenia. Depending on the content of symptoms, obsessive-compulsive disorder, body dysmorphic disorder, and posttraumatic stress disorder should also be considered.

See DSM-5 for additional disorders to consider in the differential diagnosis. Also refer to the discussions of comorbidity and differential diagnosis in their respective sections of DSM-5.

Summary

- Schizophrenia and the other psychotic disorders share the common manifestation of psychosis. Psychotic thinking is a symptom, not a diagnosis by itself, and can be a presenting symptom of other disorders not in this diagnostic class.
- Schizophrenia is a serious mental disorder affecting thinking, communication, and behavior. Psychosis is a critical element of this diagnosis; hallucinations and delusions are two of the five symptoms listed in Criterion A. The other three symptoms are disorganized speech, grossly disorganized or catatonic behavior, and negative symptoms.
- Persons must meet at least two of these Criterion A symptoms, and one must be a delusion, hallucination, or disorganized speech for at least 1 month.
- Persons must have significant disturbances in functioning secondary to the symptoms, with a wide range of functional domains possibly affected (e.g., school, work, interpersonal relationships) for at least 6 months.
- The lifetime prevalence of schizophrenia is estimated to be approximately 0.3%–0.7%.
- Age at onset is typically in the late teens and the mid-30s and is slightly younger in men than in women (mid-20s vs. late 20s).
- Morbidity data for persons with schizophrenia are often difficult to capture, but it is widely accepted that those with schizophrenia suffer from a greater burden of weight gain, diabetes, metabolic syndrome, cigarette smoking, cardiovascular and pulmonary disease, and substance abuse. A shared vulnerability for psychosis and medical disorders may explain some of these comorbidities.
- Individuals with schizophrenia have a decrease in their life expectancy.
- Psychotic symptoms tend to diminish over the life course, perhaps in association with normal age-related declines in dopamine activity. Negative symptoms are more common in males and tend to be the most persistent and tend to have a worse prognosis.
- Approximately 5%–6% of persons with schizophrenia die by suicide.

--------- **IN-DEPTH DIAGNOSIS** ---------

Brief Psychotic Disorder

Ms. Baker is a 38-year-old married woman with three children and an eleventh-grade education. Her husband abandoned her a week ago and cannot be located. She is unemployed and recently spent the last of her money paying bills. She presented to the emergency clinic with her sister. According to her sister, Ms. Baker has not been bathing or cooking meals for the last few days, and she was seen staring at a wall for hours while talking to herself. There were no prior mood disorder symptoms and no previous psychotic episodes. There is no known history of drug abuse.

On examination, Ms. Baker was alert and oriented, with intermittent eye contact. She reported no thoughts of suicide. She stated that she hears the voice of her grandmother trying to help her. Her grandmother's voice is very clear, and Ms. Baker feels her presence near her. Ms. Baker is admitted to the psychiatric hospital for observation.

Her admission drug screen and labs are all normal. On the unit she quickly recovered and, after attending groups and speaking to a social worker, was discharged. No psychotic symptoms were evident at discharge and no medications prescribed. An outpatient therapist appointment was made for follow-up care. No further psychotic episodes or mood disorder symptoms occurred in the next 6–8 months.

Ms. Baker presented with sudden hallucinations and disorganized, possibly catatonic, behavior. These symptoms occurred when she was under significant stress, because her husband left her and she faced a sudden financial crisis. It is extremely helpful that her sister can provide collateral information, especially about the recent onset of the symptoms and behavior. The psychotic symptoms did not appear to occur in the midst of a depressive or manic episode. Medical or substance causation is unlikely without a history of either and with normal labs and toxicology screens. Likewise, Ms. Baker's intact orientation effectively rules out a delirium. The presumed diagnosis at admission is brief psychotic disorder, with marked stressors. Brief psychotic disorder often responds to interventions such as supportive care with individual or group therapy. By definition, the symptoms of brief psychotic disorder must last at least 1 day and less than 1 month. If the symptoms continue past 30 days, other diagnoses must be considered.

Approach to the Diagnosis

A sudden onset or brief history of psychotic symptoms compels the clinician to consider the diagnosis of brief psychotic disorder. The first task is to confirm the presence of one or more of the diagnostic symptoms, which include all those seen in schizophrenia except negative symptoms. Often individuals are so confused by their symptoms that they cannot or will not be able to provide a detailed history. Collateral information from coworkers, friends, and family can be extremely helpful. Once the symptoms are identified, the duration must be determined. If the best estimation is less than 1 month, brief psychotic disorder remains a possibility. However, because of the brief nature of the symptoms and lack of past history, it is especially important to consider other causations. For example, any fluctuation in sensorium could indicate an intoxication or delirium. A careful evaluation of cognition, including a formal screen of cognitive capacity, can be illustrative. Reviewing past medical history, vital signs, labs, electrocardiogram, toxicology screen, and any brain imaging obtained may indicate an organic cause of the psychotic symptoms. If these are all negative, then the differential of a psychotic disorder is most likely.

Sedative medications or antipsychotic drugs may help calm any agitated person and allow more detailed history. Mood disorders with psychotic features can be seen in both mania and depression. Current and past mood episodes should be screened for carefully. Eliciting a marked stressor may help confirm the diagnosis of brief psychotic disorder, although the diagnosis is indicated without a stressor as well. Possible stressors include loss of a loved one, witnessing or personally experiencing a traumatic event, or extreme financial hardship.

As stated in DSM-5, "There appears to be an increased risk of suicidal behavior, particularly during the acute episode" (p. 95).

Getting the History

A 43-year-old woman is seen with her husband in a mental health clinic by an attending psychiatrist. She has been hearing voices for the past 3 weeks. She and her husband are baffled by her symptoms but do report that both of them have been very worried about their son who is deployed with the military overseas. The psychiatrist begins the interview by trying to empathize with the woman: "It must be very hard not to know what is happening with your son."

Next, the psychiatrist takes a brief but comprehensive approach to the history and mental status examination. She also orders labs, a thyroid test, and a drug screen. She tries to ask more questions to identify the types of symptoms present: "What did you hear? What type of voices? Did they tell you to harm yourself? How long did they last? Do you feel stressed?"

The psychiatrist next delves into questions about possible mood disorder symptoms: "Do you get depressed or sad? Do you have sleep, energy, or appetite problems? Do you get elevated levels of energy and activity? Less need for sleep? Suicidal thoughts? Has this happened to you before?" More symptoms of depression or mania could be elicited if present. To help clarify even further, the psychiatrist also asks the patient's husband about these symptoms. This helps the woman to recall even more things about her recent symptoms.

The psychiatrist also carefully inquires about substance use: "How much alcohol do you drink? Do you use marijuana, cocaine, or other substances? What medications are you taking?" This inquiry about substance use is important because substance/medication-induced psychotic disorders can commonly manifest with these presenting symptoms. Questions regarding physical health, labs, and a brief cognitive screening tool can help rule out delirium.

The psychiatrist next screens for other psychotic symptoms, such as delusions: "Does it feel as if people are talking about you? Does anything interfere with your mind or your body? Have you ever felt like communication devices were spying on you?" The woman's husband is also asked whether he has observed any of these symptoms.

When obtaining the history of brief psychotic disorder, the clinician must be cognizant of the distress these new symptoms are having on the person and his or her family. Eventually, the woman is seen in several follow-up appointments. The psychotic symptoms resolved 5 days after the initial psychiatric visit. The patient is seen over the next year and never has such symptoms again. In retrospect, the psychiatrist decides that the patient had brief psychotic disorder and determines that the son's deployment overseas was a stressor. The patient's husband agrees with this assessment.

The age at onset and duration of symptoms are important. For example, if the symptoms last longer than 1 month, brief psychotic disorder cannot be diagnosed, and the clinician may decide if another disorder, such as schizophreniform disorder, schizoaffective disorder, or schizophrenia, is more relevant to explore.

Tips for Clarifying the Diagnosis

• Consider the possibility of delirium first, because delirium can often be a serious condition.
• Obtain collateral sources of information to develop a timeline of the symptoms, stressors, and events in the person's life.

- Because mood disorders with psychotic features are much more common than other disorders characterized by psychosis, it is important to screen for these disorders, carefully taking into account the potential for suicide.
- Consider the diagnosis of schizophreniform disorder if the symptoms persist and are accompanied by negative symptoms.
- Often the diagnosis of brief psychotic disorder is made in retrospect, after an initial diagnosis of unspecified schizophrenia spectrum and other psychotic disorder.
- Note that brief psychotic disorder symptoms last from at least 1 day to a maximum of 1 month.

Consider the Case

Mrs. Norman is a 45-year-old black woman brought to the hospital by the police, who found her running through the street wearing only a nightgown at 3 A.M. She had been pounding on her neighbor's door while holding her Bible and claiming that ghosts and demons were chasing her. Her speech was reportedly rapid and nonsensical. While in the emergency department, Mrs. Norman sang hymns loudly and tried to abscond. She was given haloperidol 5 mg intramuscularly to keep her and others safe. Her toxicology screen was negative, and her initial labs and brain imaging were all unremarkable. Collateral information from her husband was obtained. The patient had no prior psychiatric history, no suicide attempts, and no acute medical problems. She was described as an emotional and anxious person who often saw her pastor at church for reassurance.

Mrs. Norman's husband stated that 2 days earlier she began praying, meditating, and "losing her mind." He stated that she has always been religious and that she has never abused alcohol or other substances. She was discharged from the hospital the next day without any medications and was given an appointment with a local psychologist for follow-up. No further symptoms were observed or reported by her. She fully recovered to her usual baseline functioning within 2 days.

Mrs. Norman was diagnosed with brief psychotic disorder, without marked stressors. She presented to the emergency department with a severe psychotic event. The presentation of the symptoms warranted an urgent workup, including a toxicology screen and laboratory studies. The collateral information was useful to help discern the possible causes of this condition. Psychotic symptoms can be seen in delirium, drug abuse, mood disorders with psychotic features, and schizophrenia. Because her psychotic symptoms resolved in 2–3 days, the diagnosis of brief psychotic disorder was made retrospectively. The examiner must rule out other possible causes as well. Her toxicology screen was negative, and she was taking no medications that could have caused the psychosis. Her previous functioning and quick full recovery to baseline functioning without mood symptoms helped rule out a manic or depressive episode with psychotic features. Consideration of a person's ethnicity or race, taking into account culturally appropriate expressions to stress, should be part of the assessment. Some data suggest a higher incidence of brief psychotic disorder in developing countries.

Differential Diagnosis

The differential diagnosis of brief psychotic disorder includes psychosis from other causes, such as schizophrenia, delusional disorder, and mood disorders such as major depressive disorder with psychotic features or bipolar I disorder, current episode manic, with mood-congruent psychotic features. The examiner should also carefully exclude substance/medication-induced psychotic disorder, delirium, factitious disorder, and malingering. Personality disorders such as paranoid personality disorder and schizotypal personality disorder should also be considered.

The time course of the development of a disorder is important to consider when formulating a differential diagnosis. For example, an acute or abrupt onset of confusion, disorientation, and bizarre behavior may indicate a delirium. Mood disorders can be recurrent and often have a positive family history. Schizophrenia and schizophreniform disorder have both positive and negative symptoms and a much longer duration of symptoms. Factitious disorder occurs when the patient tries to maintain the "sick role." In malingering, a secondary gain such as admission to a hospital for food and shelter is seen. Personality disorders such as schizotypal personality disorder and paranoid personality disorder endure throughout a person's lifespan.

See DSM-5 for additional disorders to consider in the differential diagnosis. Also refer to the discussions of comorbidity and differential diagnosis in their respective sections of DSM-5.

Summary

- The diagnosis of brief psychotic disorder requires the presence of one or more of the following symptoms: delusions, hallucinations, disorganized speech, or grossly disorganized or catatonic behavior. This list does not include symptoms that are culturally sanctioned.
- The duration is at least 1 day and less than 1 month, with a return to a premorbid level of functioning.
- A mood disorder such as depression or bipolar disorder with psychotic features is not the cause of symptoms.
- Schizophreniform disorder or schizophrenia criteria are not met, particularly the criteria for duration of symptoms.
- Delirium and substance/medication-induced psychosis are carefully screened for and ruled out.
- Symptoms are not the result of a personality disorder, malingering, or factitious disorder.
- Symptoms may occur with or without a marked stressor.

IN-DEPTH DIAGNOSIS

Delusional Disorder

Ms. Gordon is a 39-year-old woman brought to the emergency department by police for allegedly harassing a popular music star. She appeared well dressed, was tastefully made up, and was outwardly friendly. She had a college education, was single, and had no substance abuse history. She appropriately answered all questions from the nurses and doctor. When she was asked about the harassment complaints involving the musician, however, she became upset and explained that she was supposed to marry him. In addition, for the past 2 years Ms. Gordon has been writing the celebrity love letters and trying to call him; tonight she tried to approach him at the hotel where he was staying before a concert. When asked further questions about this "relationship," she explained in elaborate detail how they met online and how they were supposed to get married this night.

Her mental status examination was unremarkable, save for the fixed false belief that she was supposed to marry this celebrity. She remained calm as long as no one challenged this false belief. She was eventually given a low dose of an antipsychotic to keep her calm and help her sleep.

Her sister arrived later and provided more details. According to her sister, the family at first believed that Ms. Gordon was seeing this man but quickly realized it was not true. Her sister confirmed that aside from her preoccupation with the celebrity, Ms. Gordon had normal mood, sleep, energy, and activity levels. She lived alone and had stable employment in an advertising agency. The sister had not observed any symptoms of mania, depression, or hallucinations.

This case highlights the important aspects of delusional disorder, erotomanic type. Ms. Gordon has a fixed, false belief that she was to be married to the celebrity. The belief is rigidly held and cannot be reasoned away by others. She does not meet criteria for schizophrenia because she does not have any other symptoms from Criterion A for schizophrenia. Her speech is logical and goal directed, and she has no disorganized thoughts or behavior. Her level of functioning appears remarkably intact except for the ramifications of this circumscribed belief.

Ms. Gordon does not meet criteria for a mood disorder. She is upset that she cannot be with the celebrity, but otherwise observations by her family and her own report do not indicate either depression or manic symptoms. The term *erotomanic* should not be confused with bipolar mania. A person with mania could have such a delusion, but such a person would also have other classic manic symptoms, such as decreased need for sleep and elevated activity level.

Other possible causes of psychosis, such as intoxication from an illicit substance or a prescribed medication (e.g., steroids for asthma), delirium, and dementia, were carefully ruled out. Ms. Gordon does not have abnormal body image issues, as seen in body dysmorphic disorder.

Approach to the Diagnosis

Persons with delusions often become annoyed or even agitated if others disagree with or confront them directly. Therefore, a nonjudgmental and comforting approach is best. Discussing other areas of their lives that do not involve the delusions may help. For example, discussing family, children, or an upcoming holiday or current events may create a more trustful discourse with these individuals. Later, they may share their delusional beliefs more openly. Getting the family involved early may also be helpful.

The delusions seen in delusional disorder are not typically bizarre. For example, the bizarre, idiosyncratic belief that Martians are invading Earth is not typically seen with this diagnosis. The themes of the delusions, such as jealousy, persecution, erotomania, or having a special relationship with an important person, are typical presentations. It is important to differentiate this condition from schizophrenia or a mood disorder with psychotic features.

The diagnosis of delusional disorder is made after a careful history and examination. External informants can help, and collateral data are often needed from family members, friends, and old records. The person may not discuss his or her delusions with the examiner openly, so the symptoms may go undetected without external information.

It is important to examine carefully the person's history for mood symptoms such as manic episodes with psychosis or depression with psychosis. Manic patients often have delusions of grandeur and may inflate their importance in society, families, or peer groups. However, they also exhibit other symptoms, such as decreased need for sleep, elevated activity and energy levels, agitation, and mood cycling. People with psychotic depression often exhibit nihilistic delusions and may also have diminished interest in activities, crying spells, hopelessness, and lethargy.

A complete family and social history, as well as a medical history, should be obtained to help determine genetic and psychosocial issues in the person's life.

Getting the History

A 42-year-old woman presents to the emergency department for evaluation of a belief that her husband is having an affair with someone. Multiple family members determine that these allegations are false. Nonconfrontational questions for the woman may include the following: "When did you get suspicious about your husband's affair? How did you find out? Have you checked his phone calls, or do you have other evidence? Do you believe he is still having an affair? Can you explain more?"

In screening for other types of psychotic syndromes, such as schizophrenia, the clinician should ask questions such as the following: "Do you hear voices when you are alone or see things that other people do not see? Are things on the radio or TV or Internet directed toward you in particular? Are people trying to harm you, such as by poisoning you?"

In screening for mood disorders, the clinician might ask questions such as these: "Do you have times when you felt depressed (aside from the fact that you believe your husband is cheating on you)? Do you have trouble sleeping or eating? Do you have problems at work or school? Does your mind race fast? Do you have periods of elevated activity, spending money, or elevated energy levels (that are not your usual behaviors)? Do you get agitated? Do you feel closer to God or believe you are God or a prophet?"

In screening for substance abuse, the clinician might ask, "How much alcohol do you drink? Do you use marijuana? Cocaine? Methamphetamines? Any other substances? How often—maybe three or four times a week?"

Psychiatrists must often rely on collateral sources of data for making the proper diagnosis. Sometimes this information becomes necessary in emergencies when a person cannot communicate well or is unable to establish a discourse with the clinician. In other situations, gathering these data requires patience and written permission from the person. In either type of situation, it is helpful for the clinician to gather relevant clinical information from third parties, such as close relatives or friends. Persons with psychosis often have disorganized thoughts, delusions, or active hallucinations, which can make it difficult, if not impossible, to gather enough information to make a proper assessment. It can sometimes be a mistake to rely on the interview as the sole source of clinical information. For example, many of the diagnostic criteria for psychiatric conditions require time durations for symptoms to be present. Relying on the person's report alone can be misleading, because persons with these conditions can be so impaired as to not know the exact dates and places of previous episodes or treatments.

Tips for Clarifying the Diagnosis

- Obtain collateral sources of information, such as interviews with family members, past psychiatric records, and a comprehensive evaluation of the person's psychosocial and medical history.
- Carefully rule out common causes of psychosis, such as mania or depression with psychosis.
- Consider conducting external interviews to detect delusions because relying on only the patient interview can be misleading.
- Because confronting delusions can make people guarded and distrustful, focus in early interviews on developing a trusting relationship and rapport.
- Consider drug screening and other medical and neuroimaging tests to rule out other types of pathology, such as brain lesions or thyroid abnormalities.

Consider the Case

Ms. Watson, a 25-year-old woman with schizophrenia, is seen in an outpatient clinic with her husband and their neighbor, who is a close friend of the couple. The neighbor wants to discuss the case privately with the psychiatrist. Apparently, she is concerned about the overall situation with the couple. The psychiatrist asks the couple if this is okay, and they agree.

The neighbor explains that Ms. Watson has been taking antipsychotic medications for schizophrenia but has continuing thoughts that people are out to get her and that she is being monitored through the TV, computer, and cameras in her house. The neighbor has noticed that the husband also believes some of these strange things. For example, he helped his wife cover the windows so that "spy satellites" could not take pictures of them. He told the neighbor, "You never know—it could really be true." He also started to agree with many of Ms. Watson's strange beliefs that extraterrestrial life forms could be taking over people's bodies. The neighbor noticed that when the two were separated for a few weeks, the husband's symptoms seemed to improve. His beliefs were not nearly as strong as his wife's, but the neighbor wanted to make sure that this couple was not actually making things worse for each other. She has known the couple for many years, and in her opinion the wife has a more dominant personality.

When interviewed alone by the psychiatrist, Mr. Watson denied having active symptoms such as hallucinations and reported no other problems such as substance abuse or mood symptoms. He was well spoken, had a part-time job, and loved his wife deeply. He was passive and dependent on her in many ways emotionally. When the wife's fixed false beliefs were brought up, he agreed that she was mentally ill but also expressed belief that many of her thoughts "could be real." He has been reading books about UFOs and extraterrestrial sightings. He said that he agreed with many of her beliefs about those and other issues, such as cameras in public places. He did not bring up these topics until the psychiatrist specifically asked about them.

In 1877, Lasègue and Falret described *folie à deux* ("a madness shared by two"), in which the index or primary case has a psychotic illness such as schizophrenia. The secondary case usually has a close relationship with the index case, such as spouse or sibling. The index case usually has a more dominant personality style. The secondary case may have some vulnerability in personality or in other unknown ways.

In this case, the husband shares many of his wife's delusions. He does not meet criteria for schizophrenia because he does not have the usual symptoms of Criterion A, such as hallucinations or disorganized speech or thoughts. He only shares some of his wife's delusions in a milder, less bizarre presentation. Therefore, his diagnosis would be delusional disorder with bizarre content. In this case, the symptoms may be an acquired condition from a dominant psychotic partner. The secondary case usually improves when separated for some time from the primary case.

Differential Diagnosis

Delusional disorder should be considered when a person has a delusion that is not due to another condition. Persons with substance/medication-induced psychotic disorder, delirium, and major neurocognitive disorder should be appropriately screened. If the person meets Criterion A for schizophrenia, then delusional disorder should not be diagnosed. Delusional disorder typically produces less impairment than schizophrenia in social and occupational functioning.

It is also important to carefully screen persons with delusions for a mood disorder, because unipolar depression and bipolar disorder (either with depression or manic episodes) can have psychotic symptoms such as delusions as part of the person's presentation. For example, a grandiose delusion or erotomanic delusion could easily occur in the midst of a manic episode with mood-congruent psychosis.

Finally, persons with body dysmorphic disorder or obsessive-compulsive disorder can appear to have severely distorted thoughts that may appear as delusions. Appropriate clinical correlation and careful examination may be helpful.

See DSM-5 for additional disorders to consider in the differential diagnosis. Also refer to the discussions of comorbidity and differential diagnosis in their respective sections of DSM-5.

Summary

- The presence of a fixed false belief in a person who does not meet the other criteria for schizophrenia could lead to a diagnosis of delusional disorder.
- It is important to rule out medical conditions, major neurocognitive disorder, and delirium in any person with psychotic symptoms. Appropriate cognitive screening and testing may be helpful.
- Shared psychotic disorder (*folie à deux*) is no longer a distinct diagnosis in DSM-5. Persons who meet criteria should be diagnosed with delusional disorder even if the symptoms are apparently induced by a close and intense relationship with another person with psychosis.

- Delusions can occur in the midst of a depression or manic episode and should be considered part of the mood disorder episode instead of delusional disorder.
- External informants and collateral data are useful to determine if a patient has a delusion rather than a belief that is part of his or her culture or religion.

IN-DEPTH DIAGNOSIS
Schizoaffective Disorder

Mrs. Collins is a 30-year-old married woman with two children. She presented to the clinic with her husband for an evaluation. She described having had her first depression in her senior year in high school. She began taking medication at that time with good results. She went to a local community college, where she met her husband. She did well until she had her second child at age 27. At that time she had another episode of depression, which worsened to the point that she became isolated, had poor sleep and appetite, and began to hear the voice of a former high school teacher saying negative things about her. She believed that the teacher was going to report her to the authorities and that she would lose custody of her children. At that time she had her first hospitalization and was stabilized with both antidepressant and antipsychotic medications. She responded well and returned home to take care of her children. After a year, her psychiatrist felt that she had been doing well: her mood was euthymic, and she exhibited no symptoms of psychosis. Because of concerns of possible long-term side effects from her antipsychotic medication, she was gradually tapered off of it. For several months she seemed quite well, but then she began to hear whispers of the voices of her former teacher and of other people from her past. She did not describe any problems with her mood, and she exhibited no depressive or manic symptoms or signs. When interviewed by her psychiatrist, she reported that she had been hearing the voices for 6 weeks and thought they would pass. The psychiatrist restarted her antipsychotic medication, and the auditory hallucinations remitted. The psychiatrist and the patient decided that for the foreseeable future, she would take both antidepressant and antipsychotic medications.

This case illustrates some of the classic features of schizoaffective disorder. Mrs. Collins started with depressive symptoms earlier in life, and only after a subsequent depressive episode did she begin to have symptoms consistent with Criterion A for schizophrenia. In her case she had both hallucinations (the teacher's voice) and a delusion (paranoia that the teacher would report her to child custody authorities). At the time when she first began to exhibit the psychotic symptoms, she was in a full depressive episode. Considering her history, major depression with psychotic features seemed a likely diagnosis. The psychiatrist prudently kept her on both the antidepressant (for her recurrent depression) and the antipsychotic (for a suitably conservative period). After a year, an attempt to discontinue the antipsychotic medication seemed reasonable. In this case, however, Mrs. Collins's psychotic symptoms return while her mood is in the normal range. Because she reports hearing the voices for more than 2 weeks, she has a psychotic feature independent from her mood disorder. She has also had depression for more than 50% of the time since she first became psychotic (most of that time with successful treatment), thus meeting Criterion A for the schizoaffective disorder diagnosis.

Approach to the Diagnosis

Schizoaffective disorder is a diagnosis that must be made with the patient's clinical timeline in mind. Because it is an amalgam of periods of disordered mood and/or psychosis, determining the relative components of each is critical. The diagnosis can be made starting from either the mood disorder or the psychosis. The clinician can either start with the mood problem and then test if there has been a period of normal mood and the cardinal symptoms of schizophrenia delineated in Criterion A, or start with the schizophrenic symptoms of Criterion A and subject that diagnosis to the possibility that there is a concurrent mood disorder. In our experience, most often the mood disorder has been present for some time; most frequently the patient has depression but sometimes manic symptoms. Only when the patient's mood is stable and psychotic symptoms remain is the possibility of schizoaffective disorder or schizophrenia entertained. Differentiating the latter two diagnoses requires determining the cumulative time with a mood disorder.

It is often difficult to explain the necessity of the diagnosis of schizoaffective disorder to patients and families, who tend to categorize illnesses into either mood or psychotic disorders. In practice, however, the diagnosis is commonly used because patients often present with an admixture of symptoms. Schizoaffective disorder blends the diagnostic criteria and also suggests two distinct mechanisms of action. One analogy we use is the concept of fuel for the symptoms. Different fuels (neuroreceptors, chemical abnormalities, and the like) and unknown disease mechanisms may independently ignite the symptoms of the mood disorder and the Criterion A symptoms of schizophrenia. It is important to consider both psychosis and the Criterion A symptoms of schizophrenia. A person with schizoaffective disorder does not simply have psychosis; he or she must meet at least two of the symptoms in Criterion A. Many patients may have delusions or hallucinations in the context of their major depression or bipolar disorder but may not exhibit disorganized speech, grossly abnormal psychomotor behavior, or negative symptoms. Schizoaffective disorder is considered more common in women.

As stated in DSM-5, "The lifetime risk of suicide for schizophrenia and schizoaffective disorder is 5%, and the presence of depressive symptoms is correlated with a higher risk for suicide" (p. 109).

Getting the History

A 32-year-old man presented to the clinician's office with a chief complaint of depression. He had been sad and upset since he lost his job 6 months earlier. He has never been married and lives with his parents. In the interview, he reported that he has been a victim of "unknown forces" since he graduated high school. These forces are malevolent and keep him from succeeding at work or finding a wife. He bought heavyweight "blackout" blinds for his bedroom so these forces "can't spy on him." The man denied using alcohol or other substances and considers himself very religious and observant. He recently went to his primary care doctor for a yearly checkup and, aside from elevated cholesterol, has no active medical problems. His parents accompanied him to the psychiatric appointment, and when asked, they essentially confirmed his history. They were aware that he has been depressed but surprised about "the forces." They had assumed he put the heavy blinds on his windows to help him sleep. His father mentioned that the patient's older brother was a "wild" kid who ran away from home several times. Eventually, he was hospitalized for a "nervous breakdown," but the father did not know any further details.

This man presents a diagnostic challenge to the clinician. Here is one possible approach to obtaining the history needed to make an accurate diagnosis of schizoaffective disorder: Start with the man's presenting complaint, which in this case is depression. The clinician can say, "Depression may mean different things to different people. Can you describe your depression to me?" It is possible that a person may give a classic description of major depression; however, depression may also mean feeling flat or unfeeling. In the latter, a stronger suspicion of negative symptoms of schizophrenia should be entertained. Assuming that this man does describe many of the symptoms of major depression, eliciting the length of time each episode lasts and the total number of episodes is very helpful. If the man is unsure, ask if he can remember the worst one or one in which he either had suicidal thoughts or was hospitalized. The clinician needs to sketch in his or her mind (or even graph on paper) the approximate length of time the person has had a mood problem. This duration will be essential in making the final diagnosis.

The man in this case has no overt history of a manic episode. Sometimes this history can be elicited by referring to the person's suspicions: "Is there something special about you that may explain why someone would want to spy on you and keep you from being successful?" This question may bring out symptoms of grandiosity, which can be explored more deeply for periods of mania.

A further evaluation of the possible symptoms of Criterion A for schizophrenia is then necessary. This man described paranoid thinking, so a next question might be whether he ever hears or sees these forces. His speech seems organized, but allowing him to talk freely may draw out some disorganization. Close observation of his movements may show some abnormalities, and a discussion with him and his family may bring out negative symptoms. Finally, confirming that his suspicions and other symptoms of Criterion A occur in the absence of a mood problem is critical. Asking him, "Does the force bother you, even when you think your mood is in a pretty good state?" may help to define a period of Criterion A symptoms without the co-occurring mood disorder. A handy equation to remember is >50% mood disorder+≥2 weeks of Criterion A symptoms alone=schizoaffective disorder.

Tips for Clarifying the Diagnosis

- Start by establishing the diagnosis of major depression and/or a manic episode (bipolar disorder). Being emotional or having periods of sadness is not enough.
- Then determine whether the patient satisfies Criterion A for schizophrenia, noting that one symptom must be hallucinations, delusions, or disorganized speech.
- Next, determine if the symptoms of schizophrenia have occurred while the mood disorder is not present (it could be treated to remission).
- Last, calculate how much of the patient's treatment history has been either during a mood disorder manifestation or while being treated by medication. If that time

is greater than 50% of the total, then schizoaffective disorder should be considered the most likely diagnosis in the differential.

Consider the Case

Mr. Williams is an 18-year-old single man recently arrested for shoplifting in a local department store. He has been in trouble before, having spent time in juvenile detention centers as a minor. Although Mr. Williams was born and raised in the United States, his father is from Wales and his mother is an African immigrant. His parents are unfamiliar with much of U.S. cultural norms. Mr. Williams was considered a very intelligent boy but had difficulty concentrating and doing his assignments. His family felt he was bored at school and tried several alternative and homeschool approaches. He saw a school counselor, who believed he manifested symptoms consistent with oppositional defiant disorder and attention-deficit/hyperactivity disorder. He was referred to his pediatrician, who attempted several trials of stimulants, but the stimulants seemed to agitate him and keep him up at night. Sleep has always been a problem for Mr. Williams: he would often stay up for days playing computer games and, when he got older, hanging out with friends. He was arrested for vagrancy and smoking marijuana in public several times.

While Mr. Williams was in jail, the authorities became concerned with his behavior. He was agitated, talking rapidly, and saying that the "voices" were screaming in his head. He told his parents that he was not shoplifting, because he owned the store. The jail physician suspected a substance-induced condition, but all drug toxicology was negative. A psychiatrist was called, and after a detailed interview, believed that Mr. Williams was in a manic episode with psychosis. He prescribed both a mood stabilizer and an antipsychotic, and Mr. Williams's symptoms appeared to resolve. Mr. Williams was put on probation with the stipulation that he follow up with his psychiatrist and live with his parents.

Mr. Williams seemed a changed person while taking the medications—less agitated and labile, better focused, and able to sleep through the night. However, he complained that the medications dulled his senses, and after several months he stopped taking the antipsychotic medication. He felt less medicated and began to attend the local community college. However, a month into classes, he told his mother that he was hearing voices again, first whispers, but then full conversations. He believed that the voices were being beamed in by satellite from outer space, most likely as part of a governmental experiment. Despite the severity of his psychosis, his mood remained normal, and he did not manifest any signs or symptoms of mania or depression. The psychiatrist prescribed a different antipsychotic, one that Mr. Williams tolerated better and that significantly reduced the voices and paranoia.

Mr. Williams is an example of a more atypical case of possible schizoaffective disorder. He is relatively young, without an established diagnosis of either a mood disorder or history of Criterion A for schizophrenia. In this scenario, his erratic and defiant behavior could be due to a misdiagnosis of oppositional defiant disorder and attention-deficit/hyperactivity disorder instead of the correct diagnosis of bipolar disorder. One clue is his poor reaction to stimulant medications, which activated instead of focused him. Finally, at the point of incarceration, he is overtly grandiose, pressured, and psychotic. The psychiatrist's presumed diagnosis of bipolar disorder is very reasonable, as is the tapering of his antipsychotic medication over time. The recurrence of the patient's psychosis in the absence of mood abnormalities leads to a suspicion of an underlying, independent psychotic condition. At this point, the most likely diagnosis would be schizoaffective disorder, if the psychiatrist can presume that for most of Mr. Williams's life, he was dealing with manic symptoms and that he has developed the psychosis when his mood is under good control. Only time will tell if he maintains this diagnosis. It is possible that his mood symptoms may become a minor part of his overall illness, and then a diagnosis of schizophrenia may apply.

The clinician must also consider other factors that may affect Mr. Williams's diagnosis and/or course. A patient's ethnicity and immigrant status (as well as being the child of immigrants) can be factors to consider in assessing schizoaffective disorder. Cultural influences may explain some of the reactions to the psychosis. A highly emotional reaction to the psychotic symptoms could be confused with a manic or depressive episode. Recent immigration can increase an individual's risk of presenting with schizoaffective disorder.

Differential Diagnosis

Diagnosing schizoaffective disorder is an exercise in differential diagnosis. Embedded in the diagnosis is the presence of elements of both schizophrenia and a major mood disorder. By definition, the clinician must distinguish this diagnosis from three main diagnoses: schizophrenia, major depressive disorder with psychotic features, and bipolar disorder with psychotic features. Uncoupling the psychotic symptoms from the mood disorder and determining whether the mood disorder lasted for more than half the time are essential to the diagnosis. Of note, if the psychotic component is a newly presenting element for the patient, the same differential for schizophrenia must be considered. Thus, those with psychotic symptoms for less than 1 month may have a brief psychotic disorder, whereas those with psychotic symptoms for fewer than 6 months may have schizophreniform disorder.

The other diagnostic considerations are whether the disorder is secondary to a substance/medication-induced disorder or another medical condition. Personality disorders can sometimes be confused with schizoaffective disorder. For example, persons with borderline personality disorder with periods of mood instability and psychotic-like states can appear similar to those with schizoaffective disorder. The rapid volatility of the symptoms of borderline personality disorder can be helpful in making the correct diagnosis.

See DSM-5 for additional disorders to consider in the differential diagnosis. Also refer to the discussions of comorbidity and differential diagnosis in their respective sections of DSM-5.

Summary

- Schizoaffective disorder is an admixture of mood and schizophrenia-like symptoms. Symptoms from both diagnostic groups must be confirmed during the lifetime course of the disorder.
- Establishing an independent period of at least 2 weeks that satisfies Criterion A for schizophrenia is necessary.

- A careful calculation of how much of the person's treatment history has been either during an overt mood episode or while successfully treated by medication is critical. If that time is greater than 50% of the total, then schizoaffective disorder should be strongly considered.
- Schizoaffective disorder is considered more common in women.

─────────── SUMMARY ───────────

Schizophrenia Spectrum and Other Psychotic Disorders

The changes in the diagnosis of schizophrenia spectrum and other psychotic disorders in DSM-5 have been evolutionary, not revolutionary. The hope is that these changes will help better distinguish each disorder and provide the most valid and reliable sets of criteria.

The diagnosis of schizophrenia, considered the "anchor" diagnosis, now requires that one symptom of Criterion A be a delusion, hallucination, or disorganized speech, ensuring that all persons with this diagnosis have psychotic symptoms. The special status of bizarre delusions or complex hallucinations has been eliminated. In most clinicians' experiences, persons commonly present with more than two symptoms of Criterion A.

Brief psychotic disorder remains essentially the same and still relies on carefully determining that the illness interval is fewer than 30 days. Likewise, schizophreniform disorder remains a time-limited diagnosis that will either resolve or evolve to schizophrenia or another psychiatric disorder.

Delusional disorder continues to identify persons with unfounded beliefs that have a limited effect on overall behavior and functioning. Shared delusional disorder, historically called *folie à deux,* has been eliminated from DSM-5.

Diagnosing schizoaffective disorder has been difficult in the past because of the ambiguity of what was meant by having a mood disorder for a "substantial" period of time, which experts have described as ranging from 15% to 50%. The new criterion of "majority" of the time should help tighten the diagnosis. It will still be a challenge, however, to determine the length of treated time, because many patients remain on antidepressants whether or not they need them.

Psychotic disorders due to another medical condition or substance/medication-induced psychotic disorders are continuing reminders that psychotic symptoms may have physical or intoxicant etiologies. Finally, nearly all these diagnoses can have a catatonic specifier. The definition of *catatonia* is provided in the DSM-5 section "Catatonia Associated With Another Mental Disorder (Catatonia Specifier)," which lists a dozen symptoms, including stupor, catalepsy, mutism, and echolalia.

───────────── ■-■-■ ─────────────

Diagnostic Pearls

- Determining the presence of a psychosis, with either hallucinations or delusions, is the first task in diagnosing individuals with schizophrenia spectrum and other psychotic disorders.

- The length of time that the person has exhibited psychotic and/or negative symptoms drives the decision process for many cases: brief psychotic disorder<schizophreniform disorder<schizophrenia or schizoaffective disorder.

- Teasing out the presence and proportion of time that an individual has a diagnosable mood disorder is critical to determining whether the person has a schizophreniform disorder or a mood disorder.

- The accurate diagnosis of schizoaffective disorder requires two critical elements: a diagnosable mood disorder must exist for greater than 50% of the time (even if treated successfully), and a period of schizophrenia symptoms must last for at least 2 weeks in the absence of the mood disorder.

- In the majority of cases, even patients with severe schizophrenia spectrum disorders are oriented to person, place, and time. Disorientation is either a diagnostic warning flag for a substance/medication-induced psychosis or a result of an unrecognized or inadequately treated medical illness.

- Autism spectrum disorder can be confused with schizophrenia or schizophreniform disorder. Autism spectrum disorder usually begins at an earlier age, and individuals with autism spectrum disorder are not expected to experience long-enduring hallucinations and/or delusions.

Self-Assessment

Key Concepts: Double-Check Your Knowledge

What is the relevance of the following concepts to the various schizophrenia spectrum and other psychotic disorders?

- Psychosis
- Delusions
- Hallucinations
- Disorganized speech
- Grossly disorganized or catatonic behavior
- Negative symptoms
- Severity of effect on psychosocial function (such as work, relationships, self-care)
- Ruling out mood disorders and substance/medication-induced psychotic disorders
- Determining duration of mood and psychotic symptoms separately

Questions to Discuss With Colleagues and Mentors

1. A significant change in the diagnosis of schizophrenia is the elimination of the subtypes (e.g., paranoid, disorganized). Were these subtypes useful? Were they stable over time? Will not having them change practice?
2. How difficult is it to determine the difference among brief psychotic disorder, schizophreniform disorder, and schizophrenia? Are prodromal and attenuated symptom intervals reliably measured?

3. Will the change requiring that a mood disorder be present a "majority of the total duration" instead of a "substantial portion of the total duration" alter the frequency of diagnosing schizoaffective disorder?

4. DSM-IV allowed a single symptom from Criterion A for the diagnosis of schizophrenia if the delusions were bizarre or the hallucinations consisted of either commenting voices or two or more voices conversing. In clinical practice, how often might this exemption be problematic to making a diagnosis of schizophrenia?

Case-Based Questions

PART A

Mr. Jenkins, a 19-year-old man, is brought to the emergency department after being found incoherent by the police. According to paramedics, he was sitting on a street curb and appeared disoriented and confused. His identity was unknown. Witnesses told police that he appeared to be yelling at someone and that he acted as if someone were chasing him. Intravenous fluid was started at the scene, and the paramedics transported the man to the hospital. In the emergency department, Mr. Jenkins was drowsy, with a blood pressure of 180/98 and a heart rate of 148. His urine drug screen was positive for cocaine and cannabis. His pupils were dilated. One hour later, when a medical student was examining his dirty clothes and his neck, where he had a tattoo of a crucifix, the patient suddenly jumped up and screamed. He believed that ghosts in the hospital and dead people were trying to choke him. He tore the IV loose from his arm. The patient was immediately sedated with antipsychotic medication. He was later admitted to the intensive care unit for observation and monitoring of his unstable vital signs. He was found to be agitated due to hallucinations and delusions but was oriented to time, place, and person.

What is the most likely diagnosis for Mr. Jenkins? Do the circumstances leading to his hospitalization need to be considered?   Mr. Jenkins has signs and symptoms consistent with substance/medication-induced psychotic disorder. He was alert and oriented, which helps rule out the possibility of delirium. The patient also has autonomic symptoms and a urine drug screen consistent with cocaine and cannabis intoxication. At this point, it is not possible to distinguish whether the symptoms were preexisting or only due to the ingested substances.

PART B

Three days after admission, Mr. Jenkins was calmer and medically stable. He was transferred to the psychiatric unit at the hospital. He gradually became alert and oriented to all spheres. The hallucinations of ghosts also resolved. He watched TV on the unit and talked to other patients. His affect was mostly flat. The nurses stated that he was seen talking to himself and responding to things in the room that were not there. On the eighth hospital day, he explained to the psychiatrist, "It was now about the sixth hour, and darkness came over the whole land until the ninth hour, for the sun stopped shining. And the curtain of the temple was torn in two." Nobody understood this statement until a medical student queried the phrase on the Internet and discovered that it was a verse from the Bible. Mr. Jenkins continued to exhibit bizarre behavior and speech patterns. He stood in place for hours with a blank stare and had to be reminded to eat. He believed that he was a "prophet from the Gospels" and that he was here to "cure the evil of all men." He believed that his mind could move the sun and the moon. When asked about his past, he stated that he was born on Saturn and that Uranus was his home. He could not maintain a proper discourse for very long and laughed inappropriately while discussing the size of his feet and genitals. A nurse that used to work at another hospital stated that she knew Mr. Jenkins from a previous psychiatric hospitalization 10 months earlier and that he acted exactly like this. She is sure that he was not using drugs then. His mother was eventually located. She had never observed any manic or depressive symptoms in her son and stated that he had been psychotic for the past year and had never used drugs until now.

Is the persistence of the patient's psychotic symptoms important to making a definitive diagnosis? Mr. Jenkins remained psychotic after several days off cocaine and cannabis. Although the effects of such drugs can persist, the psychiatrist should begin to suspect an underlying psychotic mental illness, aside from the established diagnosis of substance abuse, especially given the nurse's observation that she had seen him in a similar mental state 10 months earlier. Because he has never had an episode of mania or depression and the psychotic symptoms have lasted for more than 6 months without the use of drugs, the diagnosis of schizophrenia is eventually made.

Short-Answer Questions

1. What are common substances that can cause psychotic symptoms?
2. Does it generally matter what type of hallucinations or delusions a person has in order to receive a diagnosis of substance/medication-induced psychotic disorder?
3. How can a clinician detect if a person with a substance/medication-induced psychotic disorder has another major mental illness, such as major depression or schizophrenia?
4. What are the symptoms of Criterion A for schizophrenia in DSM-5? Which Criterion A symptoms must be present for at least 1 month in order to make the diagnosis of schizophrenia? What is the diagnosis if the symptoms of Criterion A for schizophrenia last only 20 days?
5. What are the symptoms of Criterion B for schizophrenia?
6. Is hearing voices of a running commentary or experiencing third-person hallucinations diagnostic of schizophrenia?
7. What is the diagnosis if a patient has symptoms consistent with schizophrenia for several years and then suddenly has a manic episode?
8. Does the duration of the prodromal and attenuated form of schizophrenia count toward the 6 months needed for a diagnosis of schizophrenia?
9. Do the DSM-5 criteria for delusional disorder allow for bizarre delusions?
10. What are the two time criteria critical to making a diagnosis of schizoaffective disorder?

Answers

1. Common substances that can cause psychotic symptoms are cocaine, amphetamines, cathinones, LSD (lysergic acid diethylamide), mushrooms, cannabis, medications, phencyclidine (PCP), alcohol, inhalants, sedatives, hypnotics, and anxiolytics.
2. No. It does not matter what type of hallucinations or delusions a person has in order to receive a diagnosis of substance/medication-induced psychotic disorder, which can easily look like schizophrenia.

3. Generally, a clinician cannot detect another major mental illness and has to rely on outside sources, records, and informants, or wait for the substance/medication-induced state to clear first.

4. Criterion A symptoms for schizophrenia include delusions, hallucinations, disorganized speech, grossly abnormal psychomotor behavior (including catatonia), and negative symptoms (e.g., diminished emotional expression or avolition). At least one of the following Criterion A symptoms for schizophrenia must be present for at least 1 month: hallucinations, delusions, or disorganized speech. If the symptoms of Criterion A for schizophrenia last only 20 days, the diagnosis is brief psychotic disorder.

5. Criterion B for schizophrenia requires that level of functioning in one or more major areas (e.g., work, interpersonal relations, or self-care) is markedly below the level achieved before the onset.

6. No single symptom is diagnostic for schizophrenia. Other criteria are also required. The symptoms noted in the question may also occur in other types of psychosis, such as during a manic episode or from substance use.

7. Several diagnoses should be considered in the context of an enduring psychotic disorder and the emergence of a new set of symptoms consistent with a disruptive mood. Medical and substance-related factors should be explored. The possibility that the patient has schizoaffective disorder may be evaluated as a clinical hypothesis.

8. Yes. Under Criterion C, the duration of the prodromal and attenuated form of schizophrenia counts toward the 6 months needed for a diagnosis of schizophrenia.

9. Bizarre delusions by themselves do not rule out delusional disorder, but these delusions cannot have a significant effect on functioning, and behavior cannot be odd or bizarre.

10. The two time criteria critical to making a diagnosis of schizoaffective disorder are 2 weeks of symptoms from schizophrenia Criterion A without a mood disorder and greater than 50% of the time with a mood disorder (including treated intervals).

6

Bipolar and Related Disorders

Terence A. Ketter, M.D.

Shefali Miller, M.D.

"I feel like a million bucks—I can do anything!"

"When he starts talking this fast, I know he is going off…"

Bipolar and related disorders are common, recurrent, frequently debilitating, and in many instances tragically fatal illnesses, characterized by oscillations in mood, energy, and ability to function (Table 6–1).

In DSM-5, bipolar and related disorders are in their own chapter (rather than combined with depressive disorders in a unitary mood disorders chapter, as they were in DSM-IV). The bipolar and related disorders chapter appears after the schizophrenia spectrum and other psychotic disorders chapter and before the depressive disorders chapter, in recognition of the place of bipolar disorders as a bridge between the schizophrenia spectrum and the depressive disorder categories in terms of symptomatology, family history, and genetics.

Patients with bipolar I disorder have experienced at least one manic episode. Manic episodes last at least 1 week (or briefer if hospitalized) and require elevated, expansive, or irritable mood, accompanied by increased energy/activity and at least three additional symptoms (four if the mood is merely irritable), such as inflated self-esteem, decreased need for sleep, overtalkativeness, racing thoughts, distractibility, increased goal-directed activity, and impulsivity. Manic episodes are by definition severe; they entail psychosis, hospitalization, or severe impairment of occupational or psychosocial function. "Increased goal-directed activity or energy" has been added to DSM-5 as a new core mood elevation symptom.

TABLE 6–1. Episode types in selected DSM-5 mood disorders

	Manic episode	Hypomanic episode	Major depressive episode	Chronic, episodic, subthreshold mood elevation symptoms	Chronic, episodic, subthreshold depressive symptoms
Bipolar I disorder	R	C	C	C	C
Bipolar II disorder	X	R	R	C	C
Cyclothymic disorder	X	X	X	R	R
Unipolar major depressive disorder	X	X	R	X	C
Persistent depressive disorder (dysthymia)	X	X	X	X	R

Note. R=required; C=common (but not required); X=not permitted. Manic, hypomanic, and major depressive episodes may be with or without mixed features.

Patients with bipolar II disorder have experienced at least one hypomanic episode and at least one major depressive episode, but no manic episode. Hypomanic episodes are defined similarly to manic episodes, but they do not entail psychosis, hospitalization, or severe functional impairment, and they have shorter minimum duration (4 days rather than 7).

Major depressive episodes are characterized by sadness or anhedonia, accompanied by additional symptoms to yield a total of at least five pervasive symptoms for at least 2 weeks. The specific additional symptoms include the following: weight change, sleep disturbance, psychomotor agitation or retardation, poor energy, poor self-esteem/guilt, poor concentration (inability to focus), and suicidality. Although the vast majority of patients with bipolar I disorder also endure major depressive episodes, such episodes are not required for the diagnosis of bipolar I disorder.

For manic episodes (as well as for hypomanic and major depressive episodes), DSM-5 has added the specifier "with anxious distress," which is defined as the presence of at least two of the following symptoms: feeling keyed up or tense, feeling unusually restless, difficulty concentrating due to worry, fearing something awful may happen, and fearing that one may lose control of self.

DSM-5 also has replaced the "mixed episode" of DSM-IV with the specifier "with mixed features" that applies to manic, hypomanic, and major depressive episodes. A hypomanic episode with mixed features is a new designation in DSM-5. The "with mixed features" specifier for major depressive episodes is applied if nearly every day there are at least three manic/hypomanic symptoms occurring concurrently with at least five depressive symptoms.

Cyclothymic disorder is characterized by a chronic, fluctuating pattern of numerous periods of subsyndromal mood elevation and depression symptoms for at least 2 years (1 year in children and adolescents) without any interruption longer than 2 months. If a major depressive episode, manic episode, or hypomanic episode occurs during the first 2 years of the disturbance (1 year in children and adolescents), cyclothymic disorder is not diagnosed, because the chronic subsyndromal mood swings may be considered to be residual symptoms of bipolar I or bipolar II disorder. If a major depressive episode, manic episode, or hypomanic episode occurs after the first 2 years of cyclothymic disorder, the diagnosis of cyclothymic disorder may be replaced with unipolar major depressive disorder, bipolar I disorder, or bipolar II disorder.

Substance/medication-induced bipolar and related disorder is characterized by the ingestion of or withdrawal from a substance or medication. In DSM-5 (but not DSM-IV), a full manic or hypomanic episode emerging during antidepressant treatment (e.g., medication or electroconvulsive therapy) and persisting beyond the physiological effect of that treatment is sufficient evidence of a manic or hypomanic episode. Substance/medication-induced bipolar and related disorder is more common in patients with mixed features and with rapid cycling.

Bipolar and related disorder due to another medical condition is a function of the direct physiological effects of another medical condition (most often neurological or endocrine). It is more common in patients with mixed features and with rapid cycling and particularly common in older adults, due to the high prevalence of medical disorders in that age group. In some instances, concurrent, overlapping influences of treatments and their underlying medical conditions may make it challenging to definitively determine whether mood symptoms represent substance/medication-induced bipolar and related disorder or bipolar and related disorder due to another medical condition.

Other specified bipolar and related disorder and unspecified bipolar and related disorder in DSM-5 replace bipolar disorder not otherwise specified in DSM-IV and apply to individuals experiencing significant manic or hypomanic and depressive symptoms that do not meet diagnostic criteria of any other bipolar or depressive disorder and are not attributable to the direct physiological effects of a substance/medication-induced or general medical condition. The DSM-5 description of other specified bipolar and related disorder includes specific presentations that do not meet criteria for specific bipolar and related disorders, including the following:

- Major depressive episodes and short hypomanic episodes (lasting 2–3 days; i.e., with insufficient duration for full hypomanic episodes)
- Major depressive episodes and hypomanic episodes with insufficient symptom count for full hypomanic episodes
- Hypomanic episode without prior major depressive episode
- Short-duration cyclothymia (shorter than 2 years in adults or 1 year in children or adolescents)

The unspecified bipolar and related disorder designator is used in situations in which clinicians choose *not* to specify the reason that criteria are not met for a specific bipolar and related disorder and includes presentations in which there is insufficient information to make a more specific diagnosis (e.g., in emergency department settings).

Individuals with bipolar and related disorders more commonly present with depression than with mood elevation. Thus, all persons presenting with depression need to be questioned directly regarding any history of episodes of mood elevation, which they may experience as periods of irritability and agitation rather than elation. Individuals may focus mainly on periods of depression at the cost of paying sufficient attention to periods of mood elevation, because they perceive periods of depression as subjectively distressing and as driving functional impairment and may be less concerned about the subjective but significant other experiences and negative consequences of periods of mood elevation. Clinicians can foster the therapeutic alliance with these persons by acknowledging the important subjective and functional implications of periods of depression, but they need to balance this acknowledgment with eliciting and discussing corresponding information regarding periods of mood elevation from patients and their significant others; the latter may prove to be more sensitive observers of mood elevation.

IN-DEPTH DIAGNOSIS

Bipolar I Disorder and Bipolar II Disorder

Police bring Mr. Ross, a 21-year-old single man and a creative writing senior at an Ivy League university, to the emergency department after he created a disturbance at a computer store. His mood is irritable and expansive as he boastfully reports smashing a computer on the floor after the store manager refused to hire him as an advertising consultant (a job that had not been posted). Mr. Ross demonstrates pressured speech, flight of ideas, and distractibility while describing how the advertising campaign that he devised in the prior week will revolutionize not only the marketing of computers but also that of all other consumer goods. He denies drowsiness despite sleeping only 2 hours each night for the last week, but he admits that for the last few days he has been hearing the voice of Steve Jobs suggesting ideas for a computer advertising campaign. Mr. Ross admits to a month-long major depressive episode during high school, which was successfully treated with psychotherapy. He admits to a history of some binge drinking and weekend use of marijuana as a freshman but denies any use of alcohol or drugs in the last 3 months. His father was briefly hospitalized for an unspecified psychiatric disorder in his 20s and died in a single motor vehicle crash in his mid-30s.

Mr. Ross meets criteria for bipolar I disorder with a current manic episode with psychotic features. In addition to the presence of psychosis (i.e., auditory hallucinations and grandiose delusions), his behavior has been disturbed enough to result in his being transported to the emergency department by the authorities, indicating severe functional impairment and, therefore, representing a manic episode rather than merely a hypomanic episode. Male gender, onset in early adulthood, a possible family history of bipolar disorder, presence of psychotic features, and occurrence of a major depressive episode are all common but not required for a diagnosis of bipolar I disorder.

Approach to the Diagnosis

Bipolar disorders may be more often underdiagnosed (e.g., in individuals with bipolar disorders who view themselves as merely having depression) than overdiagnosed (e.g., in persons with Cluster B personality disorders who view themselves as merely having frequent mood changes). Correct diagnosis of bipolar disorders crucially depends on the ability to accurately detect episodes of mood elevation (i.e., hypomanic or manic episodes). Affected people more commonly present with, and are more sensitive observers of, symptoms of depression than symptoms of mood elevation, making distinguishing bipolar disorders from unipolar major depressive disorder (by detecting episodes of mood elevation) a particularly important challenge. Individuals may use the terms *mood swings, rapid cycling,* or even *mania* or *hypomania* with meanings that differ from the DSM-5 definitions, thus potentially causing confusion.

Manic episodes are by definition severe (i.e., they entail psychosis, hospitalization, or severe functional impairment) and must occur in bipolar I disorder (but must not occur in bipolar II disorder or unipolar major depressive disorder). A history of bankruptcy, incarceration, and multiple occupational/relationship failures related to episodes of mood elevation suggests that at least one such episode may have been severe enough to be considered manic rather than merely hypomanic.

Hypomanic episodes are by definition not severe (i.e., they do not entail psychosis, hospitalization, or severe functional impairment). They *must* occur in bipolar II disorder, they *can* occur in bipolar I disorder, but they *must not* occur in unipolar major depressive disorder. Function during hypomanic episodes may improve, rather than deteriorate, which makes detection more challenging. Decreased need for sleep ought to be distinguished from insomnia; it highly suggests episodes of mood elevation, although it is not a required symptom. Stressors that are either positive (e.g., occupational promotion, new romantic attachment) or negative (e.g., performance demands, relationship termination) can trigger episodes of mood elevation. Manic and hypomanic episodes with mixed features may be reported by some persons as depressions. Detection of past as opposed to current episodes, irritable as opposed to euphoric episodes, episodes with as opposed to without mixed features, and hypomanic as opposed to manic episodes is more challenging because patients are at greater risk to fail to recognize these.

Major depressive episodes must occur in bipolar II disorder and unipolar major depressive disorder and most often occur (but are not required) in bipolar I disorder. Distinguishing prior (and even current) major depressive episodes with mixed features (which may occur in bipolar and related disorders and unipolar major depressive disorder) from hypomanic episodes (which may occur in bipolar and related disorders but not in unipolar major depressive disorder) can be particularly challenging.

Collateral history from significant others, particularly regarding the possibility of prior manic or hypomanic episodes and the extent of mood elevation symptoms during major depressive episodes, can help enhance diagnostic accuracy.

Distinguishing episodes of mood elevation related to bipolar I disorder or bipolar II disorder as opposed to such episodes triggered by antidepressants or illicit substances can be challenging. Substance/medication-induced bipolar and related disorder tends to occur within 3 months of introduction of a substance or medication or a dose increase and not to persist beyond the physiological action after discontinuation of a potentially implicated substance or medication.

Common comorbid conditions such as anxiety, substance use, personality, eating, and pediatric disruptive behavioral (e.g., attention-deficit/hyperactivity disorder [ADHD], oppositional defiant disorder, and conduct disorder) disorders can distract clinicians, patients, and their families from detecting episodes of mood elevation.

As stated in DSM-5, "The lifetime risk of suicide in individuals with bipolar disorder is estimated to be at least 15 times that of the general population. In fact, bipolar disorder may account for one-quarter of all completed suicides (p. 131).... Approximately one-third of individuals with bipolar II disorder report a lifetime history of suicide attempt (p. 138).... A previous history of suicide attempt and percent days spent depressed in the past year are associated with greater risk of suicide attempts or completions" (p. 131).

Getting the History

> Ms. Wright, an 18-year-old college sophomore, complains of having had depression for the last month in the setting of academic stress (upcoming final examinations). The interviewer determines that Ms. Wright has pervasive sadness, anhedonia, insomnia, poor concentration (trouble focusing on schoolwork), and passive thoughts of death. Ms. Wright comments that most of these symptoms are particularly prominent in the morning and persist into the afternoon. The interviewer then asks, "Is your mood much different in the late afternoon and in the evening?" and Ms. Wright responds that she is more irritable than sad in the late afternoons and evenings. The interviewer next asks, "How do you spend your time in the evenings?" and the patient responds that she stays up late cramming on her schoolwork (i.e., has increased goal-directed activity), attempts to multitask but is not able to complete homework (i.e., has distractibility), has trouble keeping up with her thoughts (i.e., has flight of ideas), frequently gets up from her desk and paces (i.e., has psychomotor agitation), and has been spending most of the

rest of the night having sexual relations with a married graduate student (i.e., impulsivity). The interviewer then asks, "How much sleep are you getting?" and Ms. Wright responds that she is only getting 3 hours of sleep each night, which is substantially less than her baseline of 8 hours each night. The interviewer asks, "Are you sleepy during the day?" and she states that she is wide awake throughout the day and not napping (suggesting decreased need for sleep) and denies using caffeine or other substances. The interviewer asks, "How long have your late afternoons and evenings been like that?" and Ms. Wright states that this has been going on for a month. Also, in response to queries by the interviewer, she denies any lifetime history of psychosis, psychiatric hospitalization, or severe consequences related to the aforementioned symptoms of mood elevation. Finally, the interviewer asks, "Does anyone in your family have bipolar disorder or manic-depression?" Ms. Wright responds that her father had intermittently taken lithium for several years before running off with his secretary when the patient was 13 years old.

Ms. Wright presents with complaints of depression and meets criteria for a major depressive episode but also meets criteria for a hypomanic episode. With more limited assessment, a clinician might determine only a current major depressive episode (or possibly a major depressive episode with mixed features), consistent with a diagnosis of unipolar major depressive disorder. However, with additional careful questioning, it becomes apparent that Ms. Wright also meets criteria for a hypomanic episode, consistent with a diagnosis of bipolar II disorder. Mixed symptoms of depression and mood elevation may involve ultradian cycling (i.e., mood changes occurring within a day), as seen in Ms. Wright, or more continuous, simultaneous mixed symptoms. DSM-5 is silent regarding patients with concurrent major depressive and hypomanic episodes, raising the possibility of diagnosing both at the same time. In contrast, DSM-5 indicates that patients with concurrent major depressive and manic episodes, in view of the severity requirement for manic episodes, ought to be diagnosed with a manic episode with mixed features.

Tips for Clarifying the Diagnosis

- Carefully assess all patients presenting with depression for a history of prior manic or hypomanic episodes—specifically ask about episodes of mood elevation immediately preceding or following depressive episodes. Encourage patients prospectively to chart their mood symptoms to help clarify the diagnosis.
- Carefully ensure that full criteria (including the minimum 4-day duration requirement) for hypomanic episodes are met in order to limit the risk of overdiagnosing bipolar II disorder (as opposed to other specified bipolar and related disorder, unspecified bipolar and related disorder, and unipolar major depressive disorder).
- In view of overlapping symptoms, carefully distinguish major depressive episodes with mixed features (which may occur in unipolar major depressive disorder and bipolar and related disorders) from manic/hypomanic episodes (which *must* occur in bipolar I/bipolar II disorder and *must not* occur in unipolar major depressive disorder).
- Obtain collateral history from significant others, particularly regarding the possibility of prior manic or hypomanic episodes and the extent of mixed features during major depressive episodes.

Consider the Case

Ms. Lee, a 20-year-old single Asian American woman, complains of depression with prominent hypersomnia, increased appetite, and anergy, worsening since she stopped taking bupropion about 1 month ago. She reports that during the prior year, she had three similar depressive episodes, as well as three 4-day episodes of increased irritability accompanied by excessive energy, overtalkativeness, distractibility, decreased need for sleep (with 3 hours being sufficient rather than her usual 9 hours), physical agitation, and impulsivity. Ms. Lee reports a history of Hashimoto thyroiditis, occasional use of "diet pills," and worsening of mood symptoms around her menstrual periods, but denies ever being psychotic or hospitalized for psychiatric reasons. She reports a history of treatment with sertraline, during which she developed suicidal ideation, and with bupropion, during which she developed increased irritability. Her mother has bipolar I disorder with psychotic mania, and her sister has bipolar II disorder.

Ms. Lee meets criteria for bipolar II disorder with a current major depressive episode and rapid-cycling course (at least four episodes in prior year). Hypomanic episodes as compared to manic episodes have a shorter minimum duration (4 days rather than 7) and do not entail psychosis, psychiatric hospitalization, or severe social or occupational dysfunction. Diagnosis of bipolar II disorder requires the occurrence of at least one major depressive episode and at least one hypomanic episode. Compared with bipolar I disorder, bipolar II disorder has more anxiety and substance use disorder comorbidity; somewhat later onset; and in clinical samples, more association with female gender. Hypomanic episodes in women with bipolar II disorder are more likely to entail mixed features than those in men. In individuals with bipolar disorder who are undergoing rapid cycling, it is important to assess for confounding effects of substances or medications and medical disorders, which may indicate the presence of a substance/medication-induced bipolar and related disorder or a bipolar and related disorder due to another medical condition.

Ms. Lee's Asian American ethnicity could influence her presentation, because data suggest that Asian American and Hispanic American individuals with bipolar II disorder may be less likely to present at bipolar disorder specialty clinics than their white counterparts, perhaps due to stigma.

Differential Diagnosis

Because the differential diagnosis of bipolar disorder includes disorders induced by a medication or substance (e.g., alcohol or illicit drugs) or due to another medical condition (most commonly neurological and endocrine disorders), it is important to perform a careful substance use and medical assessment. Unipolar major depressive disorder is the most common misdiagnosis. Individuals presenting with depression need to be carefully assessed for a history of prior manic or hypomanic episodes (including collateral history from significant others). Depressed patients with onset before age 25 years; a history of multiple, rapidly emerging, and rapidly resolving depressions; untoward experiences with antidepressants (e.g., worsening of depression or switching into mood elevation); and a family history of bipolar disorder are at increased risk for having bipolar disorder. Because manic episodes in bipolar I disorder or major depressive episodes in bipolar I or bipolar II disorder can have psychotic features, psychotic disorders such as schizophrenia need to be ruled out—in the psychotic disorders, psychotic symptoms are more chronic and prominent than mood symptoms.

Bipolar II disorder is distinguished from bipolar I disorder primarily in that the latter, but not the former, entails severe episodes of mood elevation (with psychosis, hospitalization, or severe social or occupational dysfunction). Symptoms of cyclothymic disorder may overlap those of Cluster B personality disorders, but instability of mood is more prominent than disturbance of identity or interpersonal relationships. ADHD is most common in male children and adolescents and involves chronic (rather than episodic) problems related to disturbance of attention and behavior (rather than mood). Because anxiety can be accompanied by irritability/psychomotor activation (resembling mood elevation) and/or demoralization/psychomotor retardation (resembling depression), it is important to distinguish anxiety disorders and posttraumatic stress disorder from bipolar and related disorders. Also, use of certain substances can yield mood elevation symptoms, while discontinuation of such substances can yield depressive symptoms, making it important to distinguish substance use disorders from bipolar and related disorders.

Finally, patients with bipolar and related disorders commonly have comorbid anxiety disorder(s), ADHD, and/or substance use disorder(s), so that it is important to consider the possibility of any comorbid disorder(s).

See DSM-5 for additional disorders to consider in the differential diagnosis. Also refer to the discussions of comorbidity and differential diagnosis in their respective sections of DSM-5.

Summary

- Bipolar disorders are common and chronic and involve recurrent episodes of mood elevation and (most often) depression that can be challenging to distinguish from unipolar major depressive disorder.
- Bipolar disorder diagnoses are based on both current and past clinical phenomena.
- Individuals with bipolar disorder more commonly present with depression than with mood elevation and may have difficulty recognizing past (or even current) periods of mood elevation.
- Bipolar I disorder requires at least one manic episode, which entails psychosis, hospitalization, or severe functional impairment.
- Bipolar II disorder requires (in addition to at least one major depressive episode) at least one hypomanic episode, which does not entail psychosis, hospitalization, or severe functional impairment, and no prior manic episode.

SUMMARY

Bipolar and Related Disorders

Bipolar and related disorders are common (but not as common as unipolar major depressive disorder). Although the majority of people with depression have unipolar major depressive disorder, as many as one in four people with depression have bipolar and related disorders. Thus, it is crucial to screen all depressed patients for a lifetime history of bipolar and related disorders by detecting prior (or current) episodes of mood elevation. Patients are less likely to recognize or report episodes that occurred in the past and involved irritability, mixed features, or hypomania. They are more likely to report episodes that are current, involve euphoria or mania, and are without mixed features. Collateral information from significant others can be very valuable in detecting such prior episodes of mood elevation. Depressed patients with onset before age 25 years; a history of multiple, rapidly emerging, and rapidly resolving depressions; untoward experiences with antidepressants (e.g., worsening of depression or switching into mood elevation); and a family history of bipolar disorder are at increased risk for having bipolar disorder and thus merit particularly careful assessment for episodes of mood elevation. Because substance use and anxiety disorders commonly co-occur with mood disorders, it is also important to screen for these conditions in persons with mood problems. Other common comorbidities include pediatric disruptive behavioral disorders (e.g., ADHD, oppositional defiant disorder, and conduct disorder), Cluster B personality disorders (e.g., borderline personality disorder), and eating disorders. In patients with comorbid psychiatric disorders, bipolar disorders are commonly the current main focus for treatment, although on occasion comorbid disorders may represent more prominent current problems than bipolar disorders.

Diagnostic Pearls

- Bipolar disorder is diagnosed on the basis of both current and past clinical phenomena.
- Individuals with bipolar disorder more commonly present with depression than with mood elevation and may have difficulty recognizing past (or even current) periods of mood elevation.
- Unipolar major depressive disorder is a crucial differential diagnostic possibility and the most common misdiagnosis of people with bipolar disorder.
- During episodes of mood elevation, mood may be irritable rather than euphoric, making recognition of such episodes more challenging.
- Common comorbidities such as substance use, anxiety disorders, pediatric disruptive behavioral disorders, eating disorders, and Cluster B personality disorders can make diagnosing bipolar disorder more challenging.
- Bipolar disorders have complex, variable phenomenology, with different subtypes, mood states, courses, and age-dependent presentations.
- Collateral information from significant others can enhance accuracy in diagnosing bipolar disorder.

Self-Assessment

Key Concepts: Double-Check Your Knowledge

What is the relevance of the following concepts to the various bipolar and related disorders?

- Bipolar I disorder versus bipolar II disorder
- Manic episode versus hypomanic episode
- Major depressive episode with mixed features versus without mixed features
- Manic or hypomanic episode with mixed features versus without mixed features
- Concurrent hypomanic and major depressive episodes
- Rapid cycling and non–rapid cycling
- Bipolar family history
- Early-onset mood disorder (age <25) years
- Treatment-emergent affective switch (e.g., antidepressant-triggered hypomania/mania)

Questions to Discuss With Colleagues and Mentors

1. Do you screen all individuals with depression for bipolar and related disorders?
2. How do you distinguish bipolar and related disorders from unipolar major depressive disorder?
3. How do you distinguish bipolar I disorder from bipolar II disorder?
4. How do you distinguish bipolar and related disorders from Cluster B personality disorders?
5. How do you distinguish bipolar and related disorders from ADHD?
6. What are the diagnostic implications of antidepressant-induced hypomania or mania?
7. How important is a family history of bipolar and related disorders in a patient presenting with depression?

Case-Based Questions

PART A

Mr. Martin is a 26-year-old, single graduate student who complains of anxiety with physical discomfort when teaching. He reports increased social anxiety since becoming a teaching assistant 6 months ago. He gives a history of problems with social anxiety (e.g., shyness with girls, dreading being called on in class, avoiding parties) since age 16 that responded partially to individual psychotherapy. He states that for the past 6 months his social anxiety has been increasing, and he admits that for every class he taught during the past 2 weeks, he has dreaded receiving poor assessments from his students (some of whom are older than he is) and has been anxious to the point of physical discomfort (e.g., with flushing and sweating). He reports that he increased his individual psychotherapy to weekly a month ago and added group psychotherapy 2 weeks ago.

What other assessment is indicated at this time? Anxiety, mood, and substance use disorders commonly co-occur, and if one such disorder is detected, the possibility of the other two ought to be assessed as well. Co-occurrence of anxiety, mood, and substance use disorders is associated with earlier-onset age of mood problems and worse longitudinal outcome.

PART B

> On direct questioning (e.g., "Have you been feeling down lately? For how much of the time?"), Mr. Martin admits to subsyndromal depressive symptoms for the last 2 weeks. He admits to current pervasive anhedonia, low self-confidence, and difficulty concentrating, but he denies current sadness, insomnia, fatigue, appetite disturbance, psychomotor disturbance, and suicidal ideation. The clinician asks, "In the past have you felt down most of the time for a couple of weeks? Were your sleep, appetite, energy, concentration, and desire to live also affected?" Mr. Martin admits to a single lifetime major depressive episode at age 24 that occurred after the termination of a romantic relationship and was treated with increased psychotherapy. He denies any lifetime history of psychosis, suicide attempts, psychiatric hospitalization, or treatment with psychotropic medications. On direct questioning (e.g., "Tell me about alcohol and drug use in your teens and early 20s"), he admits to binge drinking and limited weekend use of marijuana as an undergraduate but denies any other lifetime drug use, although he admits to increasing his alcohol consumption to three drinks per day over the last 2 weeks. He reports that his mother and older brother have both struggled with social anxiety and depression and responded to citalopram. He also reports that his father struggled with alcoholism, which he managed through a 12-step program.

What other assessment is indicated at this time? Individuals with a history of a major depressive episode need to be assessed for a history of manic or hypomanic episodes. Collateral information from significant others can be very valuable, because they may be more sensitive observers of symptoms of mood elevation (e.g., irritability) and their consequences (e.g., marital tension).

PART C

> At the next visit, Mr. Martin's brother accompanies him and provides important collateral information. The brother reports that for a time when Mr. Martin was 24, he had less social anxiety and embarked on his first lifetime romantic relationship with a female classmate, but then began covertly dating her younger sister. When the classmate learned of Mr. Martin's actions, she terminated the relationship, and he "crashed" into a 3-month depression. On careful direct questioning, Mr. Martin and his brother agreed that this all happened after the patient had had a 1-month period of bright mood, increased activity, energy, self-confidence, rapid thoughts, increased social activity (joining three clubs on campus), and increased alcohol consumption (five or more alcoholic beverages each Friday and Saturday night). Mr. Martin's brother added that he had learned that their paternal grandfather had had several affairs followed by depressions.

What is Mr. Martin's diagnosis? Mr. Martin appears to have social anxiety disorder (currently the main focus of treatment), as well as bipolar II disorder, with current subsyndromal depressive symptoms. Alcohol abuse is a possibility to be ruled out.

Short-Answer Questions

1. What is the minimum duration of manic versus hypomanic episodes?
2. What are the severity criteria for manic versus hypomanic episodes?
3. What gender differences are encountered in bipolar disorders?
4. What age differences are encountered in bipolar disorders?
5. Bipolar and related disorder due to another medical condition results most often from what kind of medical disorders?
6. What type of psychiatric medications most commonly triggers substance/medication-induced bipolar and related disorder?
7. Which psychiatric disorders may include major depressive episodes with mixed features?
8. Which psychiatric disorders may include hypomanic episodes with mixed features?
9. Which psychiatric disorders may include manic episodes with mixed features?
10. How many episodes per year are required for a rapid-cycling course?

Answers

1. Seven days is the minimum duration for a manic episode (or any duration if hospitalization occurs) versus 4 days for a hypomanic episode.
2. Manic episodes require (and hypomanic episodes prohibit) psychosis, hospitalization, or severe functional impairment.
3. Women compared with men with bipolar disorder experience more depression, rapid cycling, mixed states, and possibly bipolar II disorder.
4. Children and adolescents may present with disruptive behavioral disorders (e.g., ADHD, oppositional defiant disorder, and conduct disorder), whereas older adults may present with bipolar and related disorder due to another medical condition.
5. Bipolar and related disorder due to another medical condition most often results from neurological and endocrine disorders.
6. Antidepressants most commonly trigger substance/medication-induced bipolar and related disorder.
7. Bipolar I disorder, bipolar II disorder, and major depressive disorder may include major depressive episodes with mixed features.
8. Bipolar I disorder or bipolar II disorder (but not major depressive disorder) may include hypomanic episodes with mixed features.
9. Bipolar I disorder (but not bipolar II disorder and major depressive disorder) may include manic episodes with mixed features.
10. Four episodes per year are required for a rapid-cycling course.

7

Depressive Disorders

Bruce A. Arnow, Ph.D.
Tonita E. Wroolie, Ph.D.
Sanno E. Zack, Ph.D.

"Nothing will get better. What's the use of trying?"

"He doesn't even smile at our grandson anymore."

The depressive disorders group includes major depressive disorder; persistent depressive disorder (dysthymia); premenstrual dysphoric disorder; disruptive mood dysregulation disorder, which is specific to children under 12 years old; substance/medication-induced depressive disorder, depressive disorder due to another medical condition, other specified depressive disorder, and unspecified depressive disorder.

The cardinal symptoms of major depressive disorder, the most common of these disorders, are sad or low mood and/or anhedonia. Other possible symptoms of major depressive disorder include significant weight loss or change in appetite, insomnia or hypersomnia, psychomotor agitation or retardation, fatigue or loss of energy, feelings of worthlessness or excessive guilt, impaired concentration or indecisiveness, and recurrent thoughts of death, suicidal ideation, or a suicide attempt or plan. Symptoms must be present most of the day, nearly every day, for at least 2 weeks. DSM-5 criteria for major depressive disorder require at least five symptoms, one of which must be depressed mood or anhedonia. Individuals meeting criteria for major depressive disorder must never have experienced a manic or hypomanic episode (unless the mania or hypomania is substance induced or is attributable to the physiological effects of another medical condition).

Although the symptomatic criteria of persistent depressive disorder (dysthymia) are similar to those of major depressive disorder, with depressed mood being a hallmark, the key feature of persistent depressive disorder is chronicity—that is, depressed mood must have been present over a period of at least 2 years in adults. In children, the minimum duration is 1 year and mood can be predominantly irritable. Persistent depressive disorder requires fewer total symptoms than major depressive disorder (i.e., three instead of five) and symptoms must be present for more days than not, rather than nearly every day, as in major depressive disorder. A large percentage of individuals who meet criteria for persistent depressive disorder may meet criteria for major depressive disorder during the course of illness.

Premenstrual dysphoric disorder involves mood changes in the final week before the onset of menses; these symptoms begin to improve within a few days after menses onset, becoming minimal or absent in the week postmenses. Key symptoms must include at least one of the following: affective lability; irritability, anger, or increased interpersonal conflicts; depressed mood, hopelessness or self-deprecating thoughts; and anxiety. Other symptoms may include decreased interest in usual activities, difficulty concentrating, lack of energy, changes in appetite or food cravings, hypersomnia or insomnia, a sense of being overwhelmed or out of control, or physical symptoms such as breast tenderness, bloating, or muscle pain. At least five symptoms are required to meet diagnostic criteria. Symptoms must be present for most menstrual cycles during the year preceding diagnosis.

Disruptive mood dysregulation disorder must be distinguished from other childhood disorders, including pediatric bipolar disorder. The key symptom in disruptive mood dysregulation disorder is severe, persistent irritability in response to everyday stressors. Individuals with disruptive mood dysregulation disorder present frequent (on average, three or more times weekly) temper outbursts, which may be verbal or behavioral (e.g., physical aggression toward people or property). Children must also manifest persistently negative mood between outbursts. The child must be at least age 6 years, and onset must be before age 10 years. Symptoms must be present for at least 12 months.

A diagnosis of substance/medication-induced depressive disorder is appropriate when the symptoms of depression developed in conjunction with exposure to a medication that is known to cause such symptoms or in close temporal proximity to substance intoxication or withdrawal. Depressive disorder due to another medical condition is appropriate when evidence indicates that the depressive symptoms are best explained by a medical condition (e.g., hypothyroidism).

Two other depressive disorders are included in DSM-5. Other specified depressive disorder involves symptoms of depression with accompanying clinically significant distress or impairment, without full criteria being met for any of the previously noted depressive disorders. When using this diagnosis, the clinician specifies the reason or reasons why criteria for a depressive disorder are not met (e.g., short duration of episode, insufficient number of symptoms). Finally, unspecified depressive disorder is similar to other specified depressive disorder, except that the clinician does not document a specific reason why the individual does not meet full criteria for another depressive disorder. In many instances, the clinician may not have sufficient information to specify a reason.

Among the key changes in DSM-5, the depressive disorders and the bipolar and related disorders are no longer grouped together as mood disorders, as they were in DSM-IV; they are now separate diagnostic classes. In major depressive disorder, the term "hopeless" has been added to the description of depressed mood and the exclusion for bereavement that was included in DSM-IV has been removed. Clinical judgment may permit diagnosing major depressive disorder in bereaved individuals. Additionally, disruptive mood dysregulation disorder is a new disorder in DSM-5. Disruptive mood dysregulation disorder addresses concerns about previous overdiagnosis of bipolar disorder in children; those meeting criteria for disruptive mood dysregulation disorder are more likely to develop unipolar depression or anxiety as adolescents or adults, rather than bipolar disorder. Persistent depressive disorder, which is also new to DSM-5, is similar to DSM-IV's dysthymic disorder. However, it is now designed to incorporate cases of chronic major depressive episode and includes specifiers to delineate the relationship between symptoms of persistent depressive disorder and major depression over the prior 2-year period. Premenstrual dysphoric disorder, which in DSM-IV appeared in Appendix B as a diagnosis requiring further study, is a separate diagnosis grouped with the depressive disorders in DSM-5.

IN-DEPTH DIAGNOSIS
Major Depressive Disorder

Ms. Spaulding, a 26-year-old single woman, presents to her internist complaining of insomnia. Upon interview, she reveals that she also has depressed mood, her ability to concentrate is diminished, she is not finding pleasure in activities that are usually fun for her, her energy and appetite are diminished, and she has recently been having thoughts that she would be better off dead. She denies having a suicide plan but says "if something were to happen, I don't think I would care." Symptoms had arisen 2 months ago, following a breakup with her boyfriend. She reports having been depressed in her early 20s, also following the end of a relationship with an earlier boyfriend. Ms. Spaulding notes that she is a "worrier"—that is, she is anxious about a number of issues, especially her job performance, although she has never had a negative job performance review. Medical tests are negative. Ms. Spaulding does not abuse substances and denies a history of mania or hypomania.

Individuals with depression often present to physicians with complaints such as insomnia or low energy. Although medical problems must be ruled out, it is important to ask questions that may reveal the presence of a mood disorder in patients such as Ms. Spaulding. She meets criteria for six of nine possible symptoms of depression, and among those six are the hallmark symptoms of low mood and anhedonia. The risk of depression is higher in females than in males. Although major depressive disorder may arise at any age, peak incidence is in the 20s. The patient has had one episode in the past. The presence of environmental stressors, in this case the breakup with her boyfriend, is more likely in early episodes as opposed to later or subsequent depressive episodes. Anxiety disorders are commonly comorbid with major depressive disorder, and Ms. Spaulding's self-designation as a "worrier" may or may not be an indication of co-occurring generalized anxiety disorder.

Approach to the Diagnosis

Depressed mood for brief periods of time is common in everyday life. The criteria for major depressive disorder involve a sustained (at least 2-week) period during which the individual experiences either depressed mood or diminished interest or pleasure in nearly all activities most of the day, nearly every day. Thus, it is important to establish the length of time the individual has had depressed mood. Given that the diagnosis requires at least five symptoms, including such issues as sleep difficulties, psychomotor agitation or retardation, fatigue or loss of energy, and suicidal ideation, it is helpful to inquire about each of the nine potential symptoms. Because the diagnostic criteria also require that the symptoms cause clinically significant distress or impairment in key areas of functioning, it is important to ask how the symptoms are interfering with the individual's life and in which domains (e.g., family, work, social).

Because depression is the most important risk factor in suicide, it is critical to inquire about suicidal thoughts. A suicide risk assessment should be carried out with every patient meeting criteria for major depressive disorder. Questions in such an assessment may include the following: 1) "Are you feeling hopeless about the present or the future?" 2) "Have you had thoughts of taking your life?" 3) (If yes) "How recently have you had such thoughts?" 4) "Have you ever tried to take your own life?" 5) "Do you have a specific plan to take your life?" Factors associated with high risk of suicide include social isolation, substance abuse, and availability of a lethal method.

As stated in DSM-5, "The possibility of suicidal behavior exists at all times during major depressive episodes. The most consistently described risk factor is a past history of suicide attempts or threats, but it should be remembered that most completed suicides are not preceded by unsuccessful attempts. Other features associated with an increased risk for completed suicide include male sex, being single or living alone, and having prominent feelings of hopelessness. The presence of borderline personality disorder markedly increases risk for future suicide attempts" (p. 167).

Getting the History

Ms. Allen, a 46-year-old divorced woman, arrives for an initial psychotherapy appointment, reporting depressed mood. The therapist asks, "How long have you been feeling this way?" (If a patient responds in an uncertain or vague manner, it may be helpful to go back to a salient event over the past year, such as a birthday or a holiday like Thanksgiving, and ask whether she was feeling this way then or whether her mood was different.) The therapist also asks a question to determine how persistent the depressed mood might be: "Do you feel this way every day, or is it more that the feeling comes and goes?" The therapist next asks specifically about each of the other symptoms of depression: "Since you've been feeling this way, have there been changes in your sleep pattern? Since you've been feeling this way, have there been changes in your appetite, such that you have a larger or smaller appetite? Since you began feeling depressed, have you lost or gained weight? Do you notice that you are agitated or slowed down?" For Ms. Allen to meet the criterion for psychomotor agitation or retardation, the symptoms would have to be severe enough for others to notice. In this case, she says that she feels her movement has slowed down. However, when the therapist asks whether others have noticed or commented on this, Ms. Allen says that no one has. The therapist suggests that she specifically ask her roommate during the coming week whether she has noticed such a change.

Although people often do report depressed mood, they rarely report anhedonia without prompting. The therapist may want to ask, "Are you able to enjoy the things you normally enjoy?" If a patient is unsure, the therapist can say, "Tell me about some of the activities you enjoyed when you were not feeling depressed." If the patient says, "Well, I enjoy family dinners with my children," the therapist can then ask her to think back to the most recent family dinner and to reflect on whether her enjoyment was consistent with how she felt in the past or whether there might be a change. Other recent family dinners can also be discussed to determine whether there might be a pattern consistent with anhedonia.

Tips for Clarifying the Diagnosis

- Establish that the person reports either depressed mood or loss of interest or pleasure in activities that were previously engaging or enjoyable.
- Determine whether there are at least five symptoms of depression (one of which is depressed mood or anhedonia).
- Determine whether the symptoms have persisted for at least 2 weeks.
- Learn which domains in the individual's life are affected by the depressive symptoms.
- Rule out physiological effects of a substance (e.g., drug of abuse, medication) as a cause of the symptoms.
- Rule out other medical illness (e.g., thyroid illness) as a cause of the depressive symptoms.

Consider the Case

Mr. Calhoun, a widower age 85, presented to his internist during a routine visit with slowed movement, weight loss, and diminished grooming, in contrast to his usual presentation. A variety of in-office and laboratory tests were completed, all of which were negative. At a second visit to discuss the outcome of the medical data, the patient reveals lack of pleasure in activities that had previously been enjoyable ("I don't even have fun when I see my grandchildren anymore"), despondency, hypersomnia, impaired concentration, and reduced appetite. He denies suicidal ideation or plan but indicates, "I feel that I don't have a reason to go on." He feels poorly all through the day but worse in the morning upon awakening. His wife died 3 years earlier, and he had been very sad for approximately 1 year but recovered. A number of close friends had also died in the previous 5 years. He does not have a history of depression. He is not taking any medications that would account for his symptoms.

Onset of major depression can occur at any age. Mr. Calhoun did not have a history of major depressive disorder earlier in his life. The onset of depression in late life is frequently associated with an accumulation of losses. Mr. Calhoun had lost his wife and numerous close friends. He described a lack of purpose and an absence of goals going forward, which is also common in late-life depression. Symptoms that are worse in the early morning, involve either loss of pleasure in all or almost all activities and/or lack of reactivity to normally pleasurable stimuli, combined with psychomotor retardation and weight loss, are indicative of major depressive disorder with melancholic features. Excessive or inappropriate guilt may also be observed in cases of melancholic depression. Of course, as occurred in this case, it is important to rule out medical illness that might account for such symptoms.

Differential Diagnosis

One of the most important psychiatric disorders to differentiate from major depressive disorder is bipolar disorder. Indeed, many individuals with bipolar disorder are incorrectly diagnosed with unipolar depression and do not receive appropriate treatment. People who appear depressed but who have experienced a manic or hypomanic episode should be diagnosed with bipolar disorder. Thus, any person who presents with depression should be asked whether there has ever been a period in which they experienced decreased need for sleep, pressured speech or unusual talkativeness, engaging in risky behavior that is unusual for them (e.g., buying items they cannot afford, risky sexual behavior), or other symptoms of mania or hypomania. It is also important to note that certain medications can be associated with manic-like symptoms; those individuals with symptoms that are attributable to the effects of medication would not be classified as having bipolar illness. Substance use may also be associated with symptoms similar to depression (e.g., cocaine withdrawal). If the symptoms are fully attributable to the effects of substance use or withdrawal, then another diagnosis would be appropriate. For example, in the case of depressed mood associated with cocaine withdrawal, the diagnosis would be cocaine-induced depressive disorder, with onset during withdrawal.

Moreover, major depression is frequently comorbid with other psychiatric illnesses. For example, anxiety disorders and substance use disorders commonly coexist with major depression. A person may present for treatment of panic disorder, but on interview may also meet criteria for major depressive disorder. In addition to presenting with other psychiatric illnesses, individuals with depression frequently present in medical settings with somatic symptoms, such as insomnia and fatigue. This presentation occurs in all cultures but is more widespread in cultures where it is explicitly considered more acceptable to present physical symptoms than psychiatric ones.

See DSM-5 for additional disorders to consider in the differential diagnosis. Also refer to the discussions of comorbidity and differential diagnosis in their respective sections of DSM-5.

Summary

- Hallmark symptoms of major depressive disorder involve depressed mood and/or loss of interest or pleasure in all or almost all activities. At least one of these symptoms must be experienced almost all day, nearly every day, for at least 2 weeks.

- Including at least one of the above symptoms being present, the individual must have at least five of nine symptoms of depression to qualify for a diagnosis of major depressive disorder.
- The symptoms must also cause significant distress or impairment in key social, occupational, or other areas of functioning.
- It is important to rule out general medical conditions or use of substances as a cause of depressive symptoms.

IN-DEPTH DIAGNOSIS

Disruptive Mood Dysregulation Disorder

Jack, an 8-year-old boy, is referred by his pediatrician to a child psychiatrist due to concerns regarding chronic irritability and outbursts of rage. Jack's parents report that he is constantly angry, lashing out at his parents and siblings with little provocation, and is frequently in trouble at school for whining, pushing others, and refusing to complete homework. They describe temper tantrums of multiple hours in duration, during which time Jack will scream, cry, and throw items such as schoolbooks and toys, often breaking them. At times he will hit his parents, younger brother, or family pets. These tantrums occur five to six times per week, and during the outbursts, Jack is unable to be soothed or redirected. Outbursts typically occur when Jack is asked to do nonpreferred activities, such as to complete homework or chores, and when Jack loses at games or perceives that others are being favored; the outbursts are worse when he is tired or hungry. His parents and pediatrician describe him as having been a difficult and colicky infant and report that he was diagnosed at age 4 with oppositional defiant disorder and symptoms of ADHD, but his difficulties have progressed over the past 2 years into chronic irritability and anger. Jack's parents became particularly concerned when he recently grabbed a knife during one tantrum and threatened to stab himself. There has been no history of elevated or euphoric mood and an absence of pressured speech, flight of ideas, or goal-directed activity. Sleep is unremarkable. Distractibility is chronic for Jack and not mood related.

Parents, teachers, and peers typically identify children with disruptive mood dysregulation disorder as irritable, moody, or difficult to get along with. Although problems with sad, irritable, or angry mood must present across multiple settings for diagnosis, more severe tantrums are often observed in one setting, such as the home, as is the case for Jack. Recurrent temper outbursts are frequently in response to common stressors, such as demands to complete chores or homework or conflicts with siblings or peers. However, the response is grossly disproportionate for both the situation and the child's developmental level. In this case, Jack's tantrums are excessive in both intensity and severity, lasting for hours at a time and escalating to hitting others, throwing and breaking household items, and threatening self-harm. Outside of these episodes, this child is irritable and angry on a chronic basis. Chronicity is an important distinction that helps differentiate disruptive mood dysregulation disorder from the episodic mood events that occur in bipolar disorder. Like Jack, the majority of children with disruptive mood dysregulation disorder are males, have premorbid difficulty with behavior and attention before meeting full criteria for disruptive mood

dysregulation disorder, and present to mental health clinics due to the level of severity of their symptoms and the negative impact on families and classrooms. Jack is comorbid for oppositional defiant disorder, the most common diagnostic co-occurrence
with disruptive mood dysregulation disorder, and also has historically presented
with symptoms of ADHD. Disruptive mood dysregulation disorder is most common
from ages 7 to 12 years and cannot be diagnosed before age 6.

Approach to the Diagnosis

Occasional temper outbursts are common in children, especially those who are
younger or developmentally immature. The criteria for disruptive mood dysregulation disorder require frequent outbursts (three or more times per week), which must
be grossly out of proportion in intensity and duration to the situation or provocation.
Thus, it is important to establish the frequency, duration, and intensity of the outbursts. In addition, the clinician should inquire about triggers for the child's outbursts.
In disruptive mood dysregulation disorder, triggers tend to be common stressors (e.g.,
not getting one's way, competing for attention with siblings) and occur across a variety
of domains, not only in one specific situation. Thus, it is important to ask whether outbursts occur in multiple settings, such as at home, school, sports practices, or other ex-
tracurricular activities, and whether they occur with peers. Symptoms must occur in
at least two settings, although they may be more severe in one.

When assessing any mood disorder, it is helpful to first establish an index mood and
time course. In the case of disruptive mood dysregulation disorder, there is a minimum
1-year time course characterized by chronic mood disturbance. Between temper outbursts, the child displays persistently negative affect (e.g., angry, irritable, or sad
mood). This is particularly important for distinguishing disruptive mood dysregulation disorder from bipolar disorder, which presents with episodic as opposed to chronic
mood disturbance and in which mood may be euthymic between episodes. The clinician should inquire whether the negative mood is observable to others, including family, teachers, and peers, and establish that there has been no more than 3 months
without symptoms. Because disruptive mood dysregulation disorder is a risk factor for
dangerous behavior, including aggression, suicide, and other behaviors warranting
psychiatric hospitalization, it is critical to inquire about suicidal thoughts and plans, actions that are a threat to others, or any other areas of risk or dangerous behavior. Both
the child and the child's caregivers should be interviewed. Teachers are also an important source of information.

As stated in DSM-5, "In general, evidence documenting suicidal behavior and aggression, as well as other severe functional consequences, in disruptive mood dysregulation disorder should be noted when evaluating children with chronic irritability"
(p. 158).

Getting the History

Arnold, an 8-year-old boy, is brought by his parents for an initial appointment with a
child psychiatrist due to concerns about severe mood dysregulation. The psychiatrist
asks Arnold's parents, "When did you first begin to have concerns about his mood?"

They respond by describing severe temper tantrums that began when they enrolled Arnold in kindergarten at age 6. The psychiatrist asks, "Can you describe the tantrums in detail? What does Arnold do or say? How long do the tantrums last? Has he ever hurt himself or someone else or destroyed property?" His parents answer that Arnold typically yells and screams for a half hour to an hour and will break classroom items and sometimes destroy other students' possessions. He has grabbed the classroom rabbit on one occasion, squeezing it hard. The psychiatrist asks how often these tantrums occur and learns that they typically happen "a few times per week." To clarify frequency, she asks, "How often is 'a few'? Would you say three or four? More?" The psychiatrist then assesses Arnold's mood between outbursts: "Tell me what Arnold's mood is like on the days between these outbursts." Arnold's parents clarify that he is generally sad and irritable. The psychiatrist asks Arnold if he agrees, clarifying that Arnold knows what *mad* and *sad* mean by eliciting examples. She further asks, "What sorts of things make you feel sad or mad?" explaining that "Sometimes kids get so mad that they want to yell or break things" and asking what sorts of things make Arnold this mad. The psychiatrist asks Arnold and his parents if the teachers or Arnold's friends also notice that he is sad and mad a lot. Once the psychiatrist establishes that his outbursts are severe and have occurred four times per week over the past year with sad and angry mood in between, she rules out instances of mania by asking if there has ever been a time when Arnold was "so happy or high or excited that he didn't seem like himself or he got into trouble." Both Arnold and his parents deny this happening. Given Arnold's irritable mood, the psychiatrist also inquires about other symptoms of mania (e.g., decreased need for sleep, unusual talkativeness, grandiosity).

The clinician should interview both the caregivers and the child about the child's symptoms. Caregivers are frequently better reporters of externalizing symptoms, and children and adolescents are better at reporting their internalizing symptoms. In the case of disruptive mood dysregulation disorder, however, the sad, irritable, or angry mood must be observable to others, so caregiver reports are particularly important, and corroboration by teachers is also helpful. Parental report of "tantrums" is insufficient for diagnosis. The clinician must ascertain frequency, intensity, duration, and severity, such as by asking for examples of the behaviors that occur during the temper outbursts (e.g., yelling, throwing items), the duration of these outbursts, the degree to which school and family routines are disrupted, and the consequences (including injury to others or destruction of property). Other important questions include how the outbursts end (e.g., being sent to the principal at school, hospitalization, or the parents having to restrain the child all may suggest high severity) and whether caregivers feel the outbursts are markedly more intense than those of siblings, peers, or other children. Obtaining information about the child's presenting mood between the temper outbursts is of equal importance to the diagnosis.

Tips for Clarifying the Diagnosis

- Ask the caregiver whether temper outbursts are grossly disproportionate to the situation.
- Clarify whether these outbursts occur three times per week or more and are observable to others besides the child.
- Establish whether the child's mood is persistently negative (sad, irritable, or angry) between outbursts.

- Determine whether symptoms have been present for at least 12 months with no more than 3 months without symptoms.
- Clarify whether the onset of symptoms was between ages 6 and 10 years.
- Rule out mania or hypomania lasting more than 1 day.

Consider the Case

> Cora is an 11-year-old girl whose parents bring her to the pediatrician with concerns regarding her sad and withdrawn mood, low frustration tolerance, and periodic "meltdowns" during which she will yell, destroy projects and favorite trinkets, or hit herself. Cora has had long-standing difficulties with peers as a result of poor social communication skills and negative mood, and her meltdowns are further exacerbated by social rejection from peers. In the classroom Cora is described as generally sad and withdrawn, saying little and keeping to herself. According to Cora's teachers, when peers tease her or she is unable to complete assignments to her satisfaction, she will rip up her paper, run out of the classroom, sob loudly, or scream at classmates who provoke her. This disruption occurs on average three times per week and results in considerable disturbance to the classroom. Cora's parents report similar struggles for her at home and add that if she is working on an art activity that is not coming out the way she wants, she will frequently have crying fits to the point that she is curled up on the floor, flailing, hitting herself, and calling herself stupid. If they attempt to intervene, she lashes out at them verbally. Onset is over the past year. There are no clear changes in appetite, sleep, or concentration associated with Cora's symptoms, although she does endorse low self-worth.

Disruptive mood dysregulation disorder is less common in girls than boys. For Cora, the disorder presents with signs of possible comorbid anxiety/perfectionism and depression, conditions with common onset in adolescent girls or those approaching adolescence. Cora's mood is chronically sad, and her temper outbursts are directed more at self than others. They occur when she is frustrated with projects or schoolwork not meeting her standards. Temper outbursts that are internally, as opposed to externally, oriented are more common in girls than boys. However, when provoked, Cora also lashes out at peers and her parents. Cora's behavioral manifestations are developmentally inappropriate, with running out of the classroom or curling up in a ball on the floor representing behavior typical of a younger child. The severity (e.g., hitting herself) is also beyond what would be expected for a frustrated almost-adolescent. Cora's age at diagnosis is somewhat atypical, because onset is at the upper age range for the disorder. Cora's presentation may progress to major depressive disorder as she moves into adolescence, but at this time she does not meet full criteria for major depressive disorder and her temper outbursts suggest disruptive mood dysregulation disorder.

Differential Diagnosis

The most important psychiatric disorder to differentiate from disruptive mood dysregulation disorder is bipolar disorder. Disruptive mood dysregulation disorder was added to DSM-5 in part as a response to the plethora of children referred for possible bipolar disorder who presented with chronic, as opposed to episodic, mood dysregulation. The primary difference between disruptive mood dysregulation disorder and bipolar disorder is that bipolar disorder manifests as delineated mood episodes with a discrete time period during which a change in mood is accompanied by four or more additional symptoms (e.g., increased goal-directed activity, racing thoughts, pressured speech, distractibility, engagement in high-risk activity). In bipolar disorder, as in disruptive mood dysregulation disorder, irritability may be the index mood; however, for patients with disruptive mood dysregulation disorder, the irritability is pervasive and continuous, whereas patients with bipolar disorder have periods of time between mood episodes in which mood may be euthymic. In addition, elevated or euphoric mood is characteristic of mania in bipolar disorder and is not typically seen in disruptive mood dysregulation disorder. If a child exhibits more than 1 day of manic-like symptoms, the child should not be diagnosed with disruptive mood dysregulation disorder. Thus, any child who presents with disruptive mood dysregulation disorder should be queried with his or her caregivers about whether there has ever been a period in which the child experienced decreased need for sleep, pressured speech or unusual talkativeness, or grandiosity; engaged in risky behavior that is unusual (e.g., running into the street, hypersexuality, atypical "daredevil" activities); or demonstrated other symptoms of mania or hypomania. Intermittent explosive disorder is also exclusionary for disruptive mood dysregulation disorder, because children with intermittent explosive disorder do not show persistent negative mood between outbursts.

Disruptive mood dysregulation disorder is typically comorbid with other psychiatric illnesses. Most patients presenting with disruptive mood dysregulation disorder will also meet criteria for oppositional defiant disorder, although the reverse is not true. Additional common co-occurrences are ADHD, anxiety disorders, unipolar depression, and autism spectrum disorder. It is important to identify the source that triggers temper outbursts when considering a diagnosis of disruptive mood dysregulation disorder. If these outbursts occur exclusively in a single context (e.g., medical appointments, classroom presentations, or disruption of a preferred routine), the tantrums might be better accounted for by specific phobia, social anxiety disorder, or autism spectrum disorder, respectively. However, co-occurrence of these disorders with disruptive mood dysregulation disorder is also possible.

See DSM-5 for additional disorders to consider in the differential diagnosis. Also refer to the discussions of comorbidity and differential diagnosis in their respective sections of DSM-5.

Summary

- The hallmark symptom of disruptive mood dysregulation disorder involves severe, recurrent temper outbursts.
- Outbursts can manifest verbally or behaviorally but are grossly disproportionate in intensity or duration to the situation.
- Outbursts occur three times per week or more.
- Between outbursts, mood is persistently irritable, angry, or sad, and others observe this presentation.

- Symptoms must be present at least 12 months, with no more than a 3-month absence.
- Onset must be before age 10 years but not before a developmental age of 6 years.
- At no time has there been a presentation of mania or hypomania lasting more than 1 day.

IN-DEPTH DIAGNOSIS

Persistent Depressive Disorder (Dysthymia)

Ms. Atkins is a 28-year-old woman whose boyfriend suggested that she seek a psychiatric evaluation. He told her that she seemed "down most of the time" and that she might be depressed. During the interview, Ms. Atkins reveals depressed mood "for as long as I can remember." On more detailed questioning, she dates the onset of her depression to about age 8. She denies anhedonia; she is active in recreational athletics and continues to enjoy them as well as other social activities. Some days are better than others, although she indicates that depressed mood is present more days than not. She also reports generally low self-esteem and low energy. Sometimes she has difficulty making decisions and struggles with overeating. Her family history is remarkable for the death of her mother when Ms. Atkins was 7 years old. She reports that her father raised her and she describes him as "usually depressed." She notes that it was at about age 8 when she fully grasped that her mother was "gone from my life" and that she was thus different from her peers in a way that caused her to feel deficient. She reports an episode of major depression in her late teens, which in addition to depressed mood included anhedonia, suicidal ideation, impaired concentration, and insomnia with early-morning awakenings. The symptoms lasted for as long as 2 years, but she adds that they had resolved by the time she was age 20.

A number of issues in Ms. Atkins's case are typical of presentations of persistent depressive disorder (dysthymia). Persistent depressive disorder is more common among females than among males. Ms. Atkins's case typifies early onset; indeed, a large percentage of persistent depressive disorder cases have an onset in childhood or adolescence. History of childhood adversity—in this case, parental loss—is also common among persons with dysthymia, as is family history of depression, whether major depressive disorder or dysthymia. The symptoms that Ms. Atkins presents— depressed mood, low self-esteem, low energy, overeating, and difficulty making decisions—are chronic, but their intensity is lower compared with that of major depressive disorder symptoms (e.g., depressed mood is present more days than not rather than nearly every day). At the same time, her case typifies the observation that the vast majority of individuals with persistent depressive disorder experience major depressive disorder during their lifetime. In this case, major depressive disorder preceded onset of dysthymia and subsequently resolved, whereas the symptoms of the latter persisted.

Approach to the Diagnosis

Persistent depressive disorder is by definition a chronic disorder that has persisted for at least 2 years in adults and 1 year in children or adolescents. The severity of symptoms may be milder than those of major depressive disorder. Patients cannot be free of symptoms for more than 2 months during the previous 2 years. Thus, both symptom persistence and severity are key issues in the diagnosis. People with "pure" dysthymia—that is, those who have never met criteria for major depressive disorder—are rare. The specifiers "with pure dysthymic syndrome," "with persistent major depressive episode," "with intermittent major depressive episodes, with current episode," and "with intermittent major depressive episodes, without current episode" are designed to describe the relationship between dysthymia and major depressive disorder for each patient diagnosed with persistent depressive disorder. Impairment is marked and may be seen in marital and family, interpersonal, and occupational domains. Psychiatric comorbidity is common and may include anxiety disorders, substance use disorders, personality disorders, or others.

Getting the History

> Ms. Crawford, a 33-year-old married woman, seeks a consultation for depressed mood. She reports that she functions tolerably well at work and carries out tasks expected of her within her marriage but that she feels "weighed down by sadness and depression" and is often "not at my best." She also endorses fatigue, low self-esteem, and poor concentration but denies suicidal ideation. To begin to determine how intense the symptoms are, the physician asks, "Do you feel this way every day, or is your mood more variable from day to day?" When Ms. Crawford indicates that her mood varies somewhat from day to day, the physician asks her approximately how many days per week on average she feels sad, down, or depressed. When she indicates "about 4 days," the physician then begins to inquire more closely about onset. When queried about how long she has been feeling this way, Ms. Crawford answers, "I'm not sure; it's been a really long time." The physician asks, "When was the last time you felt that you were *not* sad or depressed most of the time?" When Ms. Crawford indicates uncertainty, the physician begins to ask about prominent events in her life. She was married 6 years ago, and the physician asks whether she felt depressed at the time she was married. She answers, "No, that was a very happy time." The physician asks about other markers: "Did you feel depressed at the time of your first anniversary? How about on your first birthday after the wedding?" Upon further inquiry, Ms. Crawford begins to realize that the symptoms came on about 3 years ago when, after a year of unsuccessfully trying to conceive a child, she began to be concerned that she and her husband would not be able to conceive. Thus, onset was approximately 3 years ago.

In establishing the intensity of depressed mood, useful questions involve how variable the symptoms are from day to day and from week to week. It is often informative to ask, "On average, how many days per week do you feel this way?" If persistent depressive disorder is suspected, it is important to ask about all possible symptoms (e.g., poor appetite or overeating, sleep disturbance, hopelessness). It is also important to ask about specific symptoms of depression that are not included in the dysthymia criteria, including anhedonia and suicidal ideation, to help differentiate major depressive disorder from symptoms of persistent depressive disorder. With respect to onset, orienting the prominent events—for example, birthdays, anniversaries, and celebrated holidays—is often useful in establishing how long the symptoms have been present. A history of mania, hypomania, or mixed episode precludes diagnosis of persistent depressive disorder, and it is critical to rule out these disorders.

The symptoms also must cause distress or impairment, so it is important to ask how the symptoms affect the individual in important areas of life such as occupational, social, and family arenas.

Tips for Clarifying the Diagnosis

- Investigate whether the patient has experienced depressed mood for most of the day, more days than not, for 2 years or longer (1 year for children).
- Establish whether there has been no more than a 2-month period during the last 2 years during which the individual was free of symptoms.
- Use specifiers to describe whether and to what extent major depression has been present for the previous 2 years.
- Determine whether in addition to depressed mood, at least two other symptoms (e.g., low energy, poor concentration) are present.

Consider the Case

Mr. Murphy, a 42-year-old man, is casually dressed and moderately overweight. He sought a psychiatric consultation after reading in the newspaper about a medication study for depression and wondering whether the agent mentioned in the article might be helpful to him. He is single and works as an engineer. He reports having had depressed mood, most of the day and almost every day, for the previous 15 years. In addition, he reports pervasive feelings of hopelessness about his life, low self-esteem, and frequent insomnia with early-morning awakenings. He denies anhedonia, appetite disturbance, suicidal ideation, poor concentration, and other symptoms of major depression. He admits to drinking too much alcohol—reportedly three or four glasses of wine each evening. He denies history of tickets from driving under the influence, blackouts, or drinking alcohol during the day. He has never been married. He reports that he dated when he was younger, but that he has not done so for the past several years. He says that he functions well at work but that his social life is very limited and that his symptoms of depression have reduced his motivation for social contact. He does not think he would make a good husband, even if he were to meet "the right person." He has few friends and rarely goes out after work. He was raised in an intact family. History of abuse and loss are denied, but Mr. Murphy reports that both his mother and father were distant and not attuned to him and that he did not feel particularly close to them. He does not know if either of them suffered depression. The interview reveals at least two clear episodes of major depression, one at about age 32 and the other at age 36.

Although it occurs more commonly in females, persistent depressive disorder is also encountered in males. It is associated with significant functional limitations. Mr. Murphy was successful at work but led a socially circumscribed life. His current symptoms were not sufficient in number or severity to qualify for a diagnosis of major depressive disorder. Although there was no history of outright abuse or loss, Mr. Murphy came from an emotionally impoverished home and suffered from emotional neglect, which is not uncommon in cases of persistent depressive disorder. He has had episodes of major depressive disorder in the past. Patients with persistent depressive disorder who do not have major depressive disorder at some point in their lifetime are the exception rather than the rule. Mr. Murphy has comorbid alcohol abuse, and substance-related disorders are among those that frequently coexist with persistent depressive disorder. Underreporting of symptoms (e.g., suicidal ideation, alcohol abuse) may be observed in both men and women, but men are particularly known to underreport their symptom severity. Careful and detailed questioning is imperative in making an accurate diagnosis and assessment of risk.

Differential Diagnosis

Both major depressive disorder and persistent depressive disorder are characterized by depressed mood. Differences between the two disorders may involve number and intensity of symptoms, duration of symptoms, and/or the specific symptoms themselves. Persistent depressive disorder diagnosis requires three symptoms, whereas major depressive disorder diagnosis requires at least five. Major depressive disorder requires that depressed mood be present "nearly every day," whereas persistent depressive disorder requires "more days than not." Symptoms of major depressive disorder must be present for a minimum of 2 weeks, whereas the length of illness in persistent depressive disorder is 2 years for adults and 1 year for children and adolescents. Also, there are some differences in the symptoms that comprise the two disorders (Table 7–1).

TABLE 7–1. **Symptoms for major depressive disorder and persistent depressive disorder (dysthymia)**

Symptom	Major depressive disorder	Persistent depressive disorder
Depressed mood	X	X
Anhedonia	X	
Decreased or increased appetite	X	X
Insomnia or hypersomnia	X	X
Psychomotor agitation/ retardation	X	
Fatigue/energy loss	X	X
Feelings of worthlessness/guilt	X	
Diminished concentration	X	X
Suicidal ideation	X	
Low self-esteem		X
Hopelessness		X

Anhedonia, psychomotor agitation or retardation, feelings of worthlessness/ guilt, and suicidal ideation are not among the criteria for persistent depressive disorder. On the other hand, low self-esteem, which is among the symptoms that may be encountered in individuals with persistent depressive disorder, is not noted as a criterion for major depressive disorder. Some episodes of major depressive disorder do become chronic, that is, they last for 2 years or more. In most cases, persons with chronic major depressive disorder will meet criteria for persistent depressive disorder, with the specifier "with persistent major depressive episode."

An additional feature that distinguishes persistent depressive disorder from major depressive disorder is its insidious onset. Persistent depressive disorder often, but not always, begins before the age of 21 (early onset) and not infrequently can be traced back to childhood or adolescence.

See DSM-5 for additional disorders to consider in the differential diagnosis. Also refer to the discussions of comorbidity and differential diagnosis in their respective sections of DSM-5.

Summary

- Persistent depressive disorder is a chronic disorder in which depressed mood has been present for at least 2 years.
- The symptoms have been persistent—that is, the individual has not been free of symptoms for a period longer than 2 months over the previous 2 years.
- Onset is typically insidious.
- A minimum of three symptoms (depressed mood plus two others) is required to meet the threshold for diagnosis.
- The vast majority of patients with persistent depressive disorder meet criteria for major depressive episode sometime in their lives.

--- **IN-DEPTH DIAGNOSIS** ---

Premenstrual Dysphoric Disorder

Ms. Sawyer is a 34-year-old married mother of two children, ages 3 and 5 years. She presents with complaints of significantly increased irritability that began after the birth of her second child. She reports that before her first pregnancy, she noticed feeling more sensitive and frustrated a few days before her period. Once menses began, however, she was quickly "back to her old self." The symptoms did not interfere with her schoolwork or relationships, but she began to notice a pattern over time. Ms. Sawyer's pregnancies were uneventful; both children are healthy and she enjoys being a mother. She describes a stable marriage, ample child care, and support from friends and family. She is confused about what she calls her "Jekyll and Hyde" personality. Currently, every month she experiences intense "mood swings" that last about 10 days before her menses. She has difficulty sleeping and feels exhausted during the day. She has trouble concentrating and feels more disorganized than usual. Ms. Sawyer reports being most upset about the effect that her "monthly personality change" has on her family and her weight. She becomes extremely irritable and often feels "out of control and overwhelmed." She finds she yells at her children over minor things. She craves carbohydrates and gains 1–2 pounds per month. She is finally relieved of her symptoms 2–3 days after her menstrual flow begins. "It is as if a toxin leaves my body and then I'm back to my old self again for about 20 days."

Ms. Sawyer experiences monthly mood changes that begin during the luteal phase of her menstrual cycle and remit within the first few days after her menstrual flow begins. She experiences classic premenstrual dysphoric disorder symptoms, including carbohydrate cravings, irritability, mood lability, feeling easily overwhelmed, and low frustration tolerance. In particular, she is most distressed by how irritable she becomes and the effect this has on her behavior and relationships. Irritability is the most common symptom of premenstrual dysphoric disorder in U.S. women. Less well-known premenstrual dysphoric disorder symptoms include cognitive complaints. Ms. Sawyer has a history of premenstrual symptoms that worsened after having children. Women with premenstrual symptoms often report progression to full DSM-5 criteria of premenstrual dysphoric disorder after childbirth.

Approach to the Diagnosis

Patients with premenstrual dysphoric disorder have a distinct pattern of severe and distressing symptoms. Mood lability, irritability, dysphoria, and anxiety symptoms typically peak around the time of menses and remit around the onset of menses, or soon after. Patients may report difficulty with concentration; sleep problems, such as hypersomnia or insomnia; appetite changes, particularly overeating or food cravings; loss of interest; and lethargy. Symptoms must have been present in most menstrual cycles in the past year and cause a significant impairment in functioning for diagnostic criteria to be met. Behavioral and physical symptoms also may be present, but unless the patient has mood and/or anxiety symptoms, a diagnosis of premenstrual dysphoric disorder should not be given.

In addition to mood and/or anxiety symptoms, women with premenstrual dysphoric disorder may experience significant behavioral disturbances. They may avoid social situations due to diminished interest in their usual activities. Decreased efficiency and productivity may cause problems at work or school or in keeping up with household responsibilities. Relationships with their spouse or partner, friends, and family may be negatively affected by the behavioral manifestations of mood swings, sudden irritability, rejection sensitivity, and increased response to stress. The most frequent physical symptoms reported in patients with premenstrual dysphoric disorder are breast tenderness or swelling and bloating. Joint or muscle pain and weight gain also may be reported.

As stated in DSM-5, "The premenstrual phase has been considered by some to be a risk period for suicide" (p. 173).

Getting the History

Ms. Sawyer reports premenstrual symptoms that worsened after the birth of her children. In particular, she is distressed by her irritability and the effect it is having on her behavior and relationships. The physician explores the type and severity of her symptoms: "Do you feel as if your moods are out of control? Are you having sleep difficulties or experiencing appetite changes or cravings? Are you more tired than usual around your menstrual periods? What other symptoms do you experience?" The physician determines the level of distress and evaluates suicide risk. He inquires about the impact on Ms. Sawyer's functioning and asks, "How are your symptoms affecting your ability to carry out your usual activities?" Although rare with premenstrual dysphoric disorder, existence of psychotic symptoms is explored. The physician determines whether Ms. Sawyer is having a sustained mood episode or whether her symptoms are associated strictly with her menstrual cycle: "When do your symptoms begin? Do they stop altogether or significantly lessen after your menstrual periods start?" The physician explores whether the patient has a history of a previous mood disorder or has experienced mood symptoms with oral contraceptive use. He evaluates for risk factors for premenstrual dysphoric disorder, such as current stressors, substance use, medical disorders, and family history of affective disorders.

The physician performs a thorough evaluation of Ms. Sawyer's symptom profile and attempts to get a clear picture of the relationship between her symptoms and her menstrual cycle. Mood lability and irritability are prominent in premenstrual dysphoric disorder and may coincide with physical symptoms related to hormone changes during the menstrual cycle. Minimization or complete remission of symptoms before or shortly after menses begins is necessary for a diagnosis of premenstrual dysphoric disorder. The pattern of when symptoms are present or absent is shown to be stable across menstrual cycles in women with premenstrual dysphoric disorder, and documenting daily symptom ratings prospectively over several months will help confirm the diagnosis.

Tips for Clarifying the Diagnosis

- Assess whether symptoms clearly begin in the luteal phase of the menstrual cycle and improve or remit in the follicular phase.
- Determine whether the patient has a history of hormone sensitivity (increased symptoms with some oral contraceptives, postpartum mood disturbances).
- Ask whether there is a family history of premenstrual dysphoric disorder or mood disorders.
- Question whether symptoms improve with exercise or stress reduction.
- Find out whether alcohol worsens symptoms.

Consider the Case

Ms. Morris, a 43-year-old single woman with a family history (mother and sister) of severe, recurrent major depression, presents with complaints of mood lability for the past year. She has a long history of feeling more emotional before the onset of her menses, but in the last year, these symptoms have intensified and include feeling very depressed and very anxious, having difficulty with memory and concentration, and feeling easily overwhelmed. Currently, she experiences night sweats throughout the month that increase in frequency during the luteal phase. She also complains that all month long, her days are "ruined by constant fatigue." Ms. Morris was promoted to an executive position at work and has been under a great deal of stress over the past several months. Her gynecologist diagnosed her with perimenopause and recommended an oral contraceptive to "even out her hormones." While taking the oral contraceptive, Ms. Morris felt bloated and even more emotional, stating, "It was like I was crawling out of my skin." After 2 months, she stopped taking the oral contraceptives because she found them "intolerable." Ms. Morris states that because of the fatigue she experiences, she stopped her daily hourly aerobic exercise. She also started drinking one or two glasses of wine per night because she feels so "keyed up" before her period. In the past month, Ms. Morris has begun to feel very depressed; she experiences decreased enjoyment in her activities, guilty ruminations, memory and concentration problems, and passive suicidal ideation. These symptoms do not remit with her menstrual flow.

As in Ms. Morris's case, women with premenstrual dysphoric disorder often report increased symptoms during menopause transition, and premenstrual dysphoric disorder is a risk factor for perimenopausal depression. Family history of affective disorders is more common in women with premenstrual dysphoric disorder than in healthy control subjects. Oral contraceptives may be given to women with premenstrual dysphoric disorder to prevent ovulation, because ovulation triggers premenstrual dysphoric disorder. In addition, oral contraceptives sometimes are given to women in perimenopause as estrogen replacement therapy. However, many oral contraceptives are associated with increased premenstrual dysphoric disorder symptoms. Ms. Morris is under more stress while transitioning into menopause due to increased work demands. Because of the fatigue associated with premenstrual dysphoric disorder and menopause transition, she gave up the exercise that might help to manage her stress and instead increased her alcohol consumption to relieve her symptoms. Both stress and alcohol are shown to increase premenstrual dysphoric disorder symptoms, and Ms. Morris now also appears to meet criteria for major depressive disorder.

Differential Diagnosis

The symptoms of premenstrual dysphoric disorder are more severe and debilitating than those of premenstrual syndrome, although both are associated with hormonal changes in the menstrual cycle. Premenstrual dysphoric disorder has a short, fluctuating course that differs from the chronic symptoms of persistent depressive disorder. Several other disorders share similar symptoms with premenstrual dysphoric disorder. In major depressive disorder, the depressed mood or anhedonia—for a total of at least five symptoms of depression—lasts for at least 2 weeks and is not specifically associated with a particular menstrual phase. The most commonly reported symptom in premenstrual dysphoric disorder is mood lability and irritability, whereas in major depressive disorder depressed mood and diminished interest or pleasure are most prominent. The fact that the mood cycling in cyclothymia generally does not follow a regular menstrual pattern is a critical differential diagnostic criterion. The cyclical irritability with distractibility and sleep disturbance can resemble premenstrual dysphoric disorder, but premenstrual dysphoric disorder is not characterized by increased goal-directed activity, grandiosity, or pressured speech. Both premenstrual dysphoric disorder and binge-eating disorder are characterized by increased consumption of food (often carbohydrates), and although binge-eating disorder may increase in the luteal phase in some women, it is not confined to the luteal phase.

It is not uncommon for women with premenstrual dysphoric disorder to have a history of mood disorder or other psychiatric disorders. Mood and behavioral symptoms in affective or other psychiatric disorders may increase during the luteal phase ("premenstrual exacerbation"), but they do not remit around the onset of menstruation. Comorbid disorders such as a substance use disorder may exacerbate symptoms of premenstrual dysphoric disorder.

See DSM-5 for additional disorders to consider in the differential diagnosis. Also refer to the discussions of comorbidity and differential diagnosis in their respective sections of DSM-5.

Summary

- Premenstrual dysphoric disorder is a cyclical mood disorder that occurs in women during reproductive age.
- Mood lability, irritability, and depressive symptoms begin after ovulation and remit or lessen in the early follicular phase of the menstrual cycle each month.
- Significant distress is associated with symptoms.
- Symptoms increase with stress, lack of exercise, and alcohol consumption; after childbirth; during menopause transition; and, in some women, with oral contraceptive use.

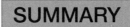

SUMMARY
Depressive Disorders

The disorders grouped under depressive disorders in DSM-5 present considerable heterogeneity in onset, chronicity, and symptom presentation. Major depressive disorder and persistent depressive disorder have the greatest overlap in symptoms; both feature depressed mood, with differences in onset, intensity, and persistence. Persistent depressive disorder is by definition a chronic disorder. Major depressive disorder, though requiring sustained symptoms for 2 weeks, can become chronic. Most patients with chronic major depression likely meet criteria for persistent depressive disorder. Premenstrual dysphoric disorder may or may not manifest with depressed mood; anxiety, irritability, and mood lability may manifest as key features of the disorder. Disruptive mood dysregulation disorder, which is characterized by chronic and severe irritability, including frequent and developmentally inappropriate temper outbursts and angry mood, is the only one of these disorders that is specifically a disorder of childhood, with an onset between ages 6 and 10. However, major depressive disorder and persistent depressive disorder may manifest during childhood.

Diagnostic Pearls

- This diagnostic class includes disorders with a chief feature of anhedonia (major depressive disorder) or depressed mood (major depressive disorder, persistent depressive disorder, premenstrual dysphoric disorder), as well as affective lability (premenstrual dysphoric disorder) and irritability (premenstrual dysphoric disorder, disruptive mood dysregulation disorder).
- Symptoms attributable to major depressive disorder must be distinguished from those caused by specific medical conditions (e.g., reduced energy in people with untreated thyroid illness, weight loss in people with untreated diabetes, fatigue with cancer).

- Major depressive disorder is also a feature of bipolar disorder in children or adults. A single episode of mania or hypomania triggers a diagnosis of bipolar disorder, rather than major depressive disorder; therefore, ruling out mania is critical for making a diagnosis of major depressive disorder.

- Persistent depressive disorder may manifest with symptoms that are less severe and intense than symptoms of major depressive disorder. However, the vast majority of people with persistent depressive disorder meet criteria for major depressive disorder at some point during their lives. Diagnosis of persistent depressive disorder includes specifiers designed to describe its relationship to major depressive disorder over the previous 2-year period.

- Symptoms of premenstrual dysphoric disorder must be minimal or absent in the week postmenses.

- The onset of disruptive mood dysregulation disorder must occur by age 10 years.

Self-Assessment

Key Concepts: Double-Check Your Knowledge

What is the relevance of the following concepts to the various depressive disorders?

- Anhedonia
- Mood lability
- Symptom peak
- Excessive or inappropriate guilt
- Severe, persistent irritability
- Recurrent thoughts of death/suicidal ideation
- Insidious onset
- Early versus late onset
- Symptom-free follicular phase

Questions to Discuss With Colleagues and Mentors

1. When a patient presents with symptoms of depression, do you screen for other medical problems that may explain the symptoms? What laboratory tests do you routinely order?
2. Do you routinely use any validated short screens for depression in your practice?
3. In cases in which premenstrual dysphoric disorder is suspected, do you incorporate prospective daily mood, anxiety, and irritability ratings across the menstrual cycle? If so, what sort of measure or log do you use?
4. What are your personal reactions to your patients who meet criteria for disruptive mood dysregulation disorder? How do you manage these reactions in yourself?

Case-Based Questions

PART A

> Ms. Frank is a 24-year-old woman whose internist refers her to a psychiatrist for treatment of depression. Her medical workup was negative. She reports that she has suffered symptoms of depressed mood for "many years" but that her mood problems exacerbated 3 months ago, when she was fired from her job. Since then, she has developed severe insomnia, awakening several hours earlier than is normal for her without being able to go back to sleep. She has experienced difficulty in enjoying activities such as social gatherings and church functions, which she previously looked forward to. She experiences reduced energy, her ability to concentrate has worsened, she feels worthless, and she now has thoughts of ending her life, although she does not have a specific plan. She has never before sought treatment or a psychiatric evaluation. The psychiatrist asks her about symptoms of mania and/or hypomania, and these are ruled out.

Given this information, does Ms. Frank meet criteria for a major depressive episode? Ms. Frank does meet criteria for a major depressive episode, with both depressed mood and anhedonia, plus insomnia, diminished energy, impaired concentration, feelings of worthlessness, and suicidal ideation. This specific episode of major depressive disorder began after she lost her job 3 months ago. There is no evidence that the episode of major depressive disorder is related to bipolar disorder, and her symptoms are not attributable to other medical illness. However, the fact that she reports having had chronically depressed mood for many years before the onset of major depression causes the psychiatrist to ask questions that would establish whether the major depression might be superimposed on persistent depressive disorder.

PART B

> The psychiatrist asks more specifically how long Ms. Frank experienced depressed mood before the onset of the major depressive episode. She is able to recall that the depressed mood began when she was a junior in high school and she experienced various social difficulties, including some rejections. She reports that along with the depressed mood, she also experienced difficulty concentrating and low self-esteem, and that although these symptoms were chronic, the insomnia, anhedonia, and suicidal ideas were not present before the last 3 months.

Given the information regarding chronicity, what is the appropriate diagnosis? Ms. Frank's previous symptoms and their chronicity are consistent with persistent depressive disorder that began before age 21. Thus, Ms. Frank meets criteria for persistent depressive disorder, early onset, with intermittent major depressive episodes, with current episode.

Short-Answer Questions

1. What is the minimum duration of the symptoms to meet criteria for major depressive disorder?
2. What is the minimum duration of symptoms for adults to meet criteria for persistent depressive disorder?
3. What is the minimum duration of symptoms for children and adolescents to meet criteria for persistent depressive disorder?

4. Define early onset and late onset for persistent depressive disorder.
5. What is the fewest number of symptoms necessary for a diagnosis of persistent depressive disorder?
6. In disruptive mood dysregulation disorder, onset must be before what age in a child?
7. How frequent must temper outbursts be to meet criteria for disruptive mood dysregulation disorder?
8. How long must temper outbursts have been present to meet criteria for disruptive mood dysregulation disorder?
9. Name the four hallmark symptoms of premenstrual dysphoric disorder; that is, the four symptoms of which at least one must be present to meet criteria for the diagnosis.
10. Describe the course of key symptoms of premenstrual dysphoric disorder during the menstrual cycle.

Answers

1. The minimum duration of the symptoms is 2 weeks to meet criteria for major depressive disorder.
2. Two years is the minimum duration of symptoms for adults to meet criteria for persistent depressive disorder.
3. One year is the minimum duration of symptoms for children and adolescents to meet criteria for persistent depressive disorder.
4. In persistent depressive disorder, early onset occurs before age 21 and late onset occurs at age 21 or older.
5. At least three symptoms are necessary for a diagnosis of persistent depressive disorder.
6. Onset of disruptive mood dysregulation disorder must be before age 10 years.
7. Temper outbursts must occur an average of three or more times weekly to meet criteria for disruptive mood dysregulation disorder.
8. Temper outbursts must have been present for at least 12 months to meet criteria for disruptive mood dysregulation disorder.
9. Mood lability, irritability, dysphoria, and anxiety are the hallmark symptoms of premenstrual dysphoric disorder.
10. In premenstrual dysphoric disorder, symptoms manifest in the final week before the onset of menses, improve after the onset of menses, and are minimal or absent in the week postmenses.

8

Anxiety Disorders

Alan K. Louie, M.D.
Laura Weiss Roberts, M.D., M.A.

"I'm going to make a fool of myself."

*"My heart suddenly goes so fast that I can't breathe,
but my doctor can't find anything wrong."*

The diagnostic class of anxiety disorders relates to the human states of fear, worry, and anxiety, which are quite familiar to most, if not all, people. Certainly, these states are, at times, key to people's survival by preparing, alerting, and mobilizing them against hazardous situations. Absence of any fear would be unhealthy—similar to the absence of pain, which would allow a person to touch a flame without flinching. Nevertheless, fear, worry, and anxiety can become too great—out of proportion or unreasonable—given the actual "hazards" of an individual's life. This reaction can negatively affect the person's ability to fulfill the roles he or she has taken on, to enjoy healthy relationships, and generally to live a complete life. For instance, a mother will commonly worry about her young child getting to school safely on the school bus. This same worry may be considered excessive as the child grows older, shaping the experience of the child and preoccupying the mother. When fear, worry, or anxiety causes unnecessary suffering and/or adversely influences how the person leads his or her life, a disorder in the anxiety disorder class may apply. Some affected individuals may seek out others, counselors, or clinicians to whom they can describe their concerns and symptoms, in hopes of reassurance, commiseration, or treatment. Others, however,

137

may be too timid or embarrassed or so limited by their anxiety that they feel they cannot disclose their symptoms to anyone, and instead, suffer in silence.

The basic emotion that is most prominent in the diagnostic class of anxiety disorders is fear. Fear is often closely associated with an external entity or physical context. Most people remember having such fears as children—for instance, fear of the dark or of particular animals. The disorder of specific phobia involves fear of a specific thing or circumstance that is severe enough in the person's life to cause suffering and to have an adverse effect on how he or she conducts life—for example, by avoiding situations in which he or she might encounter the feared thing or circumstance. Other phobic disorders may focus on more abstract situations. For instance, social anxiety disorder (social phobia) results from a fear of social encounters in which a person fears that he or she will be assessed by others. Separation anxiety disorder relates to a fear of disconnection from a place to which or people to whom the person feels close. Agoraphobia relates to a fear of being out in various public places and being away from home by oneself. With these disorders, patients experience fear when exposed to the respective entity or circumstance. As noted in the DSM-5 criteria, in the context of an anxiety disorder, fear is often coupled with behaviors that allow the person to avoid the feared entity or circumstance.

Panic attacks occurring in panic disorder also involve fear—but the hallmark in these situations is having sudden bouts of fear or the physical reactions associated with fear that then become upsetting and frightening—and at least some of these bouts of fear or the physical reactions are unpredictable and seem to occur with no clear explanation. Panic disorder is quite distinct from the anxiety disorders just described, because they require an identified entity or circumstance, external to the person, to bring on the fear. If an external factor is not required in panic disorder, then what is causing the fear symptoms? Investigators continue to research this question. Some posit that the person's fear system is firing off aberrantly, like a "false alarm," due to abnormal neuronal activity. Others have suggested that internal, not external, stimuli are inducing the panic attacks. These stimuli might be physiological sensations (e.g., shortness of breath, palpitations), with or without the patient's conscious awareness, that set off fear but that are not external or readily observed by others.

In generalized anxiety disorder, the prominent symptom is worrying. DSM-5 describes worry as "apprehensive expectation." People with generalized anxiety disorder have "apprehensive expectations" that bad things are going to happen relating to several issues and areas of daily living. This kind of relentless and widespread worrying is somewhat different from what is experienced in those who feel fear in the narrower context, for example, of a phobia. Additionally, the worry is generalized to several life issues and areas and may spread to more; therefore, it is not as circumscribed in a person's life as most specific phobias.

Some DSM-IV disorders have been removed from and others added to the anxiety disorders diagnostic class in DSM-5. For instance, obsessive-compulsive disorder, posttraumatic stress disorder, and acute stress disorder have been moved from the DSM-IV anxiety disorders class into other DSM-5 diagnostic classes. This reorganization emphasizes certain unique features, such as compulsive behaviors in obsessive-compulsive disorder and the exposure to a traumatic event in posttraumatic stress disorder. Also, separation anxiety disorder and selective mutism have been moved to the DSM-5 anxiety disorders class. They were formerly placed in the DSM-IV chapter "Disorders Usually First Diagnosed in Infancy, Childhood, or Adolescence."

Some broad trends in criteria are of note. Some of the disorders—agoraphobia, generalized anxiety disorder, separation anxiety disorder, specific phobia, and social anxiety disorder—now require symptoms to occur during a period of at least 6 months to meet diagnostic criteria in adults. This duration specification excludes more transient episodes of symptoms and results in greater consistency in DSM-5 with regard to the time requirement across diagnoses in this diagnostic class.

Changes have also been made with respect to particular criteria for some diagnoses. One example is the change in criteria for panic attacks and panic disorder. Panic attacks in DSM-5 are described as either "expected" or "unexpected." The criteria for panic disorder necessitate having repeated panic attacks that are "unexpected." Disorders other than panic disorder may also manifest with panic attacks as one of their symptoms, and adding a specifier for panic attacks may signify this circumstance. Also, panic disorder and agoraphobia are now separate and independent disorders in DSM-5 that may occur individually or together.

Additional disorders in the DSM-5 anxiety disorders diagnostic class include substance/medication-induced anxiety disorder, anxiety disorder due to another medical condition, other specified anxiety disorder, and unspecified anxiety disorder.

————— IN-DEPTH DIAGNOSIS —————
Panic Attack and Panic Disorder

Ms. Brown, a 20-year-old female soldier, presents to a military hospital complaining of "feeling like my heart is pounding" and "feeling out of breath." She is trembling and extremely scared about what is wrong with her body. She remarks that she has never had any "nervous problems." The doctor runs several tests and then tells her that she is medically fine. Ms. Brown has recently been deployed and has been away from her hometown. She has not yet been in combat, and she has not been exposed to any traumatic experiences. The symptoms came upon her rather quickly, and to her surprise, while on duty. She remarks that she cannot understand how this could be happening to her because she is in excellent shape, having just finished boot camp. She has not had problems with anxiety before and generally has not thought of herself as an excessively anxious person. She does not use alcohol or other substances or take substances/medications that may cause anxiety. She denies having homicidal and/or suicidal ideation, intent, and/or plans.

Young adults with panic attacks may present to emergency facilities with concerns that they are suffering from an acute medical problem. This interpretation of acute and extreme anxiety as a physical health complaint is a familiar presentation of panic attacks in an otherwise healthy person. Nevertheless, medical illness must be ruled out. If medical illnesses are excluded and the person meets the criteria for panic attacks, psychiatric diagnoses should be considered that are associated with panic attacks. One such condition, as expected, is panic disorder, but other diagnoses should also be considered. If Ms. Brown is later diagnosed with panic disorder, this first pre-

sentation would be consistent with this diagnosis, in that the first onset of panic attacks occurred in her early 20s and the symptoms are unpredicted. Being female
increases her risk of the diagnosis. If she has panic disorder, her reaction to and acceptance of this diagnosis in the context of the military culture should be discussed. Referral to psychiatry should be considered.

Approach to the Diagnosis

Many patients report anxiety symptoms, and some will even say they experience
"panic attacks." Encouraging uniformity, DSM-5 purposely provides criteria for use
of the term *panic attack,* defining it as symptoms that increase in minutes from low levels to a crescendo at a very high level, like a surprise attack. Purported "attacks" that
gradually build over hours (e.g., "I worked myself into a panic attack throughout the
day thinking about the evening date") do not meet the panic attack requirement for
either a sudden onset or quick crescendo. The panic attacks must manifest four or
more symptoms from a list that includes ones that are somatic (e.g., sweating) and
others that are mainly psychological (e.g., fear of dying). Some patients may have
fewer than four symptoms during attacks. These attacks, called *limited-symptom attacks* in DSM-5, may be attenuated panic attacks or progenitors and will perhaps subsequently become part of a panic disorder. DSM-5 also describes nocturnal panic
attacks that occur related to sleeping.

Bear in mind that the terms *panic attack* and *panic disorder* are not synonymous.
Panic attacks are the key symptom in panic disorder, and panic disorder requires the
presence of panic attacks. However, not everyone with panic attacks has panic disorder. The criteria for panic attacks and panic disorder are different. In DSM-5, panic attack is not a disorder but is instead a specifier that may be added to DSM-5 disorders
when panic attacks are noted in the context of a disorder. Thus, this specifier may be
added to a variety of psychiatric or general medical disorders.

DSM-5 states that at least some of the panic attacks in panic disorder must be "recurrent and unexpected." "Unexpected" refers to panic attacks that do not seem to be
produced or generated by any stimuli and thus occur without warning. Patients experiencing "unexpected" panic attacks in panic disorder often describe their attacks
as completely coming from "out of nowhere." Such spontaneous attacks have encouraged some researchers to look for an endogenous cause of the attack, including an endogenous chemical circulating in the body.

Determining whether "unexpected" panic attacks are present may be subject to
some interpretation, because every patient (and culture) has different views on the
causality of behaviors. For example, DSM-5 notes that when asked in retrospect, older
adults may be more prone than younger individuals to attribute anxiety symptoms
to various events in the environment; this may result in less reporting of "unexpected" panic attacks.

Evaluation for the panic disorder diagnosis additionally requires ascertaining if
trepidation about panic attacks and behaviors to avoid panic attacks have developed.
These are two different manifestations of panic disorder and should be seen as distinct symptoms from panic attacks.

Also of note, as stated in DSM-5, "Panic attacks and a diagnosis of panic disorder in the past 12 months are related to a higher rate of suicide attempts and suicidal ideation in the past 12 months even when comorbidity and a history of childhood abuse and other suicide risk factors are taken into account" (p. 212).

Getting the History

A 27-year-old patient reports having problems with "anxiety." The interviewer determines whether the patient has "attacks" of anxiety "that come from nowhere" and that include four of the symptoms listed in the criteria for panic attacks. The exact mix of symptoms may vary, but the patient should have at least four of the symptoms during any given attack.

The interviewer asks, "How long was the time between the start of the anxiety symptoms to their highest level? Were the anxiety symptoms set off by something, or did they seem to come spontaneously?" The patient may respond that the time was within about a few minutes. The interviewer then asks, "Do you remember the very first attack?" and then asks the patient to describe it and the context. The interviewer also asks for an estimate of the frequency and pattern of attacks since they started.

The interviewer then asks, "When you are not having a panic attack, do you have any other symptoms?" The interviewer wants to know if the patient notes anxiety about having another attack. This would be a different type of anxiety than the panic attack symptoms. The interviewer asks, "How do these symptoms affect your daily activities? Are you not doing certain things because of the symptoms?" The interviewer wants to know if the patient is not going to certain public places. The interviewer asks about the patient having homicidal and/or suicidal thoughts, intent, and/or plans; alcohol and other substance use; taking of substances/medications that may cause anxiety; and signs and symptoms of medical disorders.

The patient describes symptoms that may meet criteria for panic attacks; the patient apparently has had several attacks and some have been without warning. They are extreme, sudden in onset, and hit the highest point in minutes. The interviewer ascertains if the patient has begun to frequently have concern about when the next panic attack will strike or what will happen to the patient during an attack. The interviewer also wants to know if the patient is avoiding going places due to the panic attacks. The interviewer will want to find out how long these types of symptoms have been present subsequent to a panic attack. A medical workup, alcohol and other substance use histories, and histories relevant to suicide and homicide should be obtained. Referral to psychiatry should be considered.

Tips for Clarifying the Diagnosis

- Ask the individual who reports being "anxious" or "nervous" to describe the exact experience, including physical sensations, thoughts, feelings, and behaviors.
- Clarify the time course of the symptoms: How quickly do they start, crescendo, and then tail off?
- Question how often panic attacks occur.
- Investigate whether any of the panic attacks occur without warning or cause.
- Evaluate whether the individual has other types of anxiety, such as trepidation about having another panic attack.
- Determine whether any behaviors (e.g., not going to places) have developed to avoid panic attacks. If so, ask how long these behaviors have been occurring.

Consider the Case

Mr. Young, a 35-year-old Native American man, presents to a primary care physician in the Indian Health Service. He has had panic disorder for many years, starting in his early 20s. He sometimes has one or more panic attacks each day. The longest he has gone without panic attacks is a few months. Panic disorder has greatly affected his quality of life, and he has not been able to work or to participate in the Navajo ceremonies and dances that have been an important part of his life and role in the tribe. He has started to be concerned about when the next panic attack will strike and has stopped spending time at some public places. The places in which he feels comfortable have become progressively limited. For the past few years, he has had trouble leaving his tribal land, and now his home has become the only truly comfortable place. Recently, he has even had some panic attacks in this home. His symptoms cause him to experience low self-esteem. For the last couple of years, he has felt "depressed." His primary care physician says he is medically healthy. He denies use of substances other than alcohol or taking substances/medications that may cause anxiety. He is unclear about his alcohol use. He denies having homicidal and/or suicidal ideation, intent, and/or plans.

Beginning in early adulthood, panic disorder can be a chronic disorder that adversely affects people during what should be their most productive years. It may remit, but it often recurs. In addition to having the panic attacks, Mr. Young began to be anxious about when the next panic attack would occur. He also found that he was not going to many places because of panic attacks, and eventually he had trouble going anywhere outside his home. A comorbid major depressive disorder may now be complicating his condition. The clinician should explore Mr. Young's alcohol use further, consider the possible diagnosis of alcoholism, and continue to check regularly if Mr. Young is having homicidal and/or suicidal ideation, intent, and/or plans. Some people use alcohol to ease their panic attacks. The risk for alcoholism and suicide are of note in this case. The clinician will want to understand how Mr. Young's symptoms are viewed and managed within the dynamics of his Native American family. Referral to psychiatry should be considered.

Differential Diagnosis

The differential diagnosis of panic disorder is quite broad because the hallmark of panic disorder is having panic attacks, which may occur in the context of many other disorders. Possible diagnoses may be divided into nonpsychiatric and psychiatric disorders. The former include several general medical disorders (e.g., cardiac arrhythmias, asthma), which necessitate appropriate medical workup. Panic attacks may also be seen in many psychiatric disorders, such as other anxiety disorders. If the panic attacks occur only in relation to symptoms of another anxiety disorder, then the other anxiety disorder is given diagnostic priority. For instance, if panic attacks happen solely in social circumstances that induce fear due to social anxiety disorder, then the diagnosis of social anxiety disorder takes priority; panic attacks might be used as a specifier, and the diagnosis of panic disorder would not be recorded. In other words, these are expected panic attacks in social circumstances in a patient with social anxiety disorder.

In cases of comorbid panic disorder and another disorder that may be associated with panic attacks, the clinician would look for evidence of at least some panic attacks that are not restricted to the context of the other disorder, that are unexpected, and that are attributable solely to the panic disorder. This pattern is important because panic disorder is highly comorbid with several disorders, such as other anxiety disorders, major depressive disorder, and bipolar disorder.

As noted in DSM-5, agoraphobia may develop after panic attacks and panic disorder, as described by 30% of people with agoraphobia in community samples and at least 50% of those in clinical samples. Conversely, panic disorder may appear to follow agoraphobia in other cases. Agoraphobia is usually a long-lasting and debilitating condition.

See DSM-5 for additional disorders to consider in the differential diagnosis. Also refer to the discussions of comorbidity and differential diagnosis in their respective sections of DSM-5.

Summary

- When clinically significant anxiety symptoms are present, the clinician should determine whether the symptoms meet criteria for panic attacks and with which disorders these panic attacks might be associated.
- If panic attacks are present and some occur repeatedly and without warning, then the clinician should evaluate for panic disorder, including the patient's trepidation about subsequent panic attacks and behaviors to avoid panic attacks.
- A careful history going back to the first anxiety symptoms should be taken to assess the frequency and natural course of the symptoms.
- The differential diagnosis of panic disorder includes the careful ruling out of a wide range of psychiatric disorders (including other anxiety disorders and substance use disorders) and general medical conditions.

IN-DEPTH DIAGNOSIS

Social Anxiety Disorder (Social Phobia)

James, a 14-year-old Hispanic male, is seen for an outpatient evaluation at a pediatric clinic in the southeastern United States. He has consistently been very anxious when interacting with others. His parents encourage him to "hang out" with kids in their neighborhood, but he cannot make himself do this. Every social circumstance feels overwhelming to him, even if his parents are with him. During the evaluation, he does not have any problems with speaking. He wants to participate in high school activities and to go out with friends, but he has not pursued any of these activities for fear that he will make a fool of himself and become embarrassed. He says that he thinks he will not be seen as "macho"—he wants to be "machismo"— but thinks he will be teased for being "nervous" instead. He says he cannot be "in public." He mainly stays at home, surfs the Internet, and does his homework. He aspires to go to a professional school of some sort, but recently he has begun to worry about whether he can even finish high school because of his nervousness. He denies any physical symptoms, and his recent medical workup was normal. He does not use alcohol or other substances and does not take substances/medications that may cause anxiety. He denies having homicidal and/or suicidal ideation, intent, and/or plans.

James has always been an anxious child in social circumstances, including those with other children. Apparently, he experienced this anxiety even if his parents were present, and thus it did not seem related to separation anxiety. He never had a childhood period of not speaking in social situations and thus did not have selective mutism. Now in high school, he is finding that his life is greatly limited by his social anxiety, and he and his parents have finally sought professional help. As an adolescent, he is able to describe his major concern, which is that he will make a fool of himself in front of other adolescents, who will then reject him. The clinician might explore how his desire to be "macho" plays a role in his social anxiety and whether there is any cultural basis for it. Referral to psychiatry should be considered.

Approach to the Diagnosis

Individuals with social anxiety disorder fear assessment and disapproval by others. They fear that they will in some way appear foolish and feel shame. This fear may include concern that people will see overt signs of their social anxiety disorder, like blushing, which may serve as a tip-off symptom of this disorder. A diagnosis of social anxiety disorder involves fear that is disproportionate to the real risk of embarrassment.

People with social anxiety disorder avoid social circumstances that may be potentially embarrassing. This pattern of avoidance may result in an inability to function in social roles, such as unwillingness to go to job interviews, doctor's appointments, or family gatherings. This disorder often starts before adulthood; initial onset in adulthood is uncommon. Children may become tearful or upset when faced with going to school. When forced to attend social activities, the individual may fret in advance and report significant suffering during the activity. During the event, he or she may act bashful and reserved and hardly speak. The effects of avoiding social situations may be evidenced by difficulty with working, dating, or getting married. For these reasons, social anxiety disorder may become extremely disabling.

Getting the History

During a routine physical examination, a 20-year-old patient reports rarely leaving the house, and the primary care physician gently asks, "Why don't you leave your house?" The physician checks whether the patient fears going places or being away from home or having a panic attack in public. If the patient fears interactions with people but does not say why, the physician pursues the issue further by asking, "Are you afraid someone will hurt you?" And follows with, "Are you afraid you will embarrass yourself?" The patient quietly nods several times with shame but does not voluntarily elaborate. After a pause, the physician asks, "Are you afraid of doing things in front of other people like saying the wrong things or doing something wrong?" The physician explores if any of these fears seem delusional or if they just suggest a concern that others will be critical of the patient in social contexts.

The physician also tries to ascertain if the patient has a major depressive disorder, autism spectrum disorder, or other disorders. Further, the physician asks, "Would you have interest in leaving the house and in socializing if it weren't for these anxiety symptoms?" The physician determines how long the patient has had the symptoms and whether they have lasted longer than 6 months. The physician checks for whether the patient has homicidal and/or suicidal ideation, intent, and/or plans; criteria for alcohol and other substance use disorders; taking of substances/medications that may cause anxiety; and signs and symptoms of medical disorders.

Next, the physician carefully explores why the patient is reluctant to leave the house, bearing in mind that social anxiety may make talking about this hard for a patient (e.g., fearing the physician's disapproval). The physician tries to rule out some other psychiatric conditions that may be responsible for the symptoms, such as agoraphobia. The physician also wants to exclude the possibility that the patient stays at home because of a lack of interest in seeing other people.

The physician questions the patient about duration to determine if it meets the time criterion. If an adult patient says that the symptoms began 6 months ago, this duration would meet the criterion, but would indicate first onset in adulthood. Adult onset is unusual and would put the diagnosis of social anxiety disorder in some question. The criteria, however, are only guidelines and must always be applied in the context of good clinical common sense and judgment. Of note, the physician checks for whether the patient has homicidal and/or suicidal risk. Referral to psychiatry should be considered.

Tips for Clarifying the Diagnosis

- Establish whether the person has relatively predictable anxiety symptoms in social circumstances in which others may assess him or her and be disapproving.
- In children, determine whether the symptoms are evident in social circumstances with other children.
- Determine how long these symptoms have been occurring. (Six months is required.)
- When social anxiety only occurs in public speaking or performance circumstances, the DSM-5 "performance only" specifier may apply.

Consider the Case

Mr. Andrews is a 52-year-old single black man who seeks evaluation by a psychiatrist through a telemedicine program in the rural southern United States. His internist set up this evaluation to help with the patient's anxiety, which prevents him from going out socially. Talking over a telemedicine connection, he recollects the gradual development of relatively consistent anxiety in social circumstances—he is not sure when it began exactly. In high school, he was too anxious to socialize with everyone else. He was able to finish high school but had to keep to himself because he feared that others would laugh at him for doing or saying something wrong. He has always wanted to have friends and to be social. Now, he would like to start going out with coworkers after work but is afraid that he will make a fool of himself in various possible ways. He is only able to decrease his anxiety when interacting with people by drinking alcohol. Recently, he has been unsuccessful in trying to stop drinking several times. His internist says he is medically healthy. He does not use substances other than alcohol or take substances/medications that may cause anxiety. He denies having homicidal and/or suicidal ideation, intent, and/or plans. He has been reluctant to go to a mental health clinic because of the stigma of mental illness in his culture and the possibility that a mental health clinician will diagnosis him as "crazy."

Mr. Andrews began to have difficulties with anxiety early in life. His social anxiety had a gradual onset, as in many cases; in contrast, some people will report a precipitating event, which usually relates to embarrassment. He appears to have suffered chronic symptoms of social anxiety disorder ever since his youth, and these symptoms are still limiting his lifestyle. He very much wishes to have friends, so he is finding that the anxiety clearly is causing problems in his life. In social circumstances, he says that he intentionally drinks alcohol to lessen his social anxiety. He is having trouble stopping his drinking and needs to be assessed for alcoholism; consultation with an addiction psychiatrist should be considered. Some patients may appear to use alcohol and/or other substances to manage their social anxiety disorder. The clinician should explore whether the use of a telemedicine connection helps or hinders the interview for this socially anxious patient. The issue of stigma and the influences of rural culture and racial/ethnic identity need to be addressed.

Differential Diagnosis

DSM-5 includes many disorders in the section on differential diagnosis of social anxiety disorder. Several disorders manifest with anxiety symptoms in social circumstances. Social anxiety disorder may be parsed out by determining whether fear about potential assessment and disapproval is the primary reason for these symptoms. If present, the fear of disapproval requires examination. Such a fear may be part of normative bashfulness, often without clear impact on functioning. Concern with disapproval may indicate poor self-esteem and a major depressive disorder; in such cases, other symptoms of depression should also be present. The social anxiety disorder diagnosis is most clear when extreme fear of social assessment is central and perhaps the only symptom, occurring when exposed to potential assessment.

Many patients do experience social anxiety disorder along with other disorders. In some instances, these co-occurring disorders (e.g., major depressive disorder, substance use disorder) appear after the onset of social anxiety disorder. The relationship between avoidant personality disorder and social anxiety disorder is more complicated because of their common symptomatology.

See DSM-5 for additional disorders to consider in the differential diagnosis. Also refer to the discussions of comorbidity and differential diagnosis in their respective sections of DSM-5.

Summary

- Individuals with social anxiety disorder fear assessment and disapproval in social situations.
- Social anxiety disorder often starts before adulthood; initial onset in adulthood is uncommon.
- Social anxiety disorder can result in significant dysfunction.
- Social anxiety disorder must be differentiated from several psychiatric disorders that have an impact on socialization. Additionally, it must be separated from normative bashfulness and avoidant personality disorder.
- Social anxiety disorder may be comorbid with a number of other disorders.

IN-DEPTH DIAGNOSIS
Generalized Anxiety Disorder

Ms. Armstrong, a 35-year-old woman, is being seen in a medical clinic on a military base in the southern United States. Her husband is an active-duty serviceman. She tells her primary care physician about muscle aches and tension that inhibit her from doing many activities. Later, she also admits to worrying "day and night." She has been this way since adolescence and had assumed that everyone felt this way until her friends began to point out that she is a "worrier." She worries about anything that comes up in her daily life, and as soon as one thing turns out okay, she will move on to worry about something else. She denies symptoms of other types of anxiety disorders. She does not take substances/medications that may cause anxiety and does not use alcohol or other substances. She denies having homicidal and/or suicidal ideation, intent, and/or plans. A complete medical workup was normal, and the symptoms do not appear to be caused by a medical condition or a side effect of a medication.

After determining that she has no medical issues to produce her muscle aches and tension, the primary care physician explores whether these physical symptoms might be associated with an anxiety disorder. This line of questioning leads the patient to reveal that she has been a "lifelong worrier" and that her friends notice that she is always worrying. It is a way of life for her. Worry is ever present, associated with one life task after another, and wears her down with muscle tension and always being vigilant for peril. Further psychiatric evaluation should investigate whether she meets the full criteria for generalized anxiety disorder. The presence of a comorbid major depressive disorder should be considered. The influences of both southern and military family cultures on the perception of symptoms in this case should be explored. Referral to psychiatry should be considered.

Approach to the Diagnosis

Comparing the DSM-5 criteria for generalized anxiety disorder with that of the other anxiety disorders, readers will note an emphasis on symptoms of excessive worry, rather than fear. Worry is described in DSM-5 as "apprehensive expectation." Worrying has a pervasive nature that lingers and is always in the back of the person's mind. These qualities of the constant "worrier" are key to this diagnosis.

Getting the History

A 50-year-old patient seeing a psychotherapist complains of "nervousness." The therapist says, "People sometimes mean different things when they use that term. Tell me more about what you are experiencing." The patient with generalized anxiety disorder frequently describes varying degrees of worrying. The therapists asks, "Please give me a specific example of something you were worried about—for instance, what did you worry about this morning?" The patient might describe various everyday concerns in different areas of living that the patient magnifies in terms of the risk of adverse outcomes. The therapist asks more questions to rule out that the worrying is not focused on panic attacks; social anxiety; an obsession; separation from someone close to the patient; body image or weight; physical complaints, illness, or abnormalities; a past trauma; or other causes. The therapist needs to determine if this worry is to a delusional extent or related to other disorders, such as a mood disorder. The therapist additionally queries, "How does this worrying impact your life? Does it cause you to live in a certain way?" The patient denies having homicidal and/or suicidal ideation, intent, and/or plans. The patient does not use alcohol or other substances and does not take substances/medications that may cause anxiety. No medical problems were found by the patient's internist.

The therapist immediately establishes that the patient needs to be more specific in reporting symptoms and does not assume knowledge of what the patient means by the term *nervousness*. The therapist uses open-ended questions about the patient's experience of symptoms and then more focused ones asking for specific examples of symptoms that happened, for instance, earlier that day. Asking for specific examples of worries helps determine if they meet criteria. The therapist methodically rules out other anxiety disorders, mood disorders, psychotic disorders, and other disorders (e.g., substance/medication-induced anxiety disorder, anxiety disorder due to another medical condition) that may be the actual diagnosis. The therapist also checks whether the patient is having homicidal and/or suicidal ideation, intent, and/or plans. Finally, the therapist uses a very open-ended and nonjudgmental question to find out how the patient's life is affected and to subsequently explore for abnormal behaviors associated with the patient's trepidation. Referral to a psychiatrist should be considered.

Tips for Clarifying the Diagnosis

- Ask whether the person experiences pervasive worrying that is hard for him or her to manage.
- Find out whether the worrying involves several issues and areas of life.
- Question how long and how often the person worries.

Consider the Case

Robert, an 11-year-old boy, has been "super" nervous, so his parents made an appointment with his pediatrician. He tells the pediatrician that he feels "tense" and restless all the time. He is a terrific student, but he worries about day-to-day schoolwork, club activities, and athletic contests. He finds that he cannot stop worrying. As his pediatrician takes more history, he learns that Robert has also been quite sad and may be experiencing a major depressive episode. Robert denies having homicidal and/or suicidal ideation, intent, and/or plans. He denies use of alcohol or other substances and does not take substances/medications that may cause anxiety. A careful workup does not provide a medical diagnosis to explain the symptoms.

Although Robert possibly has generalized anxiety disorder, the diagnosis is not clear. The symptoms are relatively nonspecific, and as noted in DSM-5, the clinician must be careful about making this diagnosis too readily in children. Robert describes a number of the symptoms that may relate to generalized anxiety disorder, including feeling tense and restless and worrying about day-to-day stresses. Nevertheless, the clinician needs to be sure that these symptoms are not better explained by other conditions that may manifest with anxiety (e.g., obsessive-compulsive disorder). Robert may also be suffering from a major depressive episode, which further complicates the diagnostic picture. His anxiety symptoms may all be due to the major depressive disorder. The diagnosis of generalized anxiety disorder is not made if the anxiety symptoms occur only in the presence of a major depression—if this is the case, then the anxiety symptoms are considered part of the depressive disorder and an additional diagnosis of generalized anxiety disorder is not recorded. The generalized anxiety disorder diagnosis may be considered if there has been a time when the anxiety symptoms were present and a major depression was not. The patient is referred to psychiatry for careful evaluation and diagnosis.

Differential Diagnosis

Many disorders include symptoms of worrying. Patients with major depressive disorder, bipolar disorder, and psychotic disorders frequently experience some anxiety and worry. When the worrying is present only during episodes of these disorders, then an additional diagnosis of generalized anxiety disorder should not be made. Worrying not only is frequent in other disorders but also is a normal state from time to time for most people. Thus, generalized anxiety disorder is more likely in individuals who demonstrate more general worrying in isolation from other disorders and whose worrying is more extreme, extensive, and chronic than "normal" worry.

Generalized anxiety disorder is quite often comorbid with other disorders, such as mood disorders. To ensure the relative separateness of generalized anxiety disorder and another disorder, symptoms of generalized anxiety disorder should be seen during some periods when the other disorder is not present.

See DSM-5 for additional disorders to consider in the differential diagnosis. Also refer to the discussions of comorbidity and differential diagnosis in their respective sections of DSM-5.

Summary

- In generalized anxiety disorder, the symptoms picture emphasizes worrying of a pervasive nature about multiple issues and areas of daily life.
- Worrying is associated with certain specified symptoms (see DSM-5 criteria for generalized anxiety disorder).
- Commonly, the symptoms are chronic and not acute.
- Worrying is so frequent in both normal and pathological states that the diagnosis of generalized anxiety disorder should not be made unless its symptoms clearly depart from normal levels and cause dysfunction.
- Generalized anxiety disorder is often comorbid with mood disorders.

SUMMARY

Anxiety Disorders

Anxiety is ubiquitous—at times the experience of anxiety is expected and adaptive, and at other times the experience of anxiety can be pathological. The diagnostic class of anxiety disorders includes disorders with fear, panic attacks, worry, and/or anxiety, and may include behaviors to avoid these states. This grouping suggests some commonality across these disorders, which in DSM-5 are considered distinct from obsessive-compulsive disorder and posttraumatic stress disorder. Despite these commonalities among the disorders in this diagnostic class, they are certainly heterogeneous, for example with regard to age at onset. Some disorders in this class are relatively common, and all can cause significant suffering and impact on the person's life, along with an increased risk of suicide attempt and ideation in some.

Diagnostic Pearls

- The anxiety disorders diagnostic class includes disorders with prominent symptoms of fear, panic attacks, worry, and/or anxiety. In DSM-5, some disorders with similar symptoms (e.g., obsessive-compulsive disorder, posttraumatic stress disorder) are seen as diagnostically separate from this class and have been put in other classes.

- In separation anxiety disorder, specific phobia, social anxiety disorder, and agoraphobia, different entities or circumstances external to the individual bring on symptoms of fear and/or anxiety.

- In panic disorder, bouts of fear (panic attacks) occur repeatedly and unpredictably (without clear external cause).

- In many of these disorders, individuals frequently develop behaviors to avoid entities or circumstances that they associate with anxiety symptoms (e.g., staying away from social occasions).

- In generalized anxiety disorder, a core symptom is worrying, described in DSM-5 as "apprehensive expectation," about several issues and areas of daily living.

- Among anxiety disorders, separation anxiety disorder is the most common one in people under age 12 years.

- In selective mutism, the person does not speak in certain social circumstances, even though his or her speech is quite normal otherwise, for instance at home with family members.

- A necessary consideration is whether the symptoms of anxiety disorders may be caused by substances/medications or be due to another medical condition; each possibility has its own diagnostic code in DSM-5.

Self-Assessment

Key Concepts: Double-Check Your Knowledge

What is the relevance of the following concepts to the various anxiety disorders?

- Agoraphobic situations
- Avoidance behaviors
- Excessive worry
- Performance only
- Phobic objects and situations
- Public scrutiny and negative evaluation
- Recurrent and unexpected panic attacks
- Restlessness and muscle tension
- Selective mutism
- Worries about panic attacks

Questions to Discuss With Colleagues and Mentors

1. Do you screen all new patients for anxiety disorders, and if so, what questions do you use to screen for each disorder? For example, how do you screen for panic attacks?
2. If a patient has symptoms of fear or worry, what laboratory tests and medical workup do you pursue?
3. What are your typical reactions (e.g., feeling anxious yourself, becoming impatient, wanting to comfort) when you are with anxious people, and how do you manage your reaction in the therapeutic setting?

Case-Based Questions

PART A

> Ms. Butler, a 36-year-old woman, describes having had anxiety problems for over 10 years that have progressively worsened, and for which she has never received treatment. She is so "nervous" that she does not go out of her house. She has meals delivered to her and cannot visit her doctor. She has never been able to work. Her family doctor makes a home visit to her in a rural area of the Pacific Northwest. She tells him, "I worry all the time, and I have anxiety that lasts all day long." Her current medical workup is normal. She denies using alcohol or any other substances or taking any substances/medications that may cause anxiety. She denies having homicidal and/or suicidal ideation, intent, and/or plans. Her family doctor has asked her to see a psychiatrist.

Assuming she has one or more anxiety disorder(s), what are reasons why she does not leave the house?   With the limited history obtained at this point, the clinician might think of a variety of reasons for her not leaving the house, including having agoraphobia, being afraid of having panic attacks away from home, or fearing social anxiety if she encounters people.

PART B

Ms. Butler says she does not leave the house because she fears having a panic attack outside the house when she is by herself. Further discussion reveals that she meets DSM-5 criteria for panic disorder. Even at home, she worries all the time.

How do you ascertain if she has generalized anxiety disorder in addition to panic disorder? In generalized anxiety disorder, the concerns should not be about having another panic attack. She should have anxiety about issues and areas in daily life and have symptoms of generalized anxiety disorder during times that she does not have panic disorder symptoms.

Short-Answer Questions

1. In adults, at least how long must the duration be for a diagnosis of specific phobia, social anxiety disorder, generalized anxiety disorder, agoraphobia, and separation anxiety disorder?
2. Rank order from youngest to oldest the age at onset for panic disorder, specific phobia, and social anxiety disorder.
3. What are two characteristics required of at least some of the panic attacks in panic disorder?
4. During a panic attack, what is the typical length of time from the onset of symptoms to the maximum level of symptoms?
5. Why do social situations make patients with social anxiety disorder anxious?
6. Worrying is the cardinal feature of which of the following disorders: agoraphobia, generalized anxiety disorder, panic disorder, or social anxiety disorder?
7. In both separation anxiety disorder and agoraphobia, individuals may fear being alone. Contrast the reasons for not wanting to be alone in these two disorders.
8. List a substance that may be associated with substance-induced anxiety disorder, either during intoxication or withdrawal.
9. What is the relationship between panic disorder and suicide attempts and suicidal ideation?
10. May patients with social anxiety disorder have other DSM-5 disorders at the same time?

Answers

1. The duration must be 6 months in adults for these diagnoses.
2. The rank order for age at onset is as follows: specific phobia (7–11 years median)<social anxiety disorder (13 years median)<panic disorder (20–24 years median).
3. Panic attacks required in panic disorder are repeated and unpredicted.
4. Symptoms of a panic attack peak usually within a few minutes.
5. People with social anxiety disorder fear possible assessment and disapproval by others.
6. Worrying is a key feature of generalized anxiety disorder.
7. Individuals with separation anxiety disorder fear being disconnected from a person to whom they are close, whereas people with agoraphobia fear being where they will not be able to flee or get help.
8. The following are examples of substances that may be associated with substance-induced anxiety disorder: intoxication from alcohol, cocaine, caffeine, cannabis, hallucinogens, inhalants, and phencyclidine; or withdrawal from alcohol, opioids, cocaine, and sedatives, hypnotics, or anxiolytics.
9. A diagnosis of panic disorder is related to a greater risk of suicide attempts and suicidal ideation.
10. Yes. Not uncommonly, patients with social anxiety disorder may also meet criteria for other DSM-5 disorders, such as substance use disorders and major depressive disorder.

Obsessive-Compulsive and Related Disorders

Elias Aboujaoude, M.D., M.A.

Robert M. Holaway, Ph.D.

"I know I shouldn't but I can't stop pulling out my eyebrows."

*"His hands are raw because he washes his hands
so many times during the day."*

By introducing obsessive-compulsive and related disorders as a separate diagnostic class in DSM-5, the new nosology emphasizes repetitive thoughts and/or behaviors as an important symptom dimension that is shared across several psychiatric disorders. The list of conditions in which this dimension can feature prominently is long and would include obsessive-compulsive disorder (OCD), body dysmorphic disorder, Tourette's disorder, obsessive-compulsive personality disorder, substance use disorders, neurocognitive disorders with repetitive movements, and the DSM-IV categories of impulse control disorders not elsewhere classified (trichotillomania [hair-pulling disorder], pathological gambling, kleptomania, pyromania, intermittent explosive disorder), hypochondriasis, pervasive developmental disorders, and some sexual disorders. However, grouping such disparate conditions within the same diagnostic class would defeat the goal of increasing the clinical utility and diagnostic validity of DSM. Therefore, disorders within this class had to share, in addition to repetitive thoughts and/or behaviors, other important features, including common pathophysiology and etiology (to the extent those are understood), high comorbidity, high prevalence in first-degree relatives, and certain characteristics of assessment and treatment. This requirement resulted in the winnowing down of the DSM-5 obsessive-compulsive and related disorders class to a more practical listing that includes OCD (the organizing "anchor" and the condition that has received the most research attention), body dysmorphic disorder, hoarding disorder, trichotillomania (hair-pulling disorder), and excoriation (skin-picking) disorder. Several other diagnostic entries within the class cover presentations attributable to substance use (substance/medication-induced obsessive-compulsive and related disorder), medical etiologies (obsessive-compulsive and related disorder due to another medical condition), and atypical manifestations (other specified or unspecified obsessive-compulsive and related disorder).

Compared with DSM-IV, the obsessive-compulsive and related disorders diagnostic class in DSM-5 includes new disorders (e.g., hoarding disorder, excoriation disorder), as well as previously defined disorders that have been relocated from other sections of the manual (e.g., trichotillomania from the DSM-IV impulse-control disorders section, body dysmorphic disorder from the DSM-IV somatoform disorders section). In the case of trichotillomania, the diagnosis no longer requires "noticeable hair loss," because patients can be selective in where they pull from or can disguise missing hair. In addition, the DSM-IV criterion that hair pulling must result in pleasure has been removed.

Body dysmorphic disorder now includes a diagnostic criterion for repetitive behaviors (e.g., skin picking, hair pulling, reassurance seeking) or mental acts (e.g., social comparison) that may occur along with a preoccupation with a perceived defect in appearance and function as an attempt to correct the perceived flaw or reduce psychological distress.

A change to the diagnostic criteria that is relevant to the diagnosis of OCD, body dysmorphic disorder, and hoarding disorder is an insight specifier that ranges from "good or fair," to "poor," to "absent/delusional," allowing for greater distinction according to insight. Hoarding disorder has an additional specifier, "with excessive acquisition," to indicate when difficulty discarding possessions is accompanied by excessive collecting of unneeded items. Another new specifier that can be added to a diagnosis of OCD is "tic related," a symptom that is significant due to its implications for treatment. In addition, body dysmorphic disorder now has a "with muscle dysmorphia" specifier to designate individuals with body dysmorphic disorder who have a pathological preoccupation with muscularity.

As with any disorder, a thorough clinical assessment is crucial to effective treatment and requires a review of the various elements of the case history, including the chief complaint, history of present illness, stressors and precipitants, medical and psychiatric histories and comorbidities, current and past medications, developmental and social backgrounds, family history, review of systems, mental status examination, and distress caused by the presenting symptom—personally, academically, and professionally.

In assessing an individual with suspected OCD, specifically, it is important to recognize that although the symptoms can be highly unique and variable, they typically fall under a limited number of general themes. The most common obsessional themes include contamination fears, pathological doubt, somatic concerns, symmetry worries, and disturbing thoughts, images, or impulses of an aggressive, sexual, or religious nature. Similarly, the most common compulsive themes include checking, cleaning, counting, reassurance seeking, repeating, and mental rituals. The "Approach to the Diagnosis" section in the main discussion of OCD provides more details and specific examples.

Other obsessive-compulsive and related disorders warrant specifically tailored questions. In an individual with suspected hoarding disorder, for example, the clinician should investigate the meaning of the person's collections, the function they might fulfill, their impact on the safety and "health" of the living space, and the balance of input into and output from that space. In an individual with suspected body dysmorphic disorder, excoriation disorder, or trichotillomania, the clinician should explore whether cosmetic surgery, extreme self-grooming, and dermatological interventions are misunderstood and overvalued as shortcuts to "perfection." Inquiry into deeper self-esteem deficits that may be manifesting with a somatic fixation is also important.

While assessing for possible obsessive-compulsive and related disorders, the clinician needs to consider questions about the sociocultural context within which the problem is occurring. For example, in a religious individual who spends many hours daily in prayer, when do religious thoughts become an intrusive "symptom" and when does ritualized praying become a mental compulsion? In a superstitious individual who was raised in a superstitious culture, when does rigid avoidance of certain anxiety-producing stimuli become a treatable OCD symptom and when should it be viewed as part of that individual's cultural norm? In the person whose family survived famine and war, when does the accumulation of food and other necessities become a hoarding compulsion worthy of urgent clinical attention and when is it a self-protective and justifiable reaction to a history of loss and deprivation? Finally, given the culture's obsession with body image and saturation with body-enhancing interventions, when do individuals with heightened appearance anxiety or excessive grooming behaviors cross the threshold into pathological body dysmorphic disorder, trichotillomania, or excoriation disorder? A careful examination of the larger sociocultural space within which the repetitive thoughts or behaviors are arising, as well as attention to any associated negative consequences, helps answer these questions.

IN-DEPTH DIAGNOSIS

Obsessive-Compulsive Disorder

Ms. Hansen is a 35-year-old single woman who works as a university librarian. She presents to her first psychotherapy visit for help with intrusive thoughts focused on a form of contamination fear that she has struggled with since her early 20s. Back then, for no apparent reason, Ms. Hansen began worrying that the water supply in the house she shared with her three college roommates became contaminated by the sewer system. As a result, she started having trouble drinking the water at her house and started avoiding using the bathroom for fear she might worsen the problem and contaminate her housemates' potable water. Since then, this concern has forced Ms. Hansen to relocate numerous times, but each move would only give her a brief respite before her fears recurred, typically a few months after each move, causing significant anxiety and prompting yet another relocation. Over the years, Ms. Hansen has sought reassurance through numerous expensive consultations and inspections with plumbers, architects, and general contractors, as well as several laboratory tests meant to test water quality. None of these measures, however, provided sustained relief.

Ms. Hansen currently spends 3 hours per day worrying about cross-contamination between the clean water and waste systems in her house, or seeking reassurance that the two have not become somehow linked. She blames her preoccupation with this problem on her limited social life and absence of romantic relationships. Except for moderate depression that typically follows each move, Ms. Hansen has not suffered from other psychiatric symptoms, including tics. She has been physically healthy all her life. She drinks alcohol rarely and has never used other substances. When asked by her new therapist to describe the problem that caused her to seek help, Ms. Hansen gives this preface to her answer: "I know this is crazy and makes absolutely no sense, but I can't help worrying about it."

Based on this brief history, Ms. Hansen would appear to meet the DSM-5 criteria for OCD. She has recurrent, bothersome, intrusive thoughts focused on contamination fears (the obsession) and multiple attempts at obtaining reassurance through inspections and laboratory tests (the compulsion). Her life has been significantly affected as a direct result of her symptoms: The multiple moves have undoubtedly created much instability for Ms. Hansen, and her time-consuming preoccupations and self-reassuring actions have precluded a meaningful social or romantic life. In light of the fact that she has no other physical, psychiatric, or substance use problems that might explain her symptoms, her presentation cannot be attributed to causes other than OCD. Moreover, despite her inability to control her symptoms on her own, Ms. Hansen clearly realizes the irrationality of her symptoms. As such, she would be characterized as having "good insight" into her condition.

Approach to the Diagnosis

Most people have habits that they perform in set or unusual ways, or they may have intrusive worries that may strike another person as odd or irrelevant. Yet the overwhelming majority of individuals do not have OCD. The key to making the OCD diagnosis is to evaluate the negative effect on the person's life and how consuming these behaviors and thoughts are—not their mere presence.

A comprehensive interview should help the clinician arrive at an accurate diagnosis and implement a successful treatment plan. An empathic, nonjudgmental approach is crucial, along with a systematic effort to cover all important elements of the case, including the chief complaint, history of present illness, stressors and precipitants, medical and psychiatric histories, medication history, developmental and social backgrounds, family history, review of systems, mental status examination, and consequences of the presenting problem to the person's life.

In approaching a person with suspected OCD, the clinician needs to keep in mind that individual obsessions or compulsions can vary greatly among people but that they generally fall under a limited number of themes. Tables 9–1 and 9–2 cover common obsessional and compulsive themes seen in OCD, with examples of each. The clinician should ask questions that explore the various themes and inquire how individual obsessions and compulsions may have changed over time and whether one or more symptoms are currently occurring.

In considering a diagnosis of OCD, the clinician needs to understand individuals in their larger cultural contexts and consider what might be a culturally sanctioned

TABLE 9–1. Obsessional themes in obsessive-compulsive and related disorders

Obsessional theme	Example
Contamination fear	A young man has a consuming fear of catching a prion illness from coming across human waste.
Pathological doubt	A young woman spends several work hours daily worrying whether she has run over someone during her morning commute.
Somatic worries	A physically healthy middle-aged man frequently worries that he may spontaneously stop breathing.
Symmetry	A husband worries that if objects in his environment are not arranged symmetrically, something bad may happen to his wife.
Aggression	A law-abiding teacher with no history of violence or other psychiatric symptoms worries he may suddenly "lose control" and assault a student.
Sexuality	An adult son experiences repetitive, intrusive, and highly distressing images of him having a sexual encounter with his mother.
Religion	While in church, an observant Catholic woman experiences repetitive sacrilegious urges to desecrate a crucifix.

TABLE 9–2. Compulsive themes in obsessive-compulsive and related disorders

Compulsive theme	Example
Checking	A woman checks the locks on the front and back doors, as well as all her windows, three times before she can leave the house.
Cleaning/washing	To avoid contracting a virus, a car salesman washes his hands for 15 minutes each time he shakes hands with a customer.
Counting	A retired man who no longer drives counts the number of footsteps he takes whenever he walks anywhere.
Need to confess/seek reassurance	An administrative assistant frequently worries she may have hurt a recipient's feelings by not using the appropriate greeting in an e-mail, often prompting her to send several follow-up e-mails to seek reassurance and apologize.
Repeating	A carpenter experiences a need to have his left hand repeat all movements performed by his right hand.
Mental rituals	A nonreligious man says a silent prayer in reverse whenever he comes across the number 2 because he associates it with bad luck.

norm for the "symptom." Some cultures are considered more superstitious, for example, and some incorporate more ritualistic practices than others.

Furthermore, the content of obsessions or the details of rituals can be highly embarrassing and heavily guarded secrets, adding to the stigma many people feel about seeking psychiatric care or divulging symptoms. An open mind, nonjudgmental attitude, and empathic approach are indispensable in all areas of mental health, including the treatment of obsessive-compulsive and related disorders, if people are to feel at ease sharing their problems and if mental health professionals are to succeed in helping them.

As stated in DSM-5, "Suicidal thoughts occur at some point in as many as about half of individuals with OCD. Suicide attempts are also reported in up to one-quarter of individuals with OCD; the presence of comorbid major depressive disorder increases the risk" (p. 240).

Getting the History

> Ms. Silva is a 34-year-old woman who reports not allowing chicken meat into her kitchen because of fear of contracting salmonella. She worries that she is depriving her children and husband of a nutritious food that they might like because of her fear. To assess for any logical explanation for her worry, the physician asks, "Have you or a loved one had salmonella or other food-borne poisoning before, or do you tend to undercook food?" When Ms. Silva answers no, the exaggerated nature of the worry becomes more confirmed. The physician then asks, "Do you have decontaminating rituals that you have to perform if you think you have been exposed to chicken? Do you avoid going to, or eating in, certain places because of this?" Ms. Silva informs the physician that she relies on her husband for her grocery shopping, or if she absolutely must go to the store herself, she will skip the meat section and will engage in 2-hour showers upon her return home. She also has a special pair of shoes that she stores outside the house and reserves for trips to the grocery store, and she has unsuccessfully tried to lobby her husband to do the same. "How has this affected your marriage and family life?" the physician asks. Ms. Silva reports that her husband is very frustrated and her children have called her excessive worry "crazy." The physician then tries to find out about the onset and timeline of her symptoms, other obsessions and compulsions that she may have experienced, and any associated mood or other psychiatric symptoms. Further questions explore her medical, family, and social history.
>
> The physician carefully explores the roots of this irrational fear, its extent, and its spillover effects. He tries to elicit any associated symptoms, whether they are other obsessions and compulsions or non-OCD psychiatric symptoms. By asking about any decontaminating rituals that may be present or other avoidance behaviors, he gently allows Ms. Silva to divulge potentially embarrassing details, including her avoidance of grocery stores, her cleaning rituals, and her request that her husband wear special shoes when he goes to the store on her behalf. The interview begins by focusing on the chief complaint and then broadens in a way that elucidates it and also investigates its consequences and the presence of other linked or independent pathological findings worthy of clinical attention.

Tips for Clarifying the Diagnosis

- When a person "self-diagnoses" with OCD, investigate whether there are sufficient negative consequences to the person's life to warrant a clinical diagnosis.

- Ask these important questions: What is the time course of the symptoms? How have the symptoms changed over time? Are there symptom-free periods?
- Determine whether both obsessions and compulsions are present.
- Question whether symptom intensity correlates with stress or negative mood.
- If multiple obsessions or compulsions are present, clarify which are the most time-consuming and anxiety provoking.
- Assess how much control the person has over the symptoms. Ask what the person's success rate is when attempting to distract himself or herself from the obsession or to delay acting on the compulsion.

Consider the Case

Ms. Webb is a 75-year-old grandmother and retired university administrator who has never needed to see a mental health professional. Since the death of her husband of 50 years some 10 months earlier, Ms. Webb has become gradually withdrawn, lost weight, and developed insomnia. She has also voiced to concerned neighbors suspicions about her downstairs tenants, complaining that they mean to harm her, including by poisoning her water supply through introducing a lethal substance into the pipes supplying her house. When her neighbors try to reassure her that her tenants are good people who are upstanding members of the community, Ms. Webb questions her neighbors' motives for "covering up for them." Because of her fear, Ms. Webb now refuses to drink the water at her house and only very reluctantly uses it to shower or for cleaning purposes. As a result, she has become dehydrated, compounding the weight loss she has sustained and making her vulnerable to serious medical complications.

Ms. Webb has developed a type of contamination fear involving her water supply, and her fear has led to medically compromising avoidance behavior. However, the concomitant presence of other symptoms makes it less likely that OCD is the root cause of her problem. Social withdrawal and appetite and sleep disturbance all started after a significant loss (the death of her longtime husband) and point to a diagnosis of major depressive disorder. The fear of being poisoned by her tenants is most likely a paranoid symptom that is manifesting in the context of her mood disorder. In addition, late onset of symptoms is more commonly a feature of depression than of OCD. For all these reasons, the most likely explanation for the observed symptoms would be a depressive episode with psychotic features, rather than late-onset OCD.

This case illustrates how OCD-like symptoms can occur in a wide range of psychiatric illnesses. A broad psychiatric "review of systems" and careful history taking help delineate whether the symptoms are the result of OCD or whether an alternative diagnosis better explains them. Naturally, treatment success will highly depend on diagnostic accuracy.

Differential Diagnosis

OCD has been described as an anxiety disorder, and other anxiety disorders should be explored when an OCD diagnosis is being considered in a person who has significant worry about a particular trigger or who seeks the temporary calming effects of performing a ritual. For example, anxious avoidance of a specific location may not be provoked by OCD superstitions associated with it, but rather may result from posttraumatic stress disorder that has linked the place with a trauma in the person's history.

The particular nature of the obsession or compulsion can also point to other diagnostic possibilities. For example, in someone with rigid eating patterns as a result, perhaps, of a perceived hypersensitivity to a food ingredient, an eating disorder might be the more appropriate diagnosis. In the case of a socially withdrawn child with below-average IQ, peculiar interests, and some repetitive motor behaviors, an autism spectrum disorder might better explain the observed deficits. Similarly, in an individual with unrelenting, unnecessary checking of e-mail and social networking accounts but no other checking behaviors, compulsions, or obsessions, some pathological relationship with the digital world might best fit the clinical picture. Also, individuals with rigidly defined ways of performing tasks, who are convinced they are right, want others to adopt their patterns, and see no problem with their set ways, might be more appropriately diagnosed with obsessive-compulsive personality disorder rather than OCD. Finally, in individuals who tend to derive a pleasure or thrill from a repetitive act (e.g., skin picking, hair pulling, pathological gambling) as opposed to a temporary reduction in anxiety, the somewhat "ego-syntonic" nature of the behavior might point to a diagnosis of a behavioral addiction or impulse-control disorder rather than OCD.

Because the individual symptoms of OCD can be so variable and partially overlap with several other diagnostic categories, a broad differential diagnosis should be entertained when approaching an individual with suspected OCD, and the diagnosis of OCD should be made only after other candidate conditions have been ruled out.

See DSM-5 for additional disorders to consider in the differential diagnosis. Also refer to the discussions of comorbidity and differential diagnosis in their respective sections of DSM-5.

Summary

- OCD is a common, often disabling condition that can manifest with a great variety of obsessions or compulsions that typically fall under a limited number of themes.
- Many individuals describe performing some repetitive behaviors or having obsession-like thoughts, images, or urges. A diagnosis of OCD can be made only if symptoms are consuming and result in significant impairment.
- A careful history should be taken to assess the natural course of the symptoms, the context within which they occur, and the resulting consequences and complications.
- Making the diagnosis of OCD requires the careful ruling out of a wide range of psychiatric and other disorders that can masquerade as OCD.

─────────────── **IN-DEPTH DIAGNOSIS** ───────────────

Body Dysmorphic Disorder

Ms. Thompson is a 28-year-old married woman and former high school teacher. At age 22, following her parents' surprising divorce, she started worrying that her face was asymmetrical. More specifically, she felt that the left side of her jaw was higher than the right one by about a half inch. Ms. Thompson had sustained no injury and had no malformation that might explain this "defect." Shame over her appearance led to drastic efforts to hide the perceived asymmetry, including creative hairstyling and the use of scarves to partially cover her cheeks. When no technique worked, Ms. Thompson left her teaching job, convinced that her students were mocking her appearance, and gradually withdrew from social interactions. Reassurances by her husband that her jawline was entirely normal did not allay her anxiety, and neither did several professional consultations with dentists. Eventually, Ms. Thompson started researching oral surgeons in the hopes of finding one who could rid her of this problem by operating on her jaw.

Ms. Thompson exhibits no other psychiatric symptomatology, including any concerns about body weight or body fat composition. She has no history of medical conditions and does not use substances. She does see herself as debilitated by her symptoms but does not view the cause as psychiatric. Instead, Ms. Thompson is convinced that a jaw malformation, treatable by surgery, is at its root.

In assessing this case, it appears that Ms. Thompson is preoccupied by a nonexistent body defect and that this preoccupation has caused her severe impairment, including having to quit work and withdraw from society. Furthermore, there is no indication that she has insight into her problem: She is not relieved by reassurances from her husband or dental professionals that her jaw is normal, and she is so convinced of this flaw that she is seeking painful and potentially dangerous corrective surgery to fix it. As such, Ms. Thompson's presentation is most consistent with the DSM-5 criteria for body dysmorphic disorder with absent insight/delusional beliefs.

Approach to the Diagnosis

People with body dysmorphic disorder will often only reluctantly present for mental health evaluation and treatment. They may feel egregiously unattractive and think that only an experienced plastic surgeon or dermatologist, not a therapist or psychiatrist, can assuage their misery. This resistance to seeking care is more likely to soften if the mental health professional adopts a caring, nonjudgmental approach, fully acknowledging the distress and pain caused by the perceived defect even as he or she declines to acknowledge the presence of the defect itself.

Observing the person's appearance is crucial to ruling out the presence of a defect. In some cases where a defect can be seen, it is important to explore whether it was self-induced and resulted from an attempt to fix the perceived defect (e.g., scarring from excessive self-excoriation meant to erase a blemish). Also, anxious affect and poor eye contact can point to self-consciousness and social avoidance linked to body dysmorphic disorder. Other clues in the patient's appearance can suggest compensatory measures meant as camouflage (e.g., unusual, big, or awkward accessories or clothing, sometimes strategically positioned to hide certain areas).

In addition to the usual components of a comprehensive interview needed to make an accurate diagnosis, some questions are uniquely important when assessing a patient with suspected body dysmorphic disorder. Inquiry into the degree of "corrective" measures sought, including invasive procedures from other specialists, is crucial. Should the patient consent, contact with those specialists is important to coordinate care and provide psychoeducation: There may be little awareness of body dysmorphic disorder among professionals in other disciplines (as well as with trichotillomania and excoriation disorder) and the psychological underpinnings of some people's body-focused complaints. It is often the mental health care provider's role to educate both the person and the other providers about these conditions and how a nonpsychiatric treatment approach is rarely curative and may in fact exacerbate the condition. Collaboration with other providers serves to present a united front to patients about the primacy of mental health treatment in their situation, prevents "splitting," avoids reinforcing symptoms, and helps increase awareness.

As the clinician narrows down the diagnosis and tailors interview questions, particular attention should be paid to other conditions that share features with body dysmorphic disorder, especially other obsessive-compulsive spectrum disorders (in which repetitive behaviors or mental acts are a hallmark) and eating disorders (in which anxiety over body weight is often a defining feature).

In addition, individuals' appearance-focused symptoms should be appreciated in their larger cultural context. For example, the fixation on body mass index and biceps size in a young bodybuilder with suspected muscle dysmorphia should exceed the overall cultural dictate to work out and develop muscular physiques and should cause him or her more distress and impairment than similar avid gym goers in his or her age group.

As stated in DSM-5, "Rates of suicidal ideation and suicide attempts are high in both adults and children/adolescents with body dysmorphic disorder. Furthermore, risk for suicide appears high in adolescents. A substantial proportion of individuals attribute suicidal ideation or suicide attempts primarily to their appearance concerns. Individuals with body dysmorphic disorder have many risk factors for completed suicide, such as high rates of suicidal ideation and suicide attempts, demographic characteristics associated with suicide, and high rates of comorbid major depressive disorder" (p. 245).

Getting the History

The therapist welcomes a patient, Ms. Fleming, into his office. He is struck by her avoidant gaze and by one element in her appearance: she is sporting extremely long bangs that cover her forehead and partially her eyes. "It was my husband's idea. I don't think I need this kind of help," the 32-year-old woman tells the therapist. "I am glad to meet you, even if it seems like you hesitated about coming here," the therapist answers. "May I ask a few questions to see if I can help you?" When asked about what has been bothering her, Ms. Fleming opens up about feeling "deformed" because her eyebrows are asymmetrical. She then lifts her bangs to reveal a pair of eyebrows that appear normal and symmetrical to the therapist. "See!" the patient says as she points to her forehead, her finger anxiously trembling. "I look like a freak! I can't be seen in public looking like this! Please don't be like my husband and tell me they look normal. Give me your honest opinion!" "I'm very sorry this is causing you so much pain," the therapist answers. "My opinion is that your eyebrows look fine, but I also understand that the anxiety they cause you is very real and overwhelming, and I want to help you deal with it and help you feel better in your own skin."

Ms. Fleming presents as anxiety-ridden over the appearance of her eyebrows and as actively employing strategies that are meant to hide the embarrassing body part. She expresses reluctance about mental health care, likely due to poor insight into the psychological roots of her problem. The patient has received reassurance, at least from her husband, that her eyebrows look normal, but that seems to have done little to help her symptoms. The therapist avoids getting into a tug-of-war with Ms. Fleming about the symmetrical nature of her eyebrows, giving his honest opinion when directly asked but also focusing on the downstream effects of the patient's faulty conviction—namely, the intolerable anxiety she is feeling, which is something that both he and the patient agree on. This approach can help start a therapeutic alliance, which is absolutely crucial to getting a patient with little to no insight into her body dysmorphic disorder diagnosis to continue to accept mental health care and heed treatment recommendations.

Tips for Clarifying the Diagnosis

- Consider whether the person is preoccupied with a body part's appearance or with perceived ugliness. Preoccupation with a body part, if not focused on looks or appearance, cannot be the basis for a diagnosis of body dysmorphic disorder.
- Inquire about repetitive behaviors (e.g., mirror checking, excessive grooming, reassurance seeking) or repetitive mental acts (e.g., comparing his or her appearance to others) as a consequence of the preoccupation.
- Assess the person's level of insight, including whether he or she is completely convinced of his or her view of personal appearance. Explore any delusional dimension to the symptoms.
- Inquire about any dermatological or cosmetic interventions that were completed or that are being sought to try to remedy the perceived problem. Ask about other strategies used to hide the perceived problem (e.g., heavy makeup, particular clothes or other accessories).
- Screen for muscle dysmorphia, especially in males who engage in excessive bodybuilding or use anabolic steroids, because such males may be responding to a baseless worry that they are insufficiently muscular or too small.

Consider the Case

Ms. Thompson, the 28-year-old married woman and former high school teacher who was discussed in the first case presented in this section on body dysmorphic disorder, continued to be unhappy about her "malformed" jaw. She underwent "corrective" surgery abroad when no licensed local surgeon would agree to operate on her. Following surgery, Ms. Thompson felt self-confident and started socializing more. This self-confidence, however, proved short-lived, as a new all-consuming worry overtook her about 2 months later. For no reason and without any precipitant, Ms. Thompson started worrying that her eyebrows were significantly asymmetrical, leading her to undergo a laser procedure to remove them, followed by another procedure to permanently tattoo on a new, and in her opinion more symmetrical, pair. Around the same time, Ms. Thompson started worrying that her skin was too pale and was beginning to frequent tanning salons excessively to try to develop a darker skin tone.

This case illustrates that the feature fixated on in body dysmorphic disorder may change over time because the illness can "migrate" from one area of concern to another. It also illustrates that the desperate and expensive interventions people sometimes seek—cosmetic, surgical, dermatological, and so on—are rarely curative and can serve to validate an unnecessary worry that should instead be confronted according to established treatment guidelines. Notably, body dysmorphic disorder can affect all ethnic groups, and discomfort with skin color (e.g., "too dark," "too pale") is not an uncommon symptom. Any success derived from nonpsychiatric treatments for body dysmorphic disorder tends to be temporary, with the appearance-based anxiety often returning, either with the same focus or a different one.

Differential Diagnosis

In a society that is often described as obsessed with appearances, it is important to differentiate people's normal, culture-concordant worries about their looks from the pathological preoccupation of body dysmorphic disorder. For the diagnosis of body dysmorphic disorder to be made, the worry has to be excessive and produce clinically significant impairment in functioning. Furthermore, if a physical defect is clearly noticeable or disfiguring, the worry it generates cannot be attributed to body dysmorphic disorder.

The intrusive appearance-based thoughts of body dysmorphic disorder, and the repetitive mirror checking, grooming, or reassurance seeking that often go with them, are reminiscent of other obsessive-compulsive and related disorders, such as excoriation disorder or trichotillomania. When skin picking or hair plucking is intended as a grooming behavior meant to correct a perceived defect, a diagnosis of body dysmorphic disorder is more appropriate. The typically poorer insight seen in body dysmorphic disorder and the narrower fixation on appearance help distinguish it from OCD.

Similarly, in a person with an eating disorder, worries about being fat are more likely to be part of the eating disorder, although an eating disorder can be comorbid with body dysmorphic disorder.

Also, the poor or absent insight seen in some patients with body dysmorphic disorder can reach a delusional degree. However, the focus on appearance and the absence of disorganized thinking or hallucinations help distinguish body dysmorphic disorder from a primary psychotic illness.

See DSM-5 for additional disorders to consider in the differential diagnosis. Also refer to the discussions of comorbidity and differential diagnosis in their respective sections of DSM-5.

Summary

- Body dysmorphic disorder is an often-disabling condition characterized by a preoccupation with a nonexistent or slight body defect, repetitive actions or thoughts meant to reduce the associated anxiety, and variable degrees of insight into the psychic roots of the illness.
- The cultural message to meet certain narrow beauty standards is strong and inescapable. Patients with body dysmorphic disorder have an appearance-derived anxiety that far exceeds society's "epidemic" of unease with one's body image.
- A careful history is needed to assess the natural course of symptoms, their larger context, the resulting consequences (including depression and social withdrawal), and any complications (e.g., from personal attempts at correcting "defects" or from unnecessary dermatological or surgical interventions).

- Making the diagnosis of body dysmorphic disorder requires the careful ruling out of a wide range of psychiatric and other disorders, including OCD, eating disorders, and psychotic illnesses.

IN-DEPTH DIAGNOSIS

Trichotillomania (Hair-Pulling Disorder)

Ms. Lewis is a 28-year-old woman currently working on a doctorate in English literature. She has a 12-year history of hair pulling from her scalp and eyebrows that has waxed and waned over the years but has become progressively worse since she began working on her dissertation and studying for her comprehensive exams 3 months ago. Her first episode of hair pulling occurred at age 16, when she first began tweezing her eyebrow hairs for aesthetic purposes. She remembers continuing to pull from her right eyebrow well beyond what was aesthetically justifiable and recalls enjoying the feeling that followed plucking each hair. The initial pleasurable experience, however, was followed by shame and embarrassment, because she had to use makeup to conceal the patch of missing hair. This initial experience was followed by similar, sporadic episodes of right eyebrow hair plucking, usually using her right thumb and index fingers and most often during times of stress or other intense emotional experiences.

Over time, Ms. Lewis began pulling hair from both eyebrows and her scalp. When her parents eventually noticed the patches of missing hair, they took Ms. Lewis for evaluations with her pediatrician and a dermatologist, who determined that the hair pulling was not the result of an undiagnosed skin or other medical condition. Numerous therapists unsuccessfully focused on Ms. Lewis's "lack of self-control" and questioned whether she had body image issues for which she was attempting to compensate. Currently, Ms. Lewis has a small bald spot on the vertex of her head that she attempts to hide by pulling her hair back. She no longer goes to her usual hair salon because she fears she would have to explain her bald patch to her hairstylist or hear a lecture on how she is intentionally damaging her hair.

Although she has attempted to stop the behavior on numerous occasions, she has never been able to maintain complete cessation for more than a few weeks. She currently engages in hair pulling from her eyebrows or scalp for at least 1.5–2 hours each day, with an average of 50 hairs pulled daily. She finds that she is engaging in pulling with little awareness, usually when engrossed in reading for her comprehensive exams or when staring at her computer screen while working on her dissertation. In addition, Ms. Lewis reports that she has been "playing" with the pulled hairs. Previously, Ms. Lewis would immediately discard the pulled hairs. Now, she finds herself either "rolling" the hair between her fingers after pulling it or chewing on the root bulb. She states that she does not know exactly why she started playing with the pulled hairs but reports significant shame about these new behaviors. Because she does not want people to notice her bald spots, Ms. Lewis has been spending less time with friends, even though she acknowledges that social support would help mitigate her stress. She has also discontinued swimming, because she finds it difficult to hide the bald spot on her head when her hair is wet. Without the outlet of exercise and social activities, Ms. Lewis's mood has become increasingly depressed, which she believes further exacerbates her hair pulling and decreases her motivation to engage in alternative behaviors.

Ms. Lewis appears to meet DSM-5 criteria for trichotillomania. Her hair pulling has had a chronic course since onset, although the location and function of her pulling has changed over time. She repeatedly engages in pulling hair from her eyebrows and scalp despite efforts to control the behavior. She no longer finds the effects of pulling pleasurable, does not pull for purposes of correcting perceived imperfections, and most often engages in the behavior with little awareness. She is experiencing significant distress from her inability to control her hair pulling and from the effects the ongoing behavior is having on her physical appearance and life, and she endorses depressed mood, social withdrawal, shame, and embarrassment—all stemming from her pulling. Medical and dermatological evaluations suggest that Ms. Lewis's pulling behavior is not attributable to a medical condition. Furthermore, no other DSM-5 disorder would better explain this presentation.

Approach to the Diagnosis

Persons with trichotillomania often present for treatment with a significant amount of shame and embarrassment. They not only may be self-conscious of the effects of their pulling (bald spots, missing eyebrows) but also may feel shame and fear judgment for engaging in a behavior that family, friends, or previous providers have indicated is within their control. Thus, individuals may present as self-conscious and socially avoidant during the initial consultation. As a result, it is essential for providers during the initial assessment and throughout treatment to maintain an empathic and nonjudgmental approach and provide a supportive and understanding environment.

During a comprehensive interview, it is important to assess the nature and extent of hair-pulling behaviors with respect to location, frequency, and function. Some patients may not be completely forthcoming when reporting all the sites from which they pull hair, particularly sites that might be embarrassing to discuss, such as pubic areas. Thus, asking patients about pulling from locations they did not initially mention is important. In addition to gathering information regarding location and frequency, it is important to inquire regarding the function of the pulling behavior. For many patients with trichotillomania, pulling is experienced as an automatic and out-of-awareness activity that happens during times of stress or intense focus. Other patients report engaging in focused pulling in order to remove a coarse hair, alleviate an uncomfortable sensation or emotion, or produce a pleasurable sensation. Understanding the function of hair pulling is essential to making an accurate diagnosis. For example, hair pulling that is not excessive and functions to improve someone's appearance may be best considered normative hair removal; hair pulling that serves to correct a perceived imperfection may be better accounted for by body dysmorphic disorder; hair pulling that serves to alleviate a chronic itch or skin irritation may suggest an undiagnosed dermatological condition; and hair pulling that functions as a symmetry ritual may be best captured by OCD.

In addition to asking about the function of the hair pulling, it is important to ask what the person does with each pulled hair. For most individuals with trichotillomania, hairs are discarded following removal. Others may keep an occasional hair to roll between their fingertips or use to caress their lips or cheek. However, some people put a pulled hair in their mouth to play with it with their tongue, chew on the root bulb, or swallow. People may be reluctant to endorse such behaviors due to embarrassment. However, it is important to assess for their presence because they can result in significant health problems, including dental issues and trichobezoars (hairballs).

Getting the History

During her initial evaluation, Ms. Lowe, a 28-year-old woman, reveals that she frequently plucks individual hairs from her eyelashes or eyebrows whenever she is feeling stressed out and intensely focused on completing a homework assignment or studying for an exam. She says, "I know what you're thinking....I'm destroying my appearance and could stop—but I'm choosing not to, right?" The therapist responds, "I think what you're going through is extremely difficult, and I'm sure you've tried everything you can think of to stop pulling but have found this to be a very difficult disorder to gain control of. If you don't mind, I'd like to ask you some additional details about your pulling. What do you do with each hair after you pull it?" Ms. Lowe replies that she discards most hairs immediately after pulling them, but does frequently chew on the ends of those with large root bulbs and eventually swallows them. The therapist asks, "In addition to pulling from your eyebrows and eyelashes, do you ever pull from your scalp, arms or legs, or pubic area?" The patient expresses embarrassment, but does report occasionally pulling hair from her pubic region when using the bathroom or lying in her bed reading.

Ms. Lowe expresses an initial concern that her therapist will be critical of her hair pulling and judge her for not exercising better self-control. The therapist empathizes with how difficult it is to live with this disorder and acknowledges that the patient has probably tried everything in her power to stop pulling her hair. By taking an empathic and nonjudgmental approach, the therapist is able to gain the information necessary to make an accurate diagnosis by helping the patient to feel understood and supported and allowing her to be fully open regarding the specifics of her disorder. In addition, by developing rapport and assessing for behaviors that Ms. Lowe did not initially reveal, the therapist is able to get a thorough view of the extent of Ms. Lowe's hair pulling, including behaviors that put her at risk for possible medical problems (e.g., consuming hair).

Tips for Clarifying the Diagnosis

- Assess the frequency and location(s) of hair-pulling behaviors, including locations that may be embarrassing for individuals to discuss.
- Assess the function of the hair pulling. Does the pulling largely occur outside of awareness or feel out of control and serve the purpose of regulating an uncomfortable sensation or emotion? Does the pulling coincide with a preoccupation with the person's appearance and serve the purpose of correcting a perceived imperfection? Does the function of the hair pulling suggest that it may be better accounted for by another disorder, such as body dysmorphic disorder or OCD?
- Assess the ways in which the person has attempted to conceal the effects of hair pulling, the effect the pulling has had on his or her health, and the ways in which the behaviors have affected his or her social and occupational functioning.
- Inquire about what the person does with each hair following removal. Is each hair immediately discarded, or are the hairs sometimes consumed?
- Does the person have a medical or dermatological disorder that may cause hair pulling as a way to alleviate physical discomfort?

Consider the Case

> Ms. Davis is a 22-year-old single woman with a 10-year history of compulsively remov-
> ing hair from various locations of her body using her fingers or tweezers. In general,
> Ms. Davis reports that she finds body hair disgusting and can only tolerate hair on her
> head and face if it looks perfect. She engages in hair pulling for approximately 1 hour
> each day and commonly focuses on hair that is visible to those with whom she interacts.
> She denies having episodes of pulling that are automatic and out of her awareness;
> rather, she endorses focused pulling that serves the function of removing hairs that look
> "ugly and unattractive." She indicates that she stands in front of a mirror and pulls or
> tweezes "unsightly" hairs from her eyelashes and eyebrows almost daily to maintain
> their "perfect appearance." Several times throughout the day, especially while sitting in
> class or riding public transportation, she uses her fingers to pluck any visible hairs from
> her arms and hands, because she finds hair in these areas to be repulsive and unattract-
> ive. Although she regularly shaves her legs and armpits, she reports that she frequently
> examines these areas with her hands for new hair growth and will use tweezers to re-
> move any hairs she finds that are long enough to be pulled. In addition, she reports that
> she is intolerant of having pubic hair and frequently uses tweezers to remove any new
> hair growth.

Although Ms. Davis has a long history of engaging in focused hair pulling across a
number of sites on her body, the function of these behaviors appears to be exclusively
aesthetic and is motivated by her desire to remove unsightly hair and maintain a perfect
appearance. She finds the presence of hair in most regions of her body "ugly and unattractive" and engages in hair pulling to correct these perceived imperfections. Because
of the aesthetic function and desire to correct a perceived imperfection, Ms. Davis's hair
pulling would be better accounted for by a diagnosis of body dysmorphic disorder than
trichotillomania. This case illustrates the potential similarities in presentation among
the obsessive-compulsive and related disorders and the importance of understanding
the function of seemingly similar symptoms and behaviors during assessment in order
to determine an accurate diagnosis and treatment plan.

Differential Diagnosis

To accurately differentiate trichotillomania from other disorders, it is necessary to understand the function of the hair-pulling behavior. For example, hair pulling that is
meant to correct a perceived physical imperfection, such as "ugly" arm hair, may be
better accounted for by body dysmorphic disorder. OCD may better describe hair
pulling that functions as a superstitious ritual (e.g., a person who pulls a hair from the
top of his head whenever he hears the word *cancer* to prevent becoming sick). Hair
pulling that serves to alleviate a chronic itch, skin irritation, or other discomfort may
suggest a dermatological condition. Finally, hair pulling in response to a delusion or
command auditory hallucination is likely best explained by a psychotic disorder.

It is important to recognize that behaviors associated with trichotillomania occur
frequently in individuals who do not meet criteria for this or any other disorder. It is
common in many cultures to engage in normative hair removal for grooming purposes. For example, people may use tweezers to remove hairs from the eyebrows to
improve their appearance. It is also common for those with longer hair to play with

their hair by twisting, twirling, or tugging it. Such hair-based behaviors do not point to a pathological condition.

See DSM-5 for additional disorders to consider in the differential diagnosis. Also refer to the discussions of comorbidity and differential diagnosis in their respective sections of DSM-5.

Summary

- Trichotillomania is a serious condition characterized by the person's repeated pulling of his or her hair that often results in bald spots, hair damage, and attempts to conceal the consequences.
- Trichotillomania is associated with shame and embarrassment due to the perception that the person should be able to refrain from self-inflicted harm to his or her body.
- Trichotillomania can include focused pulling (targeting a hair due to a tactile sensation or the desire to produce a pleasurable sensation), automatic pulling (engaging in hair pulling out of the person's awareness, usually while engrossed in a specific task), or a combination.
- A careful assessment is necessary to differentiate pathological hair pulling from normative grooming and from other psychiatric disorders that share similar features, such as body dysmorphic disorder and OCD.

──────── **SUMMARY** ────────

Obsessive-Compulsive and Related Disorders

Like many psychiatric conditions, illnesses grouped in the obsessive-compulsive and related disorders diagnostic class are extreme manifestations of common, normal experiences. Exactly at what point repetition, collecting, appearance-focused anxiety, and self-grooming cross into the pathological and become clinical entities that deserve treatment is a question that mental health care providers are often called on to answer. This determination requires a deep understanding of individuals and their lives, along with consideration of empirically defined criteria, such as those offered in DSM-5, for what constitutes a diagnosis.

Repetition is an important common feature that helps unite the disparate conditions listed in the obsessive-compulsive and related disorders class—but important differences exist. For example, the contamination fear and anxious collecting seen in OCD and hoarding disorder are usually accompanied by a dysphoria and frustration that contrast with the pleasurable feelings sometimes reported by people with trichotillomania and excoriation disorder. Such distinctions and other nuances are beyond the scope of this chapter but should be pursued by interested readers (see "Recommended Readings" at the end of this chapter). More advanced reading will reveal that these conditions—diagnosable and potentially highly impairing as they are shown to be here—are also treatable in a large percentage of patients.

─────────────■-■-■─────────────
Diagnostic Pearls

- Although the obsessive-compulsive and related disorders diagnostic class is separate from anxiety disorders in DSM-5, anxiety remains a prominent feature of many conditions within this class.

- Overlap exists among conditions within the obsessive-compulsive and related disorders diagnostic class and disorders in other diagnostic classes. Careful history taking and familiarity with diagnostic criteria are necessary to clarify the diagnosis.

- The details of individuals' unusual worries and behaviors are often embarrassing to them and laden with stigma. An open mind and empathic approach are needed to put individuals at ease and maximize diagnostic accuracy and treatment success.

- Information on cultural and familial context should be elicited to help determine whether a particular concern or behavior is pathological or within the expected norm for the person being evaluated.

- There is much misunderstanding within the medical profession and society at large about obsessive-compulsive and related disorders. Increasing awareness and psychoeducation are part of the clinician's role in addressing these problems.

Self-Assessment

Key Concepts: Double-Check Your Knowledge

What is the relevance of the following concepts to the various obsessive-compulsive and related disorders?

- Intrusive thoughts, urges, or images
- Repetitive behaviors or mental acts
- Purpose of repetitive behaviors or mental acts
- Time-consuming nature of obsessions or compulsions
- Perceived body defect or flaw
- Muscle dysmorphia
- Range of insight in body dysmorphic disorder
- Trichotillomania
- Hair pulling or loss that is secondary to a medical condition

Questions to Discuss With Colleagues and Mentors

1. Do you systematically screen patients for disorders in the obsessive-compulsive and related disorders diagnostic class? If so, what questions do you use for each disorder? For example, how do you define *obsession* or *compulsion* to people in your screenings?

2. How do you manage your reaction when you are faced with disturbing symptoms of obsessive-compulsive and related disorders (e.g., hearing about an obsession to stab someone from an individual with no desire or intent to do so, or meeting a disheveled hoarder whose collections have created unsanitary conditions at home and have visibly affected his or her personal hygiene)?
3. How do you determine whether OCD (or any condition in this diagnostic class) is the "best explanation" for a person's symptoms?
4. How do you assess "insight" in patients diagnosed with a condition in the diagnostic class of obsessive-compulsive and related disorders?

Case-Based Questions

PART A

Ms. Connor is a 45-year-old woman who works as a business accountant at a software firm. While still in college at age 20, and for no apparent reason, an anxiety that struck her as peculiar suddenly hit her: Ms. Connor started worrying that she may have inadvertently stepped on a baby during her morning jog. She could not say how the baby would have materialized on the isolated riverside trail where she ran, or how she might have tripped over a baby, but her need to verify was so intense that she started to follow her jog with a slow-paced hike during which she would comb the trail for any evidence of her "crime." As a result of this time-consuming pattern, Ms. Connor had to miss morning classes, but once the ritual was completed, she could focus on afternoon lectures and on doing her homework in the evening.

Does Ms. Connor suffer from OCD? Ms. Connor's symptom can be described as a repetitive, intrusive thought that she recognizes as unusual and that involves having inadvertently hurt someone. She has associated checking behaviors meant to provide reassurance and reduce anxiety. Her life was negatively affected in that her school performance suffered. This picture is consistent with a diagnosis of OCD.

PART B

After graduating from college, Ms. Connor stopped jogging because the corporate job she chose did not accommodate late-morning starts. Two decades later, her more sedentary lifestyle has contributed to weight gain and early blood pressure problems. However, giving up on running did not eradicate the compulsions or the anxiety triggering them. Her worry changed over the years but did not go away. Ms. Connor's commute today involves a 20-minute drive from home to work. Depending on her level of anxiety, that trip is sometimes followed by another drive during which she retraces her route to ascertain that she did not run over a baby on her first attempt to get to work. On what she calls her "bad days," she even has to check her tires for additional reassurance.

What does the evolution of symptoms in this case history so far tell us about the course of OCD? OCD is often a chronic illness with a waxing and waning course. Whether the symptoms vary within the same general theme (as in this example) or take on different themes, individual symptoms often change. Their toll is cumulative over time, in this case indirectly contributing to medical problems.

PART C

> Throughout her years of struggling with OCD, Ms. Connor was able to raise two healthy children and draw reasonable satisfaction from work. Until very recently, Ms. Connor had never sought professional help for her symptoms and says she learned to "adapt" to them, setting aside a certain amount of time on some days to "calm them down."

Why did Ms. Connor delay seeking care? Although symptoms of OCD often manifest early, it is not unusual for individuals to delay treatment or not seek it at all. Reasons include lack of access to care, embarrassment about divulging symptoms, the stigma of a psychiatric diagnosis, the ability in some situations to adapt to the illness, inadequate knowledge of the pathological nature of the symptoms, and a tendency to view symptoms as peculiar personality traits.

Short-Answer Questions

1. Are both obsessions and compulsions required for a diagnosis of OCD?
2. Define obsessions in OCD.
3. Define compulsions in OCD.
4. What specifier would the clinician use for the OCD diagnosis in a person who is totally convinced that his or her fears of catching a very rare prion illness are well founded and that his or her associated cleaning rituals to prevent this outcome are entirely legitimate?
5. Would people who are preoccupied with essential body functions (e.g., adequate breathing, regular pulse rate, number of bowel movements) meet criteria for body dysmorphic disorder?
6. Could people who have an actual body defect meet criteria for body dysmorphic disorder?
7. Could patients have alcohol use disorder and receive a primary diagnosis of body dysmorphic disorder?
8. What form of body dysmorphic disorder is much more common in males?
9. Does a person's excessive twirling of his or her hair along with frequent massaging of the scalp constitute trichotillomania?
10. An elderly man is having difficulty navigating his home because of excessive clutter, which creates a risk of falling. He collects and saves unnecessary things because "he might need them some day." No other obsessions or compulsions are evident. What is the most likely diagnosis?

Answers

1. No. Obsessions and compulsions are not both required for a diagnosis of OCD.
2. OCD obsessions are recurrent and persistent thoughts, urges, or images that are experienced, at some time during the disturbance, as intrusive and unwanted and that cause marked anxiety or distress in most individuals.
3. OCD compulsions are repetitive behaviors (e.g., hand washing, ordering, checking) or mental acts (e.g., praying, counting, repeating words silently) that individuals feel driven to perform in response to an obsession or according to rules that must be applied rigidly.
4. The individual would be diagnosed with OCD with absent insight/delusional beliefs.
5. No. These people do not meet criteria for body dysmorphic disorder unless they are also preoccupied with the appearance of a body part.
6. Yes. People who have an actual body defect can meet criteria for body dysmorphic disorder, but the defect in question has to be minor and the preoccupation and distress caused by it disproportionately larger.
7. Yes. A patient can have alcohol use disorder and still receive a primary diagnosis of body dysmorphic disorder.
8. The muscle dysmorphia form of body dysmorphic disorder (i.e., the belief that the person's body build is too small or insufficiently muscular) is more common in males.
9. No. The criteria for a trichotillomania diagnosis require recurrent hair pulling with resulting hair loss.
10. The most likely diagnosis is hoarding disorder.

Recommended Readings

Aboujaoude E: Compulsive Acts: A Psychiatrist's Tales of Ritual and Obsession. Berkeley, University of California Press, 2008

Koran LM: Obsessive-Compulsive and Related Disorders in Adults: A Comprehensive Clinical Guide. New York, Cambridge University Press, 1999

Trauma- and Stressor-Related Disorders

Cheryl Gore-Felton, Ph.D.

Cheryl Koopman, Ph.D.

"I can't watch the news—the memories come flooding back."

"I am numb inside."

The trauma- and stressor-related disorders chapter is new to DSM-5 and reflects a significant shift from DSM-IV in that most disorders in this diagnostic class were previously housed in the anxiety disorders class. This change reflects empirical evidence obtained in the past decade that demonstrates the variability in responses to traumatic or stressful events. Although some individuals may respond with increased anxiety, others may respond with increased anhedonia, dysphoria, dissociation, or a combination of symptoms. To capture this heterogeneity and variability, the diagnostic class of trauma- and stressor-related disorders was created.

This diagnostic class relates to the cognitive, emotional, behavioral, physiological, and social responses to traumatic or stressful events. Exposure to a traumatic event can occur by direct experience, witnessing the event, learning that the event occurred to a close relative or close friend, or experiencing repeated contact with aversive details of the event (e.g., as for first responders). The responses to these events constitute a disorder when the stressor is extreme (i.e., exposure to actual or threatened death, serious injury, or sexual violation) and symptoms of intrusion, avoidance, negative alterations in cognitions and mood, and marked alterations in arousal begin or worsen after the traumatic event occurs. Some individuals will experience a dominance of anxiety or fear, others will experience anhedonia/dysphoria or arousal symptoms, and still others will experience a combination. Some will also experience dissociative symptoms. Importantly and as noted in DSM-5, cultural syndromes and idioms of distress may influence the way in which individuals respond to traumatic events and therefore need to be considered when establishing a diagnosis of acute stress disorder or posttraumatic stress disorder (PTSD).

The clinical expression of the reactivity to trauma varies across the lifespan. For instance, children younger than age 7 are more likely to express intrusion symptoms through play, whereas adults may experience prolonged psychological distress in response to a memory of the traumatic event. In DSM-5, separate criteria have been added for children 6 years or younger who have PTSD. Moreover, in DSM-IV, reactive attachment disorder had two subtypes, emotionally withdrawn/inhibited and indiscriminately social/disinhibited. In DSM-5, these prior subtypes now are defined as distinct disorders: reactive attachment disorder and disinhibited social engagement disorder, which result from social neglect or environments that prevent secure attachments to caregivers. Reactive attachment disorder is thought of as an internalizing disorder and is moderately associated with depression. In contrast, disinhibited social engagement disorder resembles an externalizing disorder, such as attention-deficit/hyperactivity disorder. Children with reactive attachment disorder have a lack of or incompletely formed attachments to caregiving adults, whereas children with disinhibited social engagement disorder may or may not have established attachments, including secure attachments.

Several changes were made to the criteria for PTSD in DSM-5 from the DSM-IV criteria. The events that qualify as Criterion A (the stressor criterion) are more explicit in DSM-5 as compared with DSM-IV. DSM-IV Criterion A2 (the subjective reaction) has been eliminated in DSM-5. The three major symptom clusters in DSM-IV (reexperiencing, avoidance, and arousal) have been expanded to four clusters in DSM-5 (reexperiencing, avoidance, persistent negative alterations in cognitions and mood, and alterations in arousal and reactivity). The persistent negative alterations in cognitions and mood cluster kept most of the DSM-IV numbing symptoms, but also includes newer symptoms such as persistent negative emotional states. Similarly, the arousal and reactivity cluster kept most of the DSM-IV arousal symptoms, but also includes irritable behavior or angry outbursts and reckless or self-destructive behavior. PTSD requires one or more intrusion symptoms and two or more symptoms of alterations in arousal and reactivity (e.g., hypervigilance, exaggerated startle response). For children ages 6 and younger, PTSD also requires at least one symptom of either avoidance or negative alterations in cognition and mood. For adults and children ages 7 and older, the diagnosis of PTSD requires one or more symptoms of persistent avoidance of reminders of the traumatic event, as well as two or more negative alterations in cognitions (e.g., inability to recall important aspects of the traumatic event; persistent and exaggerated beliefs or expectations about oneself, others, or the world) and in mood (e.g., persistent negative state; diminished interest or ability to experience happiness, satisfaction, or loving feelings).

The qualifying traumatic events were made explicit for acute stress disorder in DSM-5, and the criteria indicate whether the events were experienced directly, witnessed, or experienced indirectly. In addition, the DSM-IV Criterion A2 that characterized the subjective reaction to the trauma (e.g., fear, helplessness, or horror) has been eliminated. In DSM-5, acute stress disorder involves the presence of nine or more symptoms in any category of intrusion, negative mood, dissociative symptoms, avoidance symptoms, or arousal symptoms; these symptoms must be present at least 3 days after the traumatic event and can only be diagnosed up to 1 month after the event. The symptoms must cause clinically significant distress in social, occupational, or other important areas of psychosocial functioning.

In DSM-5, adjustment disorders are conceptualized as heterogeneous stress-response syndromes that occur after exposure to a distressing (traumatic or nontraumatic) event. This is in contrast to the DSM-IV conceptualization of adjustment disorders as residual categories for individuals who had clinically significant distress but whose symptoms did not meet criteria for a specific disorder. Adjustment disorders can be distinguished from acute stress disorder and PTSD in that individuals who have been exposed to a traumatic event do not meet full diagnostic criteria for acute stress disorder or PTSD. Moreover, for adjustment disorders, the type of stressor may not be considered traumatic, yet the distress is in excess of what would be considered culturally and contextually appropriate given the type of stressor that is present. As noted in DSM-5, adjustment disorders have the following specifiers: with depressed mood, with anxiety, with mixed anxiety and depressed mood, with disturbance of conduct, with mixed disturbance of emotions and conduct, and unspecified. Stressors can be single events (e.g., loss of job) or multiple events (e.g., death of a pet and marital problem). Adjustment disorders begin 3 months within the onset of a stressor and last no longer than 6 months after the termination of the stressor or its consequences. It is important to note that if the stressor or its consequences persist, the adjustment disorder may become chronic.

Other specified trauma- and stressor-related disorder is a diagnostic category including symptoms that are characteristic of trauma- and stressor-related disorders (e.g., PTSD, acute stress disorder, adjustment disorder) but that do not meet the full criteria for any of the disorders. As noted in DSM-5, this category is accompanied by the reason the symptoms do not meet the full criteria of any of the trauma- and stressor-related disorders. For example, persistent complex bereavement symptoms can be present for years after a loved one has died. Therefore, they do not meet the criteria for adjustment disorder because the symptoms are persisting for more than 6 months after the stressor or its consequences have ended.

Similar to other specified trauma- and stressor-related disorder, unspecified trauma- and stressor-related disorder causes clinically significant distress or impairment in social, occupational, or other important areas of functioning but does not meet the full criteria for any of the trauma- and stressor-related disorders. This category is used when a clinician decides not to specify the reason that the symptoms do not meet criteria for a specific disorder. Also, there may be circumstances when a clinician does not have sufficient information to provide a specific diagnosis (e.g., emergency room setting, language barriers).

Other disorders that involve clinically significant anxiety but that are not in the trauma- and stressor-related disorders diagnostic class include anxiety disorders, obsessive-compulsive and related disorders, and somatic symptom and related disorders (including illness anxiety disorder). Although there are similarities across these diagnoses, the diagnostic classes have been developed on the basis of unique characteristics of their respective disorders that set them apart from one another. For instance, panic disorder may include symptoms of avoidant behavior and fear-based anxiety; however, a person given this diagnosis has had no exposure to a traumatic event, and such exposure is required for a diagnosis of PTSD.

Working with individuals who have trauma- and stressor-related disorders requires an empathic, validating, and accepting clinical stance. For individuals who have experienced trauma, a sense of safety and control are primary psychiatric needs that affect mood, cognitions, behavior, and interpersonal relationships. For patients with a history of childhood sexual or physical abuse, interpersonal boundaries may be distorted such that relationships are too enmeshed or too disengaged. Thus, it is important for clinicians to accurately assess each individual's comfort with setting, enforcing, and maintaining healthy interpersonal boundaries across different relationships (e.g., colleagues, supervisors, children, romantic partners, parents, siblings, and strangers). A great deal of the distress that childhood trauma survivors experience occurs within interpersonal relationships as they attempt to feel safe and secure but do not know how to establish healthy boundaries with others.

IN-DEPTH DIAGNOSIS

Acute Stress Disorder and Posttraumatic Stress Disorder

Ms. Benitez, a 28-year-old married Hispanic woman who lives with her husband and 3-year-old daughter, presents to an outpatient mental health clinic with complaints of experiencing a "weird sensation, like I'm floating and not myself" whenever her husband kisses her. The sensation is so distressing that she pulls away from her husband, and at times she has even felt nauseated. During the initial evaluation, the therapist learns that 3 weeks ago, Ms. Benitez had been robbed by a man who walked up behind her in a parking lot, put a knife to her throat, and demanded her purse as she was getting into her car. Without turning around, she handed the man her purse. Upon grabbing the purse, the man licked her cheek, leaving saliva on her face. Since the incident, she has tried not to think about it and to "put it behind me." However, she has been experiencing disturbing dreams about the incident, and there were several times at work when she was bothered by "seeing the knife in my mind" while she was working on tasks that required concentration. She does not feel comfortable driving by herself anymore, and she has not gone back to the store where the incident occurred. She reports sleep disturbance and feels "jumpy all the time." Toward the end of the evaluation, she says, "Since that day, I just haven't been myself. I don't have patience with my daughter as I used to. I get angry really fast and just don't want to be around people anymore."

It is not uncommon for individuals who are victims of a violent crime to want to forget about it and avoid reminders of the incident. Ms. Benitez's symptoms are in response to a traumatic event and are within the time frame (3 days to 1 month) required to meet criteria for acute stress disorder. If her symptoms continue beyond 1 month, she should be reassessed to determine if she meets criteria for PTSD. Consistent with clinical presentation of acute stress disorder, she has a dissociative presentation (i.e., floating sensation) combined with a strong emotional and physiological reaction (i.e., pulling away from her husband when kissed and feeling nauseated) to a reminder of the traumatic event (i.e., being licked). Being both female and Hispanic increases her risk of acute stress disorder and PTSD.

Approach to the Diagnosis

As noted in DSM-5, the trauma- and stressor-related disorders chapter is new. Previously, acute stress disorder and PTSD were categorized as anxiety disorders. The change is based on the scientific literature, which indicates that the response to traumatic events is variable, with some individuals reporting symptoms consistent with anxiety and others reporting anhedonic and dysphoric symptoms or a combination. Therefore, categorizing acute stress disorder and PTSD as solely anxiety disorders was inaccurate.

When evaluating symptoms for a diagnosis of acute stress disorder or PTSD, the clinician must first make sure that a qualifying traumatic event, in accordance with DSM-5, accounts for the symptoms. Importantly, such symptoms include those that result from experiencing repeated or extreme exposure to aversive details of the event through electronic media, television, movies, or pictures, but only if the exposure is work related (e.g., for first responders, police officers). The criteria for what constitutes a traumatic event are now narrowly specified so that even if a person experiences a life-threatening illness, unless the threat to the person's life is imminent (e.g., suffocation), that threat does not meet criteria for what constitutes a traumatic event. Second, individuals no longer have to report that they experienced fear, helplessness, or horror in response to the traumatic event, so it is not necessary to validate this response during the evaluation. Third, the emphasis on dissociative symptoms in DSM-IV was found to be too restrictive, but a "with dissociative symptoms" specifier for PTSD is now included in DSM-5. To be diagnosed with acute stress disorder, an individual must endorse a minimum of nine symptoms of acute stress disorder across any of the categories of qualifying symptoms of intrusion, negative mood, dissociation, avoidance, and arousal. For PTSD, it is important to examine the number of symptoms within each category. For individuals ages 7 years and older, a PTSD diagnosis requires at least one intrusion symptom, at least one avoidance symptom, at least two symptoms of negative alterations in cognitions and mood associated with the traumatic event, and at least two symptoms of arousal and reactivity. For children ages 6 years and younger, a PTSD diagnosis requires at least one symptom of intrusion, at least one symptom of either avoidance or negative alterations in cognition, and at least two symptoms of arousal. There are some differences in how the symptom criteria are defined for children versus adults; for example, intrusion symptoms may be expressed as play reenactment in children. Also, acute stress disorder and PTSD require duration of disturbance criteria to be met, which is 3 days to 1 month for acute stress disorder and more than 1 month for PTSD.

As stated in DSM-5, "Traumatic events such as childhood abuse increase a person's suicide risk. PTSD is associated with suicidal ideation and suicide attempts, and presence of the disorder may indicate which individuals with ideation eventually make a suicide plan or actually attempt suicide" (p. 278).

Getting the History

Ms. Keane, a 28-year-old woman, is referred by her primary care physician to a psycho-therapist because of difficulty sleeping after being in a head-on car crash in which there was a fatality. Upon conducting an initial evaluation of Ms. Keane, the therapist asks, "Can you tell me when you had the car accident?" Ms. Keane responds, "Yes, 2 weeks ago." The therapist then says, "Can you tell me when you began to experience difficulty sleeping?" Ms. Keane responds, "About a week after the car accident." The therapist then replies, "I would like to understand more about your difficulty sleeping. Can you describe for me—with specific examples, if you can—what sleep difficulty you are ex-periencing?" Ms. Keane describes nightmares of reexperiencing the car accident that awaken her and disrupt her sleep. The therapist then asks more questions to under-stand what other symptoms may be present by asking if the accident has affected other parts of Ms. Keane 's life, such as the way she behaves, the way she interacts with oth-ers, the way she feels, or the way she thinks. The therapist then queries when these symptoms started and the duration of the symptoms. The therapist asks about any head trauma that may have occurred in the accident and, if the answer is yes, follows up with questions to rule out postconcussive symptoms. The therapist also asks about the history of other traumatic experiences to understand Ms. Keane's risk for ongoing trauma-related symptoms that may put her at risk to develop PTSD.

The therapist uses a combination of 1) direct, closed-ended questions to ascertain the timing of the traumatic event and the duration of symptoms and 2) open-ended questions to gain an understanding of the types of symptoms that are present and the degree to which they are interfering with Ms. Keane's psychosocial and physiological functioning. To develop an effective treatment plan, the therapist needs to rule out other comorbid diagnoses, such as depression or anxiety disorders. Given the strong emotional response that may be triggered by questions about the traumatic event, the therapist needs to pace Ms. Keane by being attentive to nonverbal responses and as-sess Ms. Keane's ability to regulate her emotional response to questions. For example, the therapist may notice Ms. Keane's breathing getting rapid as she recalls traumatic memories. The therapist may interrupt Ms. Keane and simply ask, "How are you do-ing? I noticed your breathing is getting rapid." Caretaking on the part of the therapist may also be welcomed by the patient and validates that the therapist understands how difficult the situation is for the individual. The therapist can achieve this caretak-ing by asking, "Would you care for any water?" or "Would you like to take a break?" Depending on the type of trauma experienced, the evaluation may need to occur over multiple sessions. To facilitate a safe environment for people to discuss horrific expe-riences, the therapist who works with people who have trauma-related symptoms must maintain an open, compassionate, and nonjudgmental stance.

Tips for Clarifying the Diagnosis

- Determine whether the person experienced one or more of the following events as described in DSM-5: death or threatened death, actual or threatened serious in-jury, or actual or threatened sexual violation.
- Consider whether the person experienced the traumatic event personally, witnessed the traumatic event, learned that a traumatic event happened to a close relative or

close friend in which the actual or threatened death was violent or accidental, or experienced repeated or extreme exposure to aversive details of the event.
- Assess whether the symptoms began after exposure to the traumatic event.
- Clarify whether the symptoms lasted at least 3 days and not more than 1 month (acute stress disorder) or longer than 1 month (PTSD).
- If stress reactions are in response to a stressor that is not considered severe or extreme, consider adjustment disorder as the more appropriate diagnosis.

Consider the Case

Mr. Cooper, a 32-year-old, single white man, describes an injury that he experienced while doing construction work in Iraq. He was in his office talking with coworkers and laughing at a joke one told when he heard a loud boom and sirens. He heard someone yell to get into the bunker, and then everyone started running. He was running toward the bunker when he fell to the ground, got up, and started running again. Once in the bunker he heard muffled voices, which slowly got louder, and he realized people were talking to him. He remembers saying, "I'm fine," and the next thing he knew he awoke in the hospital with bandages around his neck, arms, and legs. He had been shot multiple times, and shrapnel was embedded in his neck, affecting his ability to speak. He has had several surgeries, and a few more are scheduled, to remove the remaining shrapnel. It has been 8 months since the attack, and he reports that recently he started feeling "panicky and jumpy." He describes severe sleep disturbance with nightmares about the attack. He says everything around him seems surreal, like he is "an actor in a play" that he is watching. He finds loud noises to be particularly disturbing, causing panic attacks that make it difficult for him to leave his apartment. He reports no previous trauma history, and his childhood experiences are what would be considered normative and healthy.

Mr. Cooper describes the type and duration of symptoms that are consistent with PTSD with delayed expression. PTSD is characterized by the development of particular symptoms following exposure to events that involve threatened death, actual or threatened injury, or actual or threatened sexual violence. In this case, Mr. Cooper experienced the threat of injury and actual injury. The delay of symptoms at least 6 months after the event (i.e., 8 months in this case) is atypical. Given Mr. Cooper's complaints of derealization (e.g., he feels as if he is an actor in a play), it will be important to evaluate his symptoms for the dissociative subtype that occurs in individuals who experience high symptom severity. Additionally, it will be important to evaluate any negative alterations in cognitions and mood associated with the traumatic event that may need to be addressed in therapy. Furthermore, Mr. Cooper describes having panic attacks, but the symptoms to which he is referring are not clear. Therefore, a thorough evaluation of these symptoms is warranted, and if they occur after exposure to traumatic reminders, then the PTSD diagnosis is warranted. An additional diagnosis of panic attacks may be warranted if Mr. Cooper experiences panic attacks in circumstances other than being reminded of the traumatic event. According to DSM-5, the 12-month prevalence of PTSD is higher among adults in the United States than those in Europe and most Asian, African, and Latin American countries. Moreover, PTSD is higher among individuals whose jobs increase the risk of traumatic exposure, which is the case for Mr. Cooper.

Thus, Mr. Cooper's background and work place him at higher risk for developing PTSD. It is important to note that symptoms of intrusion vary across human development; as such, young children may start to experience nightmares that are not specific to the traumatic event.

Differential Diagnosis

Many life stressors can result in psychiatric symptoms that are acute or chronic, and not everyone who is exposed to an extreme stressor or traumatic event will meet all of the criteria for a diagnosis of PTSD or acute stress disorder. The diagnosis of adjustment disorders is used in these instances. A patient may be experiencing a high-conflict divorce that invokes feelings of panic, sleep disturbance, and dissociative symptoms. Although these symptoms are also found in individuals with PTSD and acute stress disorder, the event (i.e., divorce) does not meet the diagnostic criteria for a traumatic event.

Acute stress disorder can be differentiated from PTSD because the symptoms for acute stress disorder must occur within 4 weeks of the traumatic event, whereas PTSD is diagnosed when symptoms persist for longer than 1 month.

Other posttraumatic disorders and conditions should be considered instead of PTSD if the symptoms are not preceded by trauma exposure. Also, if the symptoms that occur in response to an extreme stressor meet criteria for another mental disorder, then the other diagnosis is given instead of or in addition to PTSD.

In obsessive-compulsive disorder, there are recurrent thoughts similar to the reexperiencing symptoms in trauma-related disorders; however, the distinguishing feature is that in obsessive-compulsive disorder, the thoughts are not related to a traumatic event. Similarly, the arousal and dissociative symptoms of panic disorder as well as the avoidance, irritability, and anxiety of generalized anxiety disorder are not associated with a specific traumatic event. In separation anxiety disorder, the symptoms associated with separation are not considered to be a traumatic event.

Major depression can be preceded by a traumatic event and should be diagnosed if other PTSD symptoms are absent. Importantly, major depressive disorder does not include Criterion B or C symptoms required for PTSD. Also, several of the Criterion D and E symptoms found in PTSD are absent in major depressive disorder.

Personality disorders may have developed or be greatly exacerbated as a result of exposure to a traumatic event or multiple traumatic events and may be indicative of PTSD. Personality disorders are expected to occur independently of trauma exposure.

Dissociative symptoms such as those seen in dissociative amnesia, dissociative identity disorder, and depersonalization/derealization disorder can be preceded by a traumatic event and may have co-occurring PTSD symptoms. When the full criteria for PTSD diagnosis are met, then PTSD with dissociative symptoms subtype should be considered.

Conversion disorder (functional neurological symptom disorder) may be better diagnosed as PTSD if the somatic symptoms occur after exposure to a traumatic event.

Flashbacks or the reexperiencing of traumatic events found in PTSD need to be differentiated from illusions, hallucinations, and other perceptual symptoms that occur in schizophrenia, brief psychotic disorder, and other psychotic disorders; depressive and bipolar disorders with psychotic features; delirium; substance/medication-induced disorders; and psychotic disorder due to a medical condition. Acute stress disorder flashbacks are directly related to the traumatic event and occur in the absence of other psychotic or substance-induced features.

In patients with bodily injury resulting in a traumatic brain injury (TBI), symptoms of acute stress disorder and PTSD may occur. Importantly, postconcussive syndromes (e.g., headaches, dizziness, memory problems, irritability, concentration problems) may occur in conjunction with acute stress disorder or PTSD. Also, patients with TBI may have dissociative symptoms (e.g., altered sense of awareness, memory problems), which are difficult to distinguish from symptoms of acute stress disorder and PTSD. Symptoms of reexperiencing and avoidance are characteristic of PTSD and acute stress disorder, whereas persistent disorientation and confusion tend to be more specific to TBI. Moreover, acute stress disorder symptoms persist for up to 1 month following trauma exposure, whereas TBI symptoms may last for years and in some cases for the rest of an individual's life.

In some persons with acute stress disorder or PTSD, dissociative symptoms or behavior that appears detached may predominate. Dissociative states may be short-lived—lasting for only a few seconds or minutes—or long lasting, persisting for days. Anger, irritability, or aggressive behavior can also be strongly manifested in persons with acute stress disorder or PTSD. The symptoms of intrusion may not be of the event itself, but may be in response to specific aspects of the event, such as reacting to seeing a sport-utility vehicle that is a reminder of where a rape occurred.

Feelings of panic are common in acute stress disorder. Panic disorder should be diagnosed only if the panic attacks are unexpected and there is anxiety about future panic attacks or the individual engages in maladaptive behavior in an effort to thwart what is thought to be disastrous consequences of a panic attack (e.g., death, severe embarrassment).

See DSM-5 for additional disorders to consider in the differential diagnosis. Also refer to the discussions of comorbidity and differential diagnosis in their respective sections of DSM-5.

Summary

- Acute stress disorder and PTSD require exposure to an event involving actual, threatened, or witnessed death, serious injury, or sexual violation. In cases of actual or threatened death of a family member or friend, the event(s) must have been violent or accidental.
- Exposure to the traumatic event can occur in one or more of the following ways: personal experience, witnessing it, learning that it occurred to a close relative or close friend, or repeated exposure to aversive details of an event that is work related.
- In acute stress disorder, nine or more symptoms occur in any of five categories: intrusion, negative mood, dissociation, avoidance, and arousal.
- In PTSD, individuals ages 7 years and older must experience one or more intrusive symptoms, one or more avoidance symptoms, two or more negative alterations in cognitions or mood, and two or more arousal symptoms. Children ages 6 and

younger must experience one or more intrusion symptoms, one or more symptoms of avoidance and/or negative alterations in cognitions or mood, and two or more arousal symptoms.

- The duration of symptoms is 3 days to 1 month for acute stress disorder, and greater than 1 month for PTSD.
- In acute stress disorder and PTSD, the symptoms cause significant distress or impairment in social, occupational, or other important psychosocial areas of functioning.
- In acute stress disorder and PTSD, the symptoms are not associated with the direct physiological effects of a substance or medical condition.
- Variability in the expression of symptoms in reaction to traumatic events may be influenced by age, cultural syndromes and idioms of distress, co-occurring traumatic brain injury, preexisting mental health disorders, and medical conditions.

—————— **IN-DEPTH DIAGNOSIS** ——————
Adjustment Disorders

Ms. Meyers, a 48-year-old married woman who was diagnosed with breast cancer 6 weeks ago, was referred to an outpatient mental health clinic for an evaluation of what her oncologist described as "anxiety symptoms." She has two children, ages 10 and 13. During the psychiatric intake evaluation, she describes difficulty she has been having with sleep since her diagnosis. She also reports experiencing a racing heart, sweating, and nausea when she has to see her oncologist, resulting in several missed appointments. When asked what stage of breast cancer she has, she is unable to answer, replying, "I don't know. There are stages?" When asked what treatment her physician is recommending, she replies, "I don't know; he said something about surgery." She has a difficult time recalling her conversations with her physician and states that she often "goes blank" when she is in his office, resulting in her not engaging with her physician regarding her care and experiencing difficulty recalling recommendations. She reports feeling "down" since the diagnosis and unable to stop thinking about having cancer. She stopped going to her job of over 15 years and has been unable to take her children to school, stating she has been "too depressed." She cannot turn to her husband for support because she does not want to upset him.

Ms. Meyers has developed emotional and behavioral (e.g., missing appointments) symptoms in response to her cancer diagnosis within 3 months of learning about it. The symptoms are clinically significant such that she is experiencing significant impairment in her occupational role (e.g., not going to work) and social relationships (e.g., disengaging from family responsibilities and from her husband emotionally). Her symptoms have features that are consistent with adjustment disorder with features of PTSD. Her experiences of "going blank" when she is in her doctor's office and not recalling her physician's recommendations can be viewed as dissociative symptoms associated with a diagnosis of PTSD, except that a diagnosis of breast cancer does not meet DSM-5 criteria for a traumatic event. Additionally, she is experiencing symptoms consistent with the depressed mood specifier. Adjustment disorders can complicate the course of illness and influence medical outcomes. In this case, Ms. Meyers is missing appointments and experiencing dissociative symptoms during visits with her physician that prevent her from engaging in her treatment.

Approach to the Diagnosis

The key to diagnosing adjustment disorder is to evaluate the presence of an identifiable stressor. The onset of emotional or behavioral symptoms must occur within 3 months of exposure to the stressor. The symptoms must meet a clinical threshold as indicated by distress that is in excess of what would be expected, and/or the patient has significant impairment in psychosocial functioning (e.g., social, occupational). It is important to determine that the stressor does not meet criteria for another specific psychiatric disorder and is not an exacerbation of a preexisting psychiatric disorder. The symptoms of adjustment disorders do not persist for more than 6 months once the stressor and its consequences are no longer present.

Adjustment disorder can be specified with depressed mood, anxiety, mixed anxiety and depressed mood, conduct disturbance, and mixed conduct and emotional disturbance. There also may be unspecified symptoms, such as physical complaints, social withdrawal, or academic problems.

Adjustment disorder can accompany many other psychiatric diagnoses, such as depressive or bipolar disorders. It can also accompany any medical illness.

An adjustment disorder is an acute form if the symptoms are present for 6 months or less or a persistent form if the symptoms persist for more than 6 months. It is important to note that symptoms cannot persist for more than 6 months after a stressor is no longer present; however, this does not mean that an initial stressor cannot lead to other stressful events, resulting in a continuous or chronic course. For example, the death of a spouse may lead to financial stress, which may in turn lead to the loss of a home; if warranted, the diagnosis of adjustment disorder can continue to be given during this sequence of events.

As stated in DSM-5, "Adjustment disorders are associated with an increased risk of suicide attempts and completed suicide" (p. 287).

Getting the History

> Darryl, a 10-year-old boy, is brought to the clinic by his mother because he has been suspended from school for vandalism. Darryl has been carving his name into the desks at school and was found using markers to write on the walls in the bathroom. He has also been talking back to his teachers, and his excessive talking is disruptive to the other students in his class. He has been picking fights with his 7-year-old sister and has been engaging in frequent angry outbursts with his mother. Darryl's mother started having discipline problems at home shortly after she and Darryl's father separated and she moved into a new home, 2 months earlier. The recent move meant that Darryl had to attend a different school across town from the friends with whom he had grown up.

When evaluating a young child, the clinician needs to conduct a comprehensive assessment of the child's medical and psychiatric history with the parents or guardians to understand the nature, duration, and scope of the emotional and behavioral problems. It is important to rule out any medical basis for the symptoms and to make sure the child's symptoms are not an exacerbation of a preexisting psychiatric diagnosis.

In Darryl's case it may be difficult to determine whether the stressor was the separation of the parents, the transfer to a new school, both, or some other related stressor. Stressors can be concurrent, and there might be multiple stressors. The stressors in this case do not meet criteria for a traumatic event; however, Darryl is definitely experiencing marked distress that is causing serious emotional and behavioral disruptions. The stressors of his parents' separation and his subsequent move have both occurred recently, so if Darryl's behavioral symptoms have arisen in reaction to one or both of these stressors, the diagnosis of adjustment disorder could be made, because the onset of the symptoms would clearly be within 3 months of the onset of the stressor(s). It would be important to inquire about the meaning of these stressors for Darryl in order to understand how they are linked to his functioning. Given Darryl's behavior at school and home, it would also be important to determine whether the criteria are met for adjustment disorder with disturbance of conduct.

Tips for Clarifying the Diagnosis

- Establish that the person's symptoms are in response to an identifiable stressor that is not considered a traumatic stressor.
- Verify that the person has developed symptoms within 3 months of the onset of the stressor.
- Assess whether the symptoms are in excess of what would be expected within the context of cultural or religious norms.
- Consider whether the symptoms persist for less than 6 months once the stressor and its consequences cease.

Consider the Case

Ms. Carter is a 32-year-old, single black woman who is seeking services at an outpatient mental health clinic, has feelings of irritability and anxiety. At times, she engages in verbal rages with coworkers and her boyfriend, followed by feelings of sadness and hopelessness. Recently, disciplinary action was administered to Ms. Carter at work for disrespectful communication and excessive absences. Ms. Carter has been working at a midsize company for the past 5 years where she has been quite successful, working her way up from an entry-level administrative position to a program manager position in a relatively short period of time. Ms. Carter states that she was recently "employee of the year" and had won numerous awards for excellence at her job. This changed 2 months ago when Ms. Carter was not selected for a director position at her company. The person who was promoted was a woman Ms. Carter had trained. Ms. Carter states that she is constantly thinking about not getting the promotion and replaying in her mind the day she found out she did not get the position. During the intake interview, Ms. Carter states that she has been thinking that "my life is falling apart, and it would be so much easier if I wasn't around." Ms. Carter is convinced that if things do not change, she will lose her job and her boyfriend.

After someone devotes a great deal of time and effort to his or her career, it is understandable that when promotions or advancements do not occur that feelings of anger, sadness, disbelief, and irritability can develop. However, when symptoms persist beyond what would be expected, causing profound impairment in social, occupational, or other important areas, the individual may have an adjustment disorder. Assessing the length of time since the stressor occurred is important, because to meet criteria for adjustment disorder, the symptoms must develop within 3 months of the onset of the stressor and persist for less than 6 months once the stressor and its consequences have ended. Additionally, the stressor is not considered a traumatic event. In this case, Ms. Carter is experiencing marked impairment in her occupational and interpersonal relationships. Her reaction is clinically significant and out of proportion to the severity or intensity of the stressor (i.e., not getting promoted). It will be important to get a thorough mental health history on Ms. Carter to make sure that her symptoms are not an exacerbation of a preexisting psychiatric disorder. The nature, meaning, and experience of the stressor by Ms. Carter will be important to understand because there may be culture-related factors (e.g., actual or perceived discrimination) that are contributing to Ms. Carter's distress. Understanding the cultural context that Ms. Carter is functioning in will assist the clinician in determining whether Ms. Carter's symptoms are beyond what would be expected.

Importantly, adjustment disorders are associated with an increased risk of suicide and suicide attempts and therefore require a thorough risk assessment and plan. This is particularly true in this case because Ms. Carter has expressed a cognitive belief consistent with suicide ideation that requires a thorough assessment, evaluation, and treatment plan to ensure her safety.

Differential Diagnosis

In DSM-5, the symptom profile for major depressive disorder, even in response to a stressor, differentiates it from adjustment disorder. Therefore, if an individual meets criteria for major depressive disorder, he or she would not be diagnosed with adjustment disorder.

Adjustment disorder can be differentiated from PTSD and acute stress disorder by the type of stressor. In adjustment disorder the stressor does not meet the Criterion A requirements found in PTSD and acute stress disorder. Moreover, adjustment disorders can be diagnosed immediately and persist up to 6 months after exposure to the stressor, whereas acute stress disorder occurs within 3 days and 1 month of a traumatic event and PTSD is diagnosed 1 month after exposure to a traumatic event. An adjustment disorder should be considered when an individual does not meet the full diagnostic requirements for PTSD or acute stress disorder.

Differentiating personality disorders from an adjustment disorder requires a thorough evaluation of lifetime psychiatric symptoms and functioning. To diagnose an adjustment disorder when a personality disorder is present, it is important to assess if the symptoms for adjustment disorder are met. Also, the distress response has to exceed what is recognized as personality disorder symptoms.

In DSM-5, psychological factors affecting other medical conditions include behaviors and other factors that exacerbate a medical condition, whereas adjustment disorder is a psychological reaction to the stressor (e.g., medical condition). Adjustment disorder can accompany any medical illness. An adjustment disorder may complicate the course of medical illness; therefore, behaviors such as missing appointments, noncompliance, and complicated interactions with medical staff may warrant an assessment of adjustment disorder.

Adjustment disorder can be distinguished from normative stress reactions by assessing the magnitude of the distress. Clinicians should evaluate whether the distress response (e.g., mood, behavior, functioning) exceeds what would normally be expected in response to the stressful event. Considerations of cultural factors are important when making determinations of normative reactions.

See DSM-5 for additional disorders to consider in the differential diagnosis. Also refer to the discussions of comorbidity and differential diagnosis in their respective sections of DSM-5.

Summary

- In adjustment disorders, symptoms develop in response to identifiable stressors that do not meet criteria for a traumatic event.
- The symptoms occur within 3 months of exposure to the stressors.
- The symptoms are characterized by marked distress in excess of what would be considered normative and culturally appropriate.
- The symptoms do not persist for more than 6 months.

--- **SUMMARY** ---

Trauma- and Stressor-Related Disorders

Reactions to traumatic events and life stress vary depending on the type of stress, the individual, and the cultural context. The diagnostic class of trauma- and stressor-related disorders includes disorders with traumatic, life-threatening stressors, as well as stressors that vary in severity. The key to these disorders is that the symptoms are in response to identifiable stressor(s). Reactive attachment disorder and disinhibited social engagement disorder are considered to be responses to having experienced a pattern of insufficient care, even if the child is currently being reared in a normative caregiving setting. Adjustment disorders occur when a person has responses to a nontraumatic event that are considered to be excessive or that cause impairment in social, occupational, or other domains of functioning. Acute stress disorder and PTSD occur in response to traumatic events.

The trauma- and stressor-related disorders have similarities with anxiety disorders and obsessive-compulsive and related disorders but differ in the course and duration of symptoms, prevalence, and age at onset. Reactive attachment disorder and disinhibited social engagement disorder are diagnosed in children and adolescents and are relatively rare. Adjustment disorders are relatively common and are associated with increased risk of suicide and suicide attempts. All of the trauma- and stressor-related disorders are serious and cause marked disruption in psychosocial functioning. For individuals with medical illness, these disorders can alter the course of their illness, thereby increasing morbidity and mortality.

--- ■ ■ ■ ---

Diagnostic Pearls

- The trauma- and stressor-related disorders diagnostic class includes disorders in which exposure to a traumatic or stressful event must precede the onset of symptoms. These disorders are no longer part of the anxiety disorders class because of the variability in response to traumatic or stressful events. For instance, some individuals may have anxiety- or fear-based symptoms, whereas others may experience anhedonic or dysphoric symptoms.

- In acute stress disorder and PTSD, traumatic events may be experienced directly or indirectly, threatened, or witnessed.

- Exposure to an event through electronic media, television, movies, or pictures does not meet criteria for an event that can trigger acute stress disorder or PTSD unless this exposure is work related.

- Acute stress disorder can be diagnosed 3 days after a traumatic event and may progress to a diagnosis of PTSD after 1 month if the symptoms persist.

- Emotional undermodulation is characterized by reexperiencing and hyperarousal in acute stress disorder and PTSD.

- The absence of necessary and appropriate caregiving during childhood is a requirement for reactive attachment disorder and disinhibited social engagement disorder. The former is expressed as an internalizing disorder with depressive symptoms and withdrawn behavior, whereas the latter is marked by disinhibition and externalizing behavior.

- Adjustment disorder can accompany any medical disorder and most psychiatric disorders.

Self-Assessment

Key Concepts: Double-Check Your Knowledge

What is the relevance of the following concepts to the various trauma- and stressor-related disorders?

- Traumatic event
- Stressors
- Avoidance
- Negative alterations in cognitions and mood
- Hypervigilance
- Sleep disturbance
- Marked distress in excess of what would be expected
- Markedly disturbed and developmentally inappropriate attachment behaviors

Questions to Discuss With Colleagues and Mentors

1. How do you determine if a response is normative or appropriate in different cultural contexts when trying to determine if a patient's symptoms meet criteria for adjustment disorder?
2. If adjustment disorder symptoms persist for more than 6 months and do not meet criteria for differential diagnoses, what diagnosis would you consider?

Case-Based Questions

PART A

Ms. Walker, a 38-year-old, HIV-positive woman, describes using alcohol and cocaine since she was in high school to "deal with stress." She describes "being on edge" all the time and "always jumping out of my skin." An uncle who came to live with her mother sexually molested her when she was between ages 5 and 9 years. She reports experiencing nightmares about her abuse and having difficulty trusting others. She often misses her medical appointments because she does not like being in a waiting room with "people I don't know." She describes her heart racing, palms sweating, and difficulty breathing when she is in the waiting room and states that this happens when she is in a closed area around people she does not know. She worries about her HIV disease and is afraid to be in a relationship because she does not want to transmit the virus to anyone. Therefore, she avoids being around people and is finding it difficult to leave her house. She is feeling hopeless and "down" about her situation.

Thinking about the stressors Ms. Walker has experienced, what diagnosis or diagnoses might best capture the symptoms and behaviors she described? Ms. Walker may have PTSD associated with her childhood sexual abuse and adjustment disorder with mixed anxiety and depressed mood associated with her HIV disease.

Ms. Walker says she is using alcohol and cocaine to cope with her stress. It will be important to understand the signs, symptoms, and causes of Ms. Walker's "stress." Ms. Walker needs to be asked directly what she means by *stress* and to describe her symptoms in detail. These questions are necessary to develop an understanding of the duration of her symptoms and the corresponding stressors that exacerbate her symptoms, as well as to appropriately diagnose her condition.

PART B

Ms. Walker's CD_4 T-cells start declining, and her viral load increases. She is hospitalized with pneumonia. Once stabilized and released from the hospital, she begins to increase her alcohol and cocaine use to cope with the fear that her hospitalization evoked. After she enters into therapy that focuses on her childhood sexual abuse, her panic symptoms subside, and she is able to go to her medical appointments. As she begins to interact with her physician and understand her HIV disease, she goes into a detox program. She finds a community organization for women living with HIV and begins attending support groups that reduce her isolation.

Given that the co-occurrence of psychiatric symptoms and medical illness can complicate the course of both, how would you begin to work with Ms. Walker? Missing medical appointments to manage her HIV compromised Ms. Walker's health. Her panic symptoms were in response to memories of her sexual abuse (i.e., being in a closed room with people she does not know reminds her of her relationship with her uncle). This case illustrates the complexity of childhood sexual abuse and comorbid medical illness. It can be difficult to know what the antecedent is to a particular stress response. A careful evaluation that explores the history of the symptoms, including the duration and contextual cues that trigger a stress response, is necessary for developing an effective course of treatment.

Short-Answer Questions

1. For acute stress disorder, what is the duration of the symptoms after exposure to the traumatic event?
2. For PTSD, what is the duration of symptoms after exposure to the traumatic event?
3. True or False: Acute stress disorder and PTSD are more common among men than women.
4. For adjustment disorder, how long can the symptoms persist?
5. Acute stress disorder symptoms occur in five categories: intrusion, negative mood, dissociation, avoidance, and arousal. How many symptoms across any of these five categories are necessary to meet criteria?
6. How many symptoms of intrusion are required for PTSD?
7. How many symptoms of avoidance are required for PTSD in individuals ages 7 years or older?
8. For adults, how many symptoms of negative alterations in cognitions and mood are required for PTSD?
9. How many symptoms of arousal and reactivity are required for PTSD?
10. Adjustment disorders often complicate medical illness. What percentage of people in a hospital psychiatric consultation setting are typically diagnosed with an adjustment disorder?

Answers

1. In acute stress disorder, the duration of the symptoms after exposure to the traumatic event is 3 days to 1 month.
2. In PTSD, the duration of symptoms after exposure to the traumatic event is longer than 1 month.
3. False. Acute stress disorder and PTSD are more common among women.
4. In adjustment disorder, symptoms can persist for no more than 6 months.
5. Nine or more symptoms across any of the five categories are necessary to meet criteria for acute stress disorder.
6. One or more symptoms of intrusion are required for PTSD.
7. One or more symptoms of avoidance are required for PTSD in individuals ages 7 years or older.
8. Two or more symptoms of negative alterations in cognitions and mood are required for PTSD in adults.
9. Two or more symptoms of arousal and reactivity are required for PTSD.
10. As many as 50% percent of people in a hospital psychiatric consultation setting may be diagnosed with an adjustment disorder.

Dissociative Disorders

David Spiegel, M.D.
Daphne Simeon, M.D.

"Sometimes I must have lapses of memory."

"Sometimes I feel as if I'm watching myself."

The dissociative disorders all reflect a disruption of the normal integration of consciousness, memory, identity, emotion, perception, body representation, motor control, and/or behavior. This diagnostic class includes dissociative identity disorder, dissociative amnesia, depersonalization/derealization disorder, other specified dissociative disorder, and unspecified dissociative disorder. Dissociative symptoms are experienced as intrusions into awareness and behavior, with loss of continuity in subjective experience (i.e., "positive" dissociative symptoms, such as identity disruption) and/or inability to access information or to control mental functions that normally are readily amenable to access or control (i.e., "negative" dissociative symptoms, such as amnesia or depersonalized detachment).

The dissociative disorders are more frequently observed in the aftermath of trauma, including childhood maltreatment, such as sexual and physical abuse. In keeping with such a history, many of the symptoms are deliberately hidden or confusing to individuals, making careful diagnostic evaluation critical. Stress often exacerbates dissociative symptoms.

Changes from DSM-IV to DSM-5 include the following:

- Dissociative identity disorder now refers to both possession and identity fragmentation, to make the disorder more applicable to culturally diverse situations within the United States and around the world than the DSM-IV version.
- Dissociative amnesia now includes dissociative fugue as a specifier, so fugue is no longer a separate disorder. Fugue is a rare condition and always involves amnesia.
- Depersonalization disorder has been revised in DSM-5 to include derealization because depersonalization and derealization often co-occur.
- In the DSM-5 chapter on trauma- and stressor-related disorders, the subtype "with dissociative symptoms" is included for posttraumatic stress disorder (PTSD), defined by the presence of depersonalization or derealization in addition to the other symptoms meeting PTSD criteria, such as dissociative flashbacks. Neuroimaging data suggest that these dissociative symptoms of PTSD involve increased frontal and inhibited limbic activity—that is, an overmodulation of affective response.

In DSM-5, dissociative identity disorder is characterized by the presence of two or more distinct personality states or an experience of possession and by recurrent episodes of amnesia for everyday events, personal information, or traumatic experiences. Individuals with dissociative identity disorder experience the following related symptoms:

- Recurrent, unexplained intrusions into their conscious functioning and sense of self (e.g., voices related to dissociated aspects of identity; dissociated actions and speech; intrusive thoughts, emotions, and impulses)
- Alterations in their sense of self (e.g., shifts in attitudes or preferences, and feeling as if their body or actions are not their own)
- Changes in perception (e.g., depersonalization or derealization, such as feeling detached from their body while cutting)
- Intermittent functional neurological symptoms

Dissociative amnesia is identified by an inability to recall autobiographical information that is inconsistent with normal forgetting. This inability may be localized (e.g., to an event or period of time), selective (e.g., to a specific aspect of an event), or generalized (e.g., to identity and life history). Dissociative amnesia may or may not involve purposeful travel or bewildered wandering. If it does, it is identified with a subtype of dissociative fugue. Although dissociative amnesia occurs in dissociative identity disorder, the type and frequency of amnesia differ between these disorders. Some individuals with dissociative amnesia notice that they have "lost time" or that they have a gap in their memory, whereas many others are unaware of their amnesias: they have amnesia for amnesia. For them, awareness of amnesia occurs only when personal identity is fragmented or when circumstances make these individuals aware that autobiographical information is missing (e.g., when they discover evidence of events they cannot recall or when others tell them or ask them about events they cannot recall).

Depersonalization/derealization disorder is defined by clinically significant chronic or recurrent depersonalization (i.e., experiences of unreality or detachment from one's mind, feelings, self, or body) and/or derealization (i.e., experiences of unreality or detachment from one's surroundings). Several types of depersonalization/ derealization symptoms include the following: numbing (emotional and/or physical), unreality of self (e.g., not having a self, feeling like a robot or a zombie), unreality of surroundings (e.g., feeling visually altered, foggy, dreamy), temporal disintegration (i.e., a distorted sense of the passing of time and connectedness to one's autobiographical memories), and perceptual alterations (e.g., visual, auditory, or tactile distortions; altered bodily sensations; out-of-body experiences). The major change from DSM-IV is that individuals with this disorder can have symptoms of depersonalization, derealization, or both; previously, individuals with derealization alone were classified separately. DSM-5 also provides a richer and fuller symptom description in the disorder's criteria.

Other specified dissociative disorder comprises four examples:

1. Chronic or recurrent mixed dissociative symptoms below the threshold for the diagnostic criteria for dissociative identity disorder
2. Identity disturbance due to prolonged and intense coercive persuasion
3. Acute dissociative reactions to stressful events
4. Dissociative trance

IN-DEPTH DIAGNOSIS

Depersonalization/Derealization Disorder

Ms. Day was a 20-year-old college freshman when she first presented to her school's mental health clinic complaining of feeling "very strange and out of it." She described that over the past 5 months she had started to feel increasingly detached from her body, as if she had no self, and her mind felt blank. She went about her daily activities like a robot, becoming less academically and interpersonally adept over time. At extreme moments she felt uncertain if she were alive or dead, as if her existence were a dream; these experiences terrified her.

When asked by the school counselor, she denied any other unusual thoughts or experiences or hearing voices or being fearful of others. She admitted to feeling depressed over a recent breakup with her boyfriend. During this time she first began to notice some feelings of numbness and unreality, but she did not pay much attention. As her low mood resolved over several months, she found herself becoming increasingly disconnected and became worried enough to finally seek help. She told the counselor that her 6-month romantic relationship with her boyfriend had been very meaningful to her and that she had been planning to introduce him to her family soon.

Ms. Day denied ever having been depressed before, any history of hypomania or psychosis, and any other past psychiatric symptoms other than a time-limited bout of extreme anxiety and panic attacks in ninth grade precipitated by the psychiatric hospitalization of her mother. When her mother returned from the hospital, all Ms. Day's symptoms cleared fairly rapidly. She also admitted to several days of transient unreality symptoms in elementary school, when her parents separated, her father left, and Ms. Day lived alone with her mother, who had paranoid schizophrenia.

Ms. Day's childhood was significant for pervasive aloneness and the sense that she not only raised herself but also had to parent her ill mother. Her mother did not abuse her but neglected Ms. Day's emotional needs and frightened her with her own limitations. Although Ms. Day largely kept to herself as a child, she did well in school and had a few close friends. She was deeply ashamed of her mother and rarely brought friends home; this boyfriend would have been the first to meet her mother. Ms. Day told the school counselor that it felt as if a switch had gone off in her brain; she was so preoccupied by the seeming physicality of her symptoms that she was referred for routine labs, otolaryngology and ophthalmology evaluations, brain magnetic resonance imaging, and electroencephalography (EEG). When all tests came back normal, she was referred to a psychiatrist. She also denied using any illicit substances, in particular cannabis, hallucinogens, ketamine, or salvia, and her urine toxicology was negative.

Ms. Day's preliminary diagnosis is depersonalization/derealization disorder. She is experiencing a variety of symptoms, such as detachment from her physical body, mind, and emotions, and she has a pervasive sense of "no self," the cardinal symptom after which the disorder is named. Although she has had two previous minor bouts of such symptoms in her lifetime, those do not qualify for the diagnosis. The first bout was too short to meet criteria for "persistent or recurrent" symptoms; although DSM-5 does not specify a minimal duration for symptoms, most clinicians follow the rough guideline of at least 1 month in duration. Ms. Day's brief bout was triggered by a severe emotional stressor, one of the more common precipitants of the disorder in large samples. The second bout of symptoms occurred in the context of escalating panic attacks probably meeting criteria for panic disorder, again precipitated by a severe emotional stressor. Although the symptoms were recurrent and occurred over a couple of months, they did not meet criteria for depersonalization/derealization disorder because they occurred exclusively in the context of another psychiatric disorder and lifted with the resolution of that disorder. In contrast, Ms. Day's third bout was of several months' duration after the resolution of the short-lived depressive episode, increasing in intensity, distress, and impairment over time, and causes from medical conditions or illicit substances were ruled out. Of note, her second bout of symptoms (during the panic disorder phase) was more heavily weighted toward derealization, whereas the third and clinically diagnostic bout was more heavily weighted toward depersonalization.

Approach to the Diagnosis

A very careful history of symptoms is central to making an accurate diagnosis of depersonalization/derealization disorder. Most patients with the disorder have been previously misdiagnosed. The symptoms are very subtle and subjective in nature, often with no observable signs, and individuals can find the symptoms very difficult to put into words. Clinicians need to encourage patients to describe their symptoms to the fullest, and address patients' fears that they sound "crazy" and that they have never heard of or known of anyone with similar experiences. For clinicians who are not readily familiar with the whole range of symptoms, a thorough assessment scale (e.g., the Cambridge Depersonalisation Scale) can be a very helpful guide. All major symptom domains need to be covered, including the sense of absence of core self and agency; the pervasive experience of unreality and detachment from self and surroundings; the numbing in the emotional and physical sphere; the disconnection and deadness of feelings; the detachment from mental content/thoughts; the perceptual alterations in all sensory modalities (visual, auditory, and tactile alterations are most common, but changes also occur in taste, smell, hunger, thirst, and libido); and the temporal disintegration (altered sense of time—past, present, and future; detachment from autobiographical memories as if they are not owned).

The onset and duration of symptoms must also be carefully assessed, as well as the frequency and duration of actual episodes and any change in all of these patterns over time. If there are psychiatric comorbidities, a thorough past and present history of the relationship of the depersonalization/derealization disorder symptoms to all other psychiatric symptoms must be assessed.

One important differential diagnosis to consider is that of a psychotic disorder or prodrome. This consideration is particularly important for Ms. Day because her mother suffered from schizophrenia. There is no suggestion, however, that Ms. Day is suffering from a schizophrenia spectrum disorder. Before the onset of her symptoms, she had a lifetime history of high academic and social functioning, unlike her mother. More important, there was no evidence of any schizophrenia spectrum symptoms at presentation, and the distortions in the experience of reality (rather than reality in and of itself) were only subjective in nature ("as if"), and Ms. Day had full cognitive awareness of this fact (intact reality testing). Finally, Ms. Day, like many others with this disorder, was initially strongly convinced about the "physical" nature of her suffering. This focus on a physical source is a common feature of the disorder's presentation, but individuals never have a delusional elaboration on the nature of the physical source. In this context, individuals commonly receive varying degrees of medical workups, often more extensive than is needed, especially if they are young with no atypical aspects to their presentation and no other pertinent risk factors. Such workups may be of value for their reassuring effect and may help individuals begin to come to terms with a psychiatric diagnosis that they may never have heard of and that is much less known than anxiety or depression.

Getting the History

The interviewer asks individuals to describe the nature of their symptoms, encouraging them to put their experiences into words and to elaborate as best they can, because the symptoms of depersonalization/derealization disorder can be very difficult to describe. After asking open-ended questions, the interviewer inquires more specifically about symptoms in all the previously described domains, including unreality of self, unreality of surroundings, physical and emotional numbing, perceptual alterations, and temporal distortions. It is important to elicit the time frame for onset of symptoms and, especially if the symptoms were initially transient as can sometimes be the case, to find out when they became clearly persistent, recurrent, and associated with significant distress and dysfunction. A goal is to obtain all other past and present psychiatric history, and to clearly ascertain the relationship of other psychiatric syndromes to the depersonalization/derealization disorder syndrome, both in the past and in the present. If it is difficult to determine whether depersonalization/derealization disorder is the primary current diagnosis, the interviewer further teases out whether the comorbid conditions are largely resolved, clearly of lesser proportion to the depersonalization/derealization disorder symptoms, or clearly secondary sequelae to the onset of depersonalization/derealization disorder. Table 11–1 provides some helpful prompts and questions, worded simply and in lay terms, to elicit more information.

TABLE 11–1.   Helpful prompts and questions for the clinical interview

I know these experiences are very hard to put into words. Do your best. You are doing a good job. Please say more.

Do you feel unreal, almost as if you no longer have a self or have lost yourself?

Do you feel detached from your feelings, as if you cannot feel, even though you know you have them?

Do you feel disconnected from your mind as if it were blank or you have no thoughts?

Do you feel detached from parts of your body or your whole body?

Does your voice sound as if it were not you speaking or choosing the words?

Do your past memories feel very remote and difficult to evoke?

Has your sense of passing time been affected?

Do you feel robotic, as though you are on automatic pilot, going through the motions?

Do your bodily sensations feel dulled?

Do things around you look as if you are seeing them through a veil or fog, or as if they are dreamy or unreal?

Do things look different visually, such as too sharp or too blurry, too two-dimensional or three-dimensional, too close up or far away, or otherwise distorted?

Does your sense of your body in space, your balance, or your movements feel somewhat off?

How do all these experiences make you feel? [After individual answers:] Sometimes people feel as if they are going crazy or losing their minds or as if they have some permanent brain damage.

Are these experiences causing you a lot of distress? In what ways?

Are these experiences affecting the way you relate to others, your interests and motivation to engage in life, or the ways you can focus and remember to do your work?

As noted earlier, the following three aspects are crucial to the diagnosis:

1. Are the depersonalization/derealization disorder symptoms the predominant picture at the present time, equally or not more so than other psychiatric syndromes? In other words, are they clearly of greater proportion than any other associated psychopathology?
2. Are the depersonalization/derealization disorder symptoms frequent and severe enough to qualify as "persistent or recurrent," associated with significant distress and/or dysfunction, and not adequately accounted for by psychiatric comorbidity?
3. Are the depersonalization/derealization disorder symptoms clearly not due to any medical or neurological condition or to ongoing use of precipitating illicit substances?

Tips for Clarifying the Diagnosis

- Determine whether the patient has clear symptoms of unreality and detachment.
- Question whether the systems are persistent or recurrent, not just transient.
- Investigate whether the symptoms cause significant distress and/or impairment.
- Consider whether the symptoms are clearly independent or out of proportion in course and presence to other psychiatric symptoms.
- Rule out other medical conditions (e.g., seizures, brain injury or lesions).
- Make sure that the symptoms are not associated with ongoing use of alcohol or other substances, including illicit drugs, such as marijuana, hallucinogens, ketamine, ecstasy, or salvia.

Consider the Case

Mr. Rogers was age 45 when he first started experiencing unusual symptoms, such as tightness in his head, tingling sensations over his scalp, "tuning out" to the extent that others thought he suddenly became noncommunicative, and experiences of his body floating and rotating in space. He denies feeling detached from his core sense of self, feelings, or agency over his actions. He does, however, admit to having his mind suddenly go blank, as if all thoughts have been sucked out. He is convinced that the cause of all his troubles is a defect in a specific right front part of his brain, which he thinks he can exactly pinpoint. The symptoms are very paroxysmal in nature and, although highly recurrent over the period of 1 year, typically last less than 1 hour. During this bout, Mr. Rogers reports no other associated symptoms. As a child he had a history of febrile seizures, which had remitted by age 7; he also had a strong family history of epilepsy on his mother's side. The episodes have no clear precipitants, such as mood or anxiety states, severe stressors, or use of alcohol or other substances. He had been a football player in high school and, during that time, had suffered one severe concussion with loss of consciousness, a 3-day hospitalization and monitoring, and weeks of residual symptoms. He denies any other psychiatric or neurological history.

Mr. Rogers requires a comprehensive medical evaluation. His case necessitates careful consideration of the medical differential diagnosis. His symptoms of depersonalization/derealization disorder are rather atypical, highly physical, and suggestive of an underlying physical cause. Their duration is also quite short; although short episodes do occur in depersonalization/derealization disorder, typically episodes are either continuous (i.e., symptoms are ongoing; in two-thirds of cases) or episodic but of longer duration (in one-third of cases). Additionally, Mr. Rogers has no identifiable acute precipitants for his symptom bouts; although lack of precipitants is not unusual for depersonalization/derealization disorder (in about one-half of cases), it does heighten the possibility of a medical differential diagnosis.

Mr. Rogers has a personal and family history of seizure disorders, and the brief duration and unusual symptoms with which he presents could suggest atypical seizures. The late age at onset of the symptoms, which rarely begin after the third decade of life in depersonalization/derealization disorder, is also suspicious. The lack of any psychiatric comorbidity is very atypical. Finally, the history of a serious concussion, although historically remote, cannot be ignored, and very late–onset sequelae can occur. For all these reasons, Mr. Rogers warrants a much more extensive workup than the usual patient presenting with depersonalization/derealization disorder. Brain imaging and a sleep-deprived encephalogram (EEG) with temporal leads are strongly indicated. If they are unremarkable, an extended ambulatory 3-day EEG recording examining the correlation between symptom bouts and brain events would assist in making a definitive diagnosis.

Differential Diagnosis

According to DSM-5, depersonalization/derealization disorder cannot be diagnosed if the symptoms occur exclusively in the context of another mental disorder. Therefore, a very thorough present and past psychiatric history must be obtained, so that the following three points become clear to the clinician:

1. If the person has had past episodes of another psychiatric disorder, such as major depressive disorder, panic disorder, social anxiety disorder, obsessive-compulsive disorder, or psychotic disorders, these episodes have been treated or spontaneously remitted to an extent that the current depersonalization/derealization disorder symptoms clearly "have a life of their own" that unequivocally extends above and beyond any such comorbidity. Similarly, patients with dissociative symptoms above and beyond depersonalization/derealization disorder would qualify for diagnosis of the respective dissociative disorder instead.
2. If the person is currently presenting with depersonalization/derealization disorder symptoms as well as symptoms of other psychiatric disorders, the depersonalization/derealization disorder symptoms must be out of proportion to the other comorbid symptoms, or the comorbid symptoms must have had clear onset after and been secondary to the symptoms of depersonalization/derealization disorder.
3. Any suspected medical or ongoing substance use that may be causing the current depersonalization/derealization disorder symptoms must be excluded. Initial substance use that acutely precipitated the symptoms but is no longer occurring is not an exclusion (e.g., patient smoked marijuana 2 months ago, had a bad trip, and has had depersonalization/derealization disorder since without any subsequent substance use).

See DSM-5 for additional disorders to consider in the differential diagnosis. Also refer to the discussions of comorbidity and differential diagnosis in their respective sections of DSM-5.

Summary

- In depersonalization/derealization disorder, a range of symptoms representing detachment and unreality from self and/or surroundings is present.
- The symptoms are persistent or recurrent; although there is no clear duration guideline in DSM-5, a minimum of 1 month is a rough guideline.
- Significant medical conditions must be ruled out, as well as comorbid psychiatric disorders. Another psychiatric disorder must never have been present; been present

but be largely remitted; be clearly secondary to the depersonalization/derealization disorder symptoms; or, if still present, be clearly lesser in associated severity, frequency, and dysfunction to the depersonalization/derealization disorder.

- The depersonalization/derealization disorder symptoms must not be due to medical conditions or ongoing drug use.
- Affected individuals must be clear about the "as-if" nature of the symptoms; psychotic elaborations must be absent.

IN-DEPTH DIAGNOSIS

Dissociative Identity Disorder

Ms. Moore, a 37-year-old divorced secretary, sought psychiatric help because of gaps in memory, suicidal thoughts, and relationship problems. She found herself unable to account for things people said she had done. She also noticed that even though she had just filled the gas tank in her car, it was half empty the next day, and miles had been added to the odometer. She was a hard worker, but her personal life was limited, and she spent much of her time alone. She was mistrusting of others and often felt taken advantage of in relationships. She was often sad but found herself able to put aside her dysphoria in the service of getting work done. Her marriage had ended at her insistence, and she had little interest in other relationships with men. She came from a family that emphasized strict religious values but in which she had felt singled out and misunderstood. It later emerged that a relative had physically and sexually abused her over a period of years. She was highly critical of herself for not having run away from home. Further examination, including measurement of hypnotizability, indicated that she was highly hypnotizable. Ms. Moore has no history of substance use of any kind. In the course of examination, she switched among several personality states, one presenting the dysphoric persona, another that was angry and critical of the former, and a third that was a childlike personality.

Key features of Ms. Moore's presentation include gaps in memory, switching among personality states, and a history of sexual abuse. To make the diagnosis, the clinician does not need to observe the changes in identity. A history of memory gaps, reports by others of changes in identity, or evidence of behavior for which the person could not account provides evidence of dissociation. A history of sexual abuse is common in such cases, and individuals with dissociative identity disorder are often dysphoric as well, but change in affect is usually a part of the dissociative process (one identity being primarily sad, another angry, and so forth). Structured shifting among identities, often facilitated with hypnosis, can help the person to understand and control the dissociation; other treatments include management of depression and suicidal ideation, psychotherapy aimed at stabilization, affect management, and then working through traumatic memories. Affected individuals are also prone to engage in activities that put them at risk for further mistreatment, so a therapeutic structure for protection is important. They also often expect further exploitation from caring figures in their life, including the therapist, so discussing and managing the "traumatic transference" are important.

Approach to the Diagnosis

The key to diagnosing dissociative identity disorder is assembling a full picture of the person's history, behavior, memories, and mood that can encompass possible discontinuities. It is useful to be open, nonjudgmental, and exploratory in assembling information about the person's pattern of interpersonal interactions, mood changes, trauma history, and history of prior diagnosis and treatment. Such individuals may exhibit puzzlement, confusion, or guardedness in revealing their histories. They may feel guilty for traumatic experiences or responsible for protecting family secrets. The information they present may be inconsistent. Persons with dissociative identity disorder are often seen for medical and psychiatric treatment for 4–10 years before the diagnosis is made. Thus, their dissociative symptoms are likely to have been overlooked or discounted by previous diagnosticians. Such individuals are not likely to change from one personality state to another during early diagnostic interviews, although this change is possible, so a careful history of the person's experiences and reports of others are useful in determining whether there is discontinuity of identity.

Standard assessments of hypnotizability, such as the Hypnotic Induction Profile or the Stanford Hypnotic Susceptibility Scale, can be useful both in the assessment of the likelihood of a dissociative disorder (high scores) and the potential for using hypnosis to identify and control the symptoms. Hypnotic and dissociative mental states are similar. Individuals with dissociative identity disorder can learn to switch among identity states using hypnosis and eventually can begin to control spontaneous switching. Overt evidence of such dissociation is not damaging but rather presents a therapeutic opportunity for the clinician to clarify the diagnosis and teach the person how to understand and control the symptoms.

Because the disorder usually occurs in the wake of sexual and/or physical abuse, affected individuals often expect mistreatment by clinicians as well, so caution and respect for the person's tolerance of distress is crucial. The clinician can distinguish himself or herself from abusers by inquiring frequently about the person's response to questions or interventions and offering to change the course of the interaction to increase the person's comfort with it. Ultimately, the clinician's job is not to proliferate but to integrate dissociated elements of the individual's personality, to view these elements as a statement of distress, keeping the focus on the whole person and constructive with the person's life story, which includes the scattered elements experienced by the person.

As stated in DSM-5, "Over 70% of outpatients with dissociative identity disorder have attempted suicide; multiple attempts are common, and other self-injurious behavior is frequent. Assessment of suicide risk may be complicated when there is amnesia for past suicidal behavior or when the presenting identity does not feel suicidal and is unaware that other dissociated identities do" (p. 295).

Getting the History

A woman reports hearing a voice that is critical of her and that provides a running commentary on her mistakes and shortcomings. Such a symptom should raise questions about the possibility of schizophrenia as well as dissociative identity disorder. Clarification of the differential diagnosis should include inquiring about the nature of the content of the hallucination: Is it bizarre or not? Does it have a consistent theme or is it disorganized? Other comorbid symptoms that would indicate schizophrenia include looseness of associations and flatness of affect. Individuals with dissociative identity disorder would have alterations in identity and episodes of amnesia. The auditory hallucination would more likely take the form of a self-critical element of an individual's own fragmented personality structure. The differential diagnosis of dissociative identity disorder from schizophrenia is especially important because the treatments are so different, and inappropriate use of neuroleptics with a dissociative disorder may not treat the target symptoms but instead flatten affect, delaying the appropriate diagnosis. Those individuals with dissociative identity disorder may come to believe that there really are multiple identities within them, which could also be misinterpreted as a psychotic delusion and therefore another symptom of schizophrenia.

Clear differential diagnosis includes a careful history regarding the onset of the disorder. A history of trauma or abuse is more likely consistent with a dissociative disorder, and history of a decline in function in late adolescence or the early 20s without a marked traumatic origin is more consistent with schizophrenia. The interviewer should carefully ask about evidence for amnesia, including lost periods of time and inability to account for activities others witnessed. Sudden changes in personality and interpersonal behavior are more consistent with dissociation, whereas social withdrawal, a decline in planning and initiation of behavior, and persistent bizarre beliefs are more consistent with schizophrenia. A careful exploration of the use of substances is essential to ensure that the symptoms are not attributable to substance intoxication or withdrawal.

Tips for Clarifying the Diagnosis

- Ask the person whether he or she or anyone else has noted sudden changes in his or her manner or identity.
- Ask whether the person finds clothing or other objects at home that he or she has apparently purchased but cannot recall buying.
- Question whether the person has noticed any gaps in his or her memory or periods of time for which he or she cannot account.
- Determine whether friends, family, or other people tell the person that he or she has said or done things that he or she cannot remember doing. Such episodes must be differentiated from substance use.
- Establish whether the person has engaged in dangerous or self-mutilative behavior that he or she cannot remember doing.
- Clarify whether the person has a history of sexual or physical abuse in childhood.

Consider the Case

Mr. Roberts is a 42-year-old man in a stable homosexual relationship who reports episodes of depression, personality change, time loss, and suicidal ideation. He has had repeated psychiatric hospitalizations and was previously diagnosed with borderline personality disorder and PTSD related to combat experiences. He has been aware for some time of his shifts in identities but views it as part of who he is and is more troubled by war-related flashbacks. He shows evidence of self-mutilation, with scars on his forearms, and he has had intermittent depressive episodes. He is unable to keep a job due to poor attendance and memory gaps.

Mr. Roberts has multiple comorbidities and is chronically impaired, but he has maintained a stable relationship. In fact, his partner enjoys Mr. Roberts's shifting of personality states and views himself as having "multiple partners." Because of his partner's perspective and Mr. Roberts's concern about symptoms other than his dissociation, treatment will focus more on stabilization, safety, and affect management. Mr. Roberts and his partner's shared sexual orientation place them in a stable relationship in a broader community that supports their bond, although they tend to be reclusive as a couple. Multiple psychiatric comorbidities present both a problem and a choice of clinical focus. In this case, Mr. Roberts, his partner, and the clinician agree to emphasize treatment of PTSD and depressive symptoms rather than resolution of the dissociative disorder.

Differential Diagnosis

The mood of individuals with dissociative identity disorder may fluctuate very rapidly in minutes or hours because of switching among different identities, which may include an active, upbeat personality state and another state that appears more depressed. Such shifts of mood can be mistaken for rapid-cycling bipolar disorder.

Psychotic disorders may appear to overlap with dissociative identity disorder. Identity fragmentation can be confused with delusional disorder, and internal communication from dissociated identities can mimic auditory hallucinations in schizophrenia. Differential diagnosis from brief psychotic disorder should be guided by the predominance of dissociative symptoms and occasional amnesia for the episode.

Other considerations in the differential diagnosis of dissociative identity disorder include the following: Posttraumatic flashbacks, amnesia, or affective blunting suggests a differential diagnosis of PTSD. Somatic symptoms involving alterations in sensory or motor functioning suggest a differential diagnosis of conversion disorder (functional neurological symptom disorder). A history of sexual abuse that results in conflicts over sexuality, body shape, and appearance may suggest a differential diagnosis of feeding and eating disorders and sexual dysfunctions. Gender confusion arising from cross-gendered identities may suggest a differential diagnosis of gender dysphoria. Dissociative identity disorder may manifest with symptoms identical to those produced by some seizure disorders, especially complex partial seizures with temporal lobe foci. Symptoms associated with the direct physiological effects of a substance can be distinguished from dissociative identity disorder by the fact that a substance (e.g., a drug of abuse or a medication) is judged to be etiologically related to the disturbance. Factitious disorder or malingering is also possible and is indicated by evidence of conscious manipulation of information about symptoms, as distinct from dissociative amnesia in regard to aspects of identity or experience.

Many individuals with dissociative identity disorder have comorbid depressive symptoms, often sufficient to meet criteria for a major depressive episode. In major depressive disorder, most or all personality states are depressed. Individuals with dissociative identity disorder often present with identities that comprise features of personality disorders, suggesting a differential diagnosis of personality disorder, especially borderline type. Comorbidity is also possible, especially when there is a severe trauma history in childhood and comorbid depression. PTSD is a common differential diagnosis and comorbid disorder. Stabilization of dissociative and posttraumatic symptoms may be necessary before diagnosing a comorbid personality disorder.

See DSM-5 for additional disorders to consider in the differential diagnosis. Also refer to the discussions of comorbidity and differential diagnosis in their respective sections of DSM-5.

Summary

- Individuals with dissociative identity disorder exhibit failure of integration of aspects of identity, memory, or consciousness.
- Individuals with dissociative identity disorder experience amnesia for daily as well as traumatic events.
- Disruption of personality or identity states occurs in individuals with dissociative identity disorder.
- Trauma history is frequent among individuals with dissociative identity disorder.

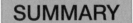

SUMMARY

Dissociative Disorders

Dissociative disorders are a failure in function rather than an aberration in mental content; they involve the loss of integration of elements of identity, personality, memory, sensation, and consciousness, as well as depersonalization/derealization (e.g., detachment from the body, sense of self, or surroundings), amnesia for traumatic or other memories, and fragmentation of identity. These disorders occur typically in the aftermath of trauma, but unlike acute stress disorder and PTSD, a traumatic stressor is not a diagnostic requirement. There is a dissociative subtype of PTSD that involves depersonalization or derealization in addition to other dissociative symptoms of PTSD, such as flashbacks and amnesia. Neuroimaging data suggest that these dissociative symptoms of PTSD involve increased frontal and inhibited limbic activity— that is, an overmodulation of affective response. Symptoms may fluctuate, and many people with the disorder have limited awareness of the extent of their disabilities. Dissociative disorders are functional disorders, meaning that the ability to integrate elements of identity, recover memories, and reintegrate perception is compromised but remains, complicating diagnosis but offering opportunities for treatment.

Diagnostic Pearls

- Dissociative disorders represent a discontinuity or failure of integration of normal mental processes, including identity, memory, perception, and consciousness.
- Dissociative symptoms can constitute an intrusion into ordinary integrated functioning, such as identity disruption, or a failure of integrated function, such as amnesia or depersonalization.

- Dissociation is often related to a history of trauma, including physical and sexual abuse in childhood, as well as emotional abuse and neglect.

- Dissociative symptoms such as amnesia, flashbacks, and depersonalization/derealization can also be part of PTSD (including a new dissociative subtype) and acute stress disorder.

- Dissociative symptoms, including pathological possession and trance, occur in many cultures around the world.

- Dissociative symptoms are often hidden or unrecognized, requiring careful and informed evaluation. They tend to be underdiagnosed or misdiagnosed.

Self-Assessment

Key Concepts: Double-Check Your Knowledge

What is the relevance of the following concepts to the various dissociative disorders?

- Dissociation and trauma
- Disintegration of identity
- Restricted memory access
- Impaired affect management
- Overmodulation of affect

Questions to Discuss With Colleagues and Mentors

1. What is the relationship between early life trauma and the development of dissociative disorders?
2. How can the clinician recognize dissociative symptoms of which the individual is not fully aware?
3. What accounts for fragmentation of identity?
4. How is dissociative identity disorder different from personality disorders?
5. How does the dysregulation of affect in dissociative disorders differ from that in mood and personality disorders?
6. What is the best way to clarify the potential role of other influences on the symptom picture, such as an emergent medical issue or effect of substances?

Case-Based Questions

PART A

Ms. Powell, age 29, is brought to the emergency department with deep lacerations on her forearm that were apparently self-inflicted. She reports having no memory of how it happened and acts in a fearful and tearful manner. She thinks she was running in the dark, tripped, and fell, cutting her arm on a piece of metal. This story, emotional but vague, does not fit the nature of the injury. She has in the past been diagnosed with bipolar disorder and antisocial personality disorder. Her presentation in the emergency department indicates some depression, no evidence of mania or hypomania, and no anger. A urine toxicology screen is negative.

What should be considered in the differential diagnosis at this point? Ms. Powell may be deliberately concealing the history of injury, either to avoid facing the consequences of self-harm or to avoid legal and interpersonal implications of accusing a family member or someone else of assault. This concealment could represent the minimization of adversity typical of mania, in which case elevated affect and pressured speech should accompany it. The appearance of anger, fear of abandonment, and manipulation may represent a demand for help coupled with interference in receiving it, which is typical of people with borderline personality disorder. If the woman has amnesia for the event, this amnesia could be due to substance use, a cognitive disorder, postconcussive syndrome, or epilepsy. The amnesia could also indicate dissociative amnesia or dissociative identity disorder. Inquiring about a recent or past trauma history can be helpful in clarifying the differential diagnosis.

PART B

> Ms. Powell agrees to assessment with hypnosis and proves to be highly hypnotizable. She is asked to relive, in hypnosis, the time just before her injury. In hypnosis, her affect and voice change markedly, and she says, "I wanted to be out, and she wouldn't let me, so I cut her so deep that she wouldn't want to be out and feel it. It was so deep that even I couldn't look at it, but it sure scared her." This dissociative picture, with amnesia, of the self-inflicted wound is consistent with a diagnosis of dissociative identity disorder rather than depression with suicidal ideation or borderline personality disorder. This diagnostic interview provides a basis for future therapeutic work, teaching Ms. Powell to control her dissociation and negotiate conflicts among her dissociated identities.

How does this information clarify the diagnosis? The fact that further information was retrievable with the assistance of hypnosis illustrates the type of amnesia typical of a dissociative disorder. A plausible explanation for Ms. Powell's wound was elicited, coupled with a sudden change in her affect and identity, which is typical of dissociative identity disorder.

Short-Answer Questions

1. Describe two effects on brain activity during response to trauma-related stimuli in the dissociative subtype of PTSD, according to recent neuroimaging studies.
2. What is the relationship between hypnotic and dissociative mental states?
3. What would confirm the diagnosis of dissociative identity disorder during a diagnostic interview?
4. For what type of events may individuals with dissociative identity disorder experience amnesia?
5. Depersonalization involves the psychological experience of feeling detached from what?
6. Derealization involves the psychological experience of feeling detached from what?

7. Dissociative fugue involves what two things?
8. What history do people with dissociative identity disorder frequently have?
9. Dissociative symptoms and substance use disorder may be comorbid diagnoses under what circumstance?
10. Can auditory hallucinations be a symptom of dissociative identity disorder?

Answers

1. Neuroimaging data suggest that dissociative symptoms in PTSD involve increased frontal and inhibited limbic activity.
2. Hypnotic and dissociative mental states are similar.
3. The occurrence of a dissociative switch during a diagnostic interview would confirm the diagnosis of dissociative identity disorder.
4. Individuals with dissociative identity disorder may experience amnesia for everyday or traumatic events.
5. Depersonalization involves the psychological experience of feeling detached from self or body.
6. Derealization involves the psychological experience of feeling detached from the surrounding world.
7. Dissociative fugue involves bewildered wandering coupled with dissociative amnesia.
8. People with dissociative identity disorder frequently have a history of physical or sexual abuse.
9. Dissociative symptoms and substance use disorder may be comorbid diagnoses if the dissociative symptoms are not better accounted for by the substance abuse.
10. Auditory hallucinations may be a symptom of dissociative identity disorder.

12

Somatic Symptom and Related Disorders

Ann C. Schwartz, M.D.
Thomas W. Heinrich, M.D.

"They tell me I'm fine, but I know I'm not."

*"None of the doctors can figure out why I have
so many things wrong with me."*

In DSM-5, the somatic symptom and related disorders diagnostic class replaces the DSM-IV somatoform disorders. The somatic symptom and related disorders all share the feature of predominant physical symptoms associated with significant distress and subsequent functional impairment. The disorders in this diagnostic class are somatic symptom disorder, illness anxiety disorder, conversion disorder (functional neurological symptom disorder), psychological factors affecting other medical conditions, factitious disorder, other specified somatic symptom and related disorder, and unspecified somatic symptom and related disorder.

Individuals with somatic symptoms are most commonly first encountered in medical rather than mental health settings. The somatic symptom and related disorders of DSM-5 differ from the somatoform disorders of DSM-IV by emphasizing the presence of distressing physical complaints coupled with abnormal thoughts and behaviors, rather than focusing on the presence of medically unexplained somatic symptoms. Individuals with somatic symptom and related disorders integrate maladaptive cognitive, behavioral, and/or emotional valence(s) with physical complaints. It is not the absence of an identified medical etiology for the individual's physical complaints that is the focus of the somatic symptom and related disorders but rather how the individual interprets these physical complaints and functions with them. Indeed, individuals may present with both a diagnosed medical condition and abnormal behaviors and thoughts related to this identified illness and its associated physical symptoms. There is a significant amount of personal distress and impairment associated with these disorders, along with increased health care utilization.

Individuals with somatic symptom and related disorders include those who have a number of maladaptive feelings, thoughts, and behaviors related to physical symptoms. These individuals typically have multiple active and distressing physical complaints, although sometimes they may present with only one severe and persistent symptom. The somatic symptoms and related maladaptive emotions, cognitions, and behaviors may or may not be associated with a medical condition. Emotionally, individuals experience significant worry and distress about their symptoms and/or illness. Cognitive features include an abnormal focus on physical symptoms and attribution of normal bodily sensations to the presence of an illness. Behavioral features of an individual with somatic symptom and related disorders may include repeated seeking of medical help and reassurance. The presence of a concurrent medical illness, which may explain the person's somatic symptoms, does not rule out the diagnosis of somatic symptom and related disorders. Individuals with somatic symptom and related disorders are usually very concerned about their somatic complaints. These individuals tend to think the worst about their health and interpret their physical complaints as excessively concerning or troublesome.

A person with illness anxiety disorder suffers from excessive concern about acquiring, or preoccupation with having, a serious yet-undiagnosed medical illness. This preoccupation exists despite a thorough medical evaluation that has failed to identify a serious medical condition that may account for the individual's concern. Although the concern may be derived from a physical sign or sensation, the individual's excessive response does not originate primarily from the somatic complaint but rather from anxiety surrounding the significance of the symptom and the potential for an adverse etiology of the complaint.

In conversion disorder (functional neurological symptom disorder), the person experiences the presence of "functional" symptoms or subjective deficits affecting the voluntary motor and sensory nervous system. In addition, there is evidence that these deficits or symptoms are inconsistent with recognized neurological and medical disease. If there is evidence of a recognized neurological, medical, or psychiatric disorder, the symptom must not be better explained by that disorder. Conversion disorder differs from the other somatic symptom and related disorders in that medically unexplained symptoms remain a key feature of this diagnosis. However, the diagnosis should not be made simply because investigations for an etiology do not uncover a clear abnormal result; there must also be evidence that the symptoms are functional in etiology, as demonstrated by internal inconsistency or incompatibility with a known disease process.

The disorder of psychological factors affecting other medical conditions, previously listed in the DSM-IV section "Other Conditions That May Be a Focus of Clinical Attention" (as psychological factor affecting medical condition), is now included in the somatic symptom and related disorders category. The essential feature of this disorder is the presence of clinically significant behavioral or psychological factors that adversely affect the management of a co-occurring medical condition, increasing the risk of poor medical or psychological outcomes.

IN-DEPTH DIAGNOSIS

Somatic Symptom Disorder

Ms. Smith is a 32-year-old woman referred to the mental health clinic for a "second opinion" from a primary care physician within the medical group. Ms. Smith endorses a multiyear history of chronic headaches, pain in multiple joints, and intermittent abdominal pain complicated by occasional nausea. She reports that she has undergone numerous studies and seen multiple specialists in an attempt to find a cause of her symptoms, but unfortunately no clear etiology has been identified to date. Nothing she does improves the chronic waxing and waning of these symptoms. She has been unable to hold a job for any length of time because of her frequent and often lengthy medical hospitalizations for nausea. The patient further explains that her immediate family has grown tired of all her physical complaints along with her intense and excessive focus on these symptoms. Despite what appears to be a very thorough medical evaluation to date, Ms. Smith feels that a few more tests may be warranted (she brought a list) to help find the medical cause of her suffering. She is very concerned that these symptoms may be a harbinger of an ominous medical condition, despite the negative workup. Although she is frustrated with the lack of explanation for her somatic complaints, she denies depression or significant anxiety unrelated to her health concerns. A careful review of her medical records reveals multiple negative studies, vague discharge summaries, numerous medication trials coupled with many medication "sensitivities," and many diagnoses from many different providers.

Ms. Smith displays multiple physical complaints, which she finds quite distressing and which interfere with her daily life—that is, the quality of her relationships with others and her ability to work. The physical symptoms of somatic symptom disorder could be related to a known medical condition or, as in this case, may be medically unexplained. The experience of somatic symptoms of unclear etiology is not in itself sufficient to make a diagnosis of somatic symptom disorder, however. These somatic symptoms must be complicated by excessive maladaptive thoughts, feelings, and behaviors.

Ms. Smith also displays persistent and excessive concern about the seriousness of her symptoms, despite a thorough medical evaluation that failed to reveal a potential etiology to her multiple somatic complaints. She displays a chronic high level of anxiety or worry related to her physical symptoms. Her family reports that she is always and overly focused on her multitude of symptoms. Her health issues appear to dominate her life, leading to significant functional and social impairment.

Approach to the Diagnosis

Astute clinicians will keep in mind somatic symptom disorder when encountering individuals with multiple somatic complaints, such as pain, sexual problems, fatigue, or gastrointestinal problems. Individuals often present dramatically with lengthy and complicated past medical and surgical histories. Evaluation of a person with possible somatic symptom disorder starts with a thorough review of the medical records for appropriate medical evaluation and confirmation of confirmed medical diagnoses. Collateral information regarding symptoms, functional disability, and previous evaluations or diagnoses (medical and psychological) should be obtained. This corroborative information is especially important during the assessment of children and older adults. Attention to the person's mental status for evidence of a mood or anxiety disorder is important, because these disorders are often comorbid with somatic symptom disorder and may complicate its presentation and subsequent treatment. The clinician should carefully assess the person's attitude toward the somatic complaints and illness-related behaviors.

Individuals with somatic symptom disorder have one or more somatic symptoms that are distressing and/or result in significant disruption of their ability to function. The symptoms may or may not be associated with an identified medical condition. The person's suffering is real, whether or not the physical symptom has a demonstrated medical explanation. Individuals with somatic symptom disorder manifest excessive worry about their symptoms and the probability of significant disease. The maladaptive thoughts, feelings, and behaviors that the individuals experience with the physical complaints tend to cause them to think the worst about their health, worry at high levels, and spend excessive amounts of time and energy devoted to their health concerns. As a consequence, it is not uncommon for the person's physical symptoms to become central to the person's personality and to contaminate important interpersonal relations (e.g., in family, professional, and health care situations).

The high level of somatically focused distress experienced by these individuals contributes to impaired health-related quality of life. The attention to somatic symptoms often leads to high utilization of health care resources; however, this high utilization does little to reduce the person's somatic complaints or health-related concerns. In addition, individuals with somatic symptom disorder often prove intolerant of various medications or other therapies meant to help address an identified pathology or the associated symptoms. As a result, they may experience their health care as frustrating and/or inadequate. As a consequence of this frustration, they often seek multiple referrals and receive care from multiple medical providers. Iatrogenic health problems may become an important feature of this complicated clinical picture.

The problems experienced by the person with somatic symptom disorder are heightened by excessive maladaptive cognitions and behaviors. The cognitive features of this disorder include a focus on physical symptoms, often with an associated misinterpretation that normal bodily sensations represent something pathological and inherently dangerous that must be addressed immediately to prevent an adverse medical outcome. Behaviorally, individuals may seek frequent medical attention for their somatic complaints, engage in excessive monitoring of health parameters (e.g., blood pressure), or seek reassurance of their health status from family and friends.

The focus on somatic symptoms leads individuals to present initially to medical services for care. It is not uncommon for individuals with somatic symptom disorder to view a referral to a mental health care provider as questionable, because the primary symptom that they experience is physical, not psychological. Some individuals presenting with somatic symptom disorder refuse to accept that there is a psychological component to the problem. For these reasons, patients with somatic symptom disorder may be commonly and exclusively encountered in medical settings.

Specifiers associated with the diagnosis of somatic symptom disorder include current severity (mild, moderate, or severe) and the course (persistent) of the disorder. In addition, if the person's somatic focus is predominantly pain, it is often most appropriately coded with the specifier "with predominant pain" (diagnosed as pain disorder in DSM-IV).

As stated in DSM-5, "Since somatic symptom disorder is associated with depressive disorders, there is an increased suicide risk. It is not known whether somatic symptom disorder is associated with suicide risk independent of its association with depressive disorders" (p. 312).

Getting the History

Ms. Adams, a 27-year-old woman, is referred from her primary care physician with multiple somatic symptoms. She is not pleased that her primary care physician has referred her to see a mental health care provider, because she believes that her problems are physical in nature. Despite a degree of defensiveness on the patient's part, the clinician determines that Ms. Adams finds these symptoms "very distressing" and that they cause a significant level of functional impairment. Her physical symptoms tend to take "center stage" during the interview, with most of her responses involving at least a mention of her somatic complaints.

The interviewer asks Ms. Adams, "Please describe your thoughts about your symptoms and what might be causing them." She answers quickly and with conviction that she feels that these symptoms are a harbinger to something very ominous and that her physicians are not taking her seriously. She adds that she is extremely frustrated with what she perceives as inadequate medical care and an unresponsive medical system. The clinician asks a question to determine whether the worrisome thoughts are excessive to her physical symptoms. Ms. Adams responds that despite many medical evaluations on both an inpatient and outpatient basis and multiple episodes of physician reassurance, her somatic worries and health-related concerns persist. She goes on to explain that these issues cause significant anxiety about the state of her health. The clinician follows up this line of questions with a query about how her somatic complaints may alter her behavior, and Ms. Adams responds by stating that she is afraid to engage in certain physical activities out of fear that she will worsen her symptoms. When the interviewer inquires about the duration of her complaints, Ms. Adams relays that she has been symptomatic for more than 6 years, although the symptoms tend to vary in quality and quantity. When she details her past medical history, she outlines a record of multiple providers, many medical tests, several medication trials, and numerous vague diagnoses and medication sensitivities.

The history provided by Ms. Adams makes somatic symptom disorder the most likely clinical diagnosis. She exhibits a greater than 6-month history of somatic symptoms that she finds very distressing and that impair her quality of life. The history

also reveals that she experiences both maladaptive thoughts (e.g., catastrophic interpretations of her symptoms) and abnormal behaviors (e.g., avoidance of certain activities) related to her physical complaints. Ms. Adams's persistent focus on her myriad
somatic symptoms is a primary feature of her presentation. Her intense attention to
her physical symptoms and illness anxiety dominate the interview and, most likely,
her social and professional relationships.

Many individuals with somatic symptom disorder may meet referral to a mental
health clinician with skepticism because they may resist accepting that there is an underlying psychological problem. The somatic symptoms they experience may or, as
in this case, may not be associated with a medical condition. But regardless of the etiology of the physical complaints, the individuals are truly distressed, often with very
high levels of health anxiety and impairment.

Tips for Clarifying the Diagnosis

- Have the person describe the somatic complaints, including organ system involvement and duration, along with aggravating and alleviating factors.
- Investigate the person's perception of the somatic symptom(s), including thoughts
  and feelings related to the physical complaint.
- Consider whether the person exhibits any maladaptive behaviors or cognitions related to the somatic complaints.
- Assess the level of health care utilization. This may include the frequency of outpatient appointments along with the number of physician referrals, emergency
  department visits, and medical hospitalizations.
- Understand how the person has responded to past reassurance, medical interventions, or pharmacotherapy.
- Determine what medical evaluation has been undertaken to date.

Consider the Case

Mr. Knight is a 42-year-old man with a medical history significant for well-controlled
hypertension and hyperlipidemia and a history of coronary artery disease and myocardial infarction. He presents to the mental health clinic on referral from his cardiologist
for evaluation of depression following a recent medical admission for chest pain. He is
somewhat disgruntled about the referral to a mental health care provider. He has presented to the emergency department several times over the last 8 months with concerns
that he may be having another "heart attack." He has recently had a cardiac catheter-
ization, which demonstrated no clinically significant occlusions. His father died from a
myocardial infarction in his "mid-40s." Mr. Knight's wife reports that he is "very focused" on his risk factors for cardiac disease and that he measures his blood pressure
multiple times a day and gets very "antsy" if he forgets a single dose of his antihyper-
tensive medication or statin. He admits that if he perceives any chest discomfort, he
races to the emergency department because otherwise it "may be too late." He denies
any affective symptoms suggestive of a major depressive disorder. He reports that he is
relieved after physician reassurance following each successive test showing that no
more "muscle has died" but that the excessive concern of progression of his heart disease gradually returns.

Individuals with somatic symptom disorder often have multiple somatic symptoms, but some individuals experience only one severe physical complaint, such as Mr. Knight's chest pain. The presence of an identified concurrent medical illness, such as coronary artery disease, does not rule out the diagnosis of somatic symptom disorder. Somatic symptom disorder differs from the DSM-IV somatoform disorders in that it does not require that the symptoms be medically unexplained. If a medical condition is present that may account for the somatic symptoms and health-related anxiety, the associated abnormal feelings, thoughts, and behaviors must be excessive. This case demonstrates the occurrence of somatic symptom disorder in a male, although the disorder is more prevalent in females. Mr. Knight demonstrates excessive maladaptive thoughts, feelings, and behaviors that are related to his complaint of chest pain and his associated health concerns of suffering another myocardial infarction. His complaints and concerns are persistent and anxiety provoking, and he spends excessive time addressing these health concerns. Cognitive distortions may include catastrophic interpretations of normal bodily sensations. Health concerns, most often surrounding the somatic complaints, may assume a central role in the individual's life, dominating interpersonal relationships and complicating psychosocial functioning. Individuals with somatic symptom disorder typically first present in the general medical setting rather than the mental health setting because their symptom focus is physical, not psychological.

Differential Diagnosis

The differential diagnosis of somatic symptom disorder is extensive and includes both other psychiatric disorders and medical conditions with nonspecific, transient, and often multisystem involvement (e.g., autoimmune disorders such as systemic lupus erythematosus). If the person's physical symptoms are better accounted for by another psychiatric disorder (e.g., the neurovegetative symptoms of major depression or the symptoms of autonomic arousal associated with panic disorder) and the diagnostic criteria for that disorder are fully satisfied, then that psychiatric disorder should be considered as an alternative diagnosis or a comorbid condition.

Psychiatric disorders to consider in the differential diagnosis of somatic symptom disorder include anxiety disorders such as generalized anxiety disorder and panic disorder, because of the predominant worry and anxiety present in somatic symptom disorder. Panic attacks are rare in somatic symptom disorder, and the anxiety in somatic symptom disorder is related to wellness concerns rather than other more general or environmental sources of anxiety. The affective symptoms such as sadness and hopelessness and the negative cognitions of guilt and suicidal thoughts are absent in somatic symptom disorder, unlike in depressive disorders. Individuals experiencing illness anxiety disorder have maladaptive anxiety about their health, but lack significant associated somatic symptoms. Conversion disorder (functional neurological symptom disorder) is defined by a loss of function, whereas in somatic symptom disorder the diagnostic focus is on somatic symptom–related distress. Somatic symptom disorder is differentiated from a delusional disorder by the fact that in somatic symptom disorder the somatic beliefs are usually realistic and not held with a delusional intensity. In somatic symptom disorder the recurrent ideas about illness or somatic symptoms do not have associated repetitive behaviors aimed at reducing anxiety, which are the hallmark of obsessive-compulsive disorder. In body dysmorphic disorder, the person is preoccupied by a perceived defect in his or her physical features, not a somatic complaint that relates to a fear of an underlying medical illness.

Somatic symptom disorder is highly comorbid with other psychiatric illnesses such as depressive disorders and anxiety disorders. If the criteria for both somatic symptom disorder and another psychiatric disorder are fulfilled in an individual, then both disorders should be coded and appropriately treated.

See DSM-5 for additional disorders to consider in the differential diagnosis. Also refer to the discussions of comorbidity and differential diagnosis in their respective sections of DSM-5.

Summary

- The individual experiences one or more somatic symptoms that he or she finds distressing and/or that result in significant disruption of daily function.
- The somatic symptoms are associated with related, excessive maladaptive thoughts, feelings, and behaviors.
- Somatic symptom disorder may occur in the presence or absence of a medical condition that accounts for the physical symptoms. However, if there is a medical condition that is responsible for the physical complaints, then the symptom-associated thoughts, feelings, and behaviors are disproportionate and excessive.
- The person experiences chronic and excessive thoughts about the seriousness of the somatic symptoms.
- The somatic complaints and health concerns contribute to the person's substantial anxiety about his or her health and/or the significance of the associated symptoms.
- The individual with somatic symptom disorder may also spend excessive time and/or energy on the physical symptoms or related health concerns.
- The person must be somatically preoccupied for >6 months. The symptoms, however, may vary throughout the course of the illness.

IN-DEPTH DIAGNOSIS

Illness Anxiety Disorder

Ms. Xavier, a 32-year-old married woman, presents to the emergency department complaining of a mild headache and "floaters" in her vision. She appears anxious and expresses concern that these are symptoms of a brain tumor. She undergoes several tests, including head imaging, and is told that the headache is likely a tension headache. She declines pain medications, stating that the pain is minimal.

Ms. Xavier has presented to the emergency department and her primary care physician at least six times in the past few months with a variety of somatic symptoms, including dizziness, headaches, and floaters in her eyes. Multiple medical evaluations have failed to identify a serious medical condition, but Ms. Xavier remains concerned that she has a brain tumor, despite reassurance from her primary care physician. She has missed a number of days of work due to medical appointments and also has difficulty completing tasks and concentrating due to anxiety. She states that the anxiety primarily revolves around her health concerns. Collateral history from her husband indicates that there has been a strain in their marriage due to her "obsession" with having a brain tumor.

Individuals with illness anxiety disorder may present to a medical setting with a high level of anxiety about having a serious illness (e.g., a brain tumor). Although Ms. Xavier is young and otherwise healthy, a complete medical workup must be completed to rule out a medical cause for the physical complaints. If medical illnesses are ruled out and she fails to respond to reassurance, illness anxiety disorder should be considered. Ms. Xavier's age (middle adulthood) is consistent with illness anxiety disorder onset. Her symptoms are chronic in nature (a minimum duration of 6 months is required for the diagnosis), and her anxiety is largely related to health issues and worries. She exhibits excessive behaviors to check for illness, including repeatedly looking up symptoms of a brain tumor on the Internet, which would be consistent with the specifier of care-seeking type. Individuals with the care-avoidant type rarely seek medical care because it can heighten their anxiety.

Approach to the Diagnosis

Individuals with illness anxiety disorder are preoccupied with and fear having a serious, undiagnosed medical illness. The minimum duration of this state of preoccupation is 6 months. A thorough medical evaluation fails to identify a serious medical condition that accounts for the individual's symptoms and concerns. Physical signs and symptoms may be present, but when they are, they are typically mild in intensity and are often either a normal physiological sensation or a bodily discomfort not generally considered indicative of disease. If a physical sign or symptom (e.g., headache) is present, the person's distress is largely from the fear of the suspected medical illness (e.g., brain tumor) rather than the physical complaint itself. If a medical condition is present, the anxiety and preoccupation are clearly excessive to the severity of the condition. Hearing about another's illness can cause anxiety because it heightens the person's health concerns.

Illness anxiety disorder has two specifiers: care-seeking type and care-avoidant type. Individuals with the care-seeking type may perform excessive behaviors (e.g., examine themselves or seek information and reassurance repeatedly) or investigate their suspected and feared disease excessively (e.g., through medical appointments, Internet searches). Individuals with the care-avoidant type may not seek medical care because it heightens their anxiety. They also may avoid situations or activities (e.g., exercise) that they fear may endanger their health.

Clinicians in medical settings may frequently encounter individuals with illness anxiety disorder who believe they are suffering from a serious medical condition; in general, these patients (particularly those with the care-seeking type) have higher utilization rates of medical services. Individuals do not respond to reassurance from physicians, family members, or negative diagnostic tests and may express dissatisfaction with medical care that they do not see as helpful. Illness concerns are prominent in their lives, and illness becomes a central feature of their identity.

Getting the History

Mr. Zimmer, a 44-year-old man, reports having a several-month history of abdominal pain and requests a repeat colonoscopy. The interviewer determines that Mr. Zimmer has had an extensive medical workup over the past few months, including physical examinations, laboratory studies, X rays, colonoscopy, and an abdominal computed tomography (CT) scan, all of which were unremarkable. The interviewer asks him to "describe the abdominal pain," and Mr. Zimmer further elaborates that his stomach feels "full" and appears to "rumble excessively." He also describes intermittent diarrhea. When the interviewer asks what he thinks is causing the symptoms, Mr. Zimmer responds, "I am certain that it is colon cancer."

The interviewer asks Mr. Zimmer about his thoughts on the negative medical workup to date, to which he responds, "The tests must have missed the tumor, but I can feel a mass in my stomach, and it is getting larger." The interviewer asks how often he palpates the "mass" and whether he has checked for illness in any other way. Mr. Zimmer responds that he presses on his stomach several times a day and also has conducted countless Internet searches on the symptoms and treatments of colon cancer. The interviewer asks, "How do these symptoms impact your daily activities, and are you avoiding doing things because of the symptoms?" Mr. Zimmer responds that he has been able to continue working as a teacher but has missed several days due to medical appointments and that he fears he will have to take additional time off in the near future to pursue treatment when he is diagnosed with cancer. He also states that he feels preoccupied during much of the day with thoughts about the cancer, which he thinks have a negative impact on his teaching. He denies excessive worrying in other areas.

Mr. Zimmer describes a high level of anxiety about his physical symptoms, including abdominal fullness and rumblings. A full medical workup should always be conducted; in this case, an extensive workup has not identified a cause for the symptoms experienced. The somatic symptoms appear to be mild and have begun to affect the patient's work (e.g., missed days for appointments and preoccupation with illness at work). His anxiety relates to the fear of having colon cancer, rather than distress from the abdominal discomfort, and also seems to revolve predominantly around concerns with illness rather than multiple domains of activities or events. Mr. Zimmer also describes excessive behaviors related to the anxiety of having colon cancer, including frequently palpating his abdomen for masses and conducting frequent Internet searches. In addition, he has sought frequent medical care for the symptoms. The interviewer will want to clarify how long these symptoms have been present—criteria require at least a 6-month duration for the state of being preoccupied with having the illness.

Tips for Clarifying the Diagnosis

- Assess whether the person is preoccupied with having or acquiring a serious illness.
- Rule out medical conditions that may account for the person's symptoms and concerns.
- Consider whether the person has been preoccupied with fears of having a serious illness for at least 6 months.
- Determine how the person responds to reassurance from physicians or tests that he or she does not have a serious medical condition.

- Investigate whether the person tends to seek out medical care and information or to avoid medical care and situations around illness because they may heighten his or her anxiety.

Consider the Case

Mrs. Best brings her 40-year-old husband to the office and reports that he is having difficulties with "anxiety." The interviewer determines that Mr. Best has episodes in which he experiences "a pounding heart," shortness of breath, difficulty swallowing, and the feeling that his heart "misses a beat." The episodes last approximately 10 minutes. The interviewer asks if there are any precipitants to these attacks. Mr. Best states that he was seen in the emergency department the previous week following an attack that started when he learned that a coworker was in the hospital with heart failure. He states that his father died of a myocardial infarction 2 years ago, and he has since felt certain that he also has cardiac problems. In a routine visit to his doctor soon after his father's death, his cardiac exam was entirely normal, although he worries that he is going to have a heart attack "any time now." Mr. Best has not returned to his primary care physician because he "just can't handle hearing any bad news." His wife reports that he is "obsessed with thoughts about having heart trouble." He previously exercised regularly but has stopped exercising because he does not want to "stress" his heart or "drop dead." He has been avoiding certain colleagues at work, stating that he "can't handle" hearing about others' health problems. He denies misuse of substances.

Mr. Best likely has illness anxiety disorder, but the case is atypical. He describes a number of symptoms of panic attacks. The attacks, however, appear to be precipitated by concerns about his heart. He is preoccupied with having cardiac disease like his father, although a medical workup to date fails to reveal cardiac issues. Individuals with illness anxiety disorder may experience panic attacks triggered by illness concerns (in this case, worry about a myocardial infarction). The case demonstrates illness anxiety disorder in a male; the prevalence of the disorder is similar in males and females. At least one-fourth of individuals with illness anxiety disorder have an anxiety disorder, and a separate diagnosis of panic disorder could be made if some of the attacks are not triggered by worries about health.

Mr. Best has features of the care-avoidant type. He avoids exercising because he fears that it might jeopardize his life. He also avoids seeing his primary care physician because he fears getting a negative report on his physical health. He is easily alarmed when he hears about others with health difficulties and avoids interactions with certain colleagues at work as a result. Clearly, a thorough medical workup is necessary to rule out a general medical disorder.

Differential Diagnosis

The first consideration in the differential diagnosis is whether an underlying medical condition exists that fully explains the clinical picture. The presence of an underlying condition does not exclude the possibility of a coexisting illness anxiety disorder, but if a medical condition is present, the health-related concerns and anxiety must be clearly disproportionate to the medical condition in order to satisfy the diagnosis of illness anxiety disorder. Individuals with illness anxiety disorder fear having or acquiring a serious medical illness. Somatic symptoms are also present in conversion disorder (functional neurological symptom disorder) and somatic symptom disorder, but persons with these disorders are primarily focused on symptom relief and less concerned about having a serious illness and getting the proper diagnosis for their symptoms. The anxiety in illness anxiety disorder is limited to health-related concerns, which helps differentiate the disorder from other anxiety disorders, such as generalized anxiety disorder, and obsessive-compulsive and related disorders. The anxiety in generalized anxiety disorder could also include anxiety related to health, but such anxiety is only one of the domains about which persons with generalized anxiety disorder worry. Individuals may experience panic attacks that are triggered by their illness concerns, and a diagnosis of panic disorder should be considered in individuals who have panic attacks that are not triggered by health concerns. Individuals with illness anxiety disorder are not delusional and are able to recognize the possibility that they do not have the feared illness. Anxiety is often a common response to medical illness. However, if the anxiety is severe enough and there is a clear relation to the onset of the medical condition, the diagnosis of an adjustment disorder should be considered by the clinician. It is only when the health-related anxiety becomes disproportionate to the related medical condition and of appropriate duration that illness anxiety disorder may be diagnosed. Persons with a major depressive episode may be preoccupied with illness, but a diagnosis of illness anxiety disorder should be considered if preoccupation with health concerns is present outside of a major depressive episode.

The exact comorbidities are unknown because illness anxiety disorder is a new disorder, but approximately two-thirds of individuals with illness anxiety disorder have at least one other comorbid major psychiatric disorder. Comorbid psychiatric disorders include anxiety disorders, such as generalized anxiety disorder or panic disorder; obsessive-compulsive disorder; and mood disorders, including major depressive disorder and persistent depressive disorder (dysthymia). In addition, individuals with illness anxiety disorder may have comorbid personality disorders.

See DSM-5 for additional disorders to consider in the differential diagnosis. Also refer to the discussions of comorbidity and differential diagnosis in their respective sections of DSM-5.

Summary

- In illness anxiety disorder, the primary feature includes preoccupation with and a high level of anxiety about having or acquiring a serious illness.
- If a medical condition is diagnosed, the individual's anxiety and preoccupation are excessive and disproportionate to the severity of the condition.
- Somatic symptoms may be present, and if present, are typically mild. The anxiety is not focused on the somatic symptoms, but rather on a suspected serious underlying medical diagnosis.
- A thorough medical evaluation fails to identify a serious medical condition that accounts for the patient's symptoms.

- The individual either performs excessive behaviors (e.g., seeking out reassurance and information) or exhibits maladaptive avoidance (e.g., avoiding doctors' appointments).
- The preoccupation may not be continuous, but the state of being preoccupied is chronic, with a minimum duration of at least 6 months.

IN-DEPTH DIAGNOSIS

Conversion Disorder
(Functional Neurological Symptom Disorder)

Ms. Omni is a 31-year-old woman brought to the emergency department by ambulance after an acute onset of right-sided weakness. An administrative assistant at a large law firm, she was at work in a meeting when she experienced numbness in her right hand and dizziness. She reports that she felt light-headed and dizzy and left the meeting to sit down. Over the next hour, her right hand became weak, and she was unable to hold her coffee cup. The weakness gradually spread to her lower extremity; on presentation, she was unable to move her right leg. On physical examination, she appears anxious and states that in the meeting she was working to complete a project with an approaching deadline. On strength testing, Ms. Omni is unable to lift her right leg. Her deep tendon reflexes are normal. While supine, she is asked to raise her left leg against resistance while the doctor's hand cups her right heel. In this maneuver, the doctor feels downward pressure with the hand under her right heel, which she was previously unable to raise (positive Hoover sign). A CT scan of the brain is completed and reveals no acute process. Ms. Omni states that she does not use alcohol or other substances.

Patients with conversion disorder (functional neurological symptom disorder) often present to emergency facilities, especially when the onset is acute. Although the symptoms appear inconsistent with medical or neurological disease, a thorough medical workup must be completed. If medical illnesses are ruled out, conversion disorder should be considered. In this case, Ms. Omni's weakness appears nonphysiological or psychogenic in that there is not a neuropathic cause and the symptoms are inconsistent in nature (e.g., positive Hoover sign, inconsistent strength in hip extension). The stressful work environment appears to have been a precipitant in symptom onset, but the presence of identifiable conflicts or stressors is not required in making the diagnosis. The peak of onset for motor symptoms is typically in the fourth decade, and the symptoms are more common in females. Substance abuse is uncommon in these individuals.

Approach to the Diagnosis

The essential feature in conversion disorder in DSM-5 is the presence of symptoms or deficits affecting motor and sensory functioning with evidence that the symptoms or deficits are inconsistent or incongruous with recognized neurological or medical conditions. The presenting symptoms can vary and may include motor symptoms, sensory symptoms, reduced or absent speech volume, or episodes resembling epileptic seizures.

The symptoms are nonphysiological or psychogenic, meaning that there is not a corresponding, recognized medical or neurological cause. An example would be a tremor that disappears with distraction when the person is asked to perform other tasks. Neurological and medical diseases must be excluded as a cause of the symptoms.

In DSM-IV, psychological factors are judged to be associated with the symptom or deficit. In DSM-5, such symptoms or conflicts may be present and may appear relevant to the development of the symptoms (e.g., a person develops dysphonia after witnessing an emotionally traumatic event); however, this is not required for this diagnosis because these stressors are not always apparent at the time of the initial diagnosis.

In DSM-IV, the diagnosis of conversion disorder required that the symptom or deficit not be intentionally produced or feigned. This criterion is not in DSM-5 because clinicians may have difficulty reliably assessing the underlying motivation behind the production of the neurological symptoms. However, if there is evidence that the symptoms are intentionally produced, the diagnosis of conversion disorder would not be made, and factitious disorder or malingering should be considered. The presence of apparent secondary gain should not be used to make the diagnosis.

Specifiers include the symptom type, course, and presence of stressors. Symptom specifiers include with weakness or paralysis, abnormal movement, swallowing symptoms, speech symptom, attacks or seizures, anesthesia or sensory loss, special sensory symptom, or mixed symptoms. The course can be described as acute or persistent. With or without psychological stressor is an additional specifier.

Getting the History

> Mr. Henry, a 24-year-old man, presents to his primary care physician and reports a new-onset tremor in both hands. The physician asks about the onset, severity, and duration of the symptoms. Mr. Henry states that the tremors started suddenly 2 months ago. The tremors are bothersome in that he is having difficulty eating and drinking. He also has had difficulty writing and typing at work and just feels "clumsy." The physician inquires about current medication, and Mr. Henry states that he is not taking any medications. The physician explores the family history, and Mr. Henry denies a family history of movement disorders. The physician asks about alcohol use, and Mr. Henry responds, "I used to have one or two beers on the weekend but haven't had anything to drink in over a month." The physician completes a physical examination, which is essentially normal except for the bilateral tremor in both hands and an occasional jerking movement in the man's right arm. Because the tremor is not typical, the physician asks Mr. Henry to tap his toes and perform other strength maneuvers. While the patient is focused on these activities, the tremor diminishes and even disappears briefly. The physician asks, "Do you recall a particular stressor or event that may have precipitated these tremors?" Mr. Henry does not recall any precipitating event or stressor. The physician continues to check for medical disorders and also orders various laboratory tests to rule out a medical source of the symptoms.

The physician carefully explores medical causes of the patient's tremor, including medication side effects, possible genetic movement disorder, and possible contribution of substances. There does not appear to be an underlying medical cause. The physician observes that the tremor is not consistent with a recognized neurological tremor and that it decreases when the patient is distracted. The physician then explores potential stressors or conflicts that may have precipitated the symptoms and also determines that the patient is having functional impairment from his symptoms. The physician should also be vigilant for clues on whether the symptoms may be produced voluntarily, because this would exclude the diagnosis of conversion disorder.

Tips for Clarifying the Diagnosis

- Assess whether the person has one or more symptoms or deficits that affect voluntary motor or sensory function.
- Consider whether the symptoms are inconsistent with a known medical or neurological disorder.
- Rule out a medical or neurological source of the symptoms.
- Determine whether there was an apparent psychological precipitant to the symptoms.
- Investigate whether there is evidence that the symptoms or deficits are purposely produced.

Consider the Case

Mr. Aarons, a 46-year-old man, is referred to the mental health clinic by the neurology clinic for a 6-month history of increasing seizures. He has a history of a seizure disorder since his 20s, but the episodes have increased to once or twice per week. He states that he has been taking his medications as prescribed. His wife has witnessed the episodes and states that the recent seizures appear different in nature. In the "new" seizures, he first gets rigid, falls to the ground, and then has thrashing movements of his extremities. He shouts out at times. They occur one to two times per week and are not associated with incontinence, as his seizures in the past have been. She stated that the last one occurred after an argument with the couple's teenage daughter when the daughter was arrested for underage drinking. The wife expresses concern that Mr. Aarons is unable to drive, but he appears indifferent to this and to the worsening of his symptoms. The neurologist has evaluated him and stated that although the patient does have a history of seizures, he is therapeutic on his antiepileptic medication and there is no epileptiform activity during video-electroencephalographic monitoring, which successfully captured one of his typical episodes. Mr. Aarons is otherwise healthy and does not drink alcohol or use illicit substances. He has been married for 19 years and has two daughters, ages 12 and 17.

Mr. Aarons has a known history of seizure disorder but presented after an increase in the frequency of his seizures despite being adherent to his medications. The recent seizures differ from his seizures in the past, and the thrashing movements and verbalizations during the seizures are inconsistent with patterns associated with known seizure phenomena. A thorough workup by his neurologist fails to find a neurological cause for the new spells. He is male and 46, which is atypical for conversion disorder, because there is a higher incidence among females and the onset of nonepileptic attacks peaks in the third decade. Mr. Aarons can have a diagnosis of conversion disorder in conjunction with his known medical history of a seizure disorder. The conflict with his teenage daughter may be a contributor to the onset and exacerbation of his nonepileptic seizures. The relative lack of concern over the increase in his symptoms *(la belle indifférence)* may be present but is not specific to individuals with this disorder.

Differential Diagnosis

Individuals with conversion disorder present with medical symptoms and deficits, so the main differential diagnosis includes neurological and medical conditions that could explain the symptoms. These individuals must have a thorough medical workup and may require repeated assessments, especially if the symptoms appear progressive. The disorder may coexist with a medical condition, but the diagnosis of conversion disorder should be made only if the symptoms are not better explained by the underlying medical condition. Other mental disorders to be considered include other somatic symptom and related disorders, dissociative disorders, body dysmorphic disorder, depressive disorders, and panic disorder. If symptoms of conversion disorder and another disorder are present, both diagnoses should be made. The distinction of whether the symptoms are voluntarily produced can be a difficult one. Individuals with functional neurological symptoms are not aware of producing the symptoms, whereas individuals with malingering and factitious disorder are deliberately and purposefully feigning the symptoms.

Comorbidities with anxiety disorders and depressive disorders are more common in individuals with neurological disease. Personality disorders are more common in patients with conversion disorder than in the general population. In addition, comorbid neurological or medical conditions may be present. Psychosis and substance use disorders are uncommon.

See DSM-5 for additional disorders to consider in the differential diagnosis. Also refer to the discussions of comorbidity and differential diagnosis in their respective sections of DSM-5.

Summary

- Individuals with conversion disorder have one or more symptoms or deficits that affect voluntary motor or sensory function.
- There is positive evidence that the symptoms are inconsistent with a recognized neurological or medical disease.
- Medical and neurological diseases have been excluded and do not explain the symptoms or deficits.
- There may be identifiable psychological precipitants in the initiation or exacerbation of the symptoms, although such a precipitant is not required for the diagnosis because clear stressors and trauma may not be identifiable.
- Positive evidence that the symptoms are voluntarily produced or feigned excludes a diagnosis of conversion disorder; however, a judgment that the symptoms are not intentionally produced is not required, because the intention may be difficult to assess.
- Symptoms and deficits vary in severity from minor to severe and, in course, from acute to chronic. The physical and mental disability can be similar to that experienced by individuals with comparable medical diseases.
- Conversion disorder must be differentiated from neurological and medical conditions and other somatic symptom and related disorders.

—————— SUMMARY ——————

Somatic Symptom and Related Disorders

The somatic symptom and related disorders all share a focus on somatic symptoms and their occurrence primarily in general medical, rather than mental health care, settings. They represent a new class of disorders in DSM-5, replacing the somatoform disorders section in previous editions of DSM. The hallmark of the disorders included in this section of DSM-5 is the prominence of distressful somatic symptoms associated with functional impairment. The new approach to disorders presenting with physical symptoms emphasizes that the diagnoses are made on the basis of troubling somatic symptoms along with associated maladaptive thoughts, feelings, and behaviors, rather than the absence of a medical explanation for the physical complaints. A number of biological, social, and psychological factors contribute to the development of somatic symptom and related disorders. Variations in the presentation of these disorders likely relates to a nonphysiological interaction of these factors. This diagnostic class acknowledges that how an individual interprets and adapts to the experience of somatic symptoms may be as important as the somatic symptoms themselves. Medically unexplained symptoms are no longer predominant features in most of the diagnostic criteria for somatic symptom and related disorders, because individuals may have maladaptive cognitive or behavioral responses to physical symptoms due to a diagnosed medical condition.

——————— ■ ■ ■ ———————

Diagnostic Pearls

- Individuals with somatic symptoms respond to the presence of physical complaints and health concerns with excessive and maladaptive thoughts, feelings, and/or behaviors.

- These disorders are commonly associated with a markedly poor, patient-rated self-assessment of health status.

- There is a significant increase in health care utilization among individuals with somatic symptom and related disorders.

- Individuals with somatic symptom and related disorders are most often found in the medical setting and less commonly encountered in mental health settings.

- It is not the absence of an identified medical etiology of the physical complaints that is the focus of the somatic symptom and related disorders but rather the way in which individuals interpret and adapt to them.

- Conversion disorder (functional neurological symptom disorder) differs from the other somatic symptom and related disorders in that a medically unexplained symptom of the voluntary motor and sensory nervous system remains a key feature of this diagnosis.

- In illness anxiety disorder, a person experiences intense concern about acquiring, or preoccupation with having, an undiagnosed medical illness.
- The essential feature of psychological factors affecting other medical conditions is the presence of clinically significant behavioral or psychological factors that adversely affect the management of a co-occurring medical condition.

Self-Assessment

Key Concepts: Double-Check Your Knowledge

What is the relevance of the following concepts to the various somatic symptom and related disorders?

- Preoccupation with somatic symptoms or illness-related concerns
- Presentation in general medical versus mental health settings
- Cognitive misinterpretations of somatic symptoms
- Comorbidity with anxiety and depressive disorders
- Medically unexplained symptoms
- Impairment in professional and personal quality of life
- Marked impairment in self-reported health status
- Elevated rates of health care utilization
- High levels of illness anxiety
- Risk of iatrogenic harm

Questions to Discuss With Colleagues and Mentors

1. What is the best way to communicate a diagnosis of a somatic symptom or related disorder to the patient?
2. How can mental health care providers serve as effective consultants to colleagues in other branches of medicine when caring for patients with somatic symptom and related disorders?
3. How does a provider determine if a person's health-related thoughts, feelings, and behaviors are excessive to the person's actual state of health or, as the case may be, illness?
4. What signs on physical examination would be suggestive of a conversion disorder (functional neurological symptom disorder)?
5. How does a provider clinically differentiate a somatic symptom and related disorder from an illness anxiety disorder?
6. What is the best way to engage individuals experiencing somatic symptom and related disorders in mental health care, given their inherent focus on physical health rather than mental health?

Case-Based Questions

PART A

Ms. Reed is a 36-year-old woman with a recent diagnosis of hypothyroidism who presents to the mental health clinic upon referral from her primary care physician for evaluation of anxiety. The referral form indicates that she has had recurrent physical complaints (e.g., fatigue, dizziness, palpitations) over the last 3 years. As a result of the workup of these symptoms, she was discovered to have clinical hypothyroidism. The hypothyroidism was successfully treated, but unfortunately the symptoms continued, largely unabated. Further medical evaluation did not reveal any etiology for these continued symptoms. Her primary care physician, however, referred her to an endocrinologist out of concern that some of her symptoms may be due to either over- or undertreatment of her hypothyroidism. The endocrinologist determined that she was clinically and physiologically euthyroid. Ms. Reed "no-showed" for her first scheduled mental health intake 2 weeks ago but arrived on time for her current appointment. She disagrees with the referral to a mental health care provider.

What aspects of her history are consistent with somatic symptom and related disorders? Ms. Reed presented initially to her primary care provider, a common occurrence for individuals with probable somatic symptom and related disorders. In addition, she has undergone a series of studies, along with a subspecialty medical referral, to determine a possible etiology of her somatic symptoms. Increased utilization of health care resources is frequently encountered in individuals with somatic symptom and related disorders. Her missed appointment may signify a hesitancy to see a mental health care provider. Individuals with somatic symptom and related disorders may resist referral to mental health care due to the somatic, rather than psychological, focus of their symptomatology.

PART B

Ms. Reed reports that the somatic symptoms are very bothersome and prevent her from engaging in many of the activities she used to enjoy. She finds herself spending a significant amount of time searching the lay press for potential etiologies of her symptoms and natural remedies. She is profoundly frustrated and somewhat angered at the medical establishment for what she perceives as substandard medical care and attention to her symptoms. She is also anxious and worried that her symptoms signify some yet-unidentified, terrible disease. Ms. Reed is very focused on her physical complaints throughout the interview. She wants to know how a mental health care provider is going to help with her "obviously physical" problems.

What aspects of Ms. Reed's presentation further support your diagnosis of somatic symptom and related disorders? Ms. Reed meets criteria for somatic symptom disorder in that she has been experiencing one or more somatic symptoms for more than 6 months. These symptoms are distressing and disrupt her daily life. She also exhibits maladaptive and excessive thoughts and behaviors associated with her physical symptoms. The presence of an underlying medical disorder that may account for her symptoms (i.e., hypothyroidism) does not rule out somatic symptom disorder. She endorses significant health-related anxiety and believes that her symptoms represent an undiagnosed and likely dangerous physical malady. As a consequence of these beliefs, she finds herself spending excessive time searching for answers to her somatic symptoms. The somatic symptoms may become a central characteristic and defining aspect of her personality.

Short-Answer Questions

1. What is required of the individual's thoughts, feelings, and beliefs related to the somatic symptoms in somatic symptom disorder if the person has a medical condition that may account for the somatic symptoms?

2. What is the minimum duration of the symptoms in somatic symptom disorder and of the health preoccupation in illness anxiety disorder?

3. What are some examples of the maladaptive thoughts and feelings related to the somatic symptom focus present in somatic symptom disorder?

4. How does a mental health care provider differentiate somatic symptom disorder from illness anxiety disorder?

5. What are some of the abnormal or excessive health-related behaviors that may be observed in individuals with somatic symptom disorder?

6. Individuals with conversion disorder (functional neurological symptom disorder) have one or more symptoms involving which parts of the nervous system?

7. How must psychological factors affect medical conditions to qualify for the diagnosis of psychological factors affecting other medical conditions?

8. The DSM-IV diagnoses of somatization disorder, hypochondriasis, pain disorder, and undifferentiated somatoform disorder have been largely subsumed under which of the somatic symptom and related disorders?

9. Which of the somatic symptom and related disorders requires that the individual purposely feign or produce symptoms or disease states?

10. What is the main differential diagnostic consideration in conversion disorder (functional neurological symptom disorder)?

Answers

1. In somatic symptom disorder, the associated maladaptive thoughts, feelings, and behaviors must be excessive.
2. Six months is the minimum duration of the symptoms in somatic symptom disorder and of the health preoccupation in illness anxiety disorder.
3. Cognitive features of somatic symptom and related disorders include intense attention to somatic symptoms, ascription of normal bodily sensations to pathological disease states, and often-intense concern about physical health status.
4. A mental health care provider can differentiate illness anxiety disorder from somatic symptom disorder by knowing that the individual with illness anxiety disorder experiences intense worries about health but his or her focus on co-occurring somatic symptoms is minimal.
5. Abnormal or excessive health-related behaviors that may be observed in individuals with somatic symptom disorder include repeated checking for health-related abnormalities, high health care utilization, and avoidance of activities that may be felt to worsen health status.
6. Individuals with conversion disorder have functional deficits in the voluntary motor or sensory nervous system.
7. The psychological or behavioral factors must have a negative impact on the individual's underlying general medical condition.
8. The DSM-IV diagnoses of somatization disorder, hypochondriasis, pain disorder, and undifferentiated somatoform disorder have been largely subsumed under somatic symptom disorder in DSM-5.
9. In factitious disorder the individual is purposely feigning or inducing symptoms and signs of disease with the aim of seeking the sick role.
10. The main differential diagnostic consideration in conversion disorder is neurological or other medical conditions.

13

Feeding and Eating Disorders

Cara Bohon, Ph.D.

"I still think I'm fat."

"My eating is out of control."

Feeding and eating disorders are characterized by the altered consumption or absorption of food that results in problems in physical health, psychological well-being, or both. This diagnostic class combines the previous DSM-IV diagnostic class of eating disorders with some of the childhood disorders, including feeding disorder of infancy or early childhood (redefined as avoidant/restrictive food intake disorder), pica, and rumination disorder. Additionally, binge-eating disorder, which was previously included as eating disorder not otherwise specified and as a category for further study, is now included as an actual diagnosis. Together with anorexia nervosa and bulimia nervosa, these diagnoses capture commonly observed patterns of eating disturbance throughout the lifespan.

Pica is characterized by the eating of nonnutritive or nonfood substances of at least 1 month in duration that is not developmentally appropriate and is not culturally normative. This diagnosis is the only one that can be made in addition to others in the diagnostic class, so someone could be diagnosed simultaneously with pica and another feeding or eating disorder. Eating disturbance in pica does not necessarily result in food restriction or weight loss, although it can, and is not related to body image or shape and weight. Many individuals with pica have intellectual disability or developmental delay, and those without intellectual problems may be embarrassed or feel ashamed about their eating.

Rumination disorder is characterized by the repeated regurgitation of food of at least 1 month in duration that is not better explained by any gastrointestinal or medical condition. All feeding and eating disorders other than pica take diagnostic precedence over rumination disorder, meaning that if the regurgitation occurs only during the course of anorexia nervosa, bulimia nervosa, binge-eating disorder, or avoidant/restrictive food intake disorder, the other disorder is diagnosed instead of rumination disorder. Rumination disorder is most commonly diagnosed in children but can have onset at any age. Like individuals with other feeding and eating disorders, individuals with rumination disorder may feel ashamed of or secretive about the disorder, making it difficult to identify.

Avoidant/restrictive food intake disorder is the expanded diagnostic term for the DSM-IV diagnosis of feeding disorder of infancy or early childhood. The change resulted in part from the prevalence of older children and adolescents who presented with similar eating disturbance and food restriction but did not meet criteria for other feeding and eating disorders. The disorder is characterized by a failure to meet nutritional or energy needs that results in significant weight loss, nutritional deficiency, dependence on oral supplements or tube feeding, or interference with psychosocial functioning. The eating disturbance is not part of an effort to control one's shape or weight, and no body image disturbance is present. The food restriction may result from an overall lack of interest in food broadly or may be based on specific sensory characteristics of food, such as texture or smell. Additionally, some individuals are worried about aversive consequences of eating, such as upset stomach. If criteria for anorexia or bulimia are met, those diagnoses take precedence over avoidant/restrictive food intake disorder. Although avoidant/restrictive food intake disorder is often seen in individuals with developmental delay, it may also occur in typically developing children and adults.

Anorexia nervosa is characterized by significantly low body weight due to food restriction, intense fear of weight gain, and disturbance in body image, such as the belief of being fat despite evidence of dangerously low weight. The fear of weight gain does not have to be explicitly articulated but could be presumed on the basis of persistent behavior that interferes with weight gain. Individuals with anorexia nervosa may or may not engage in binge-eating and purging behaviors. The diagnosis of anorexia nervosa supersedes all other eating disorder diagnoses because of the acute need for intervention. The primary difference between the DSM-IV criteria and those of DSM-5 is the removal of the requirement that postmenarcheal females have an absence of menstrual periods for three cycles. This criterion was removed in light of evidence that females not missing their periods showed equivalent levels of impairment, as well as the difficulty assessing the criterion in women taking hormonal birth control. Additionally, the DSM-5 criteria no longer suggest what constitutes low weight, which allows professionals to use clinical data better matched to the individual, such as weight and medical history, to determine what weight would be minimally expected.

Individuals presenting with bulimia nervosa engage in binge eating and compensatory behaviors at least weekly on average over the past 3 months. Additionally, they put undue emphasis on the importance of weight and shape. Binge eating occurs when an individual eats an amount of food in a discrete period of time (typically less than 2 hours) that most people would consider large under similar circumstances. Additionally, the eating is characterized by the sense of loss of control. In response to this increase in food intake, compensatory behaviors constitute an effort to counter the effects of the binge episode on weight gain. Compensatory behaviors may be self-induced vomiting, laxative or diuretic misuse, fasting, or excessive exercise. The primary change from DSM-IV is a decrease in the frequency of binge eating and compensatory behaviors required to meet a diagnosis. Research showed significant impairment when individuals engaged in these behaviors once per week, which was less than the previous frequency of twice per week.

Binge-eating disorder was previously included in DSM-IV as an eating disorder not otherwise specified until additional research could be conducted. Clinical utility and validity for the diagnosis have since been established. This diagnosis is characterized by recurrent binge eating without compensatory behaviors, at least once weekly over the past 3 months. Disturbance in body image may or may not be present. Unlike anorexia nervosa and bulimia nervosa, binge-eating disorder occurs almost equally in men and women and tends to have a later age at onset, typically in early adulthood. Individuals with binge-eating disorder are often overweight or obese and may have tried weight-loss treatments in the past with little success unless the treatment directly addressed binge-eating behavior.

DSM-5 includes two new categories to replace eating disorder not otherwise specified from DSM-IV:

- Other specified feeding or eating disorder includes specific variants of symptom presentation that do not fit the criteria for the other disorders in the diagnostic class. These include atypical anorexia nervosa (anorexia nervosa with a normal weight); bulimia nervosa of low frequency and/or limited duration (bulimia nervosa with binge eating and compensatory behaviors occurring less than once a week and/or for less than 3 months); binge-eating disorder of low frequency and/or limited duration (binge-eating disorder with binge eating occurring less than once a week and/or less than 3 months); purging disorder (recurrent purging in the absence of binge eating); and night eating syndrome (recurrent excessive eating after awakening from sleep or after the evening meal).
- Unspecified feeding or eating disorder is given as a diagnosis when symptoms of a feeding and eating disorder that cause significant distress or impairment do not meet full criteria for any other disorder in the diagnostic class. This is given if the reason that the disorder does not meet full criteria for another diagnosis is not provided or there is insufficient information available.

An overall hierarchy for diagnosing eating disorders is in place for all diagnoses except pica. The order of precedence is anorexia nervosa, bulimia nervosa, avoidant/restrictive food intake disorder, binge-eating disorder, and rumination disorder. This precedence ensures that adequate treatment is pursued on the basis of course and outcome of the different diagnoses. Because anorexia nervosa has the highest mortality rate and poses great medical risk, it is placed at the top of the hierarchy. Thus, if criteria for anorexia are met in addition to other feeding and eating disorders, only a diagnosis of anorexia is made, to emphasize the need for treatment. Similar steps follow for each disorder along the hierarchy.

IN-DEPTH DIAGNOSIS

Pica

Peter is a 6-year-old boy whose mother first noticed that erasers from all the pencils were missing. Although she had not seen Peter eat any erasers, his older sister had reported the behavior to her. Peter had been diagnosed with autism spectrum disorder at age 3, and his mother assumed that eating erasers was related to his developmental delay. She tried to keep erasers from him so that he would not eat them, but she then began to notice edges of books with bite marks, as well as missing feet from action figure toys with teeth marks along the end. Because of the communication difficulty related to his autism, his mother had trouble explaining to Peter that he should not eat these things, and when she removed various items, he seemed to find new things to eat in their place. She sought treatment for him after a few months because she realized that his obsessive urge to eat objects was becoming disruptive and seemed to be related to his lack of interest in eating meals and might be affecting his nutritional status.

Pica is often reported in children with a diagnosis of autism spectrum disorder or intellectual disability. Because these children have difficulty communicating, they often do not express concern about their eating behavior, and a parent provides information about the behavior. Siblings may have more information about the actual behavior because of their frequent proximity during play and the fact that children may hide the eating behavior from their parents for fear of discipline. Although some nonfood ingestion may be normal in the context of autism spectrum disorder, diagnosis and treatment of pica are important if the eating behavior leads to potential medical problems, such as lack of adequate nutrition, poisoning, or bowel obstruction.

Approach to the Diagnosis

Many individuals with pica present for treatment upon referral from a primary care physician after they have gastrointestinal complications from nonfood ingestion. Individuals may generally be secretive about their eating of nonfood items, because either they feel guilt and shame or (for children) they have been disciplined in the past for eating nonfood items. Because of the disorder's secretive nature, assessment should include collateral information from parents or others in the home, if available, and all diagnostic interview questions should be posed sensitively and without judgment.

Pica is diagnosed when an individual reports eating nonnutritive, nonfood substances (e.g., ice, dirt, chalk, paper, paint, hair) over a period of at least 1 month. Many individuals report that they typically ingest a primary type of nonfood, but some ingest a variety of items. It is important to ask about the duration and frequency of the nonfood eating, regardless of type. The developmental level of the individual is important to assess; as a result, pica is not often diagnosed earlier than age 2 years. Because toddlers often put objects and nonfood items in their mouths, nonfood ingestion is not considered pica until teething and oral exploration have otherwise ceased. Additionally, when assessing a potential diagnosis of pica, the clinician needs in-depth understanding of cultural practices. If the eating behavior is supported by cultural norms, such as spiritual or medicinal practices, a diagnosis of pica is not met.

Finally, the presence of other mental disorders, such as autism spectrum disorder or schizophrenia, should be considered when assessing for pica. If the eating behavior is severe enough to warrant focused treatment outside the scope of the other disorder, then pica is diagnosed. This diagnosis is generally related to the severity and frequency of the nonfood ingestion and its influence on other aspects of functioning, such as obtaining adequate nutrition.

Getting the History

> Julia, a 5-year-old girl, was referred after presenting to her primary care physician with an obstructed bowel from swallowing a sponge. In a sensitive and nonjudgmental manner, the interviewer asks whether she eats sponges often and whether she has any other things that she eats besides food. The girl appears shy and looks at her mother, who answers that she has noticed sponges missing in the last few weeks, and after doing laundry, she has noticed that the edges of Julia's blankets are frayed and chunks of the blankets are missing. After being reminded that she will not get in trouble for talking about what she had eaten, Julia admits that she ate the missing sponges and had been chewing pieces off the edge of her blankets. Because children are often poor reporters of the duration of a problem, the interviewer asks the mother to be specific about when she first noticed that sponges or pieces of blanket were missing or otherwise had suspicions about Julia's eating behavior. The interviewer asks about overall development, including language and social development, to assess for developmental delay or intellectual impairment, which is commonly comorbid with pica. The mother reports that Julia had delayed speech and did not make good eye contact. She had never been assessed for autism spectrum disorder. To determine whether nonfood ingestion is developmentally appropriate, the interviewer asks about related behaviors, such as mouthing toys. The mother reports that Julia had stopped placing other objects in her mouth approximately 2 years prior, which suggests that the current eating behavior is not developmentally appropriate. Finally, the interviewer asks about any cultural practices of the family that may include this type of eating. The mother reports that they do not have any such practices.

Because individuals with pica may not feel comfortable or be physically able due to intellectual impairments to discuss their eating behavior, information obtained from parents or other care providers is particularly important. Additionally, children may not be monitored constantly, so some nonfood ingestion may not be witnessed by others. Thus, reliance on other evidence of the behavior is important, such as missing objects or objects found in feces or by medical professionals when evaluating gastrointestinal problems. Some children may have been punished for eating objects in the past, so encouragement and reassurance that they will not be punished for talking about their behavior is important in order to obtain accurate information.

Tips for Clarifying the Diagnosis

- Evaluate the frequency and duration of ingestion of nonfood items in a sensitive manner, collecting collateral information as needed through medical records and caregiver report.
- Assess developmental level of the individual to ensure that the nonfood ingestion is not due to oral exploration or teething, which is common in toddlers and very young children.
- Evaluate the influence of cultural norms regarding eating of nonfood items.
- Explore the influence of other mental disorders on the nonfood ingestion, and evaluate whether the eating disturbance requires additional focused treatment to ensure health and adequate nutrition.

Consider the Case

> Ms. Harrington is a 25-year-old pregnant woman. She had never experienced any disordered eating in her past, but during her pregnancy she began having strong urges to eat ice. She started filling cups with ice and then chewing the ice regularly for the first few months of her pregnancy. She became concerned about her teeth from the constant crunching and felt pain from cold sensitivity. However, she did not believe she could control her urges to eat ice. She also reports cravings for dirt and sand or anything gritty against her teeth. Ms. Harrington had a typical development and was of average intellectual functioning. She does not report any other mental disorders. She denies any cultural practices involving the ingestion of nonfood objects.

Most adults with pica have intellectual disability, but pregnant women of average intelligence may also engage in ingestion of nonnutritive or nonfood items. It is unclear why pregnant women engage in nonfood ingestion, but some researchers theorize that the behavior is related to vitamin deficiencies during pregnancy. Little is known about the prevalence of pica in individuals of different ethnic backgrounds. Even if a person comes from a culture with a spiritual practice of nonfood ingestion, the behavior would qualify for a diagnosis of pica if he or she does not identify the eating behavior as equivalent to the cultural practice.

Differential Diagnosis

Pica can be diagnosed simultaneously with other disorders, except these three main conflicting diagnoses: anorexia nervosa (if the ingestion of nonfood is used by the person to control appetite), factitious disorder (if the nonfood ingestion is a means to feign symptoms of illness), and nonsuicidal self-injury (if the person swallows objects such as needles).

Pica may be diagnosed in the presence of a gastrointestinal condition, because some nonfood ingestion may lead to complications such as intestinal obstruction or mechanical bowel problems. In fact, medical complications are sometimes the way in which the disordered eating behavior is discovered. Pica is sometimes related to neglect or lack of supervision, and it is commonly associated with intellectual disability and autism spectrum disorder. It is also sometimes present in individuals with schizophrenia and obsessive-compulsive disorder. Individuals with trichotillomania (hair-pulling disorder) or excoriation (skin-picking) disorder may eat their hair or skin, resulting in pica if the nonfood eating is severe enough to warrant clinical attention. Finally, women may develop pica in response to odd cravings during pregnancy.

See DSM-5 for additional disorders to consider in the differential diagnosis. Also refer to the discussions of comorbidity and differential diagnosis in their respective sections of DSM-5.

Summary

- Pica is characterized by the eating of nonfood items that is severe enough to warrant clinical attention.
- Children younger than age 2 years are not diagnosed with pica, because eating nonfoods may be developmentally appropriate.
- Individuals with pica may have another diagnosis if the eating behavior is severe enough to warrant clinical attention directly.
- Pica is often comorbid with autism spectrum disorder and intellectual disability (intellectual developmental disorder).

––––––––– **IN-DEPTH DIAGNOSIS** –––––––––

Anorexia Nervosa

Angela is a 14-year-old Asian American girl presenting with a 20-pound weight loss over the past 3 months. She is currently in the 4th percentile for body mass index (BMI), despite being in the 25th percentile throughout most of her childhood. She denies having a problem with her eating, reporting that her eating changes have simply been an effort to be healthy. She has cut out dairy products, stating that they make her stomach upset, and has cut back on meat intake because she believes it is unhealthy. She refuses to eat what her mother prepares for dinner because it is "gross" and "greasy." Her daily food intake is often restricted to a small bowl of oatmeal, fruit, and a small salad without dressing. She runs cross-country at school but reports feeling more tired lately and unable to keep up with her team. When asked about fear of becoming fat, she denies it, but she refuses to increase her food intake, even of "healthy foods," suggesting discomfort with the prospect of weight gain.

A common presentation in anorexia nervosa is an adolescent who denies any problem with her behavior. Individuals often present for treatment with concerned parents. Having information about the person's current weight, as well as his or her weight trajectory through childhood, can help determine the presence of the low body weight criterion. The DSM-5 criterion for fear of weight gain does not require that the person express such fear verbally; the person can instead show evidence of the fear via behavior and refusal to gain to a healthy weight. Some individuals with anorexia nervosa may report gastrointestinal problems on which they blame food restriction, but the refusal to increase food intake of "safe" foods suggests that fear of weight gain is indeed present. Gastrointestinal problems are commonly cited in Asian populations to explain food restriction. Furthermore, the refusal to increase food intake is evidence that a person has not understood the seriousness of the low weight.

Approach to the Diagnosis

Individuals with anorexia nervosa often present for evaluation at the urging of parents or loved ones, rather than of their own accord. For this reason, consultation of previous records and interviews with family members or significant others are important for accurate representation of symptom presentation. Individuals must meet three specific criteria for the diagnosis, and specifiers of subtype and severity require additional information.

To assess for low body weight, the first criterion, it is important to know the person's current weight and height, lowest weight at the current height, and highest weight at the current height. Knowing the approximate dates of these weights is also helpful. If the person is still growing in height, it is important to know his or her typical growth trajectory to determine if the patterns are significantly changed. For adults, a general rule for low weight is BMI<18.5 kg/m^2, but exceptions may exist. For children and adolescents, BMI below the 5th percentile for age and gender is typically considered low weight. Severity specifiers for adults are based on body weight, as follows: mild, BMI≥17 kg/m^2; moderate, BMI 16–16.99 kg/m^2; severe, BMI 15–15.99 kg/m^2; and extreme, BMI<15 kg/m^2.

The second criterion is fear of weight gain, which can be elicited verbally and directly through questioning about the fear or can be assessed via the presence of persistent behavior that interferes with weight gain, suggesting a fear that is being alleviated through behavior. It can be helpful to ask the person how he or she would feel about gaining weight during treatment. Most individuals with anorexia nervosa will express resistance to weight gain regardless of whether they acknowledge a fear of weight gain.

The third criterion, overvaluation of shape and weight, can be assessed by inquiring where shape and weight fall in a ranking of the importance of aspects individuals use to evaluate themselves, such as work ethic and friendships. Individuals with overvaluation of shape and weight place those aspects toward the top of this ranked list. Disturbance of body image, or the lack of recognition of the seriousness of current body weight, can be assessed through questions about whether the person's current body weight is acceptable or what his or her ideal weight is. It can also be helpful to ask about body parts the person may believe are fat, despite his or her overall low weight. To determine subtype, the interviewer should ask the person to confirm the presence or absence of purging (self-induced vomiting or misuse of laxatives, diuretics, or enemas) or binge eating. If the person is hesitant to answer, family members should be asked if they have noticed bathroom trips after meals or excessive food wrappers in the trash.

As stated in DSM-5, "Suicide risk is elevated in anorexia nervosa, with rates reported as 12 per 100,000 per year. Comprehensive evaluation of individuals with anorexia nervosa should include assessment of suicide-related ideation and behaviors as well as other risk factors for suicide, including a history of suicide attempt(s)" (p. 343).

Getting the History

Jessica, a 15-year-old girl, reports weight loss but does not specify changes to eating. The interviewer asks explicitly about any changes. The patient replies that she was "really stressed out about finals and forgot to eat." The interviewer clarifies about the forgotten eating by asking if Jessica ate more at other times to make up for the missed meal. She replies, "No, I sort of liked the idea of being able to eat less. I felt in control of my hunger and could overcome it, unlike other people." The interviewer clarifies again, "So even though it seemed as if your eating changes were from stress, you kept restricting food intake because it made you feel good about yourself?" Additionally, the interviewer, needing to know about Jessica's feelings about weight and shape, asks, "Was weight loss important?" Jessica replies, "It didn't seem that way at first, but I guess I did like that I lost weight." The interviewer asks directly about the importance of the weight: "How important is your weight in dictating how you feel about yourself as a person? If you had to rank all the things you use to evaluate yourself, like how good you are at school or how good a friend you are, where would weight or shape fall in that list?" Jessica replies, "Well, I want to say that being a good friend is more important, but honestly, weight and shape matter a lot. Don't they to everyone?" The interviewer clarifies yet again: "So would you put weight and shape at the very top? If you had a scale of 0–6 and 0 meant that it didn't matter at all and 6 meant that it was the most important aspect of yourself, where would weight and shape fall?" Jessica replies, "Well, they're not the *most* important thing, but they're definitely a main aspect, so I would say 5."

When a person's initial food restriction does not obviously relate to a desire to lose weight, it is important to evaluate potential feelings about weight loss and body image. The initial weight loss may be healthy or from stress; the key is evaluating the eventual intention of weight loss to the degree of low body weight currently presenting and what sort of value the patient places on weight and shape. If a patient reports that weight and shape are main aspects of self-evaluation, then that suggests an undue influence. Furthermore, if the initial food restriction has another cause, such as stress, but subsequent food restriction is an effort to continue weight loss, it still fits the criteria of anorexia nervosa.

Tips for Clarifying the Diagnosis

- Ensure that the low weight criterion is met by consulting both normed growth charts and historical growth trajectories for the individual.
- Evaluate fear of weight gain directly and/or through questions about willingness to gain weight in treatment.
- Evaluate body image disturbance through questions about desired weight, thoughts about current weight, and level of importance of shape and weight on self-evaluation.
- For overvaluation of shape and weight, ask individuals to rank aspects of self that they use to evaluate themselves, and see where shape and weight fall in that list. If shape or weight is one of the main aspects, then this criterion is met.
- Access collateral information from significant others and past medical records.

Consider the Case

Mr. Miller is a 26-year-old man presenting for treatment after a 30-pound weight loss over the past 6 months. He denies having a history of food obsession, body image disturbance, or anxiety. He reports having changed to a vegan diet because his girlfriend was vegan and it was easier to eat with her if he changed the way he ate. He reports not liking a lot of vegan options for protein, so his diet has consisted primarily of steamed vegetables and rice. He lost weight quickly and lost energy to continue his usual hobbies, including sports. Mr. Miller reports having initially received compliments for his weight loss, which reinforced his eating changes. Over time, his eating has become more restrictive, and he has become obsessed with foods and calorie counts and has difficulty focusing on other things.

This case is atypical for a few reasons. Mr. Miller is male and his age at onset is past the prime adolescent years. Although older males with anorexia nervosa are less common, they do present for treatment and can meet criteria for the disorder. Furthermore, this man's concerns about his body and general anxiety did not precede onset of the disorder, which is a less typical order of events; however, food restriction that occurs for a non-body-related reason, such as depression, stress, or a change in dietary preference, can result in body consciousness, often through reinforcing comments from others about initial weight loss. These individuals often deny obsession with food initially but report that over time, they find it difficult to focus on other things and continually think about their next meal and how many calories to allow themselves to eat.

Differential Diagnosis

Low body weight alone could indicate a number of diagnoses, including some general medical conditions. Individuals with low weight due to a medical condition, however, are typically aware of the seriousness of their low weight and would willingly gain weight if they were able. Major depressive disorder can be associated with loss of appetite and subsequent weight loss, but again, these individuals often desire weight regain and acknowledge the low weight as a problem. Schizophrenia and substance use disorders are sometimes associated with altered eating behavior or poor nutrition, but individuals with these disorders do not endorse a fear of weight gain. Social anxiety disorder (social phobia), obsessive-compulsive disorder, and body dysmorphic disorder may have food- and body-related symptom presentations. If an individual meets criteria for anorexia nervosa and only presents the eating-related symptoms of social anxiety disorder or obsessive-compulsive disorder, the second diagnosis is not made. If the body concerns in body dysmorphic disorder are unrelated to shape and weight (e.g., the person feels his or her nose is too big), an additional diagnosis should be made. Bulimia nervosa would be the proper diagnosis if binge eating and purging are present and body weight is not low. Avoidant/restrictive food intake disorder is the proper diagnosis if food restriction is not accompanied by body image disturbance.

Individuals with anorexia nervosa may appear sluggish and withdrawn due to poor nourishment and desire to refrain from social situations where food may be present. Obsessive thinking about food and weight are common, as are desires to cook for others. Individuals with anorexia nervosa also tend to be rigid, rule bound, and harm avoidant. Some individuals present with excessive exercise, which may precede the disorder. If they do not present for treatment earlier at the urgings of family, some patients will present medically due to bradycardia, orthostatic hypotension, or frequent bone breaks due to low bone density.

See DSM-5 for additional disorders to consider in the differential diagnosis. Also refer to the discussions of comorbidity and differential diagnosis in their respective sections of DSM-5.

Summary

- Anorexia nervosa is characterized by an inability to maintain normal weight due to the restriction of food intake.
- Also present is an intense fear of weight gain or behavior that suggests an underlying fear of weight gain, such as behavior that sabotages attempts to reach a healthy weight range, even if the individual will not verbalize a fear of weight gain.
- The diagnosis of anorexia nervosa requires that the person have an overvaluation of weight and shape, which entails placing a great emphasis on weight and shape when determining self-worth.
- The weight loss in anorexia nervosa is not simply the consequence of a medical condition.
- Individuals with anorexia nervosa may or may not engage in frequent binge eating and purging.

―――――――― **IN-DEPTH DIAGNOSIS** ――――――――
Bulimia Nervosa

Samantha is a 16-year-old girl reporting obsessions about food and eating, as well as daily binge eating followed by self-induced vomiting. She reports eating breakfast and then going back for more food after her mother leaves for work. She eats, for example, five pieces of dense French toast with maple syrup. She reports vomiting afterward because of guilt over how much she ate and fear of weight gain. She eats lunch later but follows a healthy sandwich with a pint of ice cream and subsequently vomits. She reports having blood in her vomit occasionally.

As is typical, Samantha's bulimia nervosa began in late adolescence. She reports recurrent binge eating and compensatory behavior, in this case self-induced vomiting. Although she does not explicitly report shame about her eating, the fact that she waits for her mother to leave before binge eating suggests that she has some shameful feelings about it and does not want to be seen eating. Many individuals binge eat in secret or alone. The guilt feeling after a binge is often cited as the motivation to purge, as is fear of weight gain from the eating binge. The presence of blood in the vomit suggests serious potential for medical complications, such as esophageal tears, and should trigger an immediate referral for medical evaluation.

Approach to the Diagnosis

Individuals with bulimia nervosa tend to be self-critical in a number of ways, including with regard to their body image. Internalization of the thin ideal presented by Western culture is often present and may drive body dissatisfaction and negative affect. Individuals report high levels of negative affect, which often trigger binge eating. Because of their self-critical nature, they also tend to be secretive and ashamed about their eating. They often report temporary relief from negative affect during the binge, but the relief is replaced by guilt and shame over how much they ate. The guilt and shame in turn drive the urge to compensate for their eating in some way. It can be difficult to determine whether a reported binge-eating episode is objectively large for the situation described. Additionally, determining whether all binge-eating episodes are adequately large can be difficult, because individuals tend to feel shameful and/or embarrassed about their eating.

Compensatory behaviors may include vomiting, laxative or diuretic misuse, fasting, or excessive exercise. The use of fingers to induce vomiting can result in scarred hands where teeth have scraped against the hand repeatedly. As in anorexia nervosa, individuals with bulimia nervosa place undue emphasis on shape and weight. Unlike in anorexia nervosa, their weight tends to be in the normal or overweight range. When not binge eating, they tend to restrict food intake or intake of fatty foods, so they are less likely to be obese, although obesity can occur.

Medical complications are associated with bulimia nervosa, specifically related to vomiting and laxative abuse. Parotid glands may be enlarged, and damage to teeth may be evident. Menstrual irregularities or amenorrhea may be present. Esophageal tears, gastric rupture, and cardiac arrhythmias are rare, but potentially fatal, complications. Gastrointestinal problems are common, especially in individuals abusing laxatives. Some individuals may convert to bulimia from anorexia nervosa. Those with the binge-eating/purging type of anorexia who subsequently gain weight may meet criteria for bulimia nervosa. Additionally, some individuals with the restricting type of anorexia nervosa may develop subsequent binge-eating/purging behavior upon weight regain and meet criteria for bulimia nervosa.

As stated in DSM-5, "Suicide risk is elevated in bulimia nervosa. Comprehensive evaluation of individuals with this disorder should include assessment of suicide-related ideation and behaviors as well as other risk factors for suicide, including a history of suicide attempts" (p. 349).

Getting the History

When Audrey, a 17-year-old girl, initially reports binge eating, she is vague and says, "Yeah, I've done that a few times." The interviewer may decide to first get a sense of a typical episode by asking her to describe the most recent and typical eating binge that occurred. The patient replies, "Oh, I ate a bowl of cereal, then ate a bag of chips, two apples, and a few cookies." To clarify the amount eaten and ensure that this is a binge, the interviewer asks about the size of the bag of chips and the cookies. Audrey responds, "The chips were in a regular-sized bag—not the family size but not the little individual serving bags. The cookies were chocolate chip. I think I had 8 of them—whatever is in the first row of the package." When asked, "And you felt a loss of control while eating?" the patient answers, "Oh yeah, I just couldn't stop. Especially with the chips and cookies." Now that the interviewer has established a typical binge and verified that it meets criteria, the focus turns to frequency: "So how often in the past month have you had an eating binge like that?" Audrey replies, "Probably once or twice a week…so maybe six times in the last month?" The interviewer follows up by asking, "And what about the 2 months before that? Were you bingeing about once or twice per week during those months too?" Audrey responds, "Yeah, I guess it has been this way for a while. Maybe for 6 months. It started just occasionally, but then it sort of became a regular thing." To assess for compensatory behaviors, the interviewer asks Audrey directly if she engages in self-induced vomiting or laxative or diuretic use to control her shape or weight or to get rid of the calories from binge eating. Audrey answers, "I tried throwing up a few times, but I wasn't very good at it. So I figured I would just exercise more on days I ate more." The interviewer then begins to clarify whether her exercise is excessive by asking about frequency, duration, and intensity, and investigating whether there are things Audrey does not do because of exercising. The patient says, "Well, I guess on days I binge, I won't accept invitations to hang out with friends because I know I won't otherwise be able to work out and do my homework."

In evaluating a patient for bulimia nervosa, the interviewer needs first to assess whether the behaviors constitute a full episode as described in DSM-5. For binge eating, this means ensuring that the amount of food is more than most individuals would normally eat in similar circumstances and that the person feels a loss of control while eating. For compensatory behaviors, if the method of compensation is exercise, the interviewer must ensure that it is excessive and is in effort to compensate for food consumed and to prevent weight gain. Many people report exercising to lose weight generally, but for diagnosis of bulimia nervosa, this exercise must be interfering, inappropriate, or against medical advice, which expresses the drive and compulsive nature of the exercise. Finally, the interviewer must verify that the behaviors occurred at least once per week over the past 3 months.

Tips for Clarifying the Diagnosis

- Ensure that reported binge eating that meets the frequency criterion of once per week is an objective binge rather than eating that the individual believes is excessive but is actually a normal amount.
- Ensure that all binge eating that meets the frequency criterion involves the loss of control.
- To count excessive exercise as compensatory behavior, establish that it is an effort to compensate for calories consumed and that it significantly interferes with life, such as leading to canceling or missing other activities and/or continuing despite injury.
- Demonstrate compassion during assessment to increase patients' honesty in reporting their binge eating and purging behaviors, about which they are often ashamed. Additionally, keep in mind that collateral information may or may not be helpful, depending on whether others have noticed secretive behaviors.

Consider the Case

Ms. Woods is a 40-year-old black woman who recently went through a divorce. During her emotional nights, she found herself seeking comfort in food. She reports eating "whatever is around," including an entire loaf of bread one night. She began throwing up to relieve her upset stomach after feeling overly full. She denies that she threw up initially to get rid of the calories from the binge eating, but once she realized that she could indulge in food yet not suffer the weight gain, she began purging regularly. She switched from vomiting to laxative misuse after reading about dental problems related to frequent vomiting. She currently binges approximately once per week, usually when she feels lonely on a weekend, and takes 10 laxatives at a time afterward to "clear out" her body.

In Ms. Woods's case, the onset of the disorder was much later than the typical onset during late adolescence or early adulthood. However, stressful life events can trigger onset of the disorder. It is also of note that vomiting did not begin as a compensatory behavior but became one over time. Individuals with onset in adulthood may feel even more worried about consequences of weight gain if weight is something with which they have struggled. Additionally, perhaps due to a greater awareness of negative consequences of their behavior, they may deliberately change compensatory behaviors during the illness to avoid such things as tooth decay. Finally, although bulimia nervosa is more common in white women, it does occur in ethnic minority groups, including blacks.

Differential Diagnosis

Bulimia nervosa must be differentiated from other feeding and eating disorders, including anorexia nervosa, binge-eating/purging type, and binge-eating disorder. The key difference between bulimia nervosa and anorexia nervosa, binge-eating/purging type, is the current body weight. It is common for individuals to move from one diagnosis to the other depending on body weight, so evaluating current body weight and behavior is important. If binge eating and purging occur only during periods of low weight, bulimia nervosa criteria are not met. A diagnosis of binge-eating disorder may be given if regular compensatory behavior is not present. Some neurological or medical conditions, such as Kleine-Levin syndrome, can affect eating behaviors, but overvaluation of shape and weight is not present. Depressed mood is common in bulimia nervosa, and overeating is common in major depressive disorder with atypical features. However, overvaluation of shape and weight and compensatory behaviors are not as common in major depressive disorder outside of an additional diagnosis of bulimia nervosa. Binge eating may be present as an impulsive behavior in borderline personality disorder, but again, overvaluation of shape and weight is not present.

Individuals with bulimia nervosa often report higher levels of negative affect and depressed mood than do healthy individuals. They often report body dissatisfaction and may report a history of dieting attempts to control their shape or weight. Often, this unsuccessful dieting leads to patterns of disordered eating, including periods of food restriction followed by binge eating and purging. For some individuals, binge eating seems to be tightly related to their mood, and both binge eating and purging may be done to improve their mood. For others, there may be a strong craving for food or obsession about eating, followed by guilt and shame about eating and fear of weight gain. Such guilt, shame, and fear drive the motivation to engage in compensatory behavior.

See DSM-5 for additional disorders to consider in the differential diagnosis. Also refer to the discussions of comorbidity and differential diagnosis in their respective sections of DSM-5.

Summary

- Individuals with bulimia nervosa have recurrent (on average, at least once-weekly) binge eating and compensatory behaviors.
- Binge-eating episodes must constitute a large amount of food in a discrete period of time (e.g., 2 hours) and must be accompanied by a feeling of loss of control.
- Overvaluation of weight and shape must be present, which includes placing an emphasis on weight and shape in determination of self-worth.
- Compensatory behaviors may be purging, which includes self-induced vomiting or excessive laxative or diuretic use; fasting; or excessive exercise. Exercise is considered excessive when it is functionally impairing by either interrupting other social or work/school activities or resulting in medical consequences.
- All symptoms occur at least weekly on average for at least 3 months.
- The symptoms of bulimia nervosa are not present solely during an episode of anorexia nervosa; in other words, binge eating and compensatory behaviors must be present even when the individual is not underweight and meeting criteria for anorexia.

——————— SUMMARY ———————

Feeding and Eating Disorders

The category of feeding and eating disorders includes symptom presentations characterized by a disturbance in typical eating patterns. This disturbance may consist of eating nonnutritive substances, as in pica; overall restriction of food intake, as in avoidant/restrictive food intake disorder and anorexia nervosa; repetitive and abnormal regurgitation of food, as in rumination disorder; or binge eating, as in bulimia nervosa and binge-eating disorder. Some, but not all, of the disorders occur primarily in females and include disturbance of body image or overconcern with weight and shape. Most of the disorders have onset during childhood or adolescence, although adult onset can occur. Because of the nutritive impact of eating disorders, medical evaluations are important to assess for medical consequences and ensure no other medical cause for the disordered eating. Additionally, the medical complications can be quite severe and, in some cases, lead to death. Indeed, anorexia nervosa has the highest mortality rate of all psychiatric illnesses. Thus, prompt diagnosis and treatment are important.

------------------------------ ■-■-■ ------------------------------
Diagnostic Pearls

- Although eating disorders are commonly thought to affect predominantly females, this predominance is only true of anorexia nervosa and bulimia nervosa. Binge-eating disorder is only slightly more prevalent in females; and pica, rumination disorder, and avoidant/restrictive food intake disorder are equally prevalent in both genders.

- Anorexia nervosa and bulimia nervosa both include a disturbance in body image or overvaluation of shape and weight on self-evaluation. This disturbance is not present in avoidant/restrictive food intake disorder and may or may not be present in other diagnoses.

- Age at onset for all feeding and eating disorders is generally before adulthood, although there are exceptions. Onset for bulimia nervosa and binge-eating disorder is typically in late adolescence and early adulthood. Onset for anorexia nervosa is early to late adolescence; and onset for pica, rumination disorder, and avoidant/restrictive food intake disorder is often younger.

- Anorexia nervosa poses the highest mortality rate of all psychiatric illnesses. Thus, a diagnosis of anorexia nervosa supersedes diagnoses of other feeding and eating disorders to ensure adequate treatment.

- Adolescents are often secretive about their eating and may be poor reporters of their behaviors. Additionally, binge eating and compensatory behaviors may occur in secret, so parents and significant others may not be aware. It is important to get whatever collateral information is available and also attempt to remain nonjudgmental and compassionate during assessment to help reduce shame and guilt about behaviors.

Self-Assessment

Key Concepts: Double-Check Your Knowledge

What is the relevance of the following concepts to the various feeding and eating disorders?

- Overvaluation of shape and weight
- Significantly low weight
- Fear of weight gain
- Binge eating episode
- Excessive exercise

Questions to Discuss With Colleagues and Mentors

1. What laboratory tests do you use when assessing medical complications in eating disorders?
2. How do you clarify the diagnosis when individuals refuse to disclose disordered eating behaviors although other sources suggest persistent food refusal?

Case-Based Questions

PART A

Jennifer is a 14-year-old Hispanic girl who reports restricting her food intake over the past few months because of discomfort in her stomach. She reports feeling so badly that she also makes herself throw up, hoping that it will alleviate the pain. Additionally, she sometimes feels severe hunger after periods of food restriction, which leads to loss of control in eating binges followed by self-induced vomiting to prevent abdominal pain. She has lost 20 pounds in the past 2 months, which puts her overall body weight in the 3rd percentile for her age, sex, and height. She is being hospitalized for bradycardia and requires enteral feeding because of her persistent food refusal.

Which diagnoses should be considered at this point? At this point, Jennifer may meet criteria for avoidant/restrictive food intake disorder; anorexia nervosa, binge-eating/purging type; or a gastrointestinal problem. Additional information is needed to differentiate among these diagnoses.

PART B

Jennifer's medical doctors cannot find any clear medical basis for her abdominal pain. They believe that she has irritable bowel syndrome. Although the doctors offered recommendations for decreasing her discomfort, she continues to refuse food. Upon release from the hospital after gaining weight (to the 10th percentile) through enteral feeding, she resumes her pattern of food restriction and occasional binge eating and purging.

Would she meet criteria for anorexia nervosa or bulimia nervosa? Upon release from the hospital, Jennifer no longer meets the low-weight criterion for a diagnosis of anorexia nervosa. Although she is engaging in binge eating and purging behavior, it is unclear that the frequency and duration would meet diagnostic criteria for bulimia nervosa. Additionally, and relevant for both anorexia and bulimia, there is no report of body image disturbance or emphasis on body image.

PART C

After discharge from the hospital and cessation of the enteral feeding, Jennifer's weight drops again. She denies concern about shape and weight and reports that her eating patterns are entirely due to abdominal pain. However, the doctors report that most individuals with irritable bowel syndrome are able to eat normally, even if they report some discomfort.

Which diagnosis seems most appropriate? Because the persistent food restriction appears to exist beyond what would be reasonably expected given her medical condition and she continues to require enteral feeding, Jennifer meets criteria for avoidant/restrictive food intake disorder.

Short-Answer Questions

1. Which two of the feeding and eating disorders require body image disturbance or an overemphasis on weight and shape on self-evaluation?
2. What two characteristics are necessary for an eating episode to be considered binge eating?
3. What is the best way to differentiate anorexia nervosa from avoidant/restrictive food intake disorder?
4. List the order of precedence for diagnoses of the feeding and eating disorders (other than pica).
5. Which feeding and eating disorder has onset from early to late adolescence and is often preceded by an overly anxious and harm-avoidant temperament?
6. Which of the feeding and eating disorders have greater prevalence in females?
7. What is the duration of time that symptoms must be present to meet diagnostic criteria for pica and rumination disorder?
8. Which of the feeding and eating disorders can be diagnosed in addition to the others within the category?
9. How is avoidant/restrictive food intake disorder different from a gastrointestinal problem?
10. When can both anorexia nervosa and obsessive-compulsive disorder be diagnosed?

Answers

1. Anorexia nervosa and bulimia nervosa require body image disturbance or an overemphasis on weight and shape on self-evaluation.
2. Binge eating involves a large amount of food and a feeling of loss of control.
3. Individuals with anorexia nervosa also place undue emphasis on weight and shape and have disturbance in their body image.
4. The following is the order of precedence for diagnoses of the feeding and eating disorders (other than pica): anorexia nervosa, bulimia nervosa, avoidant/restrictive food intake disorder, binge-eating disorder, and rumination disorder.
5. Anorexia nervosa has onset from early to late adolescence and is often preceded by an overly anxious and harm-avoidant temperament.
6. Anorexia nervosa and bulimia nervosa and, to a lesser extent, binge-eating disorder are more prevalent in females.
7. Symptoms must be present for 1 month to meet diagnostic criteria for pica and rumination disorder.
8. Pica can be diagnosed in addition to other feeding and eating disorders.
9. Avoidant/restrictive food intake disorder can be diagnosed in the presence of a gastrointestinal disorder, but the disturbance of intake must be beyond what is directly accountable by the medical condition. Furthermore, some individuals may have lingering difficulties eating foods despite management of physical symptoms.
10. When diagnostic criteria for anorexia nervosa have been met, yet significant obsessions and compulsions not related to food or body image are also present, an additional diagnosis of obsessive-compulsive disorder is considered.

14

Elimination Disorders

Jennifer Derenne, M.D.

Kathleen Kara Fitzpatrick, Ph.D.

"My daughter still wets the bed."

"My son messes his underpants at school."

Elimination disorders typically manifest in early childhood and are often associated with significant distress and frustration for the child and family. They are some of the most common pediatric concerns, yet parents often do not report symptoms because they believe that nothing can be done.

Enuresis, commonly referred to as "wetting," is uncontrollable leakage of urine that occurs after bladder continence would generally be expected. Symptoms may be *primary,* which means that toilet training is not successful in a child over age 5 years (or an equivalent developmental level); or *secondary*, which refers to new wetting episodes after a 6-month period of complete dryness. Urinary incontinence may be continuous or intermittent and may occur exclusively at night or during daytime hours as well.

Encopresis is voluntary or involuntary fecal soiling by a child who has previously attained (or would have been expected to attain) bowel continence. Similar to enuresis, a diagnosis of encopresis is made only after a period in which bowel continence would be expected, generally over age 4 for a typically developing child, and can also be primary (failure to successfully toilet train) or secondary (developing after a period of continence). Bowel continence is expected to develop at a younger age than urinary continence, and a diagnosis is often made after age 4 years.

Both disorders involve the complex interplay of biological and psychological factors. Anatomical abnormalities and physiological factors such as chronic constipation, bladder dysfunction, diabetes (mellitus or insipidus), ineffective colon motility (such as Hirschsprung disease), and urinary tract infections must be considered in the differential diagnosis. In cases with no obvious anatomical or physiological pathology, psychological factors such as stress, child maltreatment, depression, and anxiety must be considered. Symptoms can cause extreme distress to the child, who may be teased or bullied if peers or siblings are aware of the problem. Children with elimination disorders often avoid nighttime social activities such as sleepovers, for fear of having an "accident" in front of friends.

The diagnostic criteria for encopresis and enuresis remain the same in DSM-5 as they were in DSM-IV. The major change is that both diagnoses have been removed from the section on disorders usually first diagnosed in infancy, childhood, or adolescence, and they now are part of the category of elimination disorders diagnostic class. In addition, diagnoses of other specified elimination disorder and unspecified elimination disorder have been added for symptoms characteristic of an elimination disorder that cause significant distress but do not fully meet diagnostic criteria for encopresis or enuresis.

─────────────── **IN-DEPTH DIAGNOSIS** ───────────────

Encopresis

Milo is a 10-year-old boy who was referred from his local pediatric gastroenterologist because of a history of soiling in his underwear. The specialist has ruled out medical causes of these difficulties. Currently, voiding episodes of full, hard stools most often occur in the afternoon, after a day at school, approximately twice per week. Furthermore, he has frequent fecal overflow and soiling of his underwear. He describes being teased for being "smelly" and has attempted to avoid school for fear of soiling himself on the school bus or at the end of the school day. Milo met initial toilet training milestones within normal limits, achieving nocturnal bowel continence by age 2.5 and daytime bowel continence and urinary continence at age 3. He has infrequent episodes of nocturnal enuresis, approximately once per week. Following a bout of severe stomach flu, Milo significantly restricted his intake and subsequently developed constipation. Despite efforts to maintain Milo's regular stooling with laxatives and dietary maintenance (e.g., a high-fiber diet), Milo's mother describes him as appearing to deliberately retain his feces, evidenced by sphincter tightening and toe walking. She notes that at times he does not seem aware that he needs to use the bathroom and will often deny a need to defecate despite multiple reminders. Milo reports that he often does not feel the need "to go" until he experiences an intense urge or fecal overflow. Medical evaluations have ruled out physical causes, but Milo continues to have high volumes of stool, evident on abdominal examination, and passes stools only twice per week. The family has worked to establish regular fiber in their diet and through supplements but admit that they are inconsistent and that Milo resists the increased vegetable intake. They have otherwise attempted to avoid shaming or discussing these difficulties with Milo, expecting him to deposit his feces in the toilet and place his soiled underwear in a bag in the laundry area. Milo is described by his parents and teachers as a shy, somewhat withdrawn boy who avoids his peers and has a history of school avoidance, complaining of gastrointestinal symptoms. His mother reports he had difficulty separating when younger, but this resolved with his entry to elementary school. He does not have any history of disruptive or aggressive behaviors.

Milo's presentation is fairly typical, with a history of normal stooling followed by complications resulting from constipation. The establishment of normal bowel continence is important, because it indicates that current symptoms are secondary to constipation and the reciprocal effects of withholding stool, followed by bowel impaction and fears of passing larger, more painful stools. The frequency of passage of feces outside the toilet (more than once per month), coupled by the ability to engage in regular stooling at a younger age and exclusion of physical causes for these difficulties, clearly warrants a diagnosis of encopresis. There is nothing on examination to indicate anatomical, metabolic, endocrine, or neurological abnormalities, and Milo takes no medications associated with fecal incontinence. Milo's history of shyness, separation fears, somatic complaints, and mild school refusal are all consistent with higher levels of internalizing symptoms and attention to physical symptoms that exacerbate concerns around passing more painful stools. Developmental and familial challenges in maintaining a high-fiber diet and consistent routines around toileting often interfere with efforts to establish more typical stooling patterns and are likely applicable to Milo and his family.

A consultation with his pediatric gastroenterologist would be recommended to establish whether his current constipation could be managed with medications or warrants use of enemas for more thorough evacuation of stool. Evaluation of rectal distention would also be useful to establish whether more aggressive efforts, such as the use of anal biofeedback, would be useful to assist Milo in identifying the need to stool or whether these can be managed with laxative use. It is important to assess the presence of maltreatment while keeping in mind that most children with incontinence are not suffering from abuse.

Approach to the Diagnosis

The diagnosis of encopresis is made on the basis of history, physical examination, laboratory data, and occasionally imaging studies. A thorough evaluation to rule out physical causes of fecal incontinence is critical to this diagnosis and necessary to establish the diagnosis. Specialty medical evaluations are particularly important in cases where bowel regularity has never been established (primary encopresis). Encopresis can be associated with anatomical, metabolic, endocrine, and neurological causes, as well as substance use or abuse. The most important disorder to rule out is Hirschsprung disease, in which the bowel lacks appropriate enervation and inhibits the ability both to identify the need to pass stool and to appropriately pass stools. In other cases, inflammatory bowel disorders may cause severe constipation. Effects may also be reciprocal, in that chronic and prolonged constipation can lead to bowel impaction that requires painful passage of stool. To prevent this pain, children may engage in retentive behaviors, most often tightening of the external anal sphincter muscles or tightening of gluteal muscles or pelvic muscles to prevent stool passage. Ultimately, this retention slows total transit time in the colon, which exacerbates constipation. As the colon becomes impacted (megacolon), reflexive mechanisms for stool passage become impaired, which can prevent the child from identifying the need to pass stool. A majority of children with encopresis deny feeling an urge to defecate. The longer stool is retained in the colon, the more water is absorbed from the stool and the harder stools become, making passage more painful and potentiating further restriction. A diagnosis of encopresis is not made when physical causes for fecal incontinence are identified.

Other presenting issues often prompt the referral, and screening questions around toileting can uncover issues that require more evaluation. It is important to ask about the age at which regular toileting habits were established and the presence of any "accidents" or soiling. A careful history will elicit the duration, timing, and severity of symptoms; any exacerbating and ameliorating factors; and the presence of any extended periods of fecal continence (e.g., some children may avoid toileting at school but assume more regular bowel voiding during summer break). Further questions should evaluate the extent of symptoms of constipation. The specifiers of encopresis are "with constipation and overflow incontinence" and "without constipation and overflow incontinence." DSM-5 does not define constipation, but it can be assessed with physical examination and the following questions: Does your child pass large, infrequent, or very hard stools? Does your child appear to be holding in stool (retentive posture)? Does your child pass stools that are large enough to block the toilet? How frequently does your child pass stool into the toilet? How frequently does your child pass stool into other receptacles (most often underwear)?

It is important to determine the frequency of stool passage outside of appropriate receptacles and the timing of stooling when it occurs. Most often, children and adolescents pass bowel movements in the late afternoon, after retaining stool for most of the day. Some experience the urge to pass stool during periods of more intense exercise, such as physical education classes or sports activities. It is also important to determine whether the fecal incontinence is intermittent or continuous and the conditions under which there is bowel regularity, if any, particularly in the context of constipation. Resolution of constipation itself is often an effective treatment for encopresis when efforts are maintained over 6–12 months. Important questions include the following: Other than the toilet, where does your child deposit bowel movements? How frequently does your child experience fecal soiling of the underwear (incontinence overflow)? Is there any evidence of nocturnal encopresis? Has your child ever been treated for constipation or other gastrointestinal difficulties? Has your child seen a gastroenterologist? If so, what is the maintenance routine for bowel regularity? How compliant is your child with these routines? How long have you maintained these routines? Have there been periods when your child was able to toilet regularly? How long have these periods lasted? Are there additional difficulties with enuresis (nocturnal and/or diurnal)?

Another important issue is whether the child takes any medications. In the absence of constipation, laxative use can cause encopretic behavior and may be associated with eating disorder behavior. Caregivers should be asked about their approach and attitude toward toilet training, their response to soiling, and whether there are any recent changes or stresses to the family. How is the child doing socially and academically? Are there any other developmental concerns (gross or fine motor skills, learning, speech, growth)? Are there concerns around neglect or failure to have appropriate toileting facilities available? Are there concerns around aggressive, violent, or regressive behaviors? Providers should sensitively, yet directly, ask about any maltreatment or abuse. Questions around general psychopathology are critical, given the wide range of comorbidity for this diagnosis. Specific questions should target anxiety, mood, and disruptive behavior disorders.

Getting the History

A mother reports that her 8-year-old son, Cody, has daytime soiling episodes. The interviewer starts with open-ended questions to determine the duration, frequency, and quality of symptoms. The first questions are directed to the mother: "How long has this been an issue? Does Cody pass stool outside the toilet, or does it just appear to be staining of the underwear? Is there a history of gastrointestinal difficulties, including stomach upset, vomiting, constipation, or diarrhea? How often does Cody pass stools— daily or with less frequency? Are stools large or hard? Do they cause significant pain when passing?" The interviewer then directs questions to Cody: "Have you ever been told you have constipation? If so, what did you do about it? Do you think that constipation is a problem now? How have you managed it? Have you changed your diet? Do you take any laxatives or stool softeners? How often are stools passed in the toilet? Where else do they occur (e.g., underwear, somewhere in the bedroom)? Are there places you won't go to the bathroom (e.g., public places, at school, in certain restrooms)? Why or why not? What happens when you have an accident? Do you know that you need to use the bathroom, or does stooling just 'happen'?" The interviewer also asks the parent, "Does your child seem to know when he needs to use the bathroom?" The frequency of the soiling episodes can vary, but to meet DSM-5 criteria, they must occur at least once per month for 3 consecutive months.

The interviewer should also inquire about general functioning. It is important to include both Cody and his mother in the questioning to build rapport with the child but also to get a more comprehensive sense of the issues involved. It is often helpful to do parts of the interview with the parent and child together and also to meet alone with the child or parent, particularly if the conversation appears to be causing distress. It is important to be nonjudgmental and empathic, because talking about soiling is very embarrassing to most children. The interviewer asks the parent, "How is Cody doing overall? How are things at school? How would your son's teacher describe him? How are his grades?" The interviewer asks Cody, "Do you have a best friend? What sorts of things do you like to do with your friends? Do you ever have sleepovers? Do you go? Do you play any sports? Which ones? How about at home—are there any arguments with your parents or siblings? Do you have any other areas of concern?"

As noted repeatedly in this section, rule-out of physical causes is critical. Some important questions are captured above, but others include the following: "Has your son ever had any major medical illness or injury, such as a head or spinal injury? Does he take any medications or over-the-counter supplements? How much water does he drink?"

The DSM-5 diagnosis of encopresis is relatively straightforward, despite the need for rule-out of physical causes of incontinence. The interviewer needs to determine whether the child is over age 4 years (or developmental equivalent) and must confirm the presence of symptoms at least once per month for 3 months. Unlike with enuresis, encopresis criteria do not specify frequency of symptoms or the presence of significant distress or functional impairment. Finally, the interviewer must confirm that there are not any medical illnesses or exposure to substances that may better explain the symptoms of fecal incontinence. The disorder is coded for the presence or absence of constipation, because this specification directs treatment.

Tips for Clarifying the Diagnosis

- Refer the individual to gastroenterology to rule out physical causes of fecal incontinence.
- Assuming there is no physical cause of bowel incontinence, focus on determining the presence and extent of a history of constipation.
- Evaluate constipation and routines around maintenance of bowel regularity. Assess whether the family maintains appropriate fiber, water, and (where necessary) stool-softening regimens to reduce impaction. Advise them that in many cases, simply relieving constipation for a period of 6–12 months can resolve encopresis.
- In the absence of constipation, consider behavioral difficulties and/or environmental challenges to regular toileting, such as unclean or inadequate toileting facilities. Sensitively screen for current or historical abuse.
- Use a sensitive and empathic approach to the family to obtain information that may be sensitive and difficult to discuss but is important for the care of the child. Most children, particularly older ones, experience significant shame around fecal incontinence.

Consider the Case

Connor is a 14-year-old boy with a history of oppositional defiant disorder and disruptive behaviors who presents to an outpatient child psychiatry clinic because of concerns around significant weight gain secondary to a trial of atypical antipsychotic medication. Following discontinuation of this medication, Connor has lost a majority of his excess weight but has experienced a return of more challenging disruptive behaviors and temper outbursts. On evaluation, it is discovered that Connor has also never attained regular fecal or nocturnal urinary continence. He does not experience nocturnal fecal incontinence. His parents consulted a pediatric gastroenterology specialist 3 years before the current intake and are aware that Connor is outside of expected norms of toileting but have viewed his toileting difficulties as part of the larger scope of his "defiant" behaviors. He was diagnosed with constipation at the time of the previous visit, but his parents were unclear if more significant testing was undertaken to rule out physical causes of incontinence. They were instructed to provide over-the-counter stool softeners to soften stools and did so for 1 month following their visit with the specialist. They expressed great frustration with Connor and have responded to toileting accidents with anger and privilege withdrawal, including having him wear soiled underwear as a punishment. This was discontinued when it resulted in a rash. He has recently experienced increasing periods of dryness at night, with a recent stretch of close to 10 days of dry nights, but these stretches are disrupted with any change in routine or structure. His parents used an alarm system, which they felt was unsuccessful in remediating his nocturnal enuresis. They have never engaged in any treatment to address fecal incontinence and noted that these symptoms had not been evaluated or discussed in his previous therapeutic relationship. Upon questioning, his parents note that at least one-third of the conflict at home stems from Connor's incontinence: either parental upset at these behaviors or Connor's response to punishments and privilege withdrawal.

Upon assessment, Connor presents as an active, inattentive young man who expresses great shame in describing himself, both behaviorally and in terms of toileting. He describes avoiding bathrooms at school because they are "disgusting" and other boys tease him if he enters a stall (e.g., throwing toilet paper over the door, knocking or hitting the door and calling him names). He also reports not always being aware of the need to stool, and his mother describes him as "zoning out" or "going into a trance" when he has a bowel movement. Otherwise, he feels well and denies nausea, vomiting, cramping, or painful stools. The family is instructed to take Connor for a physical examination, which reveals no presence of constipation or bowel impaction. They are also referred to follow-up with a pediatric gastroenterologist for a thorough evaluation to rule out physical causes for his encopresis and nocturnal enuresis, which yields normal findings.

Connor's presentation is complicated, though not atypical, in that his symptoms were uncovered as part of a general psychiatric evaluation but not targeted in previous treatment. The failure to establish any regular history of either fecal or urinary continence is particularly concerning and warrants more in-depth evaluation to rule out physical causes for toileting difficulties, in particular for Hirschsprung disease, inflammatory bowel disorders, and metabolic or absorption difficulties.

Differential Diagnosis

The differential diagnosis of encopresis centers on excluding the presence of medical conditions or substances that can cause fecal incontinence, including Hirschsprung disease, inflammatory bowel disorders, a range of gastrointestinal difficulties, neurological impairment, spinal injuries that impair sensation in the bowel region or control over bowel evacuation, laxative abuse or overuse, and metabolic disorders. Exposure to medications can influence encopresis, most often by increasing constipation. As such, many medications may be implicated in exacerbating encopresis.

Children with encopresis may also exhibit medical and behavioral problems at a higher rate than children without the disorder. Specific learning disorder, anxiety disorders, depressive disorders, attention-deficit/hyperactivity disorder (ADHD), and trauma- and stressor-related disorders all have high rates of comorbidity with encopresis. Encopresis should also be evaluated in children receiving treatment for other medical difficulties, particularly in hospital settings.

See DSM-5 for additional disorders to consider in the differential diagnosis. Also refer to the discussions of comorbidity and differential diagnosis in their respective sections of DSM-5.

Summary

- The diagnosis of encopresis must be made in children over age 4 years (or developmental equivalent).
- Encopresis is not diagnosed in the presence of medical illness or medication use that can result in fecal incontinence.

- Encopresis has two specifiers that are important for directing treatment: "with constipation and overflow incontinence" and "without constipation and overflow incontinence."
- Encopresis can lead to significant difficulty in the child's academic, social, and home functioning.

IN-DEPTH DIAGNOSIS

Enuresis

Sally is an 8-year-old girl who is brought to her pediatrician's office for evaluation of nighttime wetting. She was very distressed about a recent overnight trip to visit relatives; her cousin noticed that she wet the bed and began teasing her. Sally began toilet training at age 3 and seemed interested in wearing "big girl panties" featuring her favorite cartoon characters. She is dry during the day and is able to stay dry for a night or two but has wetting accidents most nights. There have been no consistent periods of nighttime dryness. Sally's parents try to be patient but admit that they are stressed with work and finances and sometimes yell when Sally has an accident. They deny corporal punishment. Disposable undergarments are expensive, and Sally's mom, who does most of the laundry, recently went back to work and does not have the time or energy to wash sheets every day. The parents do not limit fluids in the evening, and Sally likes to drink fruit juice. She is proud of drinking a big glass of milk at dinner, which is typically 2–3 hours before bed. They have tried sticker charts and point systems to reward dry nights but gave up after a few days because "it didn't seem to be working." Sally's physical examination is normal, as is her screening urinalysis.

Sally's presentation is very typical—she is dry during the day and does have some dry nights. However, she is over age 5 and has never been completely dry. Therefore, she has primary nocturnal diuresis. Nothing on examination indicates genitourinary, gastrointestinal, or neurological abnormalities. Similarly, her screening urinalysis does not reveal evidence of diabetes insipidus, diabetes mellitus, or a urinary tract infection. Her mom's return to work and the family's overall stress level are likely affecting Sally and making it difficult for her parents to be neutral, calm, and consistent with behavioral plans that would likely be effective if they gave them more time. It is important to assess whether the parents' frustration is leading to any sort of maltreatment, but it is very important to stress that most children with enuresis are not being abused.

Approach to the Diagnosis

The diagnosis of enuresis is made on the basis of history, physical examination, laboratory data, and imaging studies. A careful history will elicit the duration, timing, and severity of symptoms; exacerbating and ameliorating factors; and the presence of any extended periods of dryness. How many voids are there during the day? What is the child's bowel function like? It is important to determine whether enuresis occurs solely at night or also during the day, whether the incontinence is intermittent or continuous, and whether there are any other genitourinary, gastrointestinal, or neurological symptoms. Is there any history of urinary tract infection or other medical illness? Does the child take any medications or have access to medications stored in the home, such as diuretics, lithium, or atypical antipsychotics? Caregivers should be asked about their approach and attitude toward toilet training, their response to wetting accidents, and whether there are any recent changes or stresses to the family. How is the child doing socially and academically? Are there any other developmental concerns (gross or fine motor skills, learning, speech, growth)? Providers should sensitively, yet directly, ask about any maltreatment or abuse.

Physical examination should generally be done by the pediatrician rather than by a psychiatrist and should focus on the genitourinary, gastrointestinal, and neurological systems. The back should be examined for birthmarks or tufts of hair that could indicate underlying pathology involving the spinal cord. The abdomen should be examined for presence of a distended bladder or excessive stool, which indicates constipation and is frequently associated with enuresis.

In cases of primary nocturnal enuresis, a screening urinalysis is often the only diagnostic test necessary. If results are unremarkable, there is no need to request additional tests. However, the presence of a urinary tract infection in a boy, a febrile urinary tract infection in a girl, or repeated afebrile urinary tract infections would prompt renal and bladder ultrasonography. Abnormalities would indicate the need for further studies, such as a voiding cystourethrography.

Daytime wetting requires a bit more investigation to determine whether the underlying problem is one of storage or emptying. The clinician should request urinalysis and urine culture, as well as bladder ultrasonography to assess postvoid residual and uroflow testing to provide qualitative and quantitative assessment of the urinary stream. Certain features of the history and physical examination may signify the need for magnetic resonance imaging, intravenous pyelography, or computed tomography scan. For example, constant "dribbling" may suggest the presence of an ectopic ureter, whereas suspicious physical findings may indicate tethered cord syndrome.

Getting the History

> A mother reports that her 10-year-old son, Danny, has daytime wetting episodes. The clinician starts with open-ended questions to determine the duration, frequency, and quality of symptoms: "How long has this wetting been an issue? Are there times when you stay dry? What happens when you have an accident?" The child or parent of a child with enuresis will typically report that the child never attained complete dryness or that the child is dry during the day but continues to have wetting episodes at night. The exact frequency of the wetting episodes can vary, but to meet DSM-5 criteria, they must occur at least twice per week for 3 consecutive months *or* cause significant distress or impairment in functioning across social, academic, and home domains.
>
> The interviewer involves both Danny and his mother in the questioning to build rapport with the child but also to get a more comprehensive sense of the issues involved. The interviewer asks, "How is Danny doing overall? Danny, how are things at school? How would Danny's teacher describe him? How many friends do you have, Danny? Do you have a best friend? What sorts of things do you like to do with your friends? Do you ever have sleepovers? Do you go? How about at home? Do you have any arguments with your parents or siblings? Do you have any other areas of concern?" It is often helpful to do parts of the interview with both parent and child together as well as to meet with the child or parent alone, particularly if the conversation appears to be causing distress.

The interviewer will also need to ask specific questions about medical illnesses or medications that may cause urinary incontinence. "Does Danny have any medical illnesses? Any seizures? Diabetes? Spinal injuries? Danny, do you take any medications regularly?" The clinician should confirm with the parent that the child does not take (or have access to) diuretics, lithium, or antipsychotics.

The DSM-5 diagnosis of enuresis is relatively straightforward. The interviewer needs to determine whether the child is over age 5 years (or developmental equivalent) and must confirm that symptoms are present at least twice per week for 3 months *or* cause significant distress or functional impairment. Finally, the interviewer must confirm that there are not any medical illnesses or exposures to substances that may better explain the symptoms of urinary incontinence. However, it is important to note that a child with an acute urinary tract infection or one who takes a diuretic may also be diagnosed with enuresis, providing that symptoms were present before the introduction of medication or presence of the illness.

Tips for Clarifying the Diagnosis

- Determine whether symptoms are primary or secondary, nocturnal or diurnal, and continuous or intermittent.
- Order a screening urinalysis for information regarding urine specific gravity, which would argue for or against diabetes insipidus; urine glucose, which may indicate diabetes mellitus; and the presence of bacteria, which would dictate need for a culture to rule out infection. Each of these conditions can be associated with enuresis.
- Remember that diurnal enuresis is less common than nocturnal enuresis, is more common in girls than in boys, and is more often associated with an underlying anatomical or physiological abnormality.
- Maintain a sensitive and empathic approach to the family to obtain information that may be difficult to discuss but is important for the care of the patient. Take into consideration that it is important for the family to feel as though the clinician is being complete and ruling out potential physical causes of enuresis rather than focusing solely on stress as a causative factor.

Consider the Case

Johnny is a 13-year-old boy with a history of well-controlled type 1, insulin-dependent diabetes mellitus and ADHD, with predominantly inattentive presentation, who presents to his pediatrician with concerns about new-onset nocturnal enuresis. He is too embarrassed to tell his parents why he wanted to see the doctor. He was previously completely dry but notes that he did have some difficulty with toilet training and was not completely dry until age 10. His parents used an alarm system, which worked after a couple of months. The return of symptoms has caused him significant embarrassment, and he now goes to great lengths to hide his wetting episodes. He even bought another set of sheets and sometimes hides soiled sheets in his closet until his parents are not home and he is able to wash them in private. He actively tries to avoid fluids at night and voluntarily stopped drinking caffeinated diet soda because he recognized that it was increasing his need to urinate during the day. He reports that he is very stressed by his family's upcoming move to a new city. He describes himself as shy and interested in online gaming, and he worries about making friends in middle school. Otherwise, he feels well and denies recent weight loss, polyuria, polyphagia, or polydipsia. He reports complying with all doses of insulin, counts carbohydrates at every meal, and checks his blood sugar as he is supposed to. Physical examination is unremarkable, and urinalysis is within normal limits. His hemoglobin A1C is 6.5%.

Johnny's presentation is slightly atypical in that he is older than age 8 and he has had a period of complete dryness, which indicates a diagnosis of secondary nocturnal enuresis. However, he did initially have primary nocturnal enuresis, which resolved with alarm therapy. Enuresis appears to be more common in children and adolescents with ADHD. The pediatrician is right to be more vigilant in Johnny's case because of his insulin-dependent diabetes mellitus. Adolescents with previously well-controlled blood glucose sometimes become nonadherent in the teen years as they become more independent and struggle with being "different" from their peers. Glucose spillage into the urine could present as polyuria, with particular difficulty at night. At this age, ethnicity and race are not likely to have much impact on diagnosis or presentation; however, in some cultures, children are expected to be toilet trained at an earlier age and may therefore present to a medical provider sooner than a child of a different background. Earlier toilet training is often related to concerns about cost or lack of readily available diapers. Developmentally, Johnny (appropriately) wants to be more independent with his activities of daily living. He may feel that his parents have high expectations for him and he may not want to burden or embarrass them.

Differential Diagnosis

The differential diagnosis of enuresis centers on excluding the presence of medical conditions or substances that can cause urinary urgency or increased urine production, such as untreated diabetes insipidus or diabetes mellitus, an acute urinary tract infection, vaginal reflux, or neurogenic bladder related to spinal cord pathology (also lazy bladder syndrome, detrusor-sphincter dyssynergia, and Hinman syndrome). Exposure to medications such as atypical antipsychotics, lithium carbonate, and diuretics must also be excluded.

Children with enuresis may exhibit behavioral problems at a higher rate than other children. Developmental difficulties such as learning disabilities, speech delay, and fine and gross motor delays may be present. In children with other developmental delays, it is important to determine the child's developmental age rather than rely solely on chronological age to diagnose enuresis.

Enuresis is not diagnosed in the presence of a neurogenic bladder or a general medical condition that causes polyuria (increased urination) or urgency (e.g., untreated diabetes mellitus or diabetes insipidus), during an acute urinary tract infection, or during treatment with an antipsychotic. However, a diagnosis of enuresis is compatible with such conditions if urinary incontinence was regularly present before the development of the general medical condition or if it persists after the institution of appropriate treatment.

See DSM-5 for additional disorders to consider in the differential diagnosis. Also refer to the discussions of comorbidity and differential diagnosis in their respective sections of DSM-5.

Summary

- The diagnosis of enuresis must be made in children over age 5 years (or developmental equivalent).
- Enuresis is not diagnosed in the presence of medical illness or use of medications that can result in polyuria or urge incontinence.
- Enuresis can lead to significant difficulty in the child's academic, social, and home functioning.

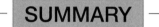
SUMMARY

Elimination Disorders

Enuresis and encopresis characteristically manifest in children and adolescents and can be extremely challenging to diagnose and treat. Because a number of medical conditions and medications can cause symptoms of bowel and bladder incontinence, it is essential that the mental health clinician work in concert with a medical provider to properly identify the biological, psychological, and social factors that contribute to the overall clinical picture. Children with elimination disorders are more likely to also have developmental delays, speech and language difficulties, learning disabilities, ADHD, and other behavioral problems.

Diagnostic Pearls

- Only a minority of elimination disorders can be traced to an underlying anatomical abnormality, malabsorption syndrome, endocrine issue, or neurological condition. Despite this, medical evaluation is a critical component of the evaluation.
- Bowel continence occurs before urinary continence, and children are expected to be consistently using the toilet for bowel voiding by age 4 (or developmental equivalent).
- Nocturnal encopresis is rare and is generally related to overflow incontinence from constipation; the majority of cases occur during the day.
- Children with ADHD have about a 30% greater chance of experiencing enuresis. This increase is likely related to a neurochemical effect rather than inattention or impulsivity.
- Nocturnal enuresis can be diagnosed on the basis of history, physical examination, and a screening urinalysis. No additional testing is required in

the absence of abnormalities, but additional testing may be required in cases of recurrent infection.

• Daytime incontinence or diurnal enuresis may be characterized as a problem of storage or emptying. In addition to a careful history and physical examination, children should also undergo urinalysis, urine culture, bladder ultrasonography, and uroflow testing.

Self-Assessment

Key Concepts: Double-Check Your Knowledge

What is the relevance of the following concepts to the various elimination disorders?

• Encopresis with and without constipation
• "Overflow" incontinence
• Relationship to comorbidity
• Physical causes of fecal incontinence
• Laxative use and contraindications for their use
• Behavioral training and biofeedback use
• Nocturnal versus diurnal enuresis
• Primary versus secondary enuresis
• Relationship between deep sleep and nocturnal enuresis
• Medical conditions and medications that may cause urinary incontinence

Questions to Discuss With Colleagues and Mentors

1. Do you screen all children and adolescents for elimination disorders, or do certain situations prompt you to take a more detailed history?
2. How do you make certain that families follow through on their child's medical prescriptions and adherence with bladder and/or bowel hygiene routines?
3. How do you overcome an individual's discomfort with talking about bladder and bowel habits?
4. Do you have an approach to working collaboratively with pediatricians and family practitioners to rule out medical causes of enuresis or encopresis before making a diagnosis?

Case-Based Questions

PART A

Delia is an 11-year-old girl who presents with her foster mother to her pediatrician with concerns about fecal smearing, as well as passage of bowel movements in a cabinet under the sink in the bathroom or into her underwear. Her early developmental history is generally unknown, but she was removed from her biological family due to concerns regarding neglect and physical abuse. Physical examinations have ruled out physical causes of fecal incontinence and are not suggestive of anal trauma. Since joining her foster family, she has never toileted appropriately with defecation and was initially enuretic, but she has responded to efforts to assist her with daytime dryness. She continues to wet several times per week. She is engaged in toilet training, and her foster parents are very patient with her. She passes regular stools and has fecal staining, which her foster mother relates to lack of wiping following bowel evacuation. The family has followed voiding schedules and incentive programs, with very limited success toward bowel continence. The family has not used stool softeners or laxatives, and currently Delia is not taking any prescription or over-the-counter medications. The doctor has ruled out constipation, and the family reports that at times Delia's bowel movements are appropriately soft and of sufficient bulk. They did not note blood in her stool but observed that some stools were soft and appeared to have a mucus-like texture or clear, foul-smelling discharge. Delia appears to know that she needs to have a bowel movement at times and will hide in the bathroom but will not use the toilet, preferring to evacuate her bowels under the sink instead. Outside of toileting concerns, Delia has been defiant and aggressive in the home, occasionally engaging in head-banging and self-scratching behaviors. She has been found to be hoarding food in her room, although not eating it but allowing it to rot. She has learning difficulties, which may be related to inconsistent education in her early years, because her family reportedly moved frequently. She has presented with some dissociative symptoms and flat affect at times, but she is responsive at other times. She can be difficult to establish rapport with, although her foster mother clearly has a caring and firm relationship with her. Delia has regressive behaviors with change, such as the foster family's older biological children returning home.

How should the pediatrician approach diagnosis in Delia's case? Because Delia is over age 4 and has no known history of constipation or physical causes for fecal incontinence, she has encopresis without constipation. Continued efforts at behavioral regulation, including a thorough diagnostic evaluation, are warranted. Additional evaluation by a pediatric gastrointestinal specialist is warranted to evaluate for physical causes of these difficulties.

PART B

Delia's physical examination is significant for the presence of areas of inflammation of the bowel, consistent with ulcerative colitis. Furthermore, tracking of her bowel habits notes sensitivities to seasonings, including garlic and hot spices, despite her preference for these flavors. Use of steroid treatment significantly improves the consistency of her stools. However, challenges in voiding appropriately continue.

How should the pediatrician proceed? The findings on examination are suggestive of physical causes for encopresis, but her behaviors continued after resolution of these difficulties. The family has been consistent with behavioral interventions, and they do not react dramatically when soiling episodes occur. They implemented a clearer bowel regimen, including having Delia assist with cleanup. With time, Delia was able to note that she had a strong preference for quiet and privacy when voiding and was able to void at home, but she had continued difficulty transitioning to toileting outside the home, necessitating additional behavioral treatment to generalize these skills to toilets at school and in public.

Short-Answer Questions

1. By what age are children typically expected to no longer have daytime bowel incontinence?
2. Which specialists should be consulted for children presenting with encopresis?
3. Which medical disorder should be strongly considered as a rule-out, particularly for children who never achieve bowel continence?
4. Name at least three psychiatric conditions that may be comorbid with encopresis.
5. By what age are children typically expected to be toilet trained and fully "dry"?
6. What tests must be ordered for children presenting with nocturnal enuresis?
7. List three medical conditions associated with urinary incontinence.
8. Name three psychiatric conditions that may be comorbid with enuresis.

Answers

1. Children typically are expected to no longer have daytime bowel incontinence by age 4 years.
2. Specialists in pediatric gastroenterology and possibly neurology and endocrinology may be consulted for children presenting with encopresis.
3. Hirschsprung disease should be strongly considered as a rule-out, particularly for children who never achieve bowel continence.
4. Psychiatric conditions that may be comorbid with encopresis include specific learning disorder, anxiety disorders, depressive disorders, ADHD, and trauma- and stressor-related disorders.
5. Children are typically expected to be toilet trained and fully "dry" by age 5 (or developmental equivalent).
6. Screening urinalysis must be ordered for children presenting with nocturnal enuresis.
7. Medical conditions associated with urinary incontinence include diabetes insipidus, diabetes mellitus, acute urinary tract infection, and neurogenic bladder.
8. Psychiatric conditions that may be comorbid with enuresis include encopresis, ADHD, and sleep disorders.

15

Sleep-Wake Disorders

Michelle Primeau, M.D.
Ruth O'Hara, Ph.D.

"I can't get to sleep."

"He snores so loud!"

Sleep disorders can manifest as a complaint of unsatisfactory sleep or as impaired daytime function or both. In the DSM-5 chapter on sleep-wake disorders, several changes have been implemented from DSM-IV. These changes were made to allow greater differentiation of the varied causes of sleep disruption, and to help identify those who require referral to a sleep specialist:

- In the past, insomnia was at times considered an independent phenomenon ("primary insomnia") or related to another condition ("secondary insomnia"). The distinction between primary and secondary insomnia is eliminated in DSM-5.
- The diagnosis of primary hypersomnia has been replaced by hypersomnolence disorder, which now includes greater specificity in the diagnostic criteria.
- Similarly, the diagnosis of narcolepsy now requires not only subjective symptoms, such as sleep "attacks" or *cataplexy* (the loss of muscle tone with maintained consciousness, triggered usually by a positive experience, such as hearing something funny), but also objective biological indicators, such as hypocretin and the occurrence of rapid eye movement (REM) sleep. Further specifiers cover other medical conditions associated with narcolepsy symptoms.
- In DSM-5, the DSM-IV diagnosis of breathing-related sleep disorder is now separated into three disorders: obstructive sleep apnea hypopnea, central sleep apnea, and sleep-related hypoventilation.

- Circadian rhythm sleep-wake disorders now include advanced sleep phase type, and the jet lag specifier has been removed.
- Disorders previously split as individual parasomnias, such as sleepwalking and sleep terrors, have now been grouped into non–rapid eye movement (NREM) sleep arousal disorders, to better reflect the clinical, etiological, and epidemiological characteristics. Nightmare disorder has been modified to include specifiers to account for associated medical, psychiatric, and sleep disorders that may co-occur, as well as for duration and severity.
- Two new diagnoses have been added to DSM-5: REM sleep behavior disorder (a parasomnia) and restless legs syndrome (RLS).
- Substance/medication-induced sleep disorder remains the same in DSM-5, except that tobacco has been added as a substance.
- The category for sleep disorders related to another mental disorder has been eliminated.
- Finally, for patients not meeting the full criteria for insomnia, hypersomnia, or another sleep-wake disorder, DSM-5 contains other and unspecified diagnoses to apply to those experiencing clinically significant distress.

Sleep complaints are common in everyday life. Most people have had the experience of having some stressful experience, such as a job interview, and being unable to sleep for a few days before the event. However, disrupted sleep may reflect an underlying sleep disorder that leads to or exacerbates an existing psychiatric or other medical condition. Sleep disturbances can reflect very different sleep disorders, many of which have established treatments. Diagnosing and targeting co-occurring sleep disorders can help alleviate psychiatric symptoms.

Some sleep-wake disorders occur only during sleep; in fact, a person may be unaware that any unusual behavior is occurring in his or her sleep. For example, children with NREM sleep arousal disorders, such as sleepwalking or sleep terrors, may not have any recollection of disruption the preceding night, even though their behavior may be quite unsettling to their parents.

Other sleep disorders are characterized by symptoms occurring during wakefulness. For example, RLS is characterized by a subjective discomfort in the legs with inactivity that is alleviated by movement.

Sleep disorders frequently co-occur with psychiatric conditions, and can reduce an individual's quality of life. Given the important interactions between sleep-wake disorders and psychiatric illness, diagnosing co-occurring sleep disorders is very important for effective long-term management of chronic, recurrent psychiatric illnesses.

─────────── **IN-DEPTH DIAGNOSIS** ───────────

Insomnia Disorder

Ms. Albers, a 32-year-old woman, presents with a complaint of insomnia; she previously had brief periods of insomnia, usually related to situational stressors or travel and relieved by a sleeping pill, but for the past 6 months, she has had increasing difficulty with falling asleep, despite taking a sleeping pill nightly. Nine months ago, she started noticing that she would wake up in the middle of the night and worry about work or her upcoming wedding, but more recently she has progressed to difficulties falling asleep at the beginning of the night. She finds that she is now worrying during the day about her inability to sleep and has come to dread the nights. She feels that her lack of sleep is causing her to be more irritable, have decreased concentration, and be ineffective at work. She has started canceling social outings and early-morning meetings to accommodate her sleep. She has become so preoccupied with her sleep that her primary care physician prescribed a benzodiazepine to help with her anxiety, but she is reluctant to take it, because "the only thing I'm worried about is my sleep."

Insomnia disorder occurs more frequently in women and tends to manifest in young adulthood. Often, individuals will report brief, prior episodes that resolved on their own. However, to meet criteria for the diagnosis of insomnia disorder, the index episode will have been maintained for at least 3 months and occur at least 3 nights per week. The key component to note in Ms. Albers's case is the significant impact that she perceives the sleep disruption to have on her daytime function and her escalating preoccupation and concern over her sleep. It is common for individuals to awaken in the middle of the night, but becoming worried or stressed, striving to sleep, and being preoccupied with daytime impairments separate an individual with insomnia. Mid–sleep period awakenings sometimes become so stressful that the individual worries about them and progresses to the point of having difficulty falling asleep at the beginning of the night. The fact that Ms. Albers presents as very anxious is evidence of the hyperarousal that is often seen in individuals with insomnia. Although they may have comorbid depression and anxiety, some individuals report that sleep is their only concern. Finally, the use of sedative-hypnotic medications is common in patients with insomnia disorder.

Approach to the Diagnosis

Many people report problems with their sleep, but it is important to remember that not all sleep problems are insomnia. The first important consideration is whether the person is *complaining* about his or her sleep. For example, an individual may report a short sleep period but may not find that period to be distressing. It is important to identify exactly what the person's complaint is—difficulty falling asleep, maintaining sleep, early-morning awakening, or some combination—because this information may indicate the presence of other sleep-wake disorders. Some people are able to identify discrete times at which they have some worsening of the complaint (e.g., "I have difficulty falling asleep every Sunday night, worrying about the coming week") or locations that affect their sleep (e.g., "I can only sleep well on vacation"), whereas others have sleeping trouble every day, no matter the situation.

Individuals with insomnia disorder frequently underestimate their actual sleep time and report more prolonged awakenings at night than are noted on objective studies of sleep. In general, the convention is to consider a sleep latency or wakefulness after sleep onset of >30 minutes to be outside of normal limits. Similarly, individuals with insomnia disorder report increased daytime symptoms, such as difficulty in concentrating or performing complex, targeted tasks; but when tested, they fre-

quently fall within normal limits. It is thought that the perceived difficulties may reflect the increased effort required to maintain the same outcomes.

Individuals with insomnia disorder are often described as "wired but tired,"
meaning that they report fatigue but they are not overtly sleepy on subjective and objective measures of sleepiness and they are unable to nap if given the chance. Individuals often report an inability to quiet their minds. Negative sleep-related cognitions
often become prominent in individuals with insomnia disorder and can help to highlight the distress individuals are having from their sleep complaints (e.g., "If I don't
sleep well tonight, then I'm going to be horrible at my meeting tomorrow"). They
may become overly attentive to the effect that losing sleep has on performance and
selectively attend to negative outcomes. The individual may make accommodations
for their sleep difficulties. For example, individuals may cancel morning meetings so
they can sleep later after a bad night or try to go to bed early to "catch up." In children,
insomnia may manifest as bedtime resistance, calling parents back to the room multiple times, and requiring caregiver assistance in returning to sleep after night awakenings. Polysomnography is not essential to make the diagnosis of insomnia, unless
other clinical correlates indicate a possible physiological sleep disorder, such as
breathing-related sleep disorders, which are frequently comorbid with insomnia.

Getting the History

A 35-year-old patient presents with the chief complaint of "insomnia." The interviewer
inquires about the duration of time that the symptoms have been present and asks the
person about any identifiable trigger at onset. Specifics as to the nature of the problem
are then obtained: Is it difficult falling asleep, staying asleep, or both? In a typical week,
how often does this occur?

Often, to get an accurate picture of the problem, the interviewer asks questions that
focus on sleep hygiene that may be targeted and guide the diagnosis. It is helpful to go
through the night chronologically: "What time do you get into bed? What time do you
turn off the TV/lights/computer and allow for sleep? How long do you feel it takes to
fall asleep? Once asleep, do you ever wake up? How long does it take to return to sleep?
At what time do you have your final awakening, and when do you get out of bed? Are
those times different on weekends? What about taking naps (intentional) or dozing (unintentional)? Do your sleep patterns bother you? What is bothersome about your
sleep?"

The answer to the following question can help point to circadian rhythm sleep-
wake disorders: "Do you consider yourself a 'night owl' or a 'morning lark'?" Several
questions can help rule out the potential contribution of substances such as caffeine, tobacco, or alcohol to the person's sleep: "Do you ever take medications for your sleep?
If so, what do you take and at what time? Do you use any substances that may affect
your sleep?" Some questions can help screen for obstructive sleep apnea hypopnea:
"Do you snore? Has anyone ever told you that you appear to stop breathing while you
are sleeping? Are you sleepy during the day?"

In insomnia evaluation, it is helpful to quantify the specifics of the sleep problem.
Individuals with insomnia usually appreciate the interviewer's attention to detail in
asking about all aspects of their night because they already have scrutinized all possible contributors to their impaired sleep and, being unable to identify a solution, are

willing to discuss their sleep in minute detail. Identifying which part of the night is more impaired can help rule in or rule out other conditions. For example, difficulties initiating sleep may also be attributed to RLS or circadian rhythm sleep-wake disorder, delayed sleep phase type. It is important to consider these other sleep disorders, because treatments are very different among them.

Tips for Clarifying the Diagnosis

- Evaluate for co-occurring sleep and psychiatric conditions that may also be present in the individual.
- Understand whether the person has complaints about an impairment in some aspect of *daytime* function.
- Assess whether the person is allowing adequate time for sleep.
- Determine whether the person has cognitions about sleep, preoccupation with the negative impact of lack of sleep, and sleep-related anxiety.

Consider the Case

> Mr. Hall, a 38-year-old Marine with a history of posttraumatic stress disorder (PTSD) secondary to combat exposure, is being evaluated for residual sleep complaints. Mr. Hall was referred for sleep evaluation after he completed a research study on prolonged exposure therapy. Although his symptoms of PTSD have resolved almost completely, he still has difficulty initiating and maintaining sleep. He reports that he never had any sleep problems before his deployment; however, while deployed he had to stand watch at night and sleep during the day, and he feels that his sleep patterns remain disorganized today. To compensate for his lack of sleep at night, he frequently naps and drinks coffee or smokes cigarettes to maintain alertness during the day. He worries about how his lack of sleep is affecting the way he relates to his children and is concerned that he will have difficulty reentering the workforce because of his sleep disruption.

Although insomnia is more frequently seen in women, it occurs often in men as well. People with psychiatric conditions also commonly have comorbid insomnia, and 40%–50% of people diagnosed with insomnia have a comorbid mental disorder. In the past, insomnia was often considered to be secondary to the psychiatric condition, but recent research has indicated that considering the diagnosis as co-occurring—without prioritizing one diagnosis over another or attributing causality—may be more accurate. In patients with major depressive disorder, insomnia is the most frequently reported residual symptom, and untreated sleep symptoms can precipitate another episode of depression.

Individuals with PTSD frequently have fragmented sleep, and Mr. Hall in particular demonstrates inadequate sleep hygiene (e.g., frequent naps) and use of stimulating substances. Further elaboration of the history could help identify whether he has another sleep disorder, such as substance/medication-induced sleep disorder (he is using a large amount of stimulants to bolster alertness) or circadian rhythm sleep-wake disorder, which might explain his disorganized sleep pattern. Insomnia is quite common in veteran populations.

Differential Diagnosis

The differential diagnosis of insomnia disorder includes normal sleep variations, such as those who physiologically require less sleep, or age-related sleep changes. Situational/acute insomnia may be brief, and precipitated by a change in life events. If occurring at least 3 nights per week, with clinically significant impairment, but not meeting the 3-month mark, a diagnosis of other specified insomnia disorder may be made.

Circadian rhythm sleep-wake disorder is the primary diagnosis to consider when evaluating a person for insomnia disorder. Frequently, individuals with circadian rhythm sleep-wake disorder, delayed sleep phase type, are mistaken for having insomnia disorder because of their difficulty initiating sleep. These individuals tend to fall asleep and stay asleep later than is considered typical and in a way that interferes with their social or occupational functioning. In individuals whose circadian phase is advanced, they may describe excessive sleepiness in the evenings and early-morning awakenings. However, when going to bed at a time better aligned with their natural rhythms, these individuals do not actually have difficulty initiating or maintaining sleep. Similarly, circadian rhythm sleep-wake disorder, advanced sleep phase type, may manifest in an older adult with early-morning awakening. These individuals tend to fall asleep earlier in the evenings than intended, awaken earlier, and be unable to return to sleep. Circadian rhythm sleep-wake disorder, shift work type, differs from insomnia disorder by the history of recent shift work.

RLS can manifest as difficulty falling asleep or returning to sleep because of intrusive discomfort, usually in the legs. Individuals with insomnia disorder often report "tossing and turning," but individuals with RLS report an inability to sit still or feeling "tingling," "creepy crawly," or "as if my legs have to sneeze," which occurs around the same time of day or with being sedentary and improves with movement.

Other sleep-wake disorders to consider in the differential diagnosis of insomnia disorder include the following: Breathing-related sleep disorder is difficult to diagnose with history alone, but indicators of risk for breathing-related sleep disorder include being obese, snoring, witnessed apneas, and excessive daytime sleepiness. Individuals with narcolepsy sometimes may have comorbid insomnia, although the condition tends to be characterized by hypersomnia. Parasomnias are characterized specifically by events occurring while the person is asleep, and individuals usually are unaware of behaviors unless they awaken from them or are told by a witness. Substance/medication-induced sleep disorder may overlap with insomnia disorder but occurs in the context of acute intoxication or withdrawal from a substance or medication and is chronologically related to substance or medication use.

Insomnia disorder may co-occur with other sleep-wake disorders and psychiatric conditions, such as depression or anxiety, and the comorbid condition often may be seen as overlapping or contributing to the insomnia disorder.

See DSM-5 for additional disorders to consider in the differential diagnosis. Also refer to the discussions of comorbidity and differential diagnosis in their respective sections of DSM-5.

Summary

- Insomnia is a common complaint, and the symptoms have an impact not only on the sleep period but also daytime functioning.
- Insomnia is frequently comorbid with other medical and psychiatric conditions.
- A thorough history of the course of symptoms and how the insomnia manifests at night gives insight into the nature of the individual's problem and can help direct future treatment.
- Diagnosis requires ruling out other sleep disorders, such as circadian rhythm sleep-wake disorder or breathing-related sleep disorder.

—————— **IN-DEPTH DIAGNOSIS** ——————

Narcolepsy

Annie, a 6-year-old girl without prior medical history, presents with her parents for evaluation of an acute change in her behavior. Her parents report that she had been her usual self until 3 months ago, when she acquired tonsillitis, and she has not been the same since. They describe that she appears unable to stay awake during the day, frequently falling sleep at school and at home, even when engaged in an activity or conversation. Her nighttime sleep period has become disrupted as well, with apparent vivid, terrifying dreams, some of which she physically reacts to, and she has had minor injuries from falling out of bed trying to run from whatever she was seeing. Her parents also note that she appears "floppy"—with her mouth dropping open—or unable to hold up her head. On one occasion, her father told a joke at dinner, and she laughed so hard that her head fell into her spaghetti. There is no family history of anything similar, and her siblings remain healthy.

Nocturnal polysomnography demonstrates an apnea hypopnea index (AHI) of 0.5 events per hour and REM sleep latency of 15 minutes. Next-day multiple sleep latency test (MSLT) had 5/5 sleep-onset REM periods with a sleep latency of 6 minutes. Lumbar puncture was not done, given the classic presentation of symptoms, but human leukocyte antigen (HLA) typing demonstrated Annie to be a carrier of *HLA-DQB1*06:02*.

Annie demonstrates the classic abrupt onset of narcolepsy. She has brief periods of excessive sleepiness that she is unable to overcome by engaging in activity, as well as classic cataplexy. Early in the condition, children often demonstrate hypotonia, with parents describing them as "floppy," or have automatisms, such as tongue thrusting, that are atypical for the child. As the condition progresses, cataplectic "attacks" may be seen. These are triggered usually by a positive emotion, such as happiness or surprise, and can be dramatic, as in Annie's case, or even cause the individual to fall to the ground. Not included in the diagnostic criteria of narcolepsy, but also suggestive, is REM sleep behavior disorder, in which the person appears to be acting out terrifying imagery from a dream. It is also common for individuals with narcolepsy to have sleep paralysis or hallucinations when falling asleep or when awakening, representing REM sleep intruding into wakefulness, which can be quite disturbing to them.

Formal testing is required to make the diagnosis of narcolepsy, according to DSM-5. Nocturnal polysomnography can rule out the presence of breathing-related sleep disorders, which are much more common than narcolepsy and may frequently be comorbid with narcolepsy. The nocturnal polysomnography may indicate a shortened REM sleep latency (≤15 minutes, instead of the typical 90–120 minutes), or the daytime MSLT must show two or more sleep-onset REM periods, with a mean sleep latency of ≤8 minutes. Ninety-nine percent of individuals who have narcolepsy are positive for *HLA-DQB1*06:02;* however, HLA typing is less specific for narcolepsy. Low hypocretin-1 levels (narcolepsy with hypocretin deficiency ≤110 pg/mL) are confirmatory for the diagnosis. Lumbar puncture is required to obtain hypocretin-1 levels.

Approach to the Diagnosis

Individuals who have narcolepsy are frequently misdiagnosed with other conditions, such as major depressive disorder or obstructive sleep apnea hypopnea, before they are correctly diagnosed and obtain adequate treatment. For a child with narcolepsy, the parents may be able to provide a discrete onset of excessive sleepiness, often following an illness or vaccination, that is accompanied by other symptoms of visual hallucinations, acting out terrifying dreams, sleep paralysis, and cataplexy. The child often sleeps through all or part of the history. Adults with narcolepsy may have more difficulty identifying the onset of symptoms, particularly if the symptoms have been present for many years. In adolescents or adults, the onset of symptoms may not be quite as dramatic as in young children. Excessive sleepiness and increased sleep are hallmarks of early narcolepsy, but over time it may be noted that the total daily hours of sleep are as expected, although the individual has difficulty maintaining sleep and wake states. Adults may describe having "sleep attacks"—in which they do not even realize they were asleep until they awaken from a nap. Nighttime sleep becomes disrupted, with insomnia or vivid, disturbing dreams that the person may physically act out. Brief daytime naps are usually refreshing, but this is not necessarily specific to narcolepsy.

Cataplexy also may be seen, although it is more prominent early in the course of narcolepsy and may not be as evident in certain populations (e.g., those who are of African descent or who take medications that suppress REM sleep). It is also thought that individuals with cataplexy learn to restrict their range of affect to limit their emotional reactions and thereby limit the cataplectic attacks they suffer. If a person with cataplexy stops taking medications that suppress REM sleep, he or she can have a flurry of rebound cataplexy (*status cataplecticus*).

Confirmation with testing is required for the diagnosis of narcolepsy and may be done either in a sleep lab or by lumbar puncture. Overnight polysomnography may show a reduced REM sleep latency (≤15 minutes), or a daytime MSLT may be performed. The latter test should be performed after an overnight MSLT and while the person is not taking psychoactive medications. The person is then given the opportunity to take five naps over the course of the day, at 2-hour intervals, for up to 20 minutes each. Each nap is evaluated for the presence of sleep and an REM period. If the person goes into REM sleep within the 20-minute nap, that nap is considered a sleep-onset REM period. Two sleep-onset REM periods and a sleep latency ≤8 minutes confirms the diagnosis of narcolepsy. Alternatively, a lumbar puncture may be performed to measure the level of hypocretin-1 present in the cerebrospinal fluid.

Getting the History

A 23-year-old man presents with a complaint of "I am tired all the time." The interviewer may wish to clarify whether the patient feels "sleepy" or "fatigued." The patient reports that he feels sleepy and has times when he feels an absolutely irrepressible need for sleep. The interviewer asks about automatic behaviors, such as writing notes without recollection and later realizing the notes made no sense, or losing time while driving. The interviewer then asks about symptoms of cataplexy: "Have you ever had times in which your muscles get weak or wobbly on you?" When the patient answers in the affirmative, the interviewer asks, "What seems to cause these symptoms?" If an emotional trigger occurs, it is important to note what type of emotion (i.e., positive or negative) and how long the symptoms last.

To elicit symptoms of sleep paralysis, the interviewer may ask, "Do you ever wake up from sleep and feel that you are paralyzed? How often does that occur?" To elicit a history of hallucinations associated with falling asleep or awakening, the clinician may ask, "Do you ever see things or hear things that others cannot see or hear? Do they occur at any particular time? Are they scary or disturbing to you?" Time course and perceived precipitants of symptoms should also be elicited, as should a thorough evaluation of sleep hours and medications. The patient should also be screened for other sleep disorders that may cause excessive daytime sleepiness.

People often report feeling tired, but this symptom is very nonspecific. It is helpful to clarify whether a person feels overtly sleepy (e.g., eyes dry, eyelids heavy, yawning, on the verge of falling asleep) or fatigued (low energy, no "get-up-and-go"), because sleepiness is associated with sleep-disordered breathing, sleep deprivation, and narcolepsy, and fatigue is associated more with insomnia or major depressive disorder. It also can be helpful to assess risk, because individuals who are excessively sleepy may have "sleep attacks" even while driving, but those who have fatigue would be unlikely to fall asleep during an activity. Automatic behaviors may sometimes be seen as an individual inadvertently falls asleep but tries to continue the activities he or she was performing. With cataplexy, focused yet open-ended questions can be helpful. Individuals will often report that when they are very angry or anxious, they feel weak in the knees or unable to hold objects in their hands, but this symptom is not typical of cataplexy, which is elicited by positive emotions. Also, cataplectic attacks typically last a few seconds, so reports of persistent weakness over hours are also not typical of cataplexy. History regarding hallucinations is typically elicited; asking about the timing may indicate whether the hallucinations occur with falling asleep or waking up. However, it is important to remember that patients with narcolepsy have instability of sleep and wake periods, and therefore may have hypnopompic or hypnagogic symptoms associated with daytime sleep episodes.

Tips for Clarifying the Diagnosis

- Determine whether the person is unable to maintain sleep and wakefulness.
- Assess whether the person has brief periods of muscle weakness triggered by positive emotions. This weakness can be manifested by dropping head or drooping eyelids or more overtly by lower-extremity weakness that requires the individual to sit down.
- Ask how often these attacks occur and how long the sleep instability has been present.

- Confirm the diagnosis with the following tests: polysomnography with REM sleep latency ≤15 minutes, MSLT with sleep latency ≤8 minutes and two or more sleep-onset REM periods, or measurement of hypocretin-1 levels in cerebrospinal fluid.

Consider the Case

Mr. Pickell is a 35-year-old black former Marine referred to the sleep clinic by his psychiatrist for persistent excessive daytime sleepiness. Mr. Pickell has been working as a long-distance truck driver and was initially referred to a psychiatrist because he reported to his primary care physician that he was experiencing occasional perceptual distortions, such as seeing a person in the road or seeing the road as distorted. The psychiatrist also noted a restricted range of affect, disrupted nocturnal sleep, and daytime fatigue.

Mr. Pickell was prescribed a variety of antidepressants, with minimal improvement in daytime symptoms. Other medication at bedtime helped improve Mr. Pickell's sleep somewhat; but although he no longer reported visual hallucinations, he remained excessively sleepy. He was then referred for an evaluation of his sleep.

On evaluation, Mr. Pickell reports no history of snoring or witnessed apneas. Despite previously having short sleep hours while working, he has been on short-term disability for the past 3 months and has been sleeping at least 8 hours per night and reports frequently taking naps as well. He denies symptoms consistent with cataplexy, sleep paralysis, or parasomnias. He was tapered off his medications before obtaining polysomnography, which demonstrated an AHI of 7.8, with REM sleep latency of 70 minutes. An MSLT the following day was positive with mean sleep latency of 7 minutes and two sleep-onset REM periods, occurring in the last two naps. Lumbar puncture was performed, and Mr. Pickell had a very low unmeasurable hypocretin level.

Mr. Pickell is an example of a patient with narcolepsy. Of key importance for this patient is safety, because of his work as a long-distance truck driver. Patients with narcolepsy are not only excessively sleepy but often may have automatic behaviors, in which they continue with an activity, even driving, while they are asleep. Once they are appropriately treated, most patients should be able to return to work, although Mr. Pickell may need to change to shorter local routes or some other form of employment. Some patients with narcolepsy are referred for psychiatric evaluation because of visual hallucinations; also, sometimes these patients are perceived to be depressed due to a restricted range of affect that may be acquired to help minimize cataplectic symptoms. When asked, however, this man denied history of cataplexy, which is not uncommon. Some evidence indicates that individuals of African descent have less manifestation of cataplexy than do other populations; however, other explanations, such as duration of illness or presence of medications suppressing REM sleep may also contribute to the presentation in this patient. Mr. Pickell's use of selective serotonin reuptake inhibitors and serotonin-norepinephrine reuptake inhibitors could also explain his lack of cataplectic symptoms. Because of the REM-suppressing effect of many psychiatric medications, it is important to coordinate care with other providers to ensure that an individual being assessed for narcolepsy with polysomnography and MSLTs is tapered off those medications, if possible. Reduced REM sleep latency on polysomnography (≤15 minutes) or on MSLT (in at least two naps) is required for the diagnosis, along with either cataplexy or hypocretin deficiency. Mr. Pickell had extremely low levels of hypocretin on lumbar puncture, confirming the diagnosis.

Differential Diagnosis

Narcolepsy must first be differentiated from hypersomnias without hypocretin deficiency. Individuals with these disorders may similarly complain of fatigue and sleepiness and may even have an MSLT with a short sleep latency and two or more sleep-onset REM periods. *HLA-DQB1*06:02* may be used to differentiate these disorders. If the HLA typing is negative, it is highly unlikely that the individual has narcolepsy; however, if it is positive, the individual may or may not have hypocretin deficiency. Lumbar puncture for hypocretin-1 in the cerebrospinal fluid would confirm the diagnosis.

Sleep deprivation and insufficient nocturnal sleep are common reasons for excessive daytime sleepiness. Sometimes sleepiness may be due to behavioral factors (e.g., a parent busy with a full-time job, schoolwork, and children and "without enough hours in the day") or a circadian misalignment (e.g., a teenager with circadian phase delay who is unable to fall asleep until 2:00 A.M. and then must be up at 6:00 A.M. for school, or a shift worker who works nights and has difficulty sleeping during the day).

Breathing-related sleep disorders (i.e., sleep apnea syndromes) are far more common than narcolepsy and can cause sleep fragmentation leading to excessive daytime sleepiness. Individuals with major depressive disorder may suffer from hypersomnia and fatigue, but they are not typically sleepy and not likely to have any of the other associated symptoms of cataplexy, sleep paralysis, or acting out of dreams. Individuals with conversion disorder (functional neurological symptom disorder) may present with prolonged, dramatic pseudocataplectic attacks, during which reflexes can be elicited. These patients also may insist that they slept on the MSLT, but such sleep is not evident on electroencephalography. In children, excessive sleepiness may be perceived as a behavioral issue or inattentiveness, although these children do not present with hyperactivity. Cataplexy, automatic behaviors, and sleep attacks could be interpreted as seizures, although when a person has a cataplectic attack, he or she is alert and conscious and less likely to become injured from the attack than is a person with seizure disorder; also, seizures are not triggered by emotional stimuli. Electroencephalography can help in ruling out seizure disorder. Chorea and pediatric autoimmune neuropsychiatric disorders associated with streptococcal infections (PANDAS) may be considered in children developing narcolepsy, particularly because narcolepsy may occur in the context of acute post–streptococcal infection. Schizophrenia may be considered in individuals with narcolepsy because of the presence of hallucinations and may be comorbid with narcolepsy, but persons with only narcolepsy will not demonstrate the thought disorder or negative symptoms characteristic of schizophrenia.

See DSM-5 for additional disorders to consider in the differential diagnosis. Also refer to the discussions of comorbidity and differential diagnosis in their respective sections of DSM-5.

Summary

- Narcolepsy is characterized by inability to maintain sleep and wakefulness and can be difficult to diagnose because of the overlap of daytime sleepiness with other disorders.

- Cataplexy—a brief period of muscle weakness precipitated by a positive emotion—is a hallmark of the disorder but may not be present in all individuals with narcolepsy.
- Overnight polysomnography demonstrating REM sleep latency of ≤15 minutes or a daytime MSLT with mean sleep latency of ≤8 minutes and two or more sleep-onset REM periods can help make the diagnosis, but could be influenced by factors such as medications or sleep deprivation.
- True confirmation of the diagnosis of narcolepsy can be done by obtaining the level of hypocretin-1 in an individual's cerebrospinal fluid.

IN-DEPTH DIAGNOSIS
Obstructive Sleep Apnea Hypopnea

Mr. Geri, a 52-year-old man with a history of obesity, hypertension, diabetes mellitus, gastroesophageal reflux disease, and erectile dysfunction, works in a building that contains a sleep lab. He decided to get evaluated for excessive daytime sleepiness. He reports that he had always been a hard worker, dedicating long hours to his job, but over the past few years he had gained increased responsibility that he has been having difficulty maintaining because he frequently is falling asleep at his computer. He enjoys his work and does not feel bored but notes that he feels unable to maintain wakefulness when he is inactive during the day. Some days, he will even take a nap in his car before driving home, because he is so tired that he fears he may fall asleep while driving. He has not had a bed partner in many years but has been told in the past that he snores and, on occasion, has "snorted" himself awake.

Physical examination demonstrates a blood pressure of 150/90 mm Hg, body mass index of 37, neck circumference of 19 inches, and modified Mallampati score of 4. On overnight polysomnography, Mr. Geri had an AHI of 54 events per hour, with his longest apnea lasting 69 seconds and desaturating to 70%.

Mr. Geri represents a classic case of obstructive sleep apnea hypopnea. He is obese, which predisposes him to having this disorder, and he has multiple comorbidities that are associated with it. Hypertension can be seen in 60% of individuals with obstructive sleep apnea hypopnea, and there is evidence that the disorder can lead to impaired insulin resistance. Gastric reflux can be caused by the increased work of breathing while sleeping, and erectile dysfunction has been linked to obstructive sleep apnea hypopnea as well. Mr. Geri has excessive daytime sleepiness, as manifested by falling asleep when inactive, and individuals may also complain of cognitive dysfunction (e.g., poor concentration, attention, executive function). Individuals with obstructive sleep apnea hypopnea may report snoring, witnessed apneas, snorting themselves awake, and difficulty sleeping in certain positions (presumably due to positional airway collapse); but if the person does not have a bed partner, obtaining history of nighttime symptoms may be difficult. Physical examination findings may be suggestive of obstructive sleep apnea hypopnea, as was the case for Mr. Geri. He demonstrates hypertension, obesity, a large neck circumference, and evidence of a crowded oral airway on the basis of his Mallampati score (which is used to assess for difficulty in intubation and risk for sleep apnea). Although the history and physical findings may suggest the diagnosis, ultimately it is confirmed by overnight polysomnography. Mr. Geri was found to have what is considered severe obstructive sleep apnea hypopnea (>30 events per hour), with significant oxygen desaturation. In an obese patient such as Mr. Geri, obesity-hypoventilation syndrome should be considered, ideally with measurement of carbon dioxide levels.

Approach to the Diagnosis

Assessing a person for obstructive sleep apnea hypopnea requires a history and polysomnography. It is possible to make the diagnosis of obstructive sleep apnea hypopnea either by report of clinical symptoms with polysomnography demonstrating an AHI of at least 5 events per hour or by an AHI of 15 or more events per hour, regardless of symptoms. Symptoms to elicit in the history include both daytime symptoms and symptoms occurring during the sleep period. Individuals may report excessive sleepiness, fatigue, and cognitive symptoms such as diminished attention. A bed partner can be helpful in reporting symptoms occurring during sleep; for example, individuals may be unaware that they snore or have pauses in their breathing while they sleep, unless another person tells them. Other symptoms that support the diagnosis but that are not included in the diagnostic criteria are diaphoresis during sleep, sleep fragmentation, frequent nocturia, morning headaches, and dry mouth. Certain comorbid conditions, particularly hypertension, cardiovascular disease, gastroesophageal reflux, asthma, or allergies, also are suggestive of obstructive sleep apnea hypopnea. Family history of obstructive sleep apnea hypopnea suggests its presence, because there is likely a genetic basis to the syndrome as well as physical characteristics that predispose an individual to breathing-related sleep disorders. Physical examination characteristics are not included in the diagnostic criteria but may be suggestive, including obesity, hypertension, evidence of nasal obstruction (septal deviation, enlarged turbinates), tonsillar hypertrophy, Mallampati score of 3 or 4, and jaw structural abnormalities leading to a smaller oronasopharynx. Gender also is important to consider, because men are at increased risk for obstructive sleep apnea hypopnea; however, when women go through menopause, the risk equalizes.

Polysomnography is required to make the diagnosis. It may be performed either in a hospital lab (usually considered an outpatient procedure) or at home by ambulatory monitoring. Polysomnography provides information on when the individual falls asleep, stages of sleep, and certain vital signs (e.g., heart rate and oxygen saturation), as well as whether there is any impairment in nasal or oral flow or in the work of breathing. Sleep and breathing events are scored according to criteria set by the American Academy of Sleep Medicine.

Getting the History

A 50-year-old patient presents with the chief complaint "I'm always tired!" First, the interviewer assesses if what the patient experiences is sleepiness (on the verge of falling asleep) or fatigue (low energy). The interviewer then asks about the duration and severity of the chief complaint. It can be helpful to have a bed partner provide collateral information, but if none is available, the interviewer asks the patient questions such as these: "Has anyone ever told you that you snore? Has anyone ever told you that you seem to stop breathing in your sleep? Do you ever wake up gasping or choking or with a feeling of needing to catch your breath? Do you ever wake up with a dry mouth? Has anyone ever told you that you sleep with your mouth open? Do you have water at your bedside because you frequently need water in the middle of the night?"

It can be helpful to review a typical night: "What time do you go to bed? How long does it take you to fall asleep? Once asleep, do you usually wake up? What is it that wakes you? How many times per night? How long does it take you to return to sleep? What time do you get up in the morning? When you wake up, do you feel refreshed or like you need to sleep longer? Do you wake with headaches? Do you ever take purposeful naps? Do you ever inadvertently doze off? Have you ever been so sleepy that you fell asleep while driving? Have you had any accidents or "close calls" because of being sleepy while driving? What do you do to prevent falling asleep while driving? For what medical illnesses do you regularly see a doctor? Do you have hypertension, coronary artery disease, gastroesophageal reflux, asthma, allergies, depression, and/or anxiety? Does anyone in your family have any problems with sleep?"

Individuals with obstructive sleep apnea hypopnea may present as either sleepy or fatigued, but the tendency to use the vernacular "tired" is nonspecific and could indicate either symptom. Classically, people with obstructive sleep apnea hypopnea are thought to be sleepy more than fatigued, although certain populations (e.g., women) may more frequently report fatigue. As with any other complaint, the interviewer needs to assess duration, severity, and functional impact. It is important to assess also the person's level of sleepiness, particularly as it relates to driving, because driving while sleepy significantly increases risk for motor vehicle crashes and is one area of particular concern for people with sleep disorders. As noted, a bed partner can be helpful in reporting symptoms observed during sleep, but even if a bed partner is not present, an individual may have been told of symptoms in the past. Reviewing a typical night for an individual can be helpful both in ruling out other possible sleep disorders, such as insomnia or circadian rhythm sleep-wake disorders, and in providing additional information to support the diagnosis of obstructive sleep apnea hypopnea. For example, if a person awakens to use the bathroom five times per night and is able to return to sleep quickly, that pattern suggests obstructive sleep apnea hypopnea. Other supporting information would include medical conditions and family history.

Tips for Clarifying the Diagnosis

- Consider obstructive sleep apnea hypopnea in any person who is obese.
- Investigate sleep-disordered breathing as a potential cause of difficulties with sleep maintenance, as well as a cause of refractory sleepiness, fatigue, or concentration or cognitive problems.
- Assess for snoring or observed pauses in breathing while a person is sleeping, which are suggestive of obstructive sleep apnea hypopnea.
- Use polysomnography to confirm the presence of obstructive sleep apnea hypopnea.

Consider the Case

Ricky is a 6-year-old boy who presents with his parents for evaluation for possible sleep apnea. They had researched the Internet on attention-deficit/hyperactivity disorder and were wondering if sleep apnea could explain Ricky's current behavioral issues. He had been diagnosed with obstructive sleep apnea hypopnea at age 3, had his tonsils removed, and had subsequent significant improvement in his sleep, until about 6 months ago. His parents note that he has very restless sleep and moves around a great deal. He also gets very sweaty while sleeping. He does not snore but has loud, labored breathing and seems to breathe only through his mouth while sleeping. He was held back in kindergarten because of disruptive and inattentive behaviors in class, even though he had been successful in meeting other requirements for grade promotion.

Upon exam, Ricky's vital signs are normal. He is excessively active, swinging between chairs in the exam room and climbing on the exam table and attempting to jump off. He requires significant intervention by his mother for redirection. He is observed to breathe through his mouth. His nasal exam reveals a midline septum with enlarged turbinates, and he has a high, arched palate, with a Mallampati score of 3. Overnight polysomnography demonstrates an AHI of 7.5, with desaturation to 92%.

Although obstructive sleep apnea hypopnea is less commonly recognized in children, it does occur in this population. Unlike adults, children usually present their sleepiness as hyperactivity rather than somnolence. Obtaining a clinical report of nighttime symptoms frequently is difficult, particularly for young children who have their own rooms; however, some parents do hear their children snore or have heavy, labored breathing. These children often move quite a bit in their sleep, sleep in unusual positions, and may become very sweaty while sleeping. They also are frequently behind their peers for height and may suffer from enuresis after having been dry. Identification of obstructive sleep apnea hypopnea and appropriate treatment can correct enuresis, lead to gains in height, and in some cases improve daytime behavioral issues. Ricky primarily breathes through his mouth, which indicates he may have nasal obstruction, either from his enlarged turbinates (likely secondary to allergies) or adenoid tissue hypertrophy. In some rare instances, a child may have regrowth of resected tonsillar tissue. The noted high, arched palate also suggests the presence of sleep-disordered breathing, because it indicates a narrower space in which to contain soft tissue structures. In children, as in adults, polysomnography must be used to confirm the diagnosis. The relative severity in children is different from that in adults, with a lower threshold for diagnosis in the number of breathing events required to qualify for obstructive sleep apnea hypopnea (≥1 event per hour).

Differential Diagnosis

Obstructive sleep apnea hypopnea should be differentiated from primary snoring and other sleep disorders. Ultimately, polysomnography will be most helpful in differentiating it from other disorders, but there are aspects of the history that may help in the consideration of other disorders. For example, a person with a history of congestive heart failure may have obstructive sleep apnea hypopnea but may also have central sleep apnea (Cheyne-Stokes breathing). Similarly, a person who takes large doses of long-acting opioids would also be at risk for having central sleep apnea.

Sleep-related hypoventilation should be considered in a person who is morbidly obese, takes sedative-hypnotics, or has neuromuscular or pulmonary conditions. Other sleep disorders that could cause excessive sleepiness should also be considered, such as narcolepsy, circadian rhythm sleep-wake disorders, or hypersomnolence disorder—although obstructive sleep apnea hypopnea may certainly be comorbid with these disorders.

Insomnia disorder is often seen with obstructive sleep apnea hypopnea; people with insomnia disorder typically complain more of fatigue and are not sleepy on objective measures of sleepiness. They also tend to demonstrate significant anxiety regarding sleep. Individuals with nocturnal panic attacks often report subjective symptoms that overlap quite a bit with obstructive sleep apnea hypopnea (gasping, choking, heart racing upon awakening); however, these attacks usually are also seen in daytime panic attacks, occur less frequently, and would be less likely to be associated with excessive sleepiness. As in the case of Ricky above, children may present with symptoms similar to attention-deficit/hyperactivity disorder (such as hyperactivity, inattentiveness and academic delays) that may improve with treatment of obstructive sleep apnea hypopnea. Substance/medication-induced symptoms may mimic obstructive sleep apnea hypopnea. For example, ingestion of alcohol before bed may cause greater muscle relaxation and airway collapse. Again, ultimately, polysomnography would be most helpful in differentiating these disorders.

See DSM-5 for additional disorders to consider in the differential diagnosis. Also refer to the discussions of comorbidity and differential diagnosis in their respective sections of DSM-5.

Summary

- Obstructive sleep apnea hypopnea is characterized by snoring, witnessed apneas (pauses in breathing), or snorting or gasping while sleeping, or excessive daytime sleepiness, fatigue, or unrefreshing sleep.
- Polysomnography is required for the diagnosis.
- Individuals may be diagnosed with obstructive sleep apnea hypopnea if they have polysomnography demonstrating an AHI of at least 5 events per hour, with symptoms of snoring, pauses in breathing, excessive sleepiness, fatigue, or unrefreshing sleep; or an AHI ≥15, regardless of symptoms.
- In persons with excessive sleepiness, it is important to screen for sleepiness while driving.

IN-DEPTH DIAGNOSIS

Restless Legs Syndrome

Ms. Sanchez is a 67-year-old postmenopausal woman with a history of coronary artery disease, hypertension, severe obstructive sleep apnea hypopnea, and anxiety, who presents with a complaint of worsening insomnia. She notes that she recently had been hospitalized for workup of a gastrointestinal bleed and that ever since she was released from the hospital, she has had difficulty falling asleep. She finds that each evening while watching the television shows she normally enjoys, she has begun to feel restless and un-settled and "can't sit still." She has difficulty making it through an entire program with-out having to get up and walk around; she will usually feel fine for about 20 minutes after getting up, but then she begins to feel restless again. This feeling continues, even once she gets into bed, until she is so exhausted that she eventually falls asleep. She is unable to ignore the sensation, describing it as nonpainful but "uncomfortable, like my legs have to sneeze." She is worried, because she had similar symptoms during her two pregnancies but to a much less severe degree. Aside from movement, she is unable to identify anything that improves or worsens the feelings. She is not aware of any family members with similar symptoms. Current medications include aspirin, an antidepres-sant, and a diuretic, and she has not had any labs checked since she was discharged from the hospital. Neurological exam is normal, and sleep apnea remains well controlled with continuous positive airway pressure.

Restless legs syndrome (RLS) may be difficult to diagnose, and the presentation of Ms. Sanchez highlights the importance of taking a thorough sleep history. Although she complains of "insomnia," greater detail demonstrates that she actually is suffering from RLS. This disorder occurs more frequently in women than in men, and that fre-quency is often attributed to increased prevalence in pregnancy. There is also an asso-ciation with iron deficiency. This observation may explain the relationship with pregnancy, but in older adults presenting with new symptoms of RLS, a source of "oc-cult" or unknown bleeding should be considered, as in Ms. Sanchez, who had a known gastrointestinal bleed. Individuals describe the symptoms in a variety of ways, usually as a discomfort that is exacerbated by inactivity and relieved by move-ment. The symptoms do not have to occur daily, but when they do occur, they tend to have a circadian rhythmicity. Family history may be positive, because RLS has a known genetic component, but this history often is not recognized unless it is specif-ically solicited. Certain medications, such as selective serotonin reuptake inhibitors, may exacerbate the symptoms of RLS, but they would likely be less of a contributing factor in this case if Ms. Sanchez had been taking fluoxetine for some time preceding the gastrointestinal bleed.

Approach to the Diagnosis

The DSM-5 diagnosis of RLS is obtained solely from history, unlike some of the other sleep-wake disorders that entail laboratory testing to make a definitive diagnosis. Ob-taining a history of RLS requires inquiry to a specific sensation of discomfort, usually in the legs, that the individual perceives as irrepressible. The discomfort should occur during periods of rest or inactivity, and movement must alleviate (at least partially) the sensation. The symptoms usually occur at a particular time of day and should oc-cur at least three times per week. It is important to separate out whether the discom-fort is due to another medical condition. For example, an individual may feel excess soreness from an increase in physical activity, which tends to improve with additional increased physical activity, or a person who has peripheral neuropathy may experi-ence lower-extremity discomfort that impairs sleep initiation, but the discomfort is constant. Also, the symptoms must cause some sort of distress or impairment in func-tioning. The symptoms of RLS can interrupt the ability to fall asleep or can even be significant enough to waken the individual from sleep. Because of the sleep disruption, the individual may report sleepiness, fatigue, and cognitive, mood, or behavioral impairment.

Information supporting the diagnosis, but not included in the DSM-5 criteria for RLS, is somewhat more concrete than the historical details required by DSM-5. Family history indicates a likelihood of the diagnosis of RLS, and certain genetic markers (e.g., *MEIS1, BTBD9, MAP2K5/LBXCOR1*) have been associated with the diagnosis, although genetic typing is not currently clinically used for diagnosis. Iron deficiency, specifically a low ferritin level, in the context of a genetically vulnerable individual may precipitate symptoms. For example, some people develop symptoms after severe anemia secondary to gynecological hemorrhage or, similarly, in pregnancy, which depletes iron stores. In other people, the symptoms of RLS may be a warning signal of otherwise unrecognized iron depletion. Although most labs consider a ferritin level of >20 μg/L to be within normal limits, a ferritin level of >50–75 μg/L is preferable in a vulnerable individual. Also helpful in supporting the diagnosis is the presence of periodic leg movements on overnight polysomnography. Most people with RLS (70%) will also have periodic leg movements on polysomnography.

Getting the History

A 42-year-old woman presents with a history of "insomnia, tossing and turning each night." The interviewer inquires as to the specificity of symptoms: "Are you having difficulties with sleep initiation, maintenance, or both? How long has this been a problem? Have you ever had something like this before? What symptoms of daytime dysfunction are present?"

In attempting to solicit symptoms specific to RLS, the interviewer may find it helpful to preface the line of questioning with a qualifying statement, such as, "Sleep disruption can come from a variety of different causes, so I'm going to ask some questions that may seem unrelated." Some people may have become preoccupied with the sleep disruption, so they minimize the symptoms of RLS. Asking the following questions in the context of unusual situations can be helpful: "Are you able to sit through an entire movie or long plane flight?" If the patient says no, the interviewer asks for further elaboration as to what causes her to get up, such as the need to use the restroom versus a need to move. More focused questioning may be required: "Some people describe a discomfort, a 'creepy crawly' feeling, or itching or burning, deep within their legs. Do you ever get anything like that?" The patient answers in the affirmative, so the interviewer solicits occurrences in other situations, such as at home, and their frequency. The interviewer also elicits information about the circadian pattern: "Do the symptoms seem to happen at any particular time of day, or is there no pattern? Are they always there?" The interviewer assesses improvement in an open-ended manner: "Does anything seem to make the symptoms feel better or go away?" If the patient is unsure or gives a vague answer, a more direct question is important, such as, "Does it get better if you move?" With women, such as this patient, the interviewer may inquire whether they had similar symptoms when pregnant and, for any patient, whether anyone in the family has experienced anything similar. It may be helpful to inquire about health status, use of medications or other substances, and diet, as well as whether the patient has ever been diagnosed with anemia or has any evident blood loss.

People often have difficulty describing symptoms of RLS. They often identify a difficulty with sleep and require careful probing to identify symptoms of RLS as the cause. As with any other disorder, description of the course of symptoms and impaired functioning should be elicited. Some individuals have become so distraught by their sleep disruption that they may appear as people with insomnia disorder would—that is, with much anxiety and sleep-related worries. In this context, asking about the occurrence of symptoms during periods of rest or inactivity (i.e., not necessarily tied to sleep) can be helpful. Some people certainly will only note their symptoms in a circadian pattern. The discomfort is often difficult for individuals to describe, so giving descriptors such as "creepy crawly," "itching," or "like jumping beans" can sometimes resonate with them. Improvement with movement is also imperative, but sometimes people also describe elaborate rituals that they perform to ease the discomfort, such as a hot bath, massage, or even self-injurious behavior. Family history, health status, and use of medications or other substances also support the diagnosis.

In pediatric cases, inquiry as to "growing pains" at night may sometimes help identify the presence of RLS.

Tips for Clarifying the Diagnosis

- Question whether the person experiences discomfort or an unpleasant sensation in the legs, occurring typically around the same time of day.
- Clarify whether movement leads to *improvement* in the symptoms (i.e., there need not be *resolution* of the symptoms).
- Investigate whether the symptoms are exacerbated at night.
- Obtain supporting information (e.g., ferritin level <50 µg/L, presence of periodic leg movements, positive family history) that may help to clarify the diagnosis.

Consider the Case

Harvey is a 13-year-old nonverbal boy with a history of autism spectrum disorder whose parents brought him to the sleep clinic for evaluation of sleep disturbance. They note that he seems to fall asleep later than their older son did at the same age and are concerned that his sleep is causing him some anxiety. At night, they notice that he starts pacing around 9:00 P.M., and if they ask him to stay in bed, he performs automatisms of rubbing his legs, which he did not do previously. Once he does fall asleep, he occasionally wakes up and performs the same behaviors. They are concerned that he does not get enough sleep for school, and his teachers have noted some days at school in which he has greater behavioral disturbances, including tantrums and aggression.

Harvey has no other medical problems but recently started taking an atypical antipsychotic because of his behavioral issues at school and sleep problems. Family sleep history is positive for both insomnia disorder and RLS in his mother and obstructive sleep apnea hypopnea in his father.

On exam, Harvey is nonverbal and makes no eye contact. He responds to direction by his parents but resists physical examination. He was able to cooperate for polysomnography, which demonstrated sleep efficiency of 50%, an AHI of 0.7, and a periodic leg movement index of 25. His serum ferritin level was 18 µg/L.

Harvey presents an exceptionally difficult-to-identify case of RLS. Notably, the diagnosis of RLS requires a description of the symptoms in the person's own words; however, in some young children or individuals who are nonverbal, that narrative may be difficult to obtain, and other supporting information may point toward the diagnosis. In support of the diagnosis of RLS are the circadian pattern of the symptoms, the family history of RLS in the mother, findings of periodic leg movements on the sleep study, and low serum ferritin. Children with autism spectrum disorders often are picky eaters, which may explain Harvey's low ferritin level. Also of note in this case is the exacerbation of daytime behaviors due to the sleep disruption from the symptoms of RLS.

Differential Diagnosis

Differentiating RLS from other pain conditions primarily in the extremities is the first important separation. Positional discomfort would occur intermittently, without an obvious circadian pattern, and would likely completely resolve with repositioning. Leg cramps may occur intermittently as well, and often patients can palpate a solid contraction of the muscle body while it is occurring. Movement can improve the cramp. Peripheral neuropathy would be suspected in a person with a history suggestive of peripheral neuropathy (e.g., a person who has diabetes mellitus or has used neurotoxic agents) and would be of a more chronic, constant nature. Neuroleptic-induced akathisia would not be expected to have circadian rhythmicity and would likely have a chronological relationship to medication initiation or increase. Other pain syndromes might be noted to worsen with inactivity but are not isolated to a certain time of day, and claudication would be precipitated by activity in an individual with peripheral vascular disease. Anxiety or insomnia may be tied to the perception of interference with sleep and can cause a feeling of restlessness that would not resolve with movement.

In pediatric cases, positional discomfort or injury should be considered in the process of arriving at the differential diagnosis. As with adults, these feelings would not likely occur with a circadian rhythmicity or awaken the child from sleep with regularity but would occur intermittently.

See DSM-5 for additional disorders to consider in the differential diagnosis. Also refer to the discussions of comorbidity and differential diagnosis in their respective sections of DSM-5.

Summary

- RLS *requires* discomfort or urge to move the legs, worsening with inactivity, occurrence with a circadian rhythmicity, and improvement with movement.
- The symptoms cause some sort of impairment to sleep or daytime functioning.
- Certain details, such as family history, comorbid medical conditions, medications, ferritin level, and presence of periodic limb movements on polysomnography, help to support the diagnosis but are not included in the DSM-5 criteria.
- The symptoms should occur three times per week, for at least 3 months.

───────── SUMMARY ─────────

Sleep-Wake Disorders

Sleep-wake disorders can lead to, accompany, or exacerbate many psychiatric disorders. The diagnosis of sleep-wake disorders is important for the evaluation and treatment of such mental disorders as depression, PTSD, and anxiety. DSM-5 gives evidence of the importance of sleep-wake disorders to psychiatric phenotypes by elevating REM sleep behavior disorder and RLS to their own diagnostic categories. The state of the science is such that certain sleep disorders, such as obstructive sleep apnea hypopnea and narcolepsy, now have available specialized testing. Increased clinical research has resulted in further refinement in DSM-5 of the subtypes of circadian rhythm sleep-wake disorders and breathing-related sleep disorders. In general, the approach to the patient with a sleep-wake complaint should include a thorough history of behaviors occurring in both sleep (e.g., snoring, sleepwalking) and wake (e.g., excessive sleepiness, substance use) states. Collateral information from a bed partner can also be helpful, because many individuals are unaware of symptoms occurring while they sleep. Ultimately, certain sleep-wake disorders, such as obstructive sleep apnea hypopnea, require specialized tests or examinations and are best referred to a sleep medicine specialist. It is important for the mental health clinician to understand how sleep may be disordered and how sleep-wake disorders affect psychiatric and other medical conditions, and to recognize when it is important to refer a person to a sleep medicine specialist.

─────── ■ ■ ■ ───────

Diagnostic Pearls

- Many people complain of sleep-related problems, but they do not all have insomnia disorder. A variety of sleep-wake disorders should be considered.

- It is important to take a thorough sleep history and consider a full sleep evaluation by a specialist in sleep medicine to assess sleep complaints.

- Some individuals with primary sleep disorders present to mental health providers because of psychiatric-type symptoms. Daytime sleepiness, fatigue, poor concentration, irritability, anxiety, and hallucinations are just some of the symptoms that people with sleep disorders may report.

- In general, any person who is obese should be screened for breathing-related sleep disorders. Individuals with symptoms of snoring, gasping for breath, or stopping breathing while sleeping, as well as sleepiness or fatigue, should be referred for a full sleep evaluation.

- Individuals presenting with excessive daytime sleepiness of any etiology should be evaluated for safety while driving, and safeguards should be put in place if they are at risk of falling asleep while driving.

Self-Assessment

Key Concepts: Double-Check Your Knowledge

What is the relevance of the following concepts to the various sleep-wake disorders?

- Sleepiness versus fatigue
- Impairment in daytime functioning
- Sleep-related anxiety
- Cataplexy
- Hypocretin deficiency
- Multiple sleep latency test
- Mean sleep latency
- REM sleep latency
- Sleep-onset REM periods
- Apnea
- Hypopnea
- Polysomnography
- Urge to move
- Circadian rhythm

Questions to Discuss With Colleagues and Mentors

1. Do you screen all patients for sleep-disordered breathing?
2. What questions do you use to help differentiate breathing-related sleep disorders from insomnia disorder or other sleep-wake disorders?
3. How do you assess for insomnia disorder versus circadian rhythm sleep-wake disorders?
4. How do you decide when to refer a patient to a specialist in sleep medicine?

Case-Based Questions

PART A

> Mr. Xue, a 45-year-old man on stable-dose, daily methadone maintenance for opioid dependence, is referred to the sleep clinic for evaluation of sleep fragmentation and daytime sleepiness. Because of concerns of central sleep apnea and sleep-related hypoventilation, he is referred for polysomnography.

What is the differential diagnosis? Although obstructive sleep apnea hypopnea is the most common form of breathing-related sleep disorders, particularly in a middle-aged man who may have other predisposing factors, it is important to evaluate for the presence of other types of breathing-related sleep disorders if he is on high-dose, long-acting opioids.

PART B

> Polysomnography reveals that Mr. Xue has obstructive sleep apnea hypopnea and sleep-related hypoventilation, which are successfully managed with continuous positive airway pressure (CPAP). After being stable on CPAP for about 1 year, Mr. Xue decides to taper off methadone with the help of his physician. A few weeks after completion of his taper, he notes increasing difficulty falling asleep, which had not previously been a problem for him. He is concerned about the potential impact on his productivity at work.

What are the potential causes of his new difficulty falling asleep? Mr. Xue seems to have developed substance/medication-induced sleep disorder, insomnia type, in the context of opioid withdrawal. Perhaps he no longer has the sedating effect of the opioid medication or, because his breathing has improved after the opioid was removed, the CPAP is interfering with his sleep. More history would be helpful in making the diagnosis.

PART C

> Upon further questioning, Mr. Xue reports that around the same time each night, he starts to get an uncomfortable feeling in his legs and cannot sit still, even to watch television. He will pace for a short period of time, which improves the symptoms, but they often return after about 20 minutes. This feeling keeps him from falling asleep.

Do these additional details change the differential diagnosis? Mr. Xue now appears to have RLS, which has been unmasked. RLS can be treated with a variety of different classes of medications, one of which is opioids.

This case demonstrates the comorbidity that exists not only among sleep-wake disorders but also with other psychiatric conditions. It highlights the importance of digging into the history, because treating Mr. Xue merely for insomnia disorder rather than RLS would not adequately address the symptoms and may impair his ability to remain off opiate medication.

Short-Answer Questions

1. Is it correct that an individual must have difficulty initiating sleep in order to be diagnosed with insomnia?
2. A teenager presents with difficulty falling asleep on school nights. Once asleep, he is able to remain asleep, but he is difficult to awaken, very tired during the day, and often falls asleep in class. What is the likely diagnosis?
3. What laboratory test can confirm the diagnosis of narcolepsy?
4. For a diagnosis of narcolepsy using polysomnography, what duration must the REM sleep latency be?
5. Is it correct that snoring can indicate the presence of obstructive sleep apnea hypopnea?
6. What medical comorbidities have been linked to obstructive sleep apnea hypopnea?
7. What sleep-wake disorder may be seen in an individual with congestive heart failure?

8. A 72-year-old woman presents for a second opinion on a diagnosis of major depressive disorder. She started taking an antidepressant for early-morning awakenings, but it has not helped to change her sleep or her mood, although she denies significant mood symptoms. What sleep-wake disorder likely explains her symptoms?

9. A 32-year-old former Marine reports frequent, vivid nightmares impairing both his sleep and that of his bed partner. He awakens quickly from the dream but has difficulty returning to sleep. What sleep-wake disorder diagnosis should be considered?

10. A 62-year-old Vietnam-era veteran presents with a complaint of "beating up my wife while sleeping." He reports that when this happens, he is often having combat-related dreams, and he feels badly that he has hurt his wife. What is the likely diagnosis?

Answers

1. No. Individuals with insomnia may have difficulty initiating sleep, difficulty maintaining sleep, early-morning awakening, nonrestorative sleep, or some combination of those symptoms.

2. The likely diagnosis is circadian rhythm sleep-wake disorder, delayed sleep phase type.

3. Testing for hypocretin deficiency can confirm the diagnosis of narcolepsy.

4. For a diagnosis of narcolepsy using polysomnography, the REM sleep latency must be ≤15 minutes.

5. Snoring may indicate the presence of obstructive sleep apnea hypopnea, but only in combination with daytime symptoms (e.g., sleepiness, fatigue, unrefreshing sleep) and ≥5 obstructive apneas and/or hypopneas per hour of sleep.

6. Medical comorbidities that have been linked to obstructive sleep apnea hypopnea include hypertension, cardiovascular disease, cerebrovascular disease, diabetes mellitus, obesity, gastroesophageal reflux, and erectile dysfunction.

7. Central sleep apnea may be seen in an individual with congestive heart failure. Although a person with congestive heart failure may suffer from obstructive sleep apnea hypopnea, insomnia disorder, or any other sleep-wake disorder, it is also important to consider the possible presence of central sleep apnea.

8. The woman likely has circadian rhythm sleep disorder, advanced sleep phase type. Individuals with this disorder go to bed and wake up earlier than they desire. Sometimes, if individuals try to stay up to watch television or attend social activities, they may go to bed later but still wake up earlier, and so may become somewhat sleep deprived, with resultant daytime sleepiness and impaired functioning.

9. Nightmare disorder should be considered; however, PTSD is an obvious consideration in a veteran who is having nightmares.

10. This man may be describing REM sleep behavior disorder, which typically consists of vocalizations or dream enactment behavior that may possibly hurt the individual or the bed partner. Symptoms occur during REM sleep, when there typically is paralysis of voluntary muscles. REM sleep behavior disorder is associated with certain neurodegenerative conditions, such as Parkinson's disease, multiple system atrophy, or dementia with Lewy bodies, and neurological assessment may be indicated as well.

16

Sexual Dysfunctions

Richard Balon, M.D.

"He has never been interested in sex."

"I can't have sex—it hurts."

Sex is one of the three basic drives, in addition to eating and sleeping. Many mental and physical disorders and diseases affect the entire human body and all three basic drives. The impairment of sexual drive could thus occur within the context of another major mental disorder or physical illness (e.g., cardiovascular disease) or without any connection to another disorder or disease. The sexual dysfunctions discussed in this diagnostic class are those without any connection to other disorders. Sexual dysfunctions are characterized by a clinically significant inability to respond sexually and/or experience sexual pleasure (which could also be due to pain in the case of genito-pelvic pain/penetration disorder). Sexual dysfunctions frequently coexist with each other, and one may be a consequence of another. In cases of more than one sexual dysfunction in a particular person, all diagnoses should be made.

The DSM-5 group of sexual dysfunctions includes the following: delayed ejaculation (delayed ejaculation or inability to ejaculate); erectile disorder (inability to attain and maintain erection); female orgasmic disorder (delayed orgasm or anorgasmia); female sexual interest/arousal disorder (lack of sexual interest/arousal); genito-pelvic pain/penetration disorder (inability to have vaginal intercourse/penetration, marked vulvovaginal or pelvic pain during vaginal intercourse/penetration); male hypoactive sexual desire disorder (lack of sexual fantasies and desire); premature (early) ejaculation (ejaculation before the person desires, within approximately 1 minute after penetration); substance/medication-induced sexual dysfunction (sexual dysfunction

291

developing after introducing a substance, increasing the dosage, or discontinuing a substance of abuse or medication; the substance and the dysfunction should be specified); and other specified sexual dysfunction or unspecified sexual dysfunction (presentations in which symptoms characteristic of sexual dysfunction that cause clinically significant distress in the individual predominate but do not meet full criteria for any of the disorders in this diagnostic class). For other specified sexual dysfunction, the clinician can note the specific reason the presentation does not meet the criteria for any specific sexual dysfunction—for example, "sexual aversion." For unspecified sexual dysfunction, the clinician chooses not to specify the reason that criteria are not met for a specific sexual dysfunction; this includes presentations for which there is insufficient information to make a more specific diagnosis.

DSM-5 introduces several significant, general changes from DSM-IV for making the diagnosis of sexual dysfunctions more specific, refined, and distinguished from transient sexual difficulties. One change is the requirement of a specific duration of impairment of at least 6 months and, for most disorders, specification of frequency (i.e., symptoms experienced on approximately 75%–100% of occasions). Another change is an introduction of severity specifiers to rate distress as mild, moderate, or severe. DSM-5 retains specifiers helpful in delineating the possible source/etiology of the sexual dysfunction, such as whether the sexual dysfunction is lifelong (i.e., present since the individual became sexually active) or acquired, and whether it is generalized (i.e., not limited to certain types of stimulation, situations, or partners) or situational (i.e., only occurring with certain types of stimulation, situations, or partners).

A number of factors may be helpful in determining the etiology and circumstances of sexual dysfunctions, such as partner factors (e.g., a partner's health status or sexual problem); relationship factors (e.g., poor communication, discrepancy in sexual desire); individual vulnerability factors (e.g., poor body image, psychiatric comorbidity such as depression, or stressors such as job loss); cultural or religious factors; and medical factors (e.g., cardiovascular disease). It is also important to incorporate age-related changes into the diagnosis of sexual dysfunction, because aging may be associated with a normative decrease of sexual desire and response. Sexual difficulties may also be related to a lack of sexual stimulation (when no diagnosis of sexual dysfunction should be made). Clinical judgment should be used in considering both age-related changes and possible lack of sexual stimulation.

DSM-5 also introduces two new diagnoses, female sexual interest/arousal disorder and genito-pelvic pain/penetration disorder. The first disorder was introduced because the distinction between phases of sexual response in women may be a bit artificial and not necessarily linear. The second disorder appears because the diagnoses of dyspareunia and vaginismus in previous versions of DSM were overlapping and thus difficult to distinguish in clinical practice. The diagnoses of sexual dysfunctions are all gender specific in DSM-5.

Finally, DSM-5 has removed sexual aversion disorder (a rare condition) as a separate diagnosis. It now could be classified as other specified sexual dysfunction.

Discussing sexual functioning could be difficult for many, if not all, people in any situation or context, including the clinical setting. The interviewing clinician should be sensitive to the fact that people may hesitate to acknowledge that they are having sexual difficulties. For some, confidentiality is a concern; for others, barriers to disclosure relate to self-esteem, fears, culture, and religion. The careful interviewer will not be satisfied with vague answers to general or specific questions. Confidentiality of the interview should always be emphasized. Questions should progress from general to specific and should take into account the sensitivity and intimacy of discussing sexuality. Sexual dysfunctions have a broader impact than clinicians usually realize—they affect the individual and his or her partner. Thus, the clinician may consider interviewing (and educating) the individual's partner in addition, if the patient agrees. The interviewing clinician should also remember that sexual functioning is intertwined and affected by various mental and physical disorders and illnesses and therefore should ask about these conditions in connection with sexual functioning.

IN-DEPTH DIAGNOSIS
Female Orgasmic Disorder

Ms. Mitchell, a 27-year-old healthy married woman, complains of inability to reach orgasm. She states that she has never experienced orgasm. She became sexually active around age 20 and had three sexual partners before she got married. She describes those sexual partners as "typical student sexual partners: we dated and had sex occasionally. I was not really invested in the relationships, and having orgasms with these guys was not that important to me." She was interested in having sex and had heterosexual fantasies. She hoped that orgasms "would come in a real relationship." She got married 2 years ago to "a great guy. I have been and still am really sexually attracted to him." They have been having sex several times a week. She states, "I love having sex with my husband. He is caring, a great lover, and he has been trying very hard to satisfy me." She hoped that she would start to have orgasms, but "it did not happen." They have tried various things, such as oral stimulation, masturbation during intercourse, and using a vibrator. "Nothing helps." Her husband started to question his abilities and then whether anything is wrong with her. The absence of orgasm has become a "sore point in their relationship." She has been afraid that "he may start to look somewhere else." She has tried to masturbate and use a vibrator on her own, "but I cannot come, no matter what." She denies substance abuse and does not take any medication.

Ms. Mitchell meets criteria for female orgasmic disorder. She has never experienced orgasm (i.e., the difficulty has been present for more than 6 months). She has tried various ways of stimulation without any success. She has had sexual fantasies and becomes aroused when with her husband and when she was with her previous sexual partners. She does not describe any other sexual problem; she does not mention any pain during sexual intercourse. She is healthy, does not take any medication, and does not use any substances. She is happily married, and her husband is caring, trying to satisfy her; their relationship has been good. She has been sexually satisfied and has had sex several times a week, yet has not been able to reach orgasm. She started to be distressed by her inability to reach orgasm and by the fact that it has become an issue, a "sore point," in her relationship with her husband.

Ms. Mitchell has never been able to reach orgasm; thus, her dysfunction started early in her life. Her orgasmic disorder should be subclassified as lifelong and generalized, because she has never experienced an orgasm under any situation, and probably of moderate severity.

Approach to the Diagnosis

For diagnosis of this disorder, a woman must be distressed over her inability to reach orgasm, or significant interpersonal difficulties should result from this sexual difficulty (e.g., her partner may be upset, she may feel inadequate, her partner may cease having sex with her and look for satisfaction elsewhere). Not all women are distressed about the inability to reach orgasm. On the other hand, some women may not report their inability to reach orgasm, though distressed about it, possibly because of being otherwise satisfied or not wanting to upset their sexual partner. They may have difficulties discussing sexual issues. It is thus very important to ask directly about a woman's ability to reach orgasm, without relying on spontaneous reporting. In a woman who is able to reach orgasm, orgasmic sensation should be consistent, occurring on most (at least 75%) occasions of sexual activity; therefore, women with female orgasmic disorder may experience orgasm up to about 25% of the time. An important factor to consider in making the diagnosis of orgasmic disorder is adequate stimulation. Not all women experience orgasm during penile-vaginal intercourse all the time. Many women may require more stimulation, such as by masturbation or a vibrator. The woman's and her partner's orgasms also do not usually occur at the same time, and the woman may require more stimulation after her partner reaches orgasm to reach her own orgasm. Female orgasmic disorder may develop at any age, from the prepubertal period to late adulthood.

The inability to experience orgasm (or having a significantly delayed orgasm) should be evaluated in a wide context of numerous issues. The clinician needs to consider whether the absence of orgasm could be explained within the frame of another mental disorder (e.g., depression); if so, a diagnosis of female orgasmic disorder would not be made. However, the presence of another sexual dysfunction (e.g., female sexual interest/arousal disorder) does not exclude the diagnosis of female orgasmic disorder.

DSM-5 provides specifiers that should help to refine the diagnosis of female orgasmic disorder and make treatment planning more precise. The diagnosis should specify whether the woman has never experienced an orgasm under any situation, whether the orgasmic disorder is lifelong or acquired (i.e., it started after a period of having orgasms, or not having any orgasmic difficulties such as delay or decreased intensity), and whether the absence or impairment of orgasm is generalized (i.e., occurring basically in all situations and with all partners, if there were more than one) or situational (i.e., occurring with certain stimulation, situations, or partners). The clinician should also specify whether the associated distress is mild, moderate, or severe.

Relying on his or her judgment, the clinician should evaluate and discuss the following topics, even though they are not included among the DSM-5 specifiers:

- Relationship factors (e.g., discrepancies in desire for sexual activity, poor communication)
- Partner factors (e.g., partner's health, partner's interest in the woman's ability to achieve orgasm, partner providing adequate stimulation)
- Individual vulnerability (e.g., the loss of a job or other stresses that may be associated with inability to achieve orgasm; a change in living arrangements, such as living in a crowded space or sleeping with a baby in the room)

- Physical illness (e.g., hypothyroidism, arthritis)
- Cultural or religious factors (e.g., sex being designated for reproductive purposes only)

Getting the History

A 25-year-old woman reports having "sexual problems. I am unable to come." The interviewer should evaluate thoroughly all aspects of her sexual functioning and then focus on her ability to reach orgasm by asking a set of questions, gradually increasing the specificity, as follows: "Do you always have difficulties reaching orgasm? Do you reach orgasm at all? Have you ever been able to reach orgasm, or have you never been able to reach it?" Once the difficulty in experiencing orgasm is established, the interviewer should ask additional questions: "How long have you had problems reaching orgasm? Do you feel upset that you cannot? Is your partner upset with you because of this problem? Do you think that you may need more stimulation to reach orgasm? Have you ever tried to masturbate to reach orgasm? Do you and your partner use a vibrator?" It is important to establish possible partner factors: "Have you asked your partner to help you by stimulating you more? Does your partner reach orgasm too quickly? Is your partner demanding that you reach orgasm at the same time? Is your partner healthy?"

The following questioning focuses on more specific issues (to establish the specifiers): "Have you always had difficulties reaching orgasm? Let me clarify—have you never reached orgasm in your life? Are you unable to have an orgasm in any situation? Have you been unable to reach orgasm with other partners too? How much does this stress you out?"

Further questions may help clarify the diagnosis and the entire problem: "Did anything happen around the time you started to have difficulties reaching orgasm? For instance, have you started taking any new medications (e.g., selective serotonin reuptake inhibitors), or were any of your prescription dosages increased? Have you been using any illicit substances? When was your last gynecological or physical examination? Do you have any pain during intercourse? Are you happy in your relationship? Do you and your partner have any problems? Have there been any problems at home or at work? Do you feel stressed? Do you feel depressed? Are you anxious? Do you have other sexual problems?"

It is always important to establish whether the woman suffers from female orgasmic disorder by asking whether she is able to reach orgasm, whether her current situation constitutes a change from her previous ability to reach orgasm, or whether she has been unable to reach orgasm from her first sexual encounter. Furthermore, the interviewer needs to ascertain that the inability to reach orgasm is not due to a lack of stimulation; thus, questions need to be asked about the adequacy of stimulation, use of vibrators, and masturbation. Once the inability to reach orgasm is firmly established and the inadequacy of stimulation is ruled out, the length of the disturbance (e.g., 6 months vs. transient, short disturbance) and distress (e.g., being upset about inability to reach orgasm, feeling inadequate, partner complaints) should be established. Focusing on specific partner issues may be helpful in treatment planning; thus, the interviewer should ask about the partner's premature ejaculation, communication problems, and difference in demands of sexual activity. Inability to reach orgasm may occur within the context of mental and physical illness or as a side effect of a medication or a consequence of substance abuse. Because many women have difficulties communicating their sexual problems, the interviewer's questions need to be sensitive yet very specific.

Tips for Clarifying the Diagnosis

- Address whether the woman has ever experienced orgasm.
- Question whether the woman has been adequately stimulated and whether she has attempted to reach orgasm through masturbation.
- Clarify whether the woman feels distressed about her inability to experience orgasm, how much distress she feels, and whether she has been sexually satisfied.
- Ask whether the woman has discussed her inability to reach orgasm with her partner and whether she is able to discuss sexual issues with her partner and her physician.
- Investigate whether lack of orgasm has been consistent for at least 6 months, or whether the problem is temporary or transient.
- Investigate whether the woman is healthy and whether she is taking any medication.

Consider the Case

> Ms. Cook, a 51-year-old woman, complains of a gradual decrease in her ability to reach orgasm over the last 1–2 years. "Most of the time I don't have any orgasm. I may have one every month or two, no matter how excited I get, no matter how wet I get." She says, "We are having sex twice a week." She has been with her partner for 3 years. They got together 2 years after her husband died. "My partner is trying, but I am also not what I used to be. I may not have the drive I used to have." She claims that her partner does "whatever I want, and at times we tried to get me excited for hours, even masturbating, and nothing happens." Ms. Cook is physically healthy. She admits being mildly depressed for the last 3 months after she was demoted at work for performance problems. She emphasizes that her orgasmic difficulties started before her work problems, although "it has been even more difficult in bed since I started to have problems at my job."
>
> Ms. Cook is upset about her inability to reach orgasm: "I love to have one, but once in a blue moon after a whole night of hard work for it is not really any pleasure."
>
> She denies any substance abuse. She takes multivitamins and occasionally zolpidem (a nonbenzodiazepine hypnotic) for sleep. Her menstrual periods ceased at age 42. She tried "hormones" for her orgasmic problems in the past, "but it did not help."

Ms. Cook's ability to reach orgasm gradually ceased relatively late, around age 50. Women usually learn to experience orgasm as they learn more about their bodies and have more experience with various stimulations. She is still able to achieve orgasm, but very rarely and after a lot of stimulation. She experiences anorgasmia on almost all occasions of sexual activity, about 90% of the time. She has been anorgasmic for about 1–2 years. She is mildly depressed—anorgasmia may occur within the context of depression and other mental disorders—however, her depression developed much later than her inability to reach orgasm. She is in menopause, but menopausal status is not consistently associated with difficulties in reaching orgasm. Also, she reached menopause before the onset of her sexual difficulties. She takes zolpidem occasionally, but this medication is not known to be associated with impaired ability to reach orgasm. She is unhappy about not having orgasms. Her presentation is a bit atypical because of the fairly late development of her inability to have orgasm and some symptomatology such as depression. Her sexual drive may be decreased, but it does not seem to reach criteria of another sexual dysfunction.

Differential Diagnosis

The differential diagnosis of female orgasmic disorder includes nonsexual mental disorders and symptoms, such as major depressive disorder, severe anxiety disorder, psychosis, or substance use disorder. However, if a woman with anorgasmia has a history of depression or another major mental disorder that does not include inability to reach orgasm in its symptomatology, then the diagnosis of both the major mental disorder (e.g., major depressive disorder) and female orgasmic disorder should be made. Similarly, if the inability to reach orgasm precedes the development of symptomatology of major mental disorder (e.g., the woman has a lifelong history of inability to reach orgasm and recently became depressed), the clinician should diagnose both female orgasmic disorder and the major mental disorder. Female orgasmic disorder may co-occur with other sexual dysfunctions (e.g., female sexual interest/arousal disorder); thus, existence of another sexual disorder does not rule out female orgasmic disorder. The differential diagnosis of female orgasmic disorder also includes another medical condition (e.g., multiple sclerosis, spinal cord injury, fibromyalgia, endocrine disease) and interpersonal factors (e.g., intimate partner violence, severe relationship distress). The impact of using illicit substances (e.g., opioids) and medications (e.g., antidepressants, antipsychotics) should be evaluated in the differential diagnosis. The clinician should consider that even an increase in prescription medication dosage might impede the ability to reach orgasm.

Women with female orgasmic disorder may develop various associated symptomatology. A woman may subsequently be less interested in engaging in sexual activity. Failing to reach orgasm and subsequent possible interpersonal difficulties surrounding this failure may lead to anxiety regarding sexual activity and depression about her inability to have orgasm. Other factors, such as her partner's demands in spite of her difficulties in reaching orgasm or her partner reaching orgasm too quickly, may affect her associated symptomatology. If a woman is distressed about her inability to reach orgasm, she may become more anxious and then less interested in sex and less aroused. In a vicious circle, this could lead to more sexual difficulties and less ability to reach orgasm (if there was any before) and even associated pain during intercourse.

See DSM-5 for additional disorders to consider in the differential diagnosis. Also refer to the discussions of comorbidity and differential diagnosis in their respective sections of DSM-5.

Summary

- The core symptom of female orgasmic disorder is a marked delay in, decreased frequency of, or inability to reach orgasm or a marked decrease in orgasmic intensity on at least 75% of occasions of sexual activity, including masturbation.
- The impairment should last at least 6 months.
- A woman has to demonstrate significant distress or impairment (e.g., interpersonal difficulties, feelings of inadequacy).

- The adequacy of sexual stimulation should always be carefully probed.
- Women may feel sexually satisfied yet still have orgasmic difficulties or be unable to reach orgasm.
- Other mental disorders (e.g., those involving depression, psychosis, anxiety, substance abuse) and side effects of medications should be ruled out as possible causes of female orgasmic disorder.
- Female orgasmic disorder may be diagnosed in the presence of other sexual dysfunctions.

IN-DEPTH DIAGNOSIS
Delayed Ejaculation

Mr. Jones, a 21-year-old physically healthy man, complains of problems being sexually satisfied during intercourse. He says he takes a very long time to ejaculate: "at least half an hour of hard work." At times, he is unable to ejaculate at all because he is exhausted by his efforts to reach ejaculation. His girlfriend has been complaining that he reaches ejaculation a long time after she achieves orgasm. She is hesitant to have sex with him because "it is not comfortable or enjoyable at times; it is just an exhausting exercise." They tried various things, such as foreplay with "a lot of oral sex," mutual masturbation, and watching erotic movies together, but "nothing helps."

The man states that he wants to have sex often, he thinks about it frequently, but he is becoming really discouraged about the difficulties. "I hope I will be able to have children." He has no problems getting an erection. He says that he has been having difficulties with ejaculating "for as long as I can remember, even the first time I masturbated, but I believed that it would get better with some training."

He denies any depression or other symptoms of mental illness with the exception of getting anxious about being able to ejaculate. He does not take any medication and denies using any drugs: "It is not in my repertoire."

Mr. Jones demonstrates typical features of early-onset delayed ejaculation. He has difficulty achieving ejaculation, and the time to ejaculation is very long. At times, he cannot ejaculate at all. He has always had this difficulty (i.e., for more than 6 months). At times, his efforts to achieve ejaculation lead to exhaustion. He has tried to ease his difficulty (e.g., implementing mutual masturbation with his girlfriend), but nothing has helped. His delayed ejaculation and inability to reach ejaculation has become distressing for him—he feels anxious and even doubts he will be able to have children. His dysfunction has also caused interpersonal difficulties with his girlfriend (e.g., she has been hesitant to have sex with him). The man's delayed ejaculation could not be explained in terms of any physical illness, mental disorder, or use of any substance.

Approach to the Diagnosis

Delayed ejaculation is the least frequent sexual dysfunction in men (less than 1% of men complain of problems with ejaculation that last more than 6 months). It could develop at any age; however, the prevalence of delayed ejaculation remains relatively constant until around age 50, when it begins to increase significantly. Taking the sexual history should always include detailed questioning about the ability to ejaculate and any delayed ejaculation. Males, especially older ones, may attempt to explain their difficulty in terms of erectile dysfunction; erectile disorder and delayed ejaculation could coexist and should be diagnosed separately if a man meets the diagnostic criteria for both. Careful attention should be paid to a man's description of ejaculatory dysfunction. At times, men may be able to ejaculate but not describe orgasmic pleasure (which has been described as anhedonic ejaculation). Ejaculation itself is a "peripheral" or genital phenomenon, whereas the experience of orgasm is a cerebral phenomenon. Thus, these two events, although usually occurring together, can occur separately. In such a case, the diagnosis is not delayed ejaculation but rather sexual dysfunction not otherwise specified (because ejaculation occurred and was not delayed).

The absence of ejaculation in the presence of adequate desire, arousal, and stimulation makes the diagnosis of delayed ejaculation clear. However, there is no definite agreement about what "delayed" ejaculation means, and in cases of delayed but present ejaculation, diagnosis of delayed ejaculation is a matter of clinical judgment. The delay in ejaculation should be present consistently over a period of at least 6 months, reported by the patient and probably his sexual partner (although the DSM-5 criteria do not require the partner's report), and distressing to the patient and/or his partner, or it could cause some impairment in the form of interpersonal difficulties, avoidance of having intercourse, or inability to conceive. Partners may feel inadequate or unattractive and may blame themselves for the man's inability to ejaculate.

Explanation in terms of other sexual dysfunction (e.g., lack of sexual desire or ability to achieve erection), comorbid mental disorder (e.g., severe major depressive disorder), physical illness (e.g., interruption of innervation of sexual organs during surgery, neurological disease such as multiple sclerosis, consequence of an illness such as diabetic neuropathy), and use of various medications (e.g., serotonergic antidepressants, antihypertensives) and substances of abuse (e.g., opioids) should be considered, especially in cases of late-onset delayed ejaculation.

The approach to the diagnosis of delayed ejaculation should thus progress from 1) the establishing of delayed or missing ejaculation and the psychological experience of orgasm for at least 6 months in the evaluator's clinical judgment, to 2) determining the existence of distress and/or impairment in terms of the man's and his partner's experience. This approach could be followed by questions about the possible etiology using the framework of the DSM-5 specifiers.

Getting the History

A 30-year-old man complains that it "takes me forever to ejaculate." The interviewer should ask about all aspects of the patient's sexual functioning and sex life, and thus should start with general inquiries as follows: "Please tell me whether you are satisfied with your sex life. If not, why not? How often do you have sex? Is your partner satisfied with the frequency and quality of your sexual encounters?" Questioning should then become more specific, focusing on particular aspects. For example, after asking about sexual desire (e.g., "Do you feel like having sex often?") and erectile disorder (e.g., "Are you getting hard enough when you have sex? Have there been any changes in your ability to get an erection?") and ejaculation ("Have you had any problems reaching orgasm/ejaculating?"), it may become clearer that the prevailing sexual problem is delayed ejaculation or inability to ejaculate. The questions should then become even more specific, as follows: "Do you ejaculate at all? Does it take you more time to come/ejaculate lately? Have you tried any additional stimulation to reach orgasm? Are you able to ejaculate when masturbating? Can you ejaculate when having sex with someone else? What sexual fantasies do you have while having sex and while masturbating? Are you upset that it takes you a long time to ejaculate or that you cannot ejaculate? Is your partner also upset? Are you taking any medication? Which one(s)? Do you use any substances? Do you feel depressed? Are you healthy? Have you had any recent medical problems?"

After the man becomes open about his sexual problem, establishing the descriptive diagnosis of delayed, less frequent, or nonexistent ejaculation may be relatively simple. The man has to feel that all the information is confidential and considered seriously, because the inability to ejaculate may be deleterious to a man's feeling about his male function and ability to conceive (especially in younger males with early-onset delayed ejaculation). It is important to determine that the impairment is continuous (i.e., almost all occasions), lasting (i.e., 6 months or longer), and not temporary (e.g., due to interpersonal difficulties). Delayed ejaculation/inability to ejaculate should also cause distress (e.g., anxiety, self-doubt) or interpersonal difficulties (e.g., partner's unhappiness, arguments) to meet the DSM-5 criteria for delayed ejaculation. The judgment about the delay in ejaculation is clinical and should be considered in a wide context, because there is no consensus about what constitutes a reasonable and generally acceptable time to reach orgasm. The DSM-5 specifiers (lifelong vs. acquired; generalized vs. situational) should be used as a framework for more specific questioning that may help clarify the possible cause or contributing factors.

Tips for Clarifying the Diagnosis

- Ask whether the man has ever had an orgasm in terms of ejaculation and experiencing orgasm at the same time.
- Question whether the ejaculation is markedly delayed or significantly less frequent in spite of adequate desire, arousal, and stimulation.
- Verify that this dysfunction has been ongoing for at least 6 months.
- Assess whether the delay in ejaculation, decreased frequency, or inability of ejaculation is causing distress or personal difficulty.
- Ask the man whether he is taking any substances that could delay ejaculation.
- Investigate whether the man suffers from other sexual dysfunctions, such as male hypoactive sexual desire disorder or erectile disorder.

Consider the Case

Mr. Wong, a 55-year-old man of Chinese origin, is brought in by his wife, who complains that "lately, at least a year or two, he is forcing me to have sex forever. I am not able to satisfy him." He admits that as he is getting older, he has been having "more difficulties ejaculating, and my erections are getting weaker."

Mr. Wong says that he has always been proud of being able to satisfy his sexual partners, although "they usually came much earlier than I did, but they liked the fact that they always came." His time to reach ejaculation was longer, but he was able to ejaculate on all occasions. However, during the last several years, his ejaculations have been significantly delayed. At times, at least once or twice a month, he is unable to ejaculate at all. His mild erectile difficulties usually happen in the context of trying to achieve ejaculation, "at the end of my effort to satisfy my wife or at the end of my trying to ejaculate while masturbating." He is upset about his wife's complaint. They have argued a lot because she has been refusing to have sex with him lately. He is fairly healthy and has been taking medication for lowering cholesterol for about 10 years and "some pills for heartburn occasionally." He has never used any illicit substances. He drinks a glass or two of wine over the weekend.

Mr. Wong gradually developed delayed ejaculation and, at times, inability to ejaculate in his early 50s. In addition to his age, he has some predisposition for developing delayed ejaculation: he is of East Asian origin (more males of East and Southeast Asian origin report delayed ejaculation), and he has always taken a longer time to reach ejaculation. However, he was not distressed about his somewhat delayed ejaculation in his earlier years, and it did not cause him reportable interpersonal difficulties. He is, however, distressed by the development of more delayed ejaculation to the point of inability to ejaculate during the last several years, and his sexual dysfunction has caused interpersonal difficulties (e.g., he and his wife argue about it). He has some associated mild erectile disorder but is fairly healthy, and his medications or consumption of wine cannot explain his sexual dysfunction, which clearly meets the delayed ejaculation criteria. His disorder could be specified as acquired and probably generalized. He seems at least moderately distressed.

Differential Diagnosis

Differential diagnosis of delayed ejaculation includes numerous factors, especially in cases of acquired delayed ejaculation. In a young healthy male, the differential diagnosis includes mainly use of medications (e.g., selective serotonin reuptake inhibitors), substances of abuse, and psychological factors (e.g., inability to ejaculate with one partner while being able to ejaculate with others; paraphilic interests; and even a consequence of prolonged infertility treatment with pressure on "performing"—i.e., ejaculating at certain times and circumstances). Differential diagnosis could also include the disjunction between ejaculation and orgasmic experience (anhedonic ejaculation).

Differential diagnosis of late-onset delayed ejaculation is probably wider and includes various medical illnesses (e.g., impaired innervation of genitals in disorders such as multiple sclerosis, diabetes mellitus, and alcoholic neuropathy, or intentional or unintentional injury of innervation during surgery); use of medications (e.g., antihypertensives, antipsychotics, selective serotonin reuptake inhibitors, painkillers [opioids]) or drugs of abuse (opioids); psychological factors (e.g., ability to ejaculate with one partner but not another of the same sex, paraphilias, other sexual dysfunctions, or major depression); and anhedonic ejaculation (or other dysfunction with orgasm, such as painful ejaculation associated with some medications).

Factors that may affect the clinical presentation of delayed ejaculation include associated depression or anxiety; other sexual dysfunction that may either precede or develop as a consequence of delayed ejaculation (e.g., lack of desire to have sex anymore, erectile dysfunction); distress due to inability to conceive or just fear of inability to conceive; history of sexual abuse; poor body image; cultural and religious influences (religious belief that man should ejaculate just for the purpose of conception and that masturbation is a sin); partner demands (more sex, no sex) and complaints (that it takes too long to get sex, which could perpetuate the difficulty due to performance anxiety; that the sex is painful or exhausting; or the man's own exhaustion during the long attempts to achieve ejaculation while not being particularly physically fit.

See DSM-5 for additional disorders to consider in the differential diagnosis. Also refer to the discussions of comorbidity and differential diagnosis in their respective sections of DSM-5.

Summary

- Delayed ejaculation is the least frequent male sexual dysfunction.
- To establish the diagnosis of delayed ejaculation, the clinician should inquire about markedly delayed ejaculation or marked decrease in frequency of ejaculation or inability to ejaculate.
- The dysfunction should be continuous, occurring in almost all or all attempts to have intercourse or masturbation, and should last at least 6 months.
- The decision about the delay of ejaculation is clinical. There is no clear consensus about what constitutes delayed ejaculation in terms of time or frequency.
- The dysfunction should cause distress or impairment (especially in a man's relationship with his partner).
- Various factors that could explain or modify the clinical picture of delayed ejaculation include those related to the man, his partner, physical illness, medical illness, and medications/substances of abuse.

IN-DEPTH DIAGNOSIS

Female Sexual Interest/Arousal Disorder and Male Hypoactive Sexual Desire Disorder

Female Sexual Interest/Arousal Disorder

Ms. Parker is a 23-year-old healthy woman who states that she has not been interested in having sex for as long as she can remember. She is attracted to men in general and has had partners, but only as "companions. I have never thought of men in sexual terms very much, and I don't have any sexual fantasies." She is not receptive to her boyfriend's attempts to start sex, although "I give up at times, to make him happy." She may get aroused ultimately, but "I don't feel much when having sex, and it is the same when I tried to masturbate per someone's suggestion." Once aroused, she has no problem reaching orgasm. She has been having arguments with her boyfriend about her lack of interest in sex. "He thinks I don't love him. He is a great, caring guy, and I do love him, but I don't care about sex." She is upset about their arguments and worried that "he may run away." She denies taking any medication or using any drugs.

Ms. Parker meets the DSM-5 criteria for female sexual interest/arousal disorder, lifelong and generalized, because she has lacked sexual desire since her first sexual encounter. She does not have any sexual fantasies and is not receptive to her boy-friend's attempts to have sex. She also reports decreased intensity of sexual sensations during sex. Thus, she clearly presents with a mixture of lack of sexual desire and some impairment of arousal. She is able to get aroused occasionally and to reach orgasm. She loves her boyfriend and is attracted to him, but not sexually. Her sexual dysfunc-tion is persistent and has lasted more than 6 months. She has been having arguments because of her "sexual problems" and is worried about losing her partner, thus meet-ing the distress criterion (probably at a moderate level). She is healthy and denies any problems or substance abuse and does not take any medications.

Male Hypoactive Sexual Desire Disorder

> Mr. Carr, a 30-year old married man, tells his doctor that his wife is complaining of his "total lack of interest in her and in having sex with her." They have been married for 3 years and have had sex "less than a dozen" times during their marriage. His wife says that she would be happy to have sex once every month or two, but "he is not inter-ested." He denies any extramarital affair and reveals that he has not ever been inter-ested in sex, and "I really never think about it." His wife bought him some testosterone gel, and he applied it a few times, without any change in his desire. He has been able to have an erection after a "lot of stimulation by my wife, and after that, ejaculation is not a problem." He is healthy, uses no substances or prescribed medications, does not drink alcohol, and denies any depression. He is getting anxious because his wife is threaten-ing to divorce him, saying that his lack of sexual interest "shows" he does not love her.

Mr. Carr has not had interest in sex for most of his life, and he meets the criteria for male hypoactive sexual desire disorder (lifelong, probably generalized). He and his wife are having sex very infrequently for their age group, and his wife would clearly like to have sex more frequently, although her demands are not excessive. Mr. Carr has had no sexual fantasies, and his lack of interest in sex does not seem to be related to the lack of testosterone (application of testosterone gel did not make any difference in his lack of sexual desire). He is able to get an erection and ejaculate during sex. His sex-ual dysfunction is causing some interpersonal difficulties (mild). He is healthy, and his lack of sexual desire does not seem to be explainable in terms of other physical or men-tal illness or use of substances or medications.

Approach to the Diagnosis

FEMALE SEXUAL INTEREST/AROUSAL DISORDER

Female sexual interest/arousal disorder is a new diagnosis in DSM-5, requiring at least three symptoms that have persisted for at least 6 months. Because this disorder in a way combines the symptomatologies of low or nonexistent sexual desire and lack of arousal, both these sets of symptoms must be carefully explored. Various combinations of symptoms are possible. In assessing the sexual interest of a female, the clinician needs to consider a possible discrepancy in sexual desire between the patient and her partner; the clinician may not include the alleged lack of sexual desire, which could be ac-counted for by "desire discrepancy," in symptomatology counted toward the diagnosis of this disorder. The normative decline in sexual desire with age should be also considered in determining the lack of sexual desire. The lack of sexual receptivity to a partner's attempt to initiate sex should be carefully evaluated with consideration of the patient's and her partner's beliefs and preferences for initiation of sex. Wide variety in expression of sexual fantasies occurs in women, and individual patterns need to be taken into account in diagnosing female sexual interest/arousal disorder because specifications for sexual fantasies, desire, and feelings are neither known nor established. For the diagnosis, the presence of three or more symptoms of impaired sexual interest/arousal must cause significant distress or impairment. Finally, clinicians should consider physical or mental illness and substance or medication use as a possible cause of female sexual interest/arousal disorder. Further considerations include partner factors (e.g., poor health, lack of interest in proper stimulation), interpersonal problems (e.g., discrepancy in sexual desire, poor communication about sex), individual vulnerability (e.g., depression, anxiety, poor body image, stress over job loss) and cultural/religious factors (e.g., religious prohibition of sex before being married).

MALE HYPOACTIVE SEXUAL DESIRE DISORDER

When making the diagnosis of male hypoactive sexual desire disorder, the clinician must establish that the lack of sexual desire and the absence of sexual thoughts or fantasies are persistent and have lasted at least 6 months. An adaptive response to an adverse life condition (e.g., partner's pregnancy, intention to terminate relationship) should also be considered. In addition, questions about a possible discrepancy in sexual desire between partners should be asked (not all men claiming low sexual desire have low sexual desire). Increased age is a significant risk factor for decreased sexual desire. Although decrease in testosterone levels is not always associated with decrease in sexual desire, a clear-cut hypogonadism is associated with low sexual desire and should be ruled out as an underlying cause of this disorder. For the diagnosis of male hypoactive sexual desire disorder to be made, low or nonexistent sexual desire must be associated with significant distress (e.g., "not being a man") or impairment (e.g., dissolution of a relationship).

A wide spectrum of risk factors for developing low sexual desire needs to be considered in diagnosing this disorder, including depression, hyperprolactinemia, alcohol use, a man's feeling about his masculinity, religiosity, paraphilic tendencies, marital alienation, extramarital affairs, intrafamilial sexual abuse, pornography addiction, poor sexual education, and early life trauma. Thus, the diagnostic process should be a very careful exploration of multiple areas of sexual and psychological functioning and personal history.

Getting the History

FEMALE SEXUAL INTEREST/AROUSAL DISORDER

A 35-year-old woman presents with a vague complaint of not satisfying her sexual partner. The interviewer begins by asking about the nature of the woman's sexual activity and sexual satisfaction: "Are you satisfied with your sexual functioning? Why not? How often do you have sex? Has there been any change in how often you have sex lately? Is your partner satisfied with your sexual encounters? Is your partner demanding more sex lately?" Once the impairment of sexual functioning is generally established, questions should focus on various aspects of sexual interest/arousal: "Do you feel like having sex often? Do you think about sex often? Why not? Do you fantasize about having sex? If not, why not? Has there been any change in your sexual fantasies and thoughts? Who initiates sex, you or your partner? How do you respond when your partner initiates sex? Does your sexual desire appear/increase when your partner tries to initiate sex? Does your partner arouse you? Do you get wet easily, or have you had problems with lubrication lately? Have you needed more sexual stimulation to get aroused lately? What about the feelings in your genitals/vagina during intercourse? Any change? Less intense? Any pain?" The interviewer then asks, "How long has this been going on? Has there been anything that may have triggered these problems? Are you upset about your sexual problems? Why? Do you feel stressed out about the problem? Any related problems with your partner?" The interviewer also asks questions about health and substance use, such as, "What about your health? What about your menstrual periods—any changes, any difficulties? Are you taking any medication? Are you drinking? Are you using any illicit substances?"

The diagnosis of female sexual interest/arousal disorder is the most symptom specific (i.e., Criterion A requires a specific number of symptoms to be present) among the diagnoses of sexual dysfunctions and basically combines the symptomatology of sexual desire/interest and arousal. Therefore, all symptoms of possibly impaired sexual desire/interest and possibly impaired sexual arousal should be carefully evaluated. Symptoms should be evaluated in relation to the individual (e.g., sexual thoughts, fantasies), the dyad (e.g., the initiator of sex, the response of the partner, discrepancy in sexual desire/demands), and subjective feelings and physiological response (e.g., genital feelings, psychological excitement, lubrication, vasocongestion). Once the symptom configuration is established, the symptoms' persistence and duration need to be ascertained (brief decreases in sexual desire and arousal may occur in various situations and may resolve). Occurrence of other sexual problems (e.g., lack of orgasm, sexual pain) should also be explored because these problems may develop as a consequence or contribute to the development of female sexual interest/desire disorder.

MALE HYPOACTIVE SEXUAL DESIRE DISORDER

A 23-year-old man states that "my partner says I am not interested in sex." As in cases of any sexual dysfunction, the interviewer first elicits responses about sexual functioning in general, by asking, "Can you tell me whether you are satisfied with your sexual functioning? If not, why not? How often do you have sex? Do you masturbate in addition to having sex with your partner? Is your partner satisfied with your sexual encounters? Is your partner more demanding, or has there been any change in your partner's demands of sex?" Then the interviewer asks more specific questions, such as, "Do you feel like having sex often? Do you think about sex often? No? Why not? Have you always had low interest/no interest in sex? Has there been any change in your interest in sex or desire to have sex? How long has it been going on? Do you have any other sexual problems? Can you get an erection? What about ejaculation? Can you ejaculate? Do you have any problems with ejaculation?" If necessary, further questioning should establish whether the lack of sexual desire is the primary sexual dysfunction: "Which of your sexual problems appeared first: lack of libido, problems with erection, or problems with ejaculation?" These questions should be followed by queries about the distress: "Are you upset about your lack of desire? Why? How much? Has it caused any problems between you and your partner?" Finally, the interviewer asks about possible contributing factors: "Have you been depressed or anxious? How has your physical health been?

Are you taking any medications? How much do you drink? Do you use any other substances? Have you been sexually involved with anybody else? Do you have similar problems in that relationship?"

The diagnostic questioning for male hypoactive sexual desire disorder focuses on establishing the existence of sexual dysfunction first and then determines what dysfunction it is by asking about all aspects of the man's sexual functioning (e.g., desire, arousal [erection], and orgasm [ejaculation]) and questioning whether the lack of desire is the primary problem. Lack of sexual desire could possibly develop as a reaction to inability to attain erection or delayed ejaculation. It is also important to establish the existence of distress, because a small minority of men may not be distressed about their lack of sexual desire and may not be really interested in sexual and/or other relationships. Finally, questions focused on possible psychological factors (e.g., depression, marital problems, emotional connection with his partner, extramarital affairs, even frequent compulsive watching of pornography) and "environmental" factors (alcohol and other substance abuse, medication, religious issues, cultural issues) are also very important. Contrary to many beliefs, hypogonadism and/or "idiopathic" male hypoactive sexual desire disorder are not the only causes of low desire in many males. Using the framework of DSM-5, specifiers and risk factors may help elucidate and specify the diagnosis further.

Tips for Clarifying the Diagnosis

FEMALE SEXUAL INTEREST/AROUSAL DISORDER

To investigate whether a woman has female sexual interest/arousal disorder, explore the following questions:

- Does the woman have low sexual desire in the form of absent or reduced interest in sexual activity? What about sexual fantasies? Does the woman become interested or aroused while talking about sex with her partner or watching a sexually explicit movie? Does she attempt to masturbate?
- Who initiates sexual activity in the couple? How is initiation of sexual activity accepted by the woman? Any resistance?
- Does the woman experience any pleasure during sexual intercourse?
- Does the woman become aroused during intercourse? Is there adequate lubrication? Do her genital feelings change during intercourse?
- Is the woman distressed about her lack of sexual interest/arousal? How much and what is the nature of her distress or impairment?
- Is the woman healthy? Does she have any signs of depression, anxiety, or substance abuse?

MALE HYPOACTIVE SEXUAL DESIRE DISORDER

To investigate whether a man has male hypoactive sexual desire disorder, explore the following questions:

- Does the man report any change in sexual desire/interest? Does he have any sexual fantasies? Is this situation different than before or has this lack of sexual desire/interest been a lifelong pattern? Is the lack of desire persistent?

- How long has sexual desire/interest been absent?
- Is the man upset or distressed about his lack of sexual desire? Has it caused any problems for him?
- Is the lack of sexual desire specific for a particular person (partner) and/or situation, or does it occur for any sexual partner or situation?
- Is the man depressed or anxious, or concerned about his body image or sexual performance?
- Does the man have any physical signs of hypogonadism or low testosterone level?

Consider the Case

FEMALE SEXUAL INTEREST/AROUSAL DISORDER

Ms. Stone, a 45-year-old married woman states that her husband has been complaining about her lack of interest in having sex with him. "I realize that he is right. The problem is that I have not been feeling much during intercourse except for a bit of pain occasionally because I don't get wet. I just do not feel excited, no matter what we try—looking at movies, oral sex, vibrator. Sex is just not pleasurable for me anymore. I don't know how it happened and when; it has been a while ago, many months. I am not interested in sex anymore. It is not my husband—he is okay. It is sex I am not interested in. It is sad—I used to love sex." Ms. Stone is nervous because her husband's behavior "has changed lately. He is not home frequently. I am afraid he found someone to have sex with." She denies any depression. She is fairly healthy, and her periods are regular, without any changes. She takes a sleeping pill occasionally and multivitamins daily. She admits smoking a small amount of marijuana weekly "since I was in college."

Ms. Stone developed sexual dysfunction several months ago after functioning sexually fairly well. She has difficulties in getting aroused and feeling any pleasure and has also lost interest in sex. She meets symptom criteria for female sexual interest/arousal disorder (at least four symptoms). She has been suspicious that her husband may be having an affair as a consequence of her lack of interest in having sex with him, and she feels distressed about it. She has not reached menopause yet. Ms. Stone is healthy and does not take any medication that would affect her sexual functioning. She has been smoking small amounts of marijuana for years, so that activity could not explain her change in sexual functioning several months ago. The duration of her sexual functioning is not clear ("several months"); however, her impairment of sexual functioning has been persistent (if the duration of dysfunction is not precisely clear, the persistence of symptomatology may ascertain the diagnosis of female sexual interest/arousal disorder). Ms. Stone's disorder could be subtyped as acquired and probably generalized and specified as severe because she is significantly distressed.

MALE HYPOACTIVE SEXUAL DESIRE DISORDER

Mr. Carpenter, a 52-year-old married man, reports that he has been having occasional problems with erection and that his sexual desire has been "fading away lately." He can still have full erections occasionally, "but I am not really interested that much." The frequency of intercourse with his wife gradually decreased to once every several months, "after we used to have sex two to three times a week less than 2 years ago." He admits that he stopped thinking about sex, and "my fantasies about other women disappeared. I don't masturbate anymore." His testosterone level is lower than before but still within normal limits. A testosterone patch did not help, and the "little blue pill" did not help

either. Mr. Carpenter is very upset about his lack of sexual interest and declining performance because his friends have been constantly teasing him after he mentioned it to
them a while ago. "I don't feel as if I am a man anymore." He exercises regularly and is
in good shape. He denies any depression. He was diagnosed with hypothyroidism several years ago and takes thyroid hormone supplement daily (his thyroid-stimulating
hormone and free thyroxine levels are within normal limits). He has been drinking a
beer or two with friends occasionally for years but does not use any illicit drugs.

Mr. Carpenter developed lack of sexual desire relatively late in his life. His decline
in sexual desire is associated with some erectile dysfunction (associated sexual dysfunction), but his erectile dysfunction does not explain his total lack of desire or interest in
sex after a long period of good sexual functioning. His testosterone level is a bit low but
not abnormally low, and because testosterone patches were not helpful, low testosterone does not seem to be the underlying cause of his lack of desire (hypogonadism
should be ruled out in all cases of low sexual desire). His sexual activity has almost
completely ceased, and he feels distressed about it. Alcohol use may increase the occurrence of male hypoactive sexual desire disorder. He drinks beer occasionally, but has
done so for a long time, so his drinking could not explain his recent decrease in sexual
desire. Mr. Carpenter has two risk factors for developing male hypoactive sexual desire
disorder: he is over age 50 and has physical illness. He has hypothyroidism, which, if
not properly treated, could explain the decrease in his sexual desire. However, in this
case, the laboratory evaluation of thyroid functioning is within normal limits.

Differential Diagnosis

FEMALE SEXUAL INTEREST/AROUSAL DISORDER

The differential diagnosis of female sexual interest/arousal disorder is fairly broad
because the symptomatology of this sexual dysfunction covers the areas of desire and
arousal. As in other sexual dysfunctions, a broad variety of mental and physical illnesses may affect sexual desire and arousal.

Nonsexual mental disorders need to be considered. For example, major depressive disorder (one of the symptoms is markedly diminished interest or pleasure in all,
or almost all, activities) and persistent depressive disorder (dysthymia; symptoms include low energy, fatigue, low self-esteem) may account for the lack of interest/
arousal or its decrease. Some anxiety disorders (e.g., posttraumatic stress disorder)
and obsessive-compulsive disorder should also be ruled out as a possible cause of
low interest/arousal. Major psychotic disorders and some personality disorders may
also be associated with lack of or reduction in sexual interest/arousal. Similarly, substance use (e.g., opioids), not only during the episode of acute intoxication, and some
medications (e.g., antihypertensives, antipsychotics, antidepressants, chemotherapeutics, hormones) may account for the lack of sexual interest/arousal.

Medical illnesses/conditions associated with the lack of or diminished sexual inter-
est/arousal include, for instance, diabetes mellitus, thyroid disease, multiple sclerosis
and other neurological diseases, and cardiovascular diseases (e.g., endothelial disease).

Clinicians should also consider other sexual dysfunctions (e.g., chronic genital pain) as an explanation of female sexual interest/arousal disorder symptomatology. Other sexual dysfunctions (e.g., female orgasmic disorder) may also coexist with this disorder.

Sexual arousal and, in some women, sexual desire may develop in response to the partner's initiation and stimulation. The discussion of presence and adequacy of sexual stimulation should be part of the patient interview. If inadequate or absent sexual stimulation is part of the clinical picture, diagnosis of a sexual dysfunction should not be made.

Finally, interpersonal factors such as interpersonal distress, intimate partner violence, partner poor health, and stresses (e.g., job loss) may also play a role in the lack of or diminished sexual interest arousal. Some of these factors may be transient and could be a secondary adaptive alteration in sexual functioning.

The differential diagnosis of female sexual interest/arousal disorder may be complicated by development of associated factors or complications, such as another sexual dysfunction (e.g., female orgasmic disorder)—in which case it is important to establish which dysfunction is the primary one—and various psychological reactions to the lack of or diminished sexual interest or arousal, such as anxiety, depression, and interpersonal difficulties (e.g., the lack of receptive response may lead to arguments, which may further reduce the lack of interest).

See DSM-5 for additional disorders to consider in the differential diagnosis. Also refer to the discussions of comorbidity and differential diagnosis in their respective sections of DSM-5.

MALE HYPOACTIVE SEXUAL DESIRE DISORDER

The differential diagnosis of male hypoactive sexual desire disorder includes a broad variety of mental and physical illnesses that may affect sexual desire. Using the framework of subtypes (i.e., lifelong, acquired) and specifiers (i.e., situational, generalized) may be helpful in considering the differential diagnosis.

Nonsexual mental disorders need to be considered. For example, major depressive disorder (for which one of the symptoms is markedly diminished interest or pleasure in all, or almost all, activities) and persistent depressive disorder (dysthymia; symptoms include low energy, fatigue, low self-esteem) may account for the lack of sexual interest or its decrease. Some anxiety disorders (e.g., posttraumatic stress disorder) may also affect sexual desire. Major psychotic disorders and some personality disorders (e.g., schizoid personality disorder) may also be associated with lack of or reduction in sexual interest.

Substance use (e.g., chronic alcohol use, use of marijuana or opioids), not only during the episode of acute intoxication, and some medications (e.g., anticonvulsants, antihypertensives, antipsychotics, antidepressants, chemotherapeutics, and drugs used in urological diseases) may also account for the lack of sexual desire.

Various medical conditions, such as hypogonadism (verified by low testosterone level), hypothyroidism, diabetes mellitus, cardiovascular diseases, epilepsy, chronic renal failure, chronic liver disease, and testicular disease (e.g., cancer, undescended testes, mumps orchitis), are frequently associated with low or nonexistent sexual interest.

Various stressors (e.g., job loss), interpersonal factors (e.g., arguments with partner, extramarital affair, partner's pregnancy, violence), and individual factors (e.g., poor body image, history of sexual trauma, self-directed homophobia in gay men) need to be ruled out as possible causes for the deficient or absent sexual desire.

Some men (1%–2%) may identify themselves as asexual. For them, male hypoactive sexual desire disorder should not be diagnosed.

The differential diagnosis of male hypoactive sexual desire disorder may be complicated by the development of associated factors or complications, such as another sexual dysfunction (e.g., erectile disorder, delayed ejaculation). Many men (up to one-half) with male hypoactive sexual desire disorder may have other sexual dysfunction(s) that may play a role in the lack of or diminished sexual interest. These dysfunctions do not necessarily rule out the diagnosis of male hypoactive sexual desire disorder. In such cases, it is important to establish which dysfunction is primary and to identify the various psychological reactions to the lack of or diminished sexual interest or arousal, such as anxiety, depression, and interpersonal difficulties.

See DSM-5 for additional disorders to consider in the differential diagnosis. Also refer to the discussions of comorbidity and differential diagnosis in their respective sections of DSM-5.

Summary

FEMALE SEXUAL INTEREST/AROUSAL DISORDER

- Female sexual interest/arousal disorder is a new diagnosis that basically combines the symptomatology of diminished/absent sexual interest and diminished/absent sexual arousal.
- The symptoms of impaired sexual interest/arousal must have persisted for at least 6 months.
- The woman must be distressed about her level of sexual interest/arousal or experience impairment in her psychological well-being or interpersonal difficulties as a consequence of it.
- Various mental disorders (particularly major depressive disorder), other medical conditions, substance/medication use, and interpersonal and individual factors should be considered in the differential diagnosis.

MALE HYPOACTIVE SEXUAL DESIRE DISORDER

- The lack of sexual or erotic thoughts and fantasies and lack of desire to have sex (including masturbation) is the hallmark of this disorder. This lack of interest is based on clinical judgment.
- The absence or diminishment of sexual desire/interest must have persisted for at least 6 months.
- The absent or deficient sexual desire/interest should cause clinically significant distress.

- The differential diagnosis of this disorder includes various mental disorders (e.g., depression), physical conditions (e.g., endocrine disease such as hypogonadism or thyroid disease), substance/medication use, and individual and interpersonal factors.
- Male hypoactive sexual desire disorder may be associated with other sexual dysfunctions (e.g., erectile disorder, delayed ejaculation). These dysfunctions may either precede it (in which case the diagnosis of male hypoactive sexual desire disorder should not be made) or develop as its consequence.
- The framework of subtypes and specifiers (i.e., acquired vs. lifelong, situational vs. generalized) will be useful in considering the differential diagnosis of this disorder.

SUMMARY

Sexual Dysfunctions

Sexual dysfunctions are fairly prevalent impairments of sexual functioning. Prevalence of sexual dysfunctions may vary among different cultures and world regions—the highest prevalence of various sexual dysfunctions was found in East and Southeast Asia.

In an effort to make diagnoses of sexual dysfunctions more precise and to decrease the likelihood of overdiagnosis, DSM-5 criteria require a minimum duration of dysfunction of at least 6 months and include more precise severity specifiers (i.e., distress being mild, moderate, or severe) and more detailed subtypes (i.e., lifelong vs. acquired) and specifiers (i.e., situational vs. generalized). Clinicians may also consider interpersonal, partner, relationship, cultural, religious, and individual vulnerability factors in considering the diagnoses and the differential diagnoses of these disorders. These specifications make it easier to distinguish the true sexual dysfunctions from transient impairment of sexual functioning that possibly relates to various interpersonal problems and stresses. For the diagnosis of a sexual dysfunction, impairment of sexual functioning must also cause distress in interpersonal relationships and possibly in other functioning. All the diagnostic criteria rely on the clinician's judgment. The diagnosis of sexual dysfunctions is no longer anchored solely in the so-called sexual response cycle and now is gender specific. Sexual dysfunctions should always be evaluated and diagnosed in the wide context of other mental disorders, substance abuse, physical illnesses, medications taken by individuals with sexual dysfunctions, individual vulnerability, partner issues, stress, religious and cultural issues, and interpersonal factors. Inadequate stimulation and discrepancy in sexual demands between partners should always be considered in clarifying the diagnosis.

DSM-5 introduces two new diagnoses—female sexual interest/arousal disorder and genito-pelvic pain/penetration disorder—and no longer includes the diagnosis of sexual aversion disorder as an individual diagnosis.

———————————— ■-■-■ ————————————
Diagnostic Pearls

- Sexual dysfunctions need to be distinguished from transient impairment of sexual functioning; thus, the duration of impairment should be at least 6 months.

- Sexual difficulties, especially in women, could result from inadequate sexual stimulation. In such cases, sexual dysfunction should not be diagnosed.

- Sexual functioning may decline with aging; therefore, age-related changes should be considered when diagnosing sexual dysfunction.

- Sexual dysfunctions are gender specific.

- Impairment of sexual functioning could be associated with various mental disorders (e.g., depression) and physical illnesses (e.g., diabetes mellitus, neurological diseases).

- Impairment of sexual functioning could result from various substances of abuse (e.g., alcohol, nicotine, opioids) and numerous psychotropic (e.g., antidepressants, antipsychotics) and nonpsychotropic (e.g., antacids, antihypertensives, beta-blockers) medications.

- Cultural, interpersonal, and religious factors may play important roles in impairment of sexual functioning and should be considered when making the diagnosis.

- Several sexual dysfunctions may occur or overlap in one person.

- The etiology of sexual dysfunctions is usually unknown; impairment of sexual functioning is frequently a result of a complex interplay of biological, psychological, and sociocultural factors.

Self-Assessment

Key Concepts: Double-Check Your Knowledge

What is the relevance of the following concepts to the various sexual dysfunctions?

- Low sexual desire
- Impaired interest or arousal
- Erectile dysfunction
- Delayed orgasm
- Anorgasmia
- Genital pain
- Sexual fantasies
- Premature (early) ejaculation
- Impaired sexual functioning due to medical illness or medications
- Impaired sexual functioning due to substance abuse

Questions to Discuss With Colleagues and Mentors

1. Do you routinely discuss sexual functioning and sexual practices, behaviors, and preferences with your patients?
2. Do you feel comfortable asking your patients about their sexuality or sexual habits, preferences, and practices? Do you avoid certain questions about patients' preferences and practices? If not, why not?
3. What questions do you ask your patients about their sexual functioning?
4. How do you conceptualize sexual functioning and its impairment? What do you think about the DSM-5 changes in that the diagnoses are now gender specific?
5. Once you establish a diagnosis of sexual dysfunction in your patient, do you explore other aspects of your patient's sexual functioning to find out whether other sexual dysfunctions are present?
6. What do you know about the impact of other mental disorders, physical conditions, medication use, and substances of abuse on sexual functioning?

Case-Based Questions

PART A

> Ms. Gonzalez, a 35-year-old woman, states that she does not enjoy sex anymore. "Actually, I haven't had sex in a long time, and we used to have sex almost daily when we got married 3 years ago. I used to think about sex on my way home from work, but that is gone. I don't think about it. My husband has been trying to get me into the mood, but I usually turn around and go to sleep. Part of the problem is that I don't feel anything anymore down there. I used to have very pleasurable feelings when penetrated. We tried a vibrator to get back to those feelings, but it did not help." She admits worrying about her recent lack of orgasm, because "that is necessary to get pregnant and we planned to have a kid or two." She states that she and her husband have been stressed by the fact that they may lose their house. "He lost his job. He got a new one, but it does not pay enough to cover the mortgage payments or the rest of our bills. We have argued about this a lot." She denies any physical illness or problems. She does not take any medication. She drinks wine occasionally, one or two glasses with dinner. She has smoked cigarettes, a pack per day, since her early 20s. She denies using any illicit substances.

What diagnosis would you consider at this point? Could substance use have an impact on her sexual functioning? Ms. Gonzalez meets the diagnostic criteria for female sexual interest/arousal disorder: she has lost her interest in sex, does not respond to her husband's sexual advances, and has lost genital feelings during intercourse. The exact duration of her dysfunction is not known, but it has been persistent. She has probably also developed female orgasmic disorder lately, possibly as a consequence of her lack of sexual interest/arousal. She is fairly healthy and does not use any illicit substances or medications. Her occasional glass or two of wine would not explain her sexual problems, and by a long while, her smoking preceded the development of her sexual dysfunctions.

PART B

> Ms. Gonzalez admits that she became depressed within the last month or so, "as it is really upsetting to me that I do not enjoy sex and am not intimate with my husband. I used to enjoy sex so much." She also admits feeling some pain upon her husband's attempts to have sex with her.

Is there any diagnosis of sexual dysfunction to add to the diagnostic consideration on the basis of the presence of pain during intercourse?   In addition to her already complex sexual problems, Ms. Gonzalez may be developing sexual pain (genito-pelvic pain/penetration disorder) and has become depressed. Her case demonstrates that several sexual dysfunctions may co-occur or develop as a consequence of another. It also demonstrates the possible role of psychological factors in the development of sexual dysfunctions and the development of psychiatric symptomatology (e.g., depression) as a possible consequence of impaired sexual functioning.

Short-Answer Questions

1. How long must any symptomatology of impaired sexual function last to meet the diagnostic criteria for sexual dysfunction?
2. Should diagnosis of sexual dysfunction be made if there is inadequate stimulation during intercourse?
3. What happens to sexual functioning with aging?
4. What are some risk factors for female orgasmic disorder?
5. How soon after vaginal penetration must ejaculation occur to meet the diagnostic criterion of premature (early) ejaculation?
6. Which major psychiatric disorder is probably most frequently associated with diminished or absent sexual interest/desire?
7. Which class of psychotropic medications is most frequently implicated in delayed ejaculation?
8. What are the differences between the previous classification of sexual dysfunctions and the DSM-5 classification regarding gender specificity and the role of the sexual response cycle?
9. True or False: Distress is a necessary criterion for making the diagnosis of sexual dysfunction.
10. What are the new diagnoses of sexual dysfunctions included in DSM-5?

Answers

1. Any symptomatology of impaired sexual function must last 6 months to meet the diagnostic criteria for sexual dysfunction.
2. Sexual dysfunction should not be diagnosed if there is inadequate stimulation during intercourse.
3. With aging, sexual function usually declines, and frequency of sexual impairment increases.
4. Poor physical health, anxiety, depression, and relationship factors are risk factors for female orgasmic disorder.
5. Ejaculation must occur within approximately 1 minute after vaginal penetration to meet the diagnostic criterion of premature (early) ejaculation.
6. Major depressive disorder is probably the most frequent major psychiatric disorder associated with diminished or absent sexual interest/desire.
7. Serotonergic antidepressants are most frequently implicated in delayed ejaculation.
8. The DSM-5 classification is gender specific, and the diagnoses no longer relate to the so-called sexual response cycle.
9. True. Distress is a necessary criterion for diagnosing sexual dysfunction.
10. Female sexual interest/arousal disorder and genito-pelvic pain/penetration disorder are new in DSM-5.

17

Gender Dysphoria

Carlos C. Greaves, M.D.

Daryn Reicherter, M.D.

"I always knew I should be a girl."

"I can't be who I am."

Gender dysphoria describes the pervasive, subjective experience of an individual for whom the gender assigned at birth (i.e., natal gender) is felt to be wrong, mistaken, or not reflective of the person's inner conviction or truth that he or she is actually of another gender. The person feels that somehow nature has made a gross mistake so that he or she was "born in the wrong body." There is a significant conceptual shift in the diagnostic category of "gender identity disorder" in DSM-IV and "gender dysphoria" in DSM-5, in that the emphasis is on the symptomatic response to the gender nonconformity in DSM-5, as opposed to the pathologizing of the condition itself in DSM-IV.

Gender dysphoria can be the source of great suffering and identity confusion, as well as shame and stigma. It may deeply affect self-concept, identity, family structure, and social adaptation. The person has a strong identification with and desire to be part of the social world of his or her desired gender, including clothing, mannerisms, general interests, games, leisure activities, occupations, and overall societal responses that are elicited by the "other" gender—that gender that is felt as "my true gender," as "that which I really am."

Gender dysphoria tends to manifest differently in different age groups and in the different genders. Prepubertal natal girls with gender dysphoria characteristically ex-

317

press the wish to be a boy and assert that they are a male or that they will grow up to be a man. They may prefer traditional boys' clothing or hairstyles and engage in traditional boy play. They often have very negative reactions to parental attempts to have them wear dresses or to have the physical appearance of a girl. Role-play, dreams, and fantasies are often more consistent with typical male themes. They often show little interest in stereotypical feminine toys and play. They may express serious concern or disgust with the prospect of developing into mature women. Prepubertal natal boys with gender dysphoria display the wish to be a girl, assert they are a female, or express the wish to grow up to be a woman. They tend to dress in girls' or women's clothes or may improvise feminine clothing. They often role-play female figures and often are interested in female fantasy figures. They often prefer traditional female toys and games and may be uninterested in or resentful toward traditional male toys and play. Some may pretend to not have a penis and insist on sitting to urinate.

In children, the gender dysphoria diagnosis requires that the child have a strong desire to be another gender (what is felt as "natural to who I really am") from the birth gender—or insistence that they are of the other gender. This desire may also occur in adolescents and adults with gender dysphoria, but is not required for the diagnosis as it is for children. In addition, the dysphoria is based on clinically significant distress or impairment in social, school, or other important areas of functioning. Distress or impairment can result from pretending to live as a member of the birth gender or the pervasive need to convince other people (parents, siblings, friends, colleagues, etc.) of the experienced gender—and from often dealing with the serious social consequences of this conviction: rejection, teasing, ridicule, opprobrium, ostracism, contempt, threats, violence, and even death.

In young adolescents with gender dysphoria, clinical features are similar to those of children or adults, usually depending on developmental level. In adolescence, a time of an acute need for peer approval, the emergence of the awareness of being of a different gender is accompanied by substantial alienation, hiding, shame, and impairment of identity formation. A need and desire for a different genital configuration, as well as disgust at the physical attributes of the birth gender, now in full development, are most acute for this group.

In adults with gender dysphoria, the discrepancy between experienced gender and natal gender is often resented to the point where they may wish to have physical changes to their body's sexual characteristics. Adults with gender dysphoria often adopt the behaviors, dressing styles, and/or mannerisms of the opposite gender. They prefer to be viewed by society as their experienced gender rather than as a member of their assigned gender.

Persons with gender dysphoria may seek hormonal treatments, hair removal or implantation, facial bone realignment surgeries, plastic surgeries in various body parts, and eventually a shift in genital anatomy (sex reassignment surgery): penectomy and the creation of a neovagina in the male-to-female case, or the closing of the vaginal cavity with the creation of a neopenis in the female-to-male situation.

A great deal of distress, including anxiety, tension, and questions about what is real and who to believe (self or others) can develop around family dynamics, school environment, interpersonal relationships, and the capacity for intimacy.

DSM-5 identifies two specific states of gender dysphoria: that experienced in children and that experienced in adolescents and adults. The defined diagnoses are similar in basic description. Both diagnoses begin with "a marked incongruence between one's experienced/expressed gender and assigned gender, of at least 6 months' duration." The child and adult variants have different specific criteria but share the common themes of strong identification with the opposite gender, desire to be recognized as the other gender, and dislike of their physical sexual characteristics.

Both diagnoses ask for a specification of whether the condition is tied to a physical syndrome (e.g., androgen insensitivity syndrome).

DSM-5 also identifies two nonspecific diagnostic categories: other specified gender dysphoria and unspecified gender dysphoria. These diagnoses are used when the full diagnostic criteria are not met for the specific disorders but the major clinical concern is related to the themes contained in the specific diagnoses.

The gender dysphoria diagnoses should not be confused with the diagnoses in the DSM-5 chapter on paraphilic disorders. For instance, the DSM-5 diagnosis of transvestic disorder may be within the differential diagnosis of a gender dysphoria diagnosis, and dressing in the clothing of the opposite gender may be a behavior of an individual with gender dysphoria; however, transvestic disorder should be easily distinguished diagnostically from any gender dysphoria diagnosis.

The prevalence of gender dysphoria is not known but is estimated to be low (<1%). There seems to be a predominance of males over females with gender dysphoria.

DSM-IV contained diagnoses very similar to gender dysphoria in the diagnostic class of sexual and gender identity disorders. A specific diagnostic class in DSM-5 has been dedicated to gender dysphoria. The gender identity disorders characterized in DSM-IV have very similar features to the gender dysphorias in DSM-5.

IN-DEPTH DIAGNOSIS

Gender Dysphoria in Children

Jill is a 16-year-old girl. Her parents brought her to consultation because they despaired for several years at her insistence that she was a boy. She wanted to dress in boy's attire and begin masculinizing hormone treatments. What they thought would be a passing whim over the years, they now realized was a deeply set conviction. The history reveals that at approximately age 3, Jill began showing a greater interest in playing with the toys that her brother, older by 7 years, had used: cars, trucks, soldiers, swords, and so on. She was uninterested in the girl-typical toys, such as dolls, house items, and cute stuffed animals, which her parents kept buying for her. At age 4 she declared that she was a boy; any attempt of telling her otherwise was met by crying protests. In kindergarten, at age 5, Jill much preferred the company of boys, with whom she would engage in competitive body-contact games. At girls' social gatherings, she kept apart, choosing aloneness rather than joining in games and other activities. She would ask, "Where are the other boys? Why am I the only one here?" For school she insisted on wearing boyish clothes, resisting more typically feminine ones. At around age 7, her favorite movies and TV shows involved some young male hero or boy-centered story with which she would identify. At home, watching medieval chivalry movies, which she loved, she would sit with a play sword across her legs, wielding it enthusiastically as her hero went into battle.

Jill was, during late childhood, active physically, enjoying soccer and competing in running and other sports. She would feel deeply hurt when a group of boys rejected her as a member of their team on account of her being a girl; in these instances she would loudly protest "but I am not, I am not a girl!" By this point she had learned not to overtly declare being a boy, given the experiences of teasing and ridicule that her assertion elicited.

As Jill entered puberty, she found herself isolating more and more. She did not fit anywhere: girls found her "strange," thus the avoidance was mutual, whereas boys tended to ignore her or tease her for being "weird." Jill felt that it was a "tragedy" not to have a penis; she hated the emergence of her breasts, which she would flatten with cloth straps. Jill was sexually and emotionally attracted to girls and thought of herself as heterosexual. When her menarche occurred at age 14, she "cried for days," experiencing then, for the first time, a 3-month-long depressive episode.

Jill has shown from early life an awareness, a conviction, that she does not belong to the gender she was assigned at birth. She has consistently preferred to play with boy's toys, rejecting girl-typical ones, and enjoys wearing boyish clothing. Her walking and gestures are strongly male-typical; she chooses to socialize with other boys and joins them in their games when accepted by them. She feels very comfortable in cross-gender roles, rejecting gender-typical ones; she engages in make-believe and fantasy games in which she is a boy hero or a dashing medieval knight. She hates not having a penis and would like to get rid of her breasts.

Approach to the Diagnosis

The diagnosis of gender dysphoria in children should be considered when the clinician is presented with a child patient, usually brought to clinical attention by his or her parents, who since early age has been suffering significant distress as a result of doubts or confusion about the nature of his or her gender or actually carries the unshakable conviction that he or she belongs to a gender other than the one assigned at birth. This doubt or conviction, per se a source of distress, has in turn brought about alienation within the family structure, affected acceptance among playmates, and/or disrupted school activities and performance.

Parents and others perceive this child as "odd," "weird," "strange," "different," "not fitting," and so on, and in reacting to this peculiarity, they reject, tease, disparage with put-downs, humiliate, or are, not infrequently, violent toward the child. In consequence, the child feels different or alien, developing a concept of the self as deviant, bizarre, damaged, and undesirable. The individual's initial perplexity at others not seeing what is obvious—that a "mistake" was made in the assignation of gender at birth—gives way to despair at the realization that, biologically, he or she was born with an anatomy that does not correspond to his or her psychological gender construct, deep conviction, and actual subjective experience of his or her "true" gender identity, the one that he or she desires to be the "real" one.

Some individuals are able to disguise this predicament, developing an elaborate "false self" that consumes a great deal of attention and vital energy, while the hidden "real self" is further separated from the outside world. Individuals in this circumstance feel tremendous distress.

It is important to emphasize the shift from the diagnosis of gender identity disorder in DSM-IV to the one of gender dysphoria in DSM-5. The psychiatric diagnosis is not based solely on the presence of a different gender identity or the wish to change genders, but includes the personal suffering, the disruption of family life, and the difficulties experienced in the social realm that this particular human variance has brought about to the individual. If even in the context of a fully accepting environment, the individual still struggles with the incongruence of his or her paradoxical nature, as in alienation from his or her genital and/or other anatomy, the diagnosis of gender dysphoria is made.

The clinician, therefore, needs to focus on the disruptions of identity formation, adaptation to the outside world, successful coping mechanisms or lack thereof, problems of integration into the social milieu, and the negative introjects the individual has embraced that would generate self-hatred, depression, anxiety, and poor performance in academic and interpersonal realms.

Getting the History

The following set of questions for parents can help elicit the diagnosis: "You are concerned for your child. What have you noticed that is troubling you? For how long has this been going on? What is the first thing you noticed? What sort of clothing does your child prefer to wear? What games, activities, and toys does your child prefer? What happens if you deny the preferred ones and insist on others? Who does your child like to be with for play and companionship? Do you have a sense of the sort of fantasy play in which your child engages? Has your child expressed dislike for his or her body or genitals? Has your child expressed a desire to be of another gender, or has your child expressed the conviction of belonging to another gender? How troublesome is this for your child? Have you noticed sadness, isolation, nervousness, or any other signs that your child is troubled? How is your child doing at school? Do you have any pertinent information from teachers or other parents? Does your child have friends? What sort of friends? Has there been a change in the way you relate to your child? Has this condition changed the way you think about your child or the degree of closeness you experience with him or her?"

In eliciting the diagnosis of gender dysphoria in children, the interviewer will be using at least two sources, the parents and child. In examining the young person, besides observing his or her constitution, presentation, mannerisms, ways of expression, movements, speech, and so on, the interviewer can adapt the above-outlined set of questions to what would be proper to ask the young person at his or her age and developmental stage.

The parents will most likely be tense, worried, and fearful about the results of the consultation. They may have postponed arranging the appointment for months, sometimes years, in the hope that the gender-atypical behaviors they have observed—the "tomboyness" in a girl or "sissiness" in a boy—are a "passing phase" or "something our child will outgrow." Only when these behaviors persist over time and are accompanied by the young person's assertions of other-gender wishes do parents become alarmed and seek consultation. Parents may confuse sexual orientation variances with a transgender condition generating dysphoria, which delays consultation and diagnosis.

Information from siblings and peers, as well as from teachers and extended family members, can help clarify the relevance of the diagnosis of gender dysphoria in children. In a diagnosis of such sensitivity as this, the clinician needs to muster as much objectivity, nonjudgmental attitude, understanding, support, and compassion as possible.

Tips for Clarifying the Diagnosis

- Establish whether the individual feels a "marked incongruence between [his or her] experienced/expressed gender and assigned gender" that causes distress or dysfunction.
- Consider whether the young person meets six of the eight criteria required to fulfill the criteria. Many of the diagnostic criteria involve the strong dislike of the physical attributes of the individual's assigned gender, as well as preferences to behave as members of the gender that is opposite to the assigned gender.
- Verify that the diagnostic criteria have been present for at least 6 months.
- Rule out differential diagnostic concepts, especially normal variants of nonconformity to gender roles, as better explanations of the observed phenomena.

Consider the Case

Po, the son of Chinese immigrants, was referred at age 14. He has felt and exhibited signs of depression for 2 years before consultation. Other than that their young son was "quiet, gentle, and obedient," his parents had not observed anything atypical about Po. When Po entered school at age 6, his teachers noticed his avoidance of the playground for a preference to being on his own. While by himself, in school or at home, Po would sweetly sing to himself, at times dancing to his music with "the most delicate and gracious movements," according to his mother. He began to explore her wardrobe, trying out garments, shoes, laces, and so on, while watching himself in the mirror; he would also experiment with mascara, lipstick, and other cosmetics. Any attempts at dissuading him from these behaviors were met with a passive, downcast, deflated attitude, followed by a sullenness lasting a few days. If allowed to do these "girlish things," Po would be "animated, talkative, and happy." He was not interested in boys' games and toys; he also was not particularly interested in girls' toys. What he did like were "colorful fabrics, pretty buttons, needles and scissors, colorful threads" with which to make skirts, blouses, and scarves. Again, when denied these, he would "go into a funk" that lasted until he got what he wanted.

Po revealed to the examiner that he had always doubted whether he was a girl or a boy, a feeling that he had never revealed to anyone, but now that it was clear to him he had been born as a boy, he wanted to be a girl because "I feel inside as if I am a girl. I love all things girlish. I always imagined myself growing up as a girl and maybe dating boys." Po was sad that he could not bear children. He disliked his penis: "It's all wrong there." For as long as Po could remember, he had felt "different," unable to relate to either boys or girls, choosing aloneness rather than risking scorn and rejection.

Po thought of himself as bisexual but "leaning toward straight"—that is, attracted more to boys. His only close friend was another boy who was also questioning his own gender. Po had given himself a girl's name that only he knows. Po had suffered from chronic depression for 2 years, that being the reason he gave his mother to bring him for a psychiatric consultation; he knew well enough that his mother would dismiss his gender issues as "stupid and irrelevant."

Po manifests behaviors, attitudes, and interests that are gender atypical for boys; he lacks certainty as to his gender: "Am I a boy or a girl?" He leans toward the latter and, in privacy, experiments by wearing his mother's clothing and cosmetic embellishments; in private, he assumes girlish postures and make-believe games; and he has given himself a secret girl's name. These behaviors and deep doubts have been ongoing for several years. Po avoids social interaction with peers because he feels he does not fit in and also wants to avoid the hassles that would descend upon him were he to show his "real girly self." He rejects his genitals, touching them only for hygiene. He experiences a pervasive desire to take on the social roles and external presentation of his desired girl identity; his inability to do so is a source of distress and low mood. Po feels that he has a great deal of disconnect and conflict with his parents as a result of their lack of acculturation. He worries that his gender dysphoria would be misconstrued by them somehow as the bad influence of American culture.

Differential Diagnosis

DSM-5 describes a typical list of behavioral and diagnostic concepts that should be considered in the differential diagnosis of gender dysphoria. The young person who is nonconforming to stereotypical gender role behavior may reject gender-typical activities and play, but there is no doubt that his or her gender matches the one assigned at birth. This nonconformity will tend to be transitory, shifting as the individual matures or is influenced by peers. Disorders of sex development may or may not be associated with gender dysphoria and need to be ruled out. In individuals with transvestic disorder, cross-dressing elicits sexual arousal and excitement and is most frequent in adolescent and adult heterosexual or bisexual men. In rare cases, cross-dressing in children can produce arousal, associated or not with gender dysphoria or transgenderism. Both diagnoses can be made if coexistent.

An individual with body dysmorphic disorder focuses on the alteration or removal of a specific body part because it is perceived as abnormally formed, not because of any gender-related issue.

Other symptomatology, such as hallucinations, paranoid delusions, and course of illness, would differentiate between an adolescent with schizophrenia or other psychosis, which includes the unusual delusion of belonging to another gender, and a child with gender dysphoria. In the absence of psychotic symptoms, insistence by a child with gender dysphoria that he or she is of another gender is not considered delusional.

Other clinical presentations include, for example, some males who seek castration and/or penectomy for aesthetic reasons or to remove the psychological effects of androgens, without changing male identity; these presentations do not meet criteria for gender dysphoria.

The clinicians should also rule out disorders of sex development such as congenital adrenogenital disorder, congenital adrenal hyperplasia, androgen insensitivity syndrome, or defective chromosomal conditions.

See DSM-5 for additional disorders to consider in the differential diagnosis. Also refer to the discussions of comorbidity and differential diagnosis in their respective sections of DSM-5.

Summary

- Gender dysphoria is considered as a diagnosis if for at least 6 months a child has had serious doubts about his or her gender or is convinced and insists that he or she belongs to another gender, resulting in tension, suffering, confusion, and general distress.
- Such an individual prefers to play, dress, fantasize, seek companionship, and assume roles that are gender atypical. In so pursuing, he or she gets into conflict with family and friends and in school.
- The individual dislikes his or her own anatomy, particularly genitals; dreads the emergence of his or her secondary sexual characteristics; and yearns for a different body configuration—one that matches the desired gender.
- Over time, the condition has disrupted the development of the individual within the family dynamics, interpersonally, and in the general social world.
- The hallmark theme of gender dysphoria in children is a "marked incongruence between one's experienced/expressed gender and assigned gender" that causes distress or dysfunction.
- Six of the eight criteria must be met to make the diagnosis.
- Many of the diagnostic criteria involve strong preferences to behave as a member of the gender that is opposite to the assigned gender.
- There are significant differences (aside from age) in the typical presentations between gender dysphoria in children and gender dysphoria in adolescents and adults.
- The differential diagnosis must be considered before ruling in gender dysphoria in children.

IN-DEPTH DIAGNOSIS

Gender Dysphoria in Adolescents and Adults

Ken is a 38-year-old male-to-female transsexual person who had gone through sex reassignment surgery a few months before consultation. Ken was the only child of a rural Midwestern white family. He was assigned the male gender at birth. Until mid-adolescence, other than a distinct, yet vague feeling that he (at the time) was "different," his childhood developed along the lines expected for boys. Ken was not enthusiastic about sports, preferring intellectual activities and discussions. When he was about age 15, an increasing sense of alienation from his maleness developed regarding his body hair, genitals, deeper voice, facial features, and so on, with a concomitant desire for female attributes.

He denied all this to himself: "I put it aside; it was too much and too complex to deal with. In my neck of the woods, I would have been kicked out of home, thrashed by others, maybe killed." Ken was attracted to women, emotionally and sexually. After a couple of short-lived affairs with girlfriends, he fell in love with a college friend, marrying her just after graduation, although he was very much aware of his gender ambiguity. Ken and his wife had three children, a boy and two girls. He completed a master's degree in business and got a good job. When alone at home, he would wear his wife's clothing and cosmetics. He imagined himself as a woman, feeling a "huge relief" from the permanent tension he had experienced at the growing realization that he was "authentically, a woman." Ken felt that in denying his early sense of being a female, he had deeply betrayed himself, his "true nature."

Though professionally successful and happy about his children, Ken was otherwise quite dysphoric: constant tension, depressive feelings, serious anxiety, increasing difficulty with sexual performance, and despairing as to what to do. Soon after the birth of their third child, Ken announced to his wife, who by now knew about his dysphoria and its origin, his intention to transition to the female gender. "I just could not handle it any longer; when suicidal thoughts entered my mind, I knew it was time to act." He began hormone treatments, at which point his wife initiated a divorce (to his chagrin); he then underwent surgeries to shave off a prominent Adam's apple, supraorbital bones, and his chin. At this point, "he" became a "she" in the social world, facing all the complexities of transitioning, and changed his name to a female one, Kelly—the one to which she had referred to herself secretly for years.

Kelly eventually underwent sex reassignment surgery. Her dysphoria significantly lessened. She learned to modulate her voice to a higher pitch, passing as a biological woman quite well. Yet in her attempt at exploring intimacy with women or men, the conflict of whether to "come out" or not became critical: a toss-up between honesty and the likelihood of rejection (or worse).

Her aging parents were unable to accept her change. Close relationships became limited to those in the transgender community who could fully understand and relate to her experience, with the exception of a couple of faithful childhood friends. She found excellent employment, where she was respected as an unusually courageous person by the few who knew of her difficult journey.

Ken's awareness of being alienated from his assigned gender emerged after puberty and manifested at first by dislike for his male physical attributes; later, by the desire to cross-dress, use cosmetics, and act in private as a woman; and eventually, by a desire to reconfigure his genitals. He fell in love, had sex, and married a woman, subjectively experiencing the relationship not as his wife's male counterpart but as an essentially kindred entity, physically, emotionally, and spiritually; contiguity with his wife offered him a vicarious identification with his desired gender. Paternity did not shift the other-gender conviction, which was fully developed by this time. Ken's dysphoria about this paradoxical ambiguity became intense and constant, to the point that embracing his "true gender" and pursuing sex reassignment surgery overrode considerations of marriage, fatherhood, family of origin, friendships, and social and work environments, as well as the fears, mysteries, and major adjustments of an uncertain future.

Posttransition challenges (i.e., after sex reassignment surgery) resulted in a different quality of dysphoria, involving issues of disclosure, family dynamics, intimacy, and physical adaptations to a new anatomy. In the next few years, Kelly experienced a relative narrowing of the social world, the result of misunderstandings and misalignments to the worldview of the majority. Kelly eventually found a comfortable identity in the desired gender with meaningful employment, a small group of friends, and a loving companion.

Approach to the Diagnosis

With an adolescent or young adult, usually the parents seek consultation. They are concerned about the recent (or longer) development of symptoms of unease, withdrawal, depression, isolation, tension, and stress in their adolescent or young adult, or they complain about fearful and confusing acting-out behaviors, with the possible abuse of alcohol and/or illicit drugs. The parents have also noticed disruptions in their child's socializing with friends or at school, excessive use of the computer, sullenness, and poor communication, with angry responses or evasion, even upon the gentlest of questioning.

The individual may or may not have revealed the source of the dysphoria. Not infrequently, it comes to light indirectly, when a parent discovers Web sites on a computer or clothing, objects, books, magazines, and so on, hidden in a drawer or attic or under the bed, which tips them off that there is something "not right" or "very disturbing" related to gender. The adolescent or young adult, once he or she is able to trust the clinician, may request that what is disclosed be kept confidential, making the specific questioning of the parents not possible.

The individual will reveal the gender nonconformity by expressing a deeply felt dislike for his or her anatomy, secondary sex characteristics, and the roles and social expectations associated with the assigned gender at birth. The individual will express the conviction that he or she belongs to another gender, that somehow "this body is all wrong," and that he or she must become the desired gender in order to feel "whole" or "at peace" or "to right a wrong," "to become what I am."

Such individuals also may vehemently insist that these changes occur soon, so as to avoid further traits, physical and social, of belonging to the rejected birth gender. They will greatly worry about what seems an impossibly difficult and costly process, which without parental support will be unattainable for "who knows how many years...and I can't wait that long!"

Adults are typically self-referred. After explaining their gender nonconformity, the duration, their development, and their difficulties with their experience, some will ask for counsel on how to proceed with the transitioning process, if they have not already done so; for support for the completion of a course of action they have already decided upon; or for help in dealing with how to adapt to and process the complex posttransition realities. Others are uninterested in either supportive or insight-oriented psychotherapy and instead ask for a formal diagnosis so they can undergo hormone treatments or genital and/or other surgeries.

As stated in DSM-5, "Adolescents and adults with gender dysphoria before gender reassignment are at increased risk for suicidal ideation, suicide attempts, and suicides. After gender reassignment, adjustment may vary, and suicide risk may persist" (p. 454).

Getting the History

Sam, a 30-year-old man, presents for evaluation of "some mild depression." He is dressed in traditional women's clothing, has a hairstyle traditionally seen in females, and is wearing makeup. He introduces himself with a woman's name, Sarah, that is not consistent with the male name on the medical chart. He quickly clarifies that he is transgendered and is in the process of legally reassigning his gender from male to female. He reports that he is also in the process of "pretreatment" for a pending gender reassignment surgery.

Although the stated purpose of the visit is depression, he begins by explaining the gender issue that seems to be the context around his mood symptoms. He describes a long history of incongruence between his experienced/expressed gender and his as-signed gender, beginning in childhood. He clearly describes distress as a result through-out his life. These gender issues have led to significant interpersonal stressors. He reports having grown up in a strictly religious family in which his gender issue was ignored or met with disdain. He dated girls in high school as a result of the pressure to "be normal" but found it repulsive to engage in any sexual behavior with females.

The interviewer asks, "Why are you planning to have the gender reassignment sur-gery?" He responds, "So I can just have the body I should have been born with. I am a woman, really. I think like a woman, feel like a woman. And I have been living in the body of a man for all my life. It's time to become who I always have been."

The interviewer asks about the transition: "How do you like to be addressed? Your stated name is different from the name in your medical (legal) chart." The patient laughs at the question, initially. Then he responds, "People think I am a freak or a 'cross-dresser' or something. I'm really not. I have been living as a woman for years now. I am in the process of getting all this worked out 'technically.' Once I legally change my name to Sarah and have the surgery, there won't be any more confusion. Thank God!" The interviewer nods with understanding. The patient responds, "Please call me Sarah. It's a better fit."

This case clearly fits the themes in the diagnosis of gender dysphoria in adoles-cents and adults. The key features are clear. The individual meets at least two of the six criteria and has for 6 months or more. Social dysfunction and distress have been present for this person for many years.

This case not only meets criteria for the diagnosis but also meets the stated criteria for the specifier "posttransition." Even though the individual has not undergone the medical procedure or the legal change in name, he has changed gender role from male to female and has lived in a "posttransitional" state for years, per the history.

With adults, a cohesive, processed, and integrated picture will most likely be of-fered without much questioning. Once the transgender profile has been exposed and the concomitant dysphoria elucidated, the examiner ought to address the differential diagnosis and to refine an understanding of the peculiarities and uniqueness of this person's experience/situation.

Getting the history from an adolescent may require more finesse. The following are examples of helpful comments: "I am here to understand and help you, not to judge you"; "Whatever it is that you are or want to be is fine, as long as you don't hurt your-self or others"; "I realize you have been suffering a great deal; let us work together to understand what is happening to you and to alleviate your suffering." Questions about the actual phenomena the youth is experiencing internally and externally are important: "What is it that you feel you are? For how long has this been so? What are the things you'd like to do if you were free to do as you wish? How would you like to dress? What kind of person would you like others to see you as, and how do you want to come across to others? Tell me, how do you feel about your body? What is it that you feel is not right with it? And how do you feel about your genitals?"

Once answers to these and similar questions have been ascertained, a more in-depth set of questions involving the youth's hoped-for world can provide valuable diagnostic information: "How do you imagine yourself to be? What sort of images of yourself seem right and fitting for you? How are you pictured in your dreams? How would you like to be, say, 5 or 10 years from now? What sort of love partner would you like to have and of which gender? Describe for me, please, the type of body you would like to have. Do you imagine having different genitalia? How often? How do you imagine your life would be if you were to change your gender? What do you imagine the reaction would be to that change from your family, your friends, and society at large? How does all of this make you feel: good, bad, happy, sad, scared, frustrated, angry, anxious? Have you entertained suicidal thoughts? What is going on now between you and your friends? How does your situation fit with your values, religious teachings, principles, and ideal vision of yourself? Did you have any inkling of all this in your childhood? By what name would you like me to call you? Is there anything I have not asked you about that is important to you?"

Tips for Clarifying the Diagnosis

Consider the diagnosis of gender dysphoria in adolescents and adults in the following situations:

- They experience a consistent, persevering conviction that they belong to another gender.
- They dislike or feel aversion to the external identifiers of their assigned birth gender, which may or may not include the wish for a change in genital anatomy.
- They yearn for the social status, roles, and attitudes of another gender and wish to be perceived, thought of, and/or reacted to as a member of the desired gender.
- They have been experimenting with cross-dressing, sometimes going out in public or to specially accepting public venues and "passing" as a member of the desired gender.
- Their situation has brought about significant stress, tension, anxiety, depression, or anger and disturbances of family, intimate, and social relationships. Academic or work performance may or may not have been affected.

Consider the Case

Mr. O'Rourke was 60 years old when he came for consultation. He was born in New England, the fourth child of an established, intact, wealthy Irish-Italian family. He had three older brothers and a younger sister. His mother was still alive. He remembers his mother saying to him at some point in early childhood that she wished he had been a girl (8 years later, she had her desired daughter). Mr. O'Rourke thought of himself as having been a "sissy boy" who later, in adolescence, was able to "man up" because he had forced upon himself an aggressive and confrontational presentation to others: "my older brothers taught me to be tough." The softer, more sensitive inner self of his childhood was masked, finding expression in poetry and violin playing. Mr. O'Rourke went through high school and college feeling, acting, and being accepted as any other young man on campus. He was attracted to women, had several girlfriends, and was "competent" sexually.

Mr. O'Rourke did very well in law school, specializing in courtroom prosecution, where he excelled as a "tough, smart, even-headed lawyer." He had a son from a first marriage and a daughter from a second. Throughout his adult life, he experienced a nagging feeling that something core and essential to him was missing, not being fulfilled, which he described as a "hole," a "sad emptiness." Not until age 45, after studying the work of Carl Jung and coming across the concept of "anima" (the feminine side of a man's psyche), did Mr. O'Rourke understand his feelings: "It struck me like a lightning bolt; it all fell into place. What was missing was the woman in me: that care of my hair and nails; the detail of my clothing, always with a colorful flair; the subtle but deep identification with the culture's iconic females; my frequent dressing as a woman for Halloween parties and, in regular parties, hanging out with women's groups; my love of cooking, arranging flowers, my highly romantic and expressive violin playing—it was all there, yet I was not seeing it."

Soon after, gender dysphoria began to bother him. He felt he had to divorce his second wife, because the vicarious moments in which he began to cross-dress, color his lips and cheeks, use a large wig, and "act like Bette Davis or Marilyn Monroe" in a rented room were "just not quite enough. I had to go all the way, every day." The tension of "performing a manly professional role during the day and living my womanly self at night was seriously getting to me."

Through Internet dating, he began looking for a companion and found a 65-year-old woman who spent her very private life dressed in male attire, tending a nearby farm, and "hauling hay like the best of them boys." She was not transgendered, was heterosexual, and had not experienced any significant gender dysphoria.

For Mr. O'Rourke, the revelation of gender nonconformity occurred at a mature age. His sense of being female rapidly overwhelmed his previous male identification, which he then came to see as a defensive construct against, up to then, a barely perceived female nature. At this point, gender dysphoria ensued full force. This late onset of gender dysphoria is uncommon. Logistical and pragmatic considerations made full transitioning to the female gender not an option, but as a more realistic acceptance of a dual lifestyle developed and was actualized, Mr. O'Rourke's dysphoria was reduced to a minimum.

The clinician ruled out transvestic disorder, because Mr. O'Rourke could achieve sexual arousal regardless of clothing or the role he was performing and his strong desire to live as a woman, including considerations for a shift in sexual anatomy and general presentation through hormonal treatments.

Differential Diagnosis

For adolescents and adults, several possibilities on the differential diagnosis should be considered and ruled out before diagnosing gender dysphoria. Nonconformity to gender roles is the situation wherein an individual feels disturbed, angry, contemptuous, and disaffected and/or is critical of the roles culture and society impose on either gender. In this instance, the individual has no desire to be a different gender from the natal gender and feels no alienation from his or her anatomy or current external gender traits.

Sexual arousal and performance obtained through the act of cross-dressing, in mostly a heterosexual male who is perfectly content with his gender and anatomy, is known as transvestic disorder and should be distinguished from gender dysphoria.

Body dysmorphic disorder is characterized by an individual's focus on the alteration or removal of a specific body part because it is perceived as abnormally formed, not because it represents a repudiated assigned gender.

Schizophrenia and other psychotic disorders, as well as obsessive-compulsive disorder, are considered part of the differential diagnosis. Some personality disorders can manifest with gender themes but should be distinguishable from gender dysphoria.

For a homosexually oriented adolescent who is deeply homophobic, the idea of changing genders, in spite of all its complexities, might seem preferable to the rejection and shame of being gay or lesbian. Changing genders would provide sanction from family, religion, and society for the now "acceptable" heterosexual orientation. Such a preference for changing genders, however, does not reflect a pervasive sense or conviction that he or she belongs to a gender that is different from the one assigned at birth.

Some adults, usually homosexual or bisexual, enjoy cross-dressing and assuming the roles of another gender for the purposes of entertainment, leisure, or plain fun (e.g., "drag queens and kings") without any desire to change the birth gender.

See DSM-5 for additional disorders to consider in the differential diagnosis. Also refer to the discussions of comorbidity and differential diagnosis in their respective sections of DSM-5.

Summary

- The hallmark theme of gender dysphoria in adolescents and adults is a "marked incongruence between one's experienced/expressed gender and assigned gender" that causes distress or dysfunction.
- The adolescent or adult consistently experiences the certainty of belonging to a gender other than the one given at birth.
- This desire is accompanied by dislike of or aversion to the individual's own body in that it is felt as alien and wrong, with a desire to have the body and attributes of another gender, including or not including altered genital anatomy.
- There is an attraction for and desire to experience life as a member of another gender, to be seen and acknowledged as such, and to be treated accordingly.
- The gender dysphoria results in great pressure, tension, mood changes, anxiety, discomfort, and alterations in the interpersonal sphere of the person.
- A great deal of time and energy is spent in fantasizing how life would be if lived as the desired gender, thus bringing a sense of completion and fulfillment to the person.

———————— **SUMMARY** ————————

Gender Dysphoria

The diagnosis of gender dysphoria is applicable when an individual has a pervasive sense or conviction that he or she is a member of a gender that is different from the one assigned at birth. As a result, the person must have been experiencing, for at least 6 months, a few or several of the following symptoms: distress, anxiety, tension, affective disturbances, alteration in family dynamics, personal doubts and confusion, alienation from others, and disruptions in school, work, or social settings in general.

These individuals have a subjective certainty that something went amiss in their biological development, resulting in their being born in a body that does not fit the gender to which they know they belong. This predicament creates, in an individual, an intense desire to "fix what is wrong"—thus, in children, to play, dress, and be with those of their desired gender; in adolescents, to get rid of any observable traits that would identify them, to themselves and others, as belonging to the birth gender—particularly their "mismatched" genitals—and to live, work, socialize, be intimate, and find fulfillment in life as a member of the desired gender later in adulthood.

At some point in its development, the transgender consciousness, which is not considered to be delusional, will meet obstacles. In childhood, this is demonstrated in resistance to the joys of naturally chosen play, companionship, and dress. Later, in adolescence and adulthood, obstacles include the necessary redefinitions of self-concept, bodily configuration, and family and peer structures; having to master failed social expectations; building compensations for the shame of disapproval, hostility, and rejection; creating an effective masking to achieve survival; and coping with financial hardships—all this as the necessary cost of achieving a sense of wholeness. In consequence, the transgender consciousness relates throughout to the unavoidable symptomatology of gender dysphoria.

It is also a condition that imposes great challenges for parents, family, friends, and acquaintances as they attempt to position themselves vis-à-vis the transgendered person. They will also suffer from a form of derivative "gender dysphoria," the symptomatic response to witnessing this paradoxical condition in their loved one, either because of empathy, sympathy, compassion, opposition, fear, rejection, confusion, violence, ignorance, or the anticipated financial challenges ahead.

------------------ ■-■-■ ------------------

Diagnostic Pearls

- Gender dysphoria is an experienced disconnect between an individual's physical sex and experienced gender role.

- Gender dysphoria is not a sexual dysfunction or paraphilic disorder.

- Hallmark features of gender dysphoria center around the distress caused by the incongruence between the person's experienced/expressed gender and assigned gender.

- Because features may manifest differently in various stages of development, DSM-5 has two distinct diagnostic criteria sets: gender dysphoria in children and gender dysphoria in adolescents and adults.

- Gender dysphoria must be present for more than 6 months, but in most cases this time criterion will be easily met, because the experience tends to be chronic.

- Gender dysphoria diagnoses have qualifiers that inform whether a physical or medical issue is related to the diagnosis. DSM-5 asks clinicians to clarify whether the gender dysphoria is associated with "a disorder of sex development (e.g., a congenital adrenogenital disorder such as congenital adrenal hyperplasia or androgen insensitivity syndrome)." This specifier may be important in the formulation of an individual overall.

Self-Assessment

Key Concepts: Double-Check Your Knowledge

What is the relevance of the following concepts to gender dysphoria?

- Difference between natal gender and experienced gender
- Lack of relationship to sexual dysfunctions or paraphilic disorders
- Distress caused by experienced gender incongruence
- Different presentation in various stages of development
- Distinct diagnostic criteria sets for children and for adolescents and adults
- Duration of at least 6 months
- Medical specifier in the overall formulation

Questions to Discuss With Colleagues and Mentors

1. Why is gender dysphoria not considered as resulting from a delusional disorder?
2. What is the relationship of societal views regarding gender identity to the manifestations of gender dysphoria? Would there be such a thing as gender dysphoria if society ascribed equal value to all forms of gender expression?
3. How do we understand the fact that although there are two manifestations of biological sex—that is, male and female—there are many forms of gender expression?
4. Can there be gender dysphoria in people who do not question the gender they were assigned at birth? Do other forms of dysphoria relate to gender?
5. If a child clearly has an atypical gender identity and is a nonconformist regarding gender role, what factors should the clinician consider before diagnosing gender dysphoria in the child?
6. How should gender be defined and referred to in a person with a diagnosis of gender dysphoria?
7. Should the presence of a "disorder of sex development" influence the way that a case of gender dysphoria is handled clinically? If yes, why? If no, why not?

Case-Based Questions

PART A

Maria was assigned the female gender at birth; she was the third child of a West Coast, upper-middle-class family. Her father, an engineer, came from a liberal tradition of several generations of Midwestern settlers; her mother's family, originally from Mexico, had been in the United States for four generations. Neither family was religiously inclined. At the time of her birth, Maria's two older sisters were ages 5 and 7, her father was 45, and her mother was 39. Postpartum complications and age made her mother unable to bear any more children.

Since her earliest recollections Maria thought of herself as different from other children and her sisters. She was active, curious, and willful, whereas her sisters were "placid and obedient." In kindergarten she preferred to play "boy games" with the boys, rejecting the company and play toys of the girls. At home she was given the toys she preferred: cars, trains, balls of different sorts, toy soldiers, and cowboy hats and boots; she thought that dolls were "silly." Wishing to differentiate herself from her sisters, Maria favored masculine attire, which her parents indulged because they found all of this "cute and different."

Only on the basis of the information given so far, can the diagnosis of gender dysphoria be made? No. Although some information is consistent with a theme of gender dysphoria, full criteria have not been met in the information given.

PART B

In later childhood, Maria engaged in rough play with boys in her neighborhood and at school, and she began to assert with increasing vehemence that she was a boy. These assertions were met with dismissive smiles from her parents and close family members, but at school she was ridiculed. During puberty and early adolescence, at her insistence, Maria was allowed to cross-dress at home and began to use a boy's name (which became her "nickname" among intimates), and she began to wear boyish clothing to school. She dreaded and eventually hated her breasts, covering them as best she could; her menarche was a great disappointment.

From that time on, she expressed the desire to change into the male gender. She was eager for the secondary sex characteristics of maleness and found out about hormone treatments through the Internet, where she became aware of transgenderism and began to correspond with other youths experiencing similar predicaments. Her parents did not oppose this wish but asked her to wait "so that you are sure this is really what you want." She was consistently attracted to other girls, sexually and romantically, since early adolescence, and "never to boys."

At age 16, she insisted everyone call her by her chosen male name, Marcus, and, with parental sanction, began androgenic hormone treatments. At age 17, she underwent surgical breast reduction (actual elimination of all breast tissue) and developed facial and body hair; her voice deepened considerably.

By the time Marcus went to college, he had transitioned completely into the male gender. There he played sports just like any other young man on the teams; he avoided locker rooms but used men's bathrooms, adducing "pee shyness" to justify the avoidance of urinals. His main problem was in dating women, to whom at some point he had to disclose his preoperative transgender status; in all but one instance (with a declared bisexual peer woman), he was rejected as an unsuitable sexual partner. Academic difficulties plus this ongoing conflict led Marcus to drop out of college; his parents helped him financially through a few years of various jobs. Since age 17, he had worked out and exercised regularly, so that now, at age 24, though short in stature, he was quite muscularly developed. He applied to and was accepted into the fire department of a major West Coast city. By the time of consultation, at age 32, Marcus had been a firefighter for 8 years; at work, no one knew he was a biological female.

After Marcus became comfortable with his life as a man, did he meet criteria for gender dysphoria? No. Marcus is living happily (without distress or dysfunction) as a transgendered individual.

Short-Answer Questions

1. What is gender dysphoria?
2. What are the separate criteria sets of gender dysphoria?
3. What are the key features of gender dysphoria in children?
4. What are the key features of gender dysphoria in adolescents and adults?

5. What is meant by "hormone treatments" in this context?
6. What is the minimum necessary duration of symptoms for the diagnosis of gender dysphoria?
7. What are important attitudes in the examiner?
8. If a male-gendered child identifies as female but does not experience any dysfunction or distress, should gender dysphoria be diagnosed?
9. What is the prevalence of gender dysphoria?
10. What is the differential diagnosis for gender dysphoria in adolescents and adults?

Answers

1. Gender dysphoria refers to a complex set of symptoms that result when an individual experiences his or her gender identity to be at odds with the gender assigned at birth.
2. The separate criteria sets of gender dysphoria are gender dysphoria in children and gender dysphoria in adolescents and adults.
3. Key features of gender dysphoria in children are a consistent pattern of preferring the play toys, attire, company, games, make-believe fantasies, and activities that are typical of a gender other than the one given at birth. The sense of belonging to the other gender, the feeling of being in the wrong body, the dreading of the external bodily attributes of the assigned gender, and the wish for the primary and/or secondary sex characteristics of the desired gender bring about gender dysphoria symptoms.
4. Key features of gender dysphoria in adolescents and adults include a pervasive conviction that they are a member of another gender from the one assigned at birth; a strong desire to get rid of the primary and/or secondary sex characteristics of the birth gender; a strong desire to possess the primary and/or secondary sex characteristics of the desired gender; a subjective sense that their thoughts and feelings are similar to those of the desired gender; and a wish to be seen and treated as typically expected for a member of the desired gender.
5. Hormone treatments involve the administration of either estrogenic or androgenic hormones to achieve a feminization or masculinization of the individual.
6. Six months is the minimum necessary duration of symptoms for the diagnosis of gender dysphoria.
7. The examiner adapts to the age of the patient and exudes attitudes of warmth, understanding, acceptance, empathy, lack of judgment, openness, support, and encouragement.
8. No. Gender dysphoria should not be diagnosed in a male-gendered child who identifies as female but does not experience any dysfunction or distress.
9. The prevalence of gender dysphoria is less than 1%.
10. The differential diagnosis for gender dysphoria in adolescents and adults includes nonconformity to gender roles, transvestic disorder, body dysmorphic disorder, schizophrenia and other psychotic disorders, and other clinical presentations.

18

Disruptive, Impulse-Control, and Conduct Disorders

Whitney Daniels, M.D.
Hans Steiner, M.D.

"He just explodes."

*"It seems he always has to do exactly the opposite
of what I tell him."*

The disruptive, impulse-control, and conduct disorders, previously listed across a variety of diagnostic classes in DSM-IV, are now grouped together in DSM-5 and include the following: oppositional defiant disorder; intermittent explosive disorder; conduct disorder; antisocial personality disorder; pyromania; kleptomania; other specified disruptive, impulse-control, and conduct disorder; and unspecified disruptive, impulse-control, and conduct disorder. The core feature of these conditions is persistent dissocial patterns of individuals apparent across a variety of developmental stages. Although the disorders are placed in a new location within DSM-5, the diagnostic criteria have undergone only relatively minor changes with regard to time and age requirements of certain diagnoses.

In assessing individuals to clarify the presence of a diagnosis, a thorough history, including details about symptoms, timing, and age, are highly important. In addition, collateral historical information is imperative to fully grasp the nature of the symptoms, their presentation, and the contribution of the symptoms to the level of dysfunction for the individual.

In DSM-IV, antisocial personality disorder was included only in the personality disorders diagnostic class. In DSM-5, this diagnosis occurs both in personality disorders and in disruptive, impulse-control, and conduct disorders. Overall, this diagnosis manifests with significant disruptions in self and interpersonal functioning, resulting from a focus on primary gain to self and lack of empathy or desired emotional attachment with others. Please see Chapter 21 later in this volume for a discussion of personality disorders.

This chapter focuses in-depth on two disorders: oppositional defiant disorder and intermittent explosive disorder:

- Oppositional defiant disorder involves a persistent pattern of aggression, irritability, and anger, coupled with defiant and vindictive behaviors. This disorder typically manifests before adolescence but in some cases can manifest later. One of the keys to this disorder is the presence of symptoms that exceed what is normative for the age range. In the approach to a possible diagnosis of oppositional defiant disorder, taking a thorough history—including gathering of collateral information—is of uppermost importance. Clinicians assessing for this diagnosis should inquire about symptoms that are pervasive across multiple settings and environments, although symptoms need only occur in one setting to meet criteria for the diagnosis.
- Intermittent explosive disorder is characterized by recurrent behavioral outbursts during which the individual does not control his or her aggressive impulses. These recurrent behavioral outbursts are beyond what might be expected for the stimulus.

IN-DEPTH DIAGNOSIS

Oppositional Defiant Disorder

The mother of Adam, a 7-year-old boy, brings him to a suburban outpatient clinic for evaluation and possible treatment because of disruptive behavior at school. His mother, a single mother of four children (ages 2–15), works full time outside the home and reports that she is seeking help because she feels as though Adam's behavior has become unmanageable at home and is beginning to manifest at school. His mother reports excessive arguments at home between Adam and his siblings, both younger and older; Adam often talks back and does not follow rules at home or school. His mother recalls that he has been the most challenging to manage of her children, starting when he was between ages 3 and 4. She felt the immediate need to seek assistance when the school notified her because security guards had been called for the second time in 3 weeks in response to Adam's behavior. The most recent incident involved Adam climbing onto the roof of one of the school buildings and taunting the teachers and security guard as they tried to get him to come down safely. He reports that he climbed up there because he thought hiding from his teacher was fun and because she deserved it, and he did not care if he got in trouble.

Adam's case is a very common presentation of oppositional defiant disorder: a young child with long-standing behavioral concerns noted across multiple settings. It is most typical that the child's behavior is tolerated by the parent(s) at home from a very young age and is met with discord when the child attends school and has difficulty with peers, figures of authority, and following the rules. In addition to better understanding Adam's home environment, it is also important to screen for any other disorders that may have a similar presentation or have high risk of comorbidity, such as mood disorders or attention-deficit/hyperactivity disorder (ADHD).

Approach to the Diagnosis

When approaching the diagnosis of oppositional defiant disorder, the clinician needs to consider the criteria for this and other disorders very carefully. As demonstrated in the vignette, one of the most critical parts of the oppositional defiant disorder diagnosis is ruling out other diagnoses such as a mood disorder or ADHD. A clinician should understand the age of the child and his or her current developmental stage, consider the complaint from the parents, and corroborate the information in a collaborative approach, working with the parents to contact other caregivers, teachers, and school officials if possible. Outside information may provide insight into recent environmental or relationship changes for the child.

Once the child's context is clearly understood, the clinician can begin to align confirmed symptoms with assigned criteria to determine if they corroborate the diagnosis. Isolating the single diagnosis of oppositional defiant disorder can be difficult, given that this diagnosis is often accompanied by what are referred to as "internalizing" and "externalizing." DSM-5 has attempted to address this difficulty by outlining categories under Criterion A to guide clinicians in assessing the presence of angry/irritable mood, argumentative/defiant behavior, and level of vindictiveness, if appropriate.

The DSM-5 criteria are specific in that the pattern of behavior needs to be persistent and have a particular frequency, based on whether the child is under age 5, or age 5 or older. If the child is under age 5, the behavior is required to be persistent on "most days" for at least 6 months. If the child is age 5 or older, the behavior must occur at least once per week for at least 6 months. Thorough understanding of the nature and number of settings where the behavior is observed will provide severity classification of the disorder as mild, moderate, or severe.

As stated in DSM-5, "Oppositional defiant disorder has been associated with increased risk for suicide attempts, even after comorbid disorders are controlled for" (p. 464).

Getting the History

A mother comes to the clinic with Michael, her 9-year-old son, just before the New Year's holiday, concerned that he will not behave well and "will ruin everybody's vacation by being bad." She goes on to report that she has done some of her own research online at home, and she found some Web sites about children who have oppositional defiant disorder who "sound exactly like him." The interviewer then asks the mother to share more about what she has read that fits what she has experienced with her son. The mother reports that since his third birthday, Michael "has broken every rule possible." She describes symptoms such as irritability, teasing others ("to the point where it really is awful and he won't stop!"), blaming his sister "for everything," being "cranky all the time," and not going to bed in the evenings even when reminded several times.

The interviewer then attempts to obtain an accurate time frame of the symptoms: "You mentioned that you feel as if this difficulty started around his third birthday. Do you feel as if these symptoms that you just mentioned have happened since before the start of this school year, perhaps in the summer?" The mother replies, "Absolutely!" The interviewer then asks for data regarding frequency: "How often does he get in trouble because of not following the rules? Is it every day after school? Is it mostly on the weekends? What do you think?" The mother replies, "I feel as if I'm taking his video games away almost every day now." The examiner continues, "How often do you hear feedback from the teacher?" The mother responds, "Well, now the teacher has taken to sending me a weekly e-mail about Michael's behavior, because it is so frequent that he is arguing with one of his friends or getting a referral to the principal's office."

The interviewer continues to determine if any recent environmental or social changes have occurred for Michael and also elicits his academic and medical history.

Michael's case represents a very typical presentation of oppositional defiant disorder, when the parent has observed a child's defiant behaviors from a very young age and is prompted to seek assistance when the child's academic and social function has become impaired. It is very common for a parent to present having previously "diagnosed" the child via Web sites. It is the interviewer's responsibility to clarify the symptoms and take a thorough history. The interviewer clarifies symptoms, determining that Michael has more than the required number (four) from Criterion A. The interviewer then verifies the temporal pattern. Parents often feel as though their child has "always been like this" and have difficulty specifying exact time intervals. Typically, providing a timeframe for parents and/or children as benchmarks in their memory can help elicit a more distinctive temporal history. To further understand the frequency, the interviewer asks about the number of times the child has been disciplined not only at home but also at school. This line of inquiry provides salient information, covering more than just frequency. Additional information to acquire is whether this behavior is observed by others at school, affects the child socially, and ultimately occurs at least once weekly. As always, the context of the child should be examined, and any medical diagnosis that may be contributing to the child's presentation should be ruled out.

Tips for Clarifying the Diagnosis

- Clarify that the child has at least four symptoms from these three categories: angry/irritable mood, argumentative/defiant behavior, and vindictiveness.
- Be very clear on the persistence and frequency based on the age of the child (i.e., younger than age 5, or age 5 or older).
- Understand the level of dysfunction and disruption for the child that is causing impairment.
- Consider whether the behavior may be accounted for by any other disorder, and verify that it does not occur exclusively during the course of another disorder.

Consider the Case

Tina is a 5-year-old girl whose parents have brought her to the clinic for assistance with her behavior at home. Her mother, father, and stepfather report that they have recently caught her lying more, cheating at family board games, and fighting and arguing with her older sister. Her teachers have sent reports home about similar behavior happening at school and during her after-school program. Tina has a few friends at school, but her parents have witnessed her threatening and bullying her friends when they do not play games she wants to play or play according to her rules. Her mother recalls noticing this behavior worsening since Tina was age 3, when Tina had difficulty following directions. She recently has become more irritable. She has always been known to be fidgety and has never been known to remain seated to complete homework or leisure activities at home. Tina refuses to do her homework, among other tasks that she is asked to complete both at home and at school, and feels as though she is always getting in trouble for situations that are not her fault.

Tina's parents are bringing her in for care at a younger age than would typically be expected. Tina is apparently experiencing complex symptoms that relate to two diagnoses, oppositional defiant disorder and ADHD. At times, children who have difficulty following instructions or seem as though they are not listening may appear to be defiant. In Tina's case, she has displayed symptoms across diverse settings—that is, at home, school, and after-school care. Tina has been defiant despite identifying that she has heard and understands instructions, and she frequently blames her behavior on others. In addition, she has had difficulties with friendships, not only blaming her friends for her argumentative behavior, but also forcing them to play in certain ways, cheating on games, and planning schemes with ill outcomes toward her friends and sister. Tina's history is also suggestive of ADHD, given that she is described as fidgety, having difficulty sitting still, impulsive, and appearing to not listen at times. Questions that might confirm a comorbid diagnosis of ADHD include whether Tina frequently loses things, forgets instructions and activities, and/or has difficulty waiting for her turn.

Differential Diagnosis

The differential diagnosis for oppositional defiant disorder includes conditions such as conduct disorder, ADHD, depressive and bipolar disorders, disruptive mood dysregulation disorder, intermittent explosive disorder, intellectual disability (intellectual developmental disorder), language disorder, or social anxiety disorder (social phobia). Oppositional defiant disorder and ADHD often co-occur. Clinicians should rely on the characterization of symptoms, including the timing and setting, to establish whether criteria have been met. It is important to define the age at onset of symptoms, contextual presence of the symptoms, and the temporal relationship, including examination of a continual nature versus intermittent symptoms. Disruptive behavior noted with ADHD is a result of the inattention and impulsivity of the disorder, and thus should not be considered a diagnosis of co-occurring oppositional defiant disorder unless it is clear that the criteria for both diagnoses have been met. Furthermore, if an individual resists completing tasks, it should be made clear that the tasks do not demand sustained attention and effort, which would be more indicative of an ADHD diagnosis.

Oppositional defiant disorder is best differentiated from conduct disorder by the impulsivity of mood and irritability that is characteristic of oppositional defiant disorder. Conduct disorder is more severe in that it also includes the criteria of aggression toward people or animals, destruction of property, or a pattern of theft or deceit. It is also possible to observe the manifestation of aggression and/or irritability in the context of a depressive disorder or episode. The time frame of disruptive behavior may help in discerning the correct diagnosis or diagnoses. Furthermore, the irritability manifested in oppositional defiant disorder is characterized by defiant behavior and possible vindictive behavior. To further identify the presence of a distinct mood episode or mood disorder, a clinician would rely on the required neurovegetative criteria met for a mood episode, in addition to the differences in required time intervals.

See DSM-5 for additional disorders to consider in the differential diagnosis. Also refer to the discussions of comorbidity and differential diagnosis in their respective sections of DSM-5.

Summary

- Oppositional defiant disorder is characterized by the presence of persistent, non-episodic patterns of angry/irritable mood, defiant behavior, or vindictiveness for at least 6 months.
- The presence of oppositional behavior creates a significant disruption in a variety of settings, such as school and/or home.
- The severity of oppositional defiant disorder can be specified as mild, moderate, or severe, depending on the number of settings.
- The diagnosis of oppositional defiant disorder requires that other diagnoses in this class be ruled out, as well as medical and neurodevelopmental disorders.

————— IN-DEPTH DIAGNOSIS —————
Intermittent Explosive Disorder

Mr. Peters is a 28-year-old software engineer who presents at the request of a recent court order for mandatory anger management treatment. He reports that he was charged with domestic violence after a physical altercation with his wife of 2 years. He endorses a distant history of school expulsion on two separate occasions in middle school and high school, each for a physical fight. He reports that as a young boy he witnessed a significant degree of domestic violence between his parents, who both had alcoholism. He feels that over the years he has been able to control his anger and his rage, except every now and then when it has become more difficult and resulted in mild to moderate destruction of his own property. On further examination, Mr. Peters expresses an overwhelming amount of guilt and shame about his outbursts, reporting that he knows his anger is often not warranted. He says he loves his wife more than himself, and he recognizes that the punishment he inflicts on her does not fit the "crime." He is now fearful of the dissolution of his marriage and the loss of his job and benefits.

Intermittent explosive disorder is characterized by repeated serious outbursts and aggressiveness that are grossly out of proportion to the situation or to known precipitants. The outbursts are impulsive and not calculating or premeditated. They are very upsetting to the individual and to others who are affected or witness to them. Intermittent explosive disorder is not due to another disorder or condition; for example, the expansiveness or irritability seen in bipolar disorder or the behavioral dysregulation after head injury.

It is not uncommon for an individual with intermittent explosive disorder to present for treatment long after symptoms have started and as the consequences of behavioral problems have accumulated. Intermittent explosive disorder often is most evident at a stage in life when social, vocational, and/or occupational demands are placed on an individual. For Mr. Peters, the disorder manifested itself most distinctly and jarringly in the threat of dissolution of his marriage and occupation. Mr. Peters's report regarding his childhood is relevant to the diagnosis. He recalls school expulsion on more than one occasion spanning between middle and high school, indicating a likely adolescent onset. He identifies that his symptoms have been a chronic problem for him, resulting in physical damage to objects and people and, ultimately, causing extreme dysfunction in a variety of areas. Most important, he is able to identify that his reactions to certain minor provocations are also greater than what others might expect. As with all disruptive, impulse-control, and conduct disorders, it is important to understand the temporal relationship of his symptoms, to rule out any episodic nature of them that might be more indicative of a mood disorder diagnosis. Intermittent explosive disorder can be diagnosed in children over age 6 years and in adolescents, as well as adults.

Approach to the Diagnosis

Making the diagnosis of intermittent explosive disorder can be difficult, given the strict criteria outlined and the symptoms of other disorders that may appear to manifest as intermittent explosive disorder. A thorough history will reveal whether the specific time requirements for the diagnosis have been met. In addition, the quality of the outbursts must be accurately assessed to determine whether criteria are met. Parents and families will often present clear descriptions of a specific tantrum or outburst. It is important to determine whether the outburst is outside the realm of what might be a typical or expected response to an environmental provocation.

One key indication that an outburst response is out of proportion to the stimulus is destruction of property. If the nature of the outbursts tends to include destruction of property, investigating the frequency of outbursts is appropriate, determining whether there has been one in the recent 3 months and how many have occurred in the past 12 months. The quality of the outburst can be more difficult to assess when it consists of verbal altercation or assault, without destruction of property or physical assault. Even in this case, it is appropriate to screen for additional qualifiers, such as cruelty toward an animal or another human being or physical aggression.

Age at onset is critical to the diagnosis of intermittent explosive disorder. Symptoms can begin at any time throughout the lifespan, with onset often found to be within childhood (at least age 6) or adolescence, but rarely after age 40. Once the age at onset is understood, it is important to understand that the course of symptoms may be episodic in nature, following a chronic and persistent course.

Intermittent explosive disorder outbursts can be triggered by what appear to be very small matters, producing unexpected results. Regardless of the provocation, the outbursts are generally frequent with rapid onset, lasting less than 30 minutes. The character of the outbursts may be either in the form of low-intensity verbal or physical aggression without resulting damage or destruction, averaging twice weekly for 3 months, or in the form of high-intensity physical aggression with physical injury or destruction of property three times within 1 year.

Care should be taken during historical and diagnostic interview to clarify and confirm the presence or absence of a major mood disorder, episode of psychosis, direct physiological effects of a substance, or a general medical condition. In the context of these disorders, the diagnosis of intermittent explosive disorder should not be made. The presence of a childhood history of a disruptive behavior disorder of childhood is not uncommon (i.e., ADHD, oppositional defiant disorder, conduct disorder).

Getting the History

> Mr. Fields, age 42 years, presents to a clinician's office reporting that he needs help with anger management. The clinician proceeds by asking about his most recent complaints and why he feels he needs to manage his anger. Mr. Fields reports a story from the previous week, when he became enraged at his coworker who interrupted him in a meeting, which prompted Mr. Fields to abruptly end the meeting by yelling and storming out. The clinician asks Mr. Fields to consider how many times these "enraged" moments happen to him in a given week. Mr. Fields replies that some weeks it does not happen, but other weeks it may happen nearly every day, so "on average three to four times each week." The interviewer then investigates the quality of the outbursts: "Does that enraged feeling you get ever become so great that you end up physically throwing things, damaging property, or hurting others?" Mr. Fields reports that although he feels as if the outbursts could get to that point, he somehow has been able to refrain from hurting anyone and breaking things.
>
> The interviewer then asks, "Do you remember when you first started noticing feeling like your anger was out of control?" In an effort to clarify the amount of functional impairment Mr. Fields currently experiences, the interviewer asks, "How long have you been at your current job?" The man reports that he started at his current company 3 months ago, after having been terminated from his previous company the year prior. He continues on to say that this is his third job in 3 years, with the common feedback that he is "difficult to work with." Mr. Fields recalls that he felt "these anger impulses" during college. He stopped drinking and started "working out" more and going to church regularly. He felt that these efforts helped, and he has continued these "good habits" to help him manage his outbursts—"but still it's such a problem for me!" The clinician is prompted to delve further into Mr. Fields's childhood history, asking, "Did either of your parents or anyone in your family ever complain about your anger when you were in, say, middle school or high school?" The man reports that he rarely got in trouble during his school years and often made the honor roll.

The interviewer allows Mr. Fields to lead with his initial broad complaint before targeting specifics of the described symptoms. The interviewer makes sure to elicit the time of onset of symptoms, investigates whether the symptoms occurred earlier in childhood, and seeks to determine the presence of other disorders during childhood. The interviewer further investigates the quality of Mr. Fields's outbursts by highlighting the presence or absence of property destruction and the frequency of the outbursts. To qualify for the diagnosis of intermittent explosive disorder, verbal aggression should occur approximately twice per week, on average, for at least 3 months. The interviewer would also want to investigate very carefully the presence of other disorders, such as major mood or psychotic disorders, a general medical condition, or substance intoxication or withdrawal.

Tips for Clarifying the Diagnosis

- Question when the symptoms began.
- Determine the time course of the symptoms.
- Establish the intensity of the symptoms. Learn whether there is damage or destruction to people or property.
- Find out whether the outbursts are provoked and in what situation(s).
- Determine whether it is possible to predict when an outburst is going to occur.

Consider the Case

> Gary is a 15-year-old boy whose grandmother is concerned about his behavior at home and school. She reports that he recently spent one night at the juvenile detention center after the police were called to his school for verbal threats he was making toward his teacher. Gary and his grandmother report that his outbursts have been an increasing problem since he was in first grade; however, this is the first time the police have been called to a public place for his behavior. Gary migrated to the United States with his father and grandparents approximately 6 months ago. Gary's grandmother reports that since age 6, Gary has had extreme temper tantrums on numerous occasions, throwing his toys and often destroying his small handheld electronics. Recently, he has begun breaking objects in his room, such as a lamp and his dresser drawer. Once he punched a hole in his wall. She recalls that since he was 12 years old, not a month has gone by when she hasn't seen a serious tantrum resulting in property destruction in some way.

Gary's case shows an onset of symptoms dating back to at least age 6, as documented by his grandmother's history. To qualify for the diagnosis of intermittent explosive disorder, an individual must be at least age 6 years. Gary meets criteria on the basis of the degree of his symptoms and their frequency, in that his grandmother notes a history of property destruction during his tantrums, occurring on a monthly basis over several years. Most recently his outburst was at school and resulted in verbal assault of his teacher and involvement of law enforcement. His symptoms demonstrate reactions that are outside of the expected social norm, with excessive consequence severity. Given the timing of Gary's presentation for care, not long after coming to a new country, an element of adjustment may be playing a role. Because Gary is now presenting 6 months after his immigration, the diagnosis of intermittent explosive disorder is appropriate. In addition, he has a history of symptoms documented back to an early age, supporting the diagnosis.

Differential Diagnosis

Because of the low prevalence of intermittent explosive disorder, the clinician should consider the presence of another mental disorder during assessment. Irritable and aggressive behavior that is thought to be related to intermittent explosive disorder may, in fact, be a manifestation of a general medical condition, substance abuse/intoxication, mood disorder, personality disorder, or psychotic disorder, among other possibilities. It is important for clinicians to understand the temporal relationship of symptoms and to rule out any episodic quality of the symptoms that may be more characteristic of a mood disorder, as well as the presence of a substance or medication or withdrawal from a substance that may be causing a direct psychological effect on the individual. This evaluation occurs by a thorough clinical interview and examination, as well as, when indicated, a blood or urine toxicology screen. The presence of a general medical condition precludes the diagnosis of intermittent explosive disorder. Ruling out other mental disorders or general medical conditions is best accomplished by a thorough psychiatric and neurological exam.

Aggression that is well thought out, motivated, or vindictive in nature does not meet criteria for intermittent explosive disorder. The presence of a personality disorder, such as borderline personality disorder or antisocial personality disorder, does not rule out the presence of intermittent explosive disorder. The disorders should each be carefully considered, including the symptom and temporal pattern of each, and both diagnoses may be made if criteria are met. Most often, the personality disorder is an established diagnosis, with a new persistent change in the quality of intermittent impulsive aggression.

See DSM-5 for additional disorders to consider in the differential diagnosis. Also refer to the discussions of comorbidity and differential diagnosis in their respective sections of DSM-5.

Summary

- Intermittent explosive disorder is a diagnosis that may be considered when clinically significant aggression is present.
- Before making the diagnosis of intermittent explosive disorder, it is important for the clinician to rule out a general medical condition, substance intoxication or withdrawal, or another mental disorder that may account for the symptoms.
- A thorough clinical and neurological examination should be completed as part of the symptom assessment.
- Symptom severity should be assessed on the basis of the functional impairment that the symptoms are causing.

SUMMARY

Disruptive, Impulse-Control, and Conduct Disorders

The disruptive, impulse-control, and conduct disorders are among the most frequent disorders seen by child and adolescent mental health professionals. The underlying symptom that brings all of these disorders together under one diagnostic umbrella is the nature of self and interpersonal dysfunction that occurs. Oppositional defiant disorder initially manifests within the family, disrupting those relationships, and is most often brought to clinical attention once the child reaches school age and is beginning to demonstrate difficulties at school with peers and authority figures. Intermittent explosive disorder often begins in adolescence but is most likely to present to clinical attention when dysfunction affects a young adult's peer relationships and occupational endeavors.

Behavioral dysregulation is an underlying commonality in this diagnostic class. Nevertheless, each diagnosis is distinct and has specific diagnostic criteria. It is important to understand the temporal relationship of symptoms, in addition to understanding when the symptoms may have first manifested in a person's history and how consistent or persistent the symptoms have remained. With intermittent explosive disorder, for example, the timing of explosive behaviors, including the length of time and the frequency, is imperative information to glean in arriving at the correct diagnosis or diagnoses. As always, for each of these disorders, keeping the individual's appropriate expected developmental stage in the forefront is essential for clarity in understanding the diagnosis.

---■-■-■---

Diagnostic Pearls

- Across this diagnostic class, all disorders involve the violation of some aspect of social norms and individual rights.

- The disruptive, impulse-control, and conduct disorders create clinically significant disturbance and impairment in social, educational, and vocational activities, as well as in interpersonal and intrapersonal relationships.

- All diagnoses (except kleptomania) included in the disruptive, impulse-control, and conduct disorders diagnostic class share, but do not require, the common symptom of increased rate of anger.

- Although high rates of aggression are commonalities across all diagnoses in this class (except kleptomania), the types of aggression are distinctly different across the diagnoses, specifically regarding premeditated aggression for secondary gain versus impulsive aggression.

- When evaluating for these diagnoses, it is imperative to be mindful of psychosocial context, because certain environments, such as impoverished backgrounds or war-laden areas, may make the presentation normative.

Self-Assessment

Key Concepts: Double-Check Your Knowledge

What is the relevance of the following concepts to the various disruptive, impulse-control, and conduct disorders?

- Social norms
- Sequelae of behavioral disruption
- Consequence severity

- Interpersonal functioning
- Expected developmental stage
- Irritability
- Comorbid diagnoses
- Severity of aggression

Questions to Discuss With Colleagues and Mentors

1. What is the core concept that ties this diagnostic class together?
2. How much do you, or can you, rely on the collateral data from sources such as teachers, parents, employers, and spouse to inform your diagnostic approach when you are evaluating a new patient with a disruptive, impulse-control, or conduct disorder?
3. Given the common co-occurrence of other disorders, how do you clarify the diagnoses in this diagnostic class?
4. How do you think about gender and cultural considerations in this diagnostic class?
5. When a person presents with symptoms of intermittent explosive disorder, what laboratory or other testing is appropriate?

Case-Based Questions

PART A

> Mr. Hill is a 42-year-old man who reports a history of being "moody" since he was in college. He reports that he has been so moody at times in the past that he has lost a few friends and been divorced three times. His occupational history has been one of instability, and he wonders if he'll ever be able to hold a job longer than a year. He reports that when he was about age 35, he began using alcohol to help him calm down in the evenings, because he was afraid he would just absolutely explode on somebody. He denies any other substance use or abuse, and his medical workup is negative.

What is the most striking aspect of Mr. Hill's history with which a clinician should be first concerned?   Mr. Hill is describing significantly impaired self-control and interpersonal functioning, a hallmark for disruptive, impulse-control, and conduct disorders.

PART B

> Mr. Hill mentions that most days he is "fine" and can remain calm, but he has always lived in fear that he is going to explode on anyone at any moment. He says he never has a stretch of days when he is "moody" or "down," but rather that "it is just kind of unpredictable, and so random. Things that should only make me a little upset or cranky make me lose my mind it seems!"

Could Mr. Hill possibly have a mood disorder?   Given that Mr. Hill says his symptoms are random, not episodic, and do not last for a significant period of time, a mood disorder diagnosis is less likely.

PART C

> Mr. Hill, given the opportunity to talk about his childhood, reports that in retrospect "I wasn't necessarily moody as a kid, but I had a couple of times when I got in trouble at school and got in a few fights in middle school."

Which diagnosis should most likely remain at the top of the differential for Mr. Hill? Mr. Hill is describing symptoms that are most consistent with intermittent explosive disorder, with a slight history of disruptive behavior dating back to childhood. The level of dysfunction is concerning, especially because it has persisted for quite some time, in that he has been through three marriages and multiple jobs.

Short-Answer Questions

1. For a child under age 5 to be diagnosed with oppositional defiant disorder, how often must the symptoms occur?
2. For a child age 5 or older to be diagnosed with oppositional defiant disorder, how often must the symptoms occur?
3. What are the key categorical components of oppositional defiant disorder behavior that must be evidenced for diagnostic qualification?
4. How often must vindictive or spiteful behavior occur for oppositional defiant disorder?
5. What is the required time criterion for an individual to manifest aggressive impulses for the diagnosis of intermittent explosive disorder?
6. What is the youngest age for which intermittent explosive disorder may be diagnosed?
7. What is the typical age at onset for intermittent explosive disorder?

Answers

1. Generally, symptoms must occur on most days for a period of at least 6 months for a child under age 5 to be diagnosed with oppositional defiant disorder.
2. Generally, symptoms must occur at least once per week for at least 6 months for a child age 5 or older to be diagnosed with oppositional defiant disorder.
3. The key categorical components of oppositional defiant disorder behavior that must be evidenced for diagnostic qualification are angry/irritable mood, argumentative/defiant behavior, and vindictiveness.
4. Vindictive or spiteful behavior must occur at least twice within the past 6 months for oppositional defiant disorder.
5. For the diagnosis of intermittent explosive disorder, the individual must manifest verbal or physical aggression twice weekly, on average, for the past 3 months (without damage or destruction to property or physical injury to animals or other individuals), *or* three behavioral outbursts involving damage or destruction of property and/or physical assault involving physical injury to animals or other individuals within a 12-month period.
6. The youngest chronological age for which intermittent explosive disorder may be diagnosed is 6 years (or equivalent developmental level).
7. The typical age at onset for intermittent explosive disorder is childhood or adolescence.

19

Substance-Related and Addictive Disorders

Kimberly L. Brodsky, Ph.D.

Michael J. Ostacher, M.D., M.P.H., M.M.Sc.

"I don't want to start drinking again, but then
I do and I just can't stop."

"I always think I can stop heroin on my own, and for a while
I can…but soon I'm back to shooting up and
I don't even know how I got there."

The substance-related and addictive disorders include difficulties associated with 10 classes of drugs—alcohol; caffeine; cannabis; hallucinogens (including phencyclidine); inhalants; opioids; sedatives, hypnotics, and anxiolytics; stimulants; tobacco; and other (or unknown) substances—and gambling. The diagnosis of these disorders is based on a pathological pattern of behaviors in which the essential feature is the continued use of a substance or behavior despite significant problems related to it. This class of disorders has undergone significant changes in DSM-5, most notably the elimination of the distinction between substance abuse and dependence. This change was made in part because of epidemiological data suggesting overlap between abuse and dependence and lack of clear differences in harm related to each disorder in DSM-IV.

The DSM-5 criteria for substance use disorders fit within four overall groupings: impaired control, social impairment, risky use, and pharmacological criteria. Now included as a symptom of impaired control is craving, which previously was not included in the diagnosis of any substance use disorder. Two symptoms within a 12-month period are required to establish the diagnosis of a substance use disorder, a significant change from the three symptoms required for dependence in DSM-IV. With the abuse/dependence distinction gone, severity (designated as mild, moderate, or severe) is now used as a specifier instead.

Common to all substance-related disorders in this diagnostic class is the resulting activation of the brain reward system from consumption of a substance. The brain reward system involves the reinforcement of behaviors and the production of memories; substances with abuse potential short-circuit this system by directly activating the reward system, most often producing feelings of pleasure. This short circuit results in a more intense activation of the reward system than through adaptive behaviors and can result in a lack of attention to and engagement in normal activities. With the exception of hallucinogens, each class of drugs produces behavioral effects that could be described as a "high." With hallucinogens, curiosity is often a motivating factor in their use, rather than a desire for a euphoric experience. Although the term *dependence* has been removed from this category to avoid overlap with pharmacological tolerance and withdrawal, it is important to highlight the physiological aspect of these disorders. Behaviors associated with substance use disorders can often be mistakenly viewed as volitional or manipulative; however, it is important to understand these behavioral patterns as a result of alterations in reward pathways, often tied to physiological dependence and logical sequelae of the disorders themselves.

Gambling disorder is included in this diagnostic class, given evidence suggesting that gambling behavior activates the brain reward system in a similar way to drugs of abuse. The addition of gambling disorder is considered controversial by some because it is a *behavior* rather than an exogenous substance; however, the consensus was that the biological evidence merited its inclusion.

The diagnostic class of substance-related and addictive disorders is divided into two subgroups: substance-related disorders and non-substance-related disorders. Each of the substance-related disorders is further separated into substance use disorder (e.g., alcohol use disorder); intoxication (e.g., caffeine intoxication); withdrawal (e.g., cannabis withdrawal); other (e.g., other inhalant-related disorder); and unspecified (e.g., unspecified opioid-related disorder). Hallucinogen-related disorders also include phencyclidine-related disorders. In addition, substance-related disorders include tobacco-related disorders (tobacco use disorder and tobacco withdrawal) and substance/medication-induced mental disorders. Gambling disorder is the only disorder listed under non-substance-related disorders.

Substance-induced disorders comprise substance intoxication, substance withdrawal, and substance/medication-induced mental disorders included elsewhere in DSM-5 (e.g., substance/medication-induced psychotic disorder, substance/medication-induced depressive disorder). Many substances or medications can cause disorders that resemble other diagnoses, with the caveat that typically these symptoms last only temporarily. These disorders are different from substance use syndromes, in which a mix of cognitive, behavioral, and physiological symptoms are identified and contribute to the continued use of the substance, despite significant substance-related problems in functioning. These substance/medication-induced mental disorders are listed in their relevant sections of DSM-5 (e.g., depressive disorders, neurocognitive disorders). Symptoms of withdrawal and tolerance can occur during medical treatment involving prescriptive medications. Tolerance and withdrawal are normal, expected reactions to repeated doses of substances, and when these reactions occur during the course of medical treatment, they should not be counted toward the diagnosis of a substance use disorder. However, tolerance and withdrawal can be important pharmacological signs of the severity of a substance use disorder; furthermore, when prescription medications are used inappropriately or in excess of what is prescribed and other symptoms are present, a diagnosis of a substance-related disorder can be made.

In the clinical approach to an individual who has a substance-related or addictive disorder, it is important to understand that there is often ambivalence about use and its consequences and that this ambivalence can be used to motivate change. Evidence suggests that behavior change is complex and that the locus of change is in the individual with the disorder. This approach is somewhat of a departure from a medicalized approach to care in which the diagnosis is made and then prescriptions for treatment are given. Instead, individuals are led to discuss reasons to change that are within themselves, because most people with substance-related and addictive disorders "know" that they have a "problem"—yet knowing is rarely sufficient to engender change. The shame and stigma of a substance-related or addictive disorder frequently interferes with getting treatment, and although relapses should be an expected part of treatment, individuals (and treatment providers) often view themselves as failures when relapse occurs. Negative views of patients and their behaviors are common in providers and likely interfere with the alliance with the patient—and consequently decrease, rather than increase, the likelihood that the patient will engage in treatment and behavioral change.

Many individuals may use substances as an attempt to cope with severe psychosocial stressors or the symptoms of another illness (e.g., major depressive disorder, posttraumatic stress disorder, chronic pain). Although this short-term coping mechanism may in fact be quite effective at alleviating distressing feelings of physical or emotional pain, in the long term the sequelae of negative consequences associated with the substance use disorder and the physiological need for the substance take on lives of their own.

──────── **IN-DEPTH DIAGNOSIS** ────────

Alcohol-Related Disorders

A 63-year-old man, Mr. James, comes to the clinic requesting services to assist with stopping drinking. He was recently arrested for driving under the influence (DUI) and states that his marriage is "on the rocks." He reports a long-standing history of alcohol use, starting in his teens. He says that he began drinking more frequently in his 30s after his first divorce. He states that he stopped drinking around the time of his second marriage and maintained sobriety for 5 years. However, after his son died in a car crash, Mr. James began drinking again and reports that his use quickly escalated. He states that currently he drinks about 12 beers per day and often will get to sleep with a few additional shots of hard alcohol. He reports frequent blackouts and was told by his doctor that his liver is damaged. He admits that he has had three previous DUIs and is concerned about the possibility of jail time associated with this most recent charge. Mr. James reports that he has worked "on and off" doing landscaping and other odd jobs; however, he struggles financially. His children will not speak to him any longer, and his wife recently kicked him out of the house when he came home intoxicated. He says that although he knows that alcohol has created many problems for him and he cannot really afford the way he drinks, he feels that he cannot stop on his own. He reports that when he tries to stop drinking, he gets the shakes and feels sick to his stomach.

This case highlights the legal and interpersonal ramifications often associated with alcohol use disorder. It also underscores the tolerance and withdrawal frequently associated with alcohol use disorder, including physiological symptoms and relapse associated with alleviation of these symptoms. Individuals often will be able to stop using for a period of time; however, once they began drinking again, their use escalates quickly.

Approach to the Diagnosis

Tolerance and withdrawal are two physiological aspects of alcohol-related disorders to which clinicians often pay special attention. Tolerance develops with continued use of a substance such that greater dosages are required to achieve the same effect. Alcohol withdrawal is characterized by symptoms that develop approximately 4–12 hours after the reduction of prolonged heavy alcohol consumption. Withdrawal symptoms are often intensely uncomfortable; therefore, individuals will continue to imbibe alcohol to avoid or reduce these symptoms, despite adverse consequences. In this vicious cycle, individuals continue to use alcohol despite psychological and physical consequences (e.g., depression, loss of employment, estrangement from loved ones, liver disease, homelessness). Some symptoms of withdrawal (e.g., sleep disturbances) are thought to last up to months and to contribute significantly to relapse. Severe complications of withdrawal, such as delirium and grand mal seizures, affect less than 5% of individuals with alcohol use disorder.

Individuals may use alcohol in hazardous circumstances (e.g., driving while under the influence of alcohol), and they may continue to use alcohol despite the knowledge that sustained consumption will result in significant psychosocial difficulties. Individuals who decide to stop drinking often will have successful periods of abstinence; however, once they begin drinking again, their consumption likely will escalate rapidly and severe difficulties will reemerge. Failed attempts to diminish the amount of alcohol they consume, the need for an alcoholic beverage in the morning to relieve withdrawal symptoms, feelings of guilt or being criticized regarding alcohol consumption, and feelings of needing to cut back on consumption can all indicate an alcohol-related disorder and are important things to query about in a diagnostic interview. In addition, major areas of functioning are likely to be affected, resulting in, for example, alcohol-related accidents, school and job problems, interpersonal difficulties, legal problems, and health problems. Unspecified alcohol-related disorder can be diagnosed when an individual presents with symptoms characteristic of an alcohol-related disorder that cause significant distress or functional impairment; however, the symptoms do not meet the full criteria for any specific alcohol-related disorder.

The severity of alcohol use disorder is determined by the number of symptoms endorsed. Having two or three symptoms yields a diagnosis of mild alcohol use disorder, and having six or more symptoms yields a diagnosis of severe alcohol use disorder. In general, the more symptoms an individual endorses, the more severe the alcohol use disorder. Severe alcohol use disorder, especially in individuals with antisocial personality disorder, is often associated with criminal acts. For example, more than half of all individuals who commit homicide are believed to have been intoxicated at the time of the event. Severe alcohol use also contributes to feelings of sadness, irritability, and hopelessness, which can contribute to suicidal behaviors.

Alcohol use disorder frequently co-occurs with other substance use disorders; individuals may use alcohol to alleviate unwanted effects of these substances or to substitute for them when other substances are not as easily available. Individuals may also use alcohol to mask the symptoms of other illnesses, as a way of coping (e.g., posttraumatic stress disorder, depression). Symptoms of depression, anxiety, insomnia, and conduct problems frequently co-occur with heavy drinking and can precede it as well.

First alcohol intoxication most often occurs during the mid-teens. The majority of individuals who develop alcohol-related disorders do so by their late 30s. Key to the diagnosis of alcohol use disorder is the use of heavy amounts of alcohol with resulting repeated and significant distress or impairment in functioning. Although many individuals who drink consume enough to become intoxicated, only a minority of them ever develop alcohol use disorder. This discrepancy is an important part of the assessment in diagnostic interviewing.

As stated in DSM-5, "Alcohol use disorder is an important contributor to suicide risk during severe intoxication and in the context of a temporary alcohol-induced depressive and bipolar disorder. There is an increased rate of suicidal behavior as well as of completed suicide among individuals with the disorder (p. 493).... Alcohol intoxication is an important contributor to suicidal behavior. There appears to be an increased rate of suicidal behavior, as well as of completed suicide, among persons intoxicated by alcohol" (p. 498).

Getting the History

Interviewer: When did you begin drinking?
Patient (age 53 years): When I was 12 years old.
Interviewer: How much were you drinking at that time?
Patient: On the weekends with friends.
Interviewer: When did your drinking increase?
Patient: In my 20s I was drinking about a fifth of vodka a day.
Interviewer: How much and how often do you currently drink?
Patient: I'd say about two fifths per day.
Interviewer: Have you noticed that you need more alcohol to feel the same effects?
Patient: Yes.
Interviewer: How much time do you spend obtaining, using, and recovering from the use of alcohol?
Patient: Basically all of my time. I wake up in the morning and immediately need a drink to feel okay. Then I spend the day drinking and trying to get alcohol.
Interviewer: When you are not drinking, do you have cravings to use alcohol?

Patient: I can't stop thinking about it.

Interviewer: Have you ever used alcohol in a physically dangerous situation?

Patient: Yes, when I'm drunk I've gotten into fights, had my belongings stolen, and gotten arrested for public drunkenness.

Interviewer: Do you feel the need to cut back on your drinking?

Patient: That's why I'm here.

Interviewer: Have you ever tried to cut back, and how did that work?

Patient: A few times, but I always start again.

Interviewer: When you try to stop drinking, what happens?

Patient: I get the shakes, become nauseous, and can't sit still.

Interviewer: Has drinking gotten in the way of work or relationships?

Patient: Definitely. I haven't been able to keep a job, I'm homeless, and my family is fed up with me.

Interviewer: So you feel alcohol has led to some bad things but you still drink?

Patient: Part of me wants to stop so badly, but another part just can't. After all this time, how could I begin to face all of these things?

This interview highlights the key diagnostic criteria for alcohol use disorder. Initial questions seek to obtain necessary information regarding age at onset, volume of alcohol consumed, and tolerance (determined by inquiring about the need for more alcohol to produce the same effects over time). Symptoms of withdrawal are determined by inquiring about physical signs and symptoms when consumption of alcohol is reduced or the individual has tried to stop drinking. Information is also obtained about the amount of time spent consuming, obtaining, and recovering from the effects of alcohol. The interviewer also inquires whether the individual experiences cravings for alcohol and has made unsuccessful attempts to reduce or stop drinking; whether the individual has used alcohol in hazardous situations (e.g., driving under the influence); and whether the person has experienced negative consequences of alcohol consumption and continued drinking despite awareness of these consequences. Ambivalence regarding stopping drinking is a common experience among people who have alcohol-related disorders, because the alcohol is often serving some function (e.g., escape from negative emotions, numbing, coping with physical pain), and attempts to stop may have resulted in intense physiological discomfort associated with withdrawal. Clinicians often expect that individuals will present for evaluation sure of their desire to stop drinking; however, ambivalence about change is often a natural aspect of modifying any behavior. If this ambivalence is present, recognizing it as a natural aspect of recovery is crucial during an evaluation, for the clinician and client. This recognition and acceptance enhances rapport and puts in perspective a client's prior failures with previous attempts at treatment.

Tips for Clarifying the Diagnosis

- Determine answers to the following questions: Is the use of alcohol causing clinically significant impairment in the individual's ability to function? Has it impaired the person's ability to perform at work or school? Has it negatively affected interpersonal relationships?
- Question whether the individual has made unsuccessful attempts to cut back the volume of his or her drinking.

- Investigate whether there is evidence of a need for increased consumption of alcohol to produce the same effects (tolerance).
- Establish whether physical symptoms of withdrawal have occurred when the individual has reduced or stopped drinking.
- Determine whether the individual has engaged in physically hazardous activities while drinking (e.g., driving under the influence).

Consider the Case

Mr. Kim, a 21-year-old Korean male college student, presents for treatment, struggling with his grades and concerned about the possibility of failing out of college. He states that he began drinking alcohol when he and his parents moved to the United States from Korea during his high school years. He found it difficult to fit in and felt that alcohol helped him to make friends and talk to strangers. His drinking escalated during college, partially to cope with the stress associated with classes and the part-time job he works to pay for college and help out his parents at home. Mr. Kim reports that he gets intoxicated easily and that people often tell him that his face becomes flushed when he is drinking. He states that sometimes when he drinks alcohol, his heart will begin to beat rapidly. He states that the first few times he drank, he became so physically ill that he didn't drink again right away, but despite these physical symptoms he always returned to drinking.

Mr. Kim is somewhat unique in having developed an alcohol use disorder given that his reports are consistent with those of individuals, often Asians, who have polymorphisms of genes for two alcohol-metabolizing enzymes, alcohol dehydrogenase and aldehyde dehydrogenase, which affect the response to alcohol. Individuals with these gene variations experience a flushed face and palpitations, which can often be severe enough to prevent further use of alcohol. His treatment is complicated further by the cultural context in which his alcohol use is occurring: he was born in Korea to Korean parents, and is now immersed in a distinctly U.S. phenomenon of college-age drinking. Clinicians need to be aware of important cultural differences, including the specific meaning of alcohol misuse in Korean culture, and the expectations put upon Mr. Kim by his family; these areas need to be explored carefully by treaters and consultation obtained, if necessary.

Differential Diagnosis

The differential diagnosis of alcohol-related disorders includes consideration of the following:

- **Alcohol use disorder:** nonpathological use of alcohol; sedative, hypnotic, or anxiolytic use disorder; conduct disorder in childhood and adult antisocial personality disorder
- **Alcohol intoxication:** other medical conditions (e.g., diabetic acidosis, cerebellar ataxia, multiple sclerosis); sedative, hypnotic, or anxiolytic intoxication
- **Alcohol withdrawal:** other medical conditions (e.g., hypoglycemia, diabetic ketoacidosis, essential tremor); sedative, hypnotic, or anxiolytic withdrawal
- **Unspecified alcohol-related disorder**

Alcohol use disorder is seen in the majority of individuals with antisocial personality disorder. Because antisocial personality disorder is associated with an early onset of alcohol use disorder and a worse prognosis, it is important to establish both diagnoses. The signs and symptoms of alcohol use disorder are similar to those seen in sedative-, hypnotic-, or anxiolytic-related disorders; however, the course is often different, particularly concerning associated medical problems. Thus, it is important to distinguish between the two. Individuals with alcohol use disorder can develop patterns of use that create legal and disciplinary consequences; such patterns should be carefully distinguished from the difficulty with authority and behavioral patterns associated with conduct disorder. Part of the association between depression and alcohol use disorder may be due to temporary depressive symptoms associated with the acute effects of intoxication or withdrawal; therefore, a diagnosis of major depressive disorder should be made with extreme caution until the individual can be assessed outside the context of acute effects of alcohol.

A key element of alcohol use disorder involves the large volume of alcohol consumed, which results in repeated and significant distress or impaired functioning. Most individuals who drink alcohol consume enough to feel intoxicated; however, less than one-fifth of them ever develop alcohol use disorder. Many cultures and age groups encourage drinking at certain events (e.g., college and fraternity events, religious events). Drinking, even daily, and intoxication do not by themselves qualify an individual for diagnosis of alcohol use disorder. Alcohol use disorder can be diagnosed with or without physiological dependence; however, physiological dependence is not a requirement for the diagnosis of alcohol use disorder. Endorsing two or three symptoms signifies mild alcohol use disorder, and endorsing six or more symptoms indicates severe alcohol use disorder. In general, the greater the number of symptoms endorsed and the earlier the age at onset, the more severe the alcohol use disorder is likely to be.

See DSM-5 for additional disorders to consider in the differential diagnosis. Also refer to the discussions of comorbidity and differential diagnosis in their respective sections of DSM-5.

Summary

- Alcohol-related disorders are the most prevalent of the substance-related disorders in the United States.
- First alcohol intoxication most often occurs during the mid-teens. The majority of individuals who develop alcohol-related disorders do so by their late 30s.
- Polymorphisms of genes for alcohol-metabolizing enzymes are often seen in Asians and affect their response to alcohol. Individuals with these gene variations experience flushed face and palpitations that may be severe enough to limit the future consumption of alcohol and diminish the risk for the development of alcohol-related disorders.
- Alcohol withdrawal is characterized by symptoms that develop approximately 4–12 hours after the reduction of prolonged heavy alcohol consumption. With-

drawal symptoms are often intensely uncomfortable, and individuals may continue to imbibe alcohol to avoid or reduce these withdrawal symptoms, despite adverse consequences.

IN-DEPTH DIAGNOSIS

Cannabis-Related Disorders

A 27-year-old man, Mr. Clark, presents with anxiety and insomnia. Questioning reveals that he has been using 1–2 grams of marijuana daily for the past 7 or 8 years. He began using intermittently as a teenager but became a daily user as an undergraduate in college. He denies that his grades were affected by his marijuana use but says he decided not to return to school after his sophomore year because his work in a small café would better help him achieve his goal of running a restaurant. He has been working at several restaurants since, initially as a server but then he became the assistant manager of a local lunch and dinner restaurant. He decided that "being a waiter is better—I like being in touch with the customers and I get to make my own hours." He often works late, coming home after 2 A.M., and he has found that smoking marijuana before going to bed helps him sleep. If he does not use any cannabis, he reports, he generally cannot sleep at all. He smokes upon awakening because it helps him "chill." He reports that he has had periods of trying to stop in the past year because of the cost, but "it's the only thing that helps with my anxiety, and there's no way I can sleep without it." He is not currently in a relationship but lives with three coworkers in a shared apartment.

Cannabis-related disorders are much more likely in adults whose use began in early adolescence. The acceptance of cannabis use is increasing (along with legalized use in some states), and because it is perceived to be less addicting than other substances, even daily use may not be recognized as problematic. School and work performance may be decreased in chronic users, who may achieve less than expected in social and occupational functioning. It is quite difficult for chronic users to stop because of withdrawal effects; people with cannabis-related disorders may believe that withdrawal symptoms such as anxiety, irritability, and insomnia relieved by use may represent a benefit of the use of the drug for those symptoms.

Approach to the Diagnosis

As with all substance use (but especially cannabis), the clinician must be aware of either negative or positive feelings about the use of the drug. Cannabis use disorder is difficult to diagnose, in part because of beliefs among both patients and clinicians that the drug is less likely to lead to use disorders than other substances, intoxication is less obvious than for other substances, and the development of dependence is often slower than for other substances. The notion persists that cannabis is less dangerous than alcohol, opiates, stimulants, sedatives, hypnotics, and even nicotine. Nevertheless, for some people the drug has a strong negative effect in terms of functioning and ability to control use, and clinicians must be attuned to this. Unspecified cannabis-related disorder can be diagnosed when an individual presents with symptoms characteristic of a cannabis-related disorder that cause significant distress or functional impairment; however, the symptoms do not meet the full criteria for any specific cannabis-related disorder.

Cannabis is most commonly smoked via a variety of methods: pipes, water pipes (bongs), cigarettes (joints), and hollowed-out cigars (blunts). It is sometimes ingested orally by mixing it with food. More recently, devices vaporize cannabis, which involves heating the plant to release psychoactive cannabinoids for inhalation. Smoking and vaporization typically produce more rapid onset and more intense experiences.

Pharmacological and behavioral tolerance to most of the effects of cannabis has been reported in individuals who use it chronically. Generally tolerance is lost when cannabis use is discontinued for a significant period of time. The abrupt cessation of daily use often results in cannabis withdrawal syndrome, which includes symptoms of irritability, anger, anxiety, depressed mood, restlessness, sleep difficulty, and decreased appetite or weight loss. Though not as severe as opiate or alcohol withdrawal, cannabis withdrawal can cause significant distress and contribute to relapse.

Although medical uses of cannabis remain controversial and equivocal, its use for medical purposes should be considered before making a diagnosis; symptoms of tolerance and withdrawal naturally occur within the context of a prescription for a medical condition and should not be the primary criteria for diagnosis.

Cannabis use may continue despite knowledge of physical or psychological problems associated with it. Individuals with cannabis use disorder may use cannabis throughout the day over a period of months or years and may spend many hours a day under the influence. Others may use it less frequently, but their use causes recurrent problems related to family, school, work, or other important activities. Periodic cannabis use and intoxication can negatively affect behavioral and cognitive functioning and thus interfere with optimal performance. Arguments with relatives over the use of cannabis in the home are common. Use of cannabis on the job or while working at a place that requires drug testing can also be a sign of cannabis use disorder. It is important to query for these signs and symptoms in diagnostic interviews.

Individuals who regularly use cannabis often report that it helps them cope with mood, sleep, pain, and so on. Many individuals will not report spending an excessive amount of time under the influence, despite being intoxicated the majority of the day. An important marker supporting a diagnosis is continued use despite clear risk of negative consequences to other valued activities or relationships. It is important to recognize and assess for these common signs and symptoms of cannabis use to better assess the extent of usage. Experienced users of cannabis develop behavioral and pharmacological tolerance. Signs of acute and chronic use include red eyes, yellowing of fingertips, chronic cough, and exaggerated craving and impulse for specific foods.

Cannabis use has been related to a reduction in prosocial, goal-directed activity, which some have labeled amotivational syndrome, manifesting in poor school performance and employment problems.

Getting the History

Interviewer: When did you begin smoking marijuana?
Patient (age 32 years): I was 14 years old.
Interviewer: How much were you smoking at that time?

Patient: On the weekends with friends.
Interviewer: When did your smoking increase?
Patient: Around my sophomore year in college, I started smoking during the day before classes.
Interviewer: How much and how often do you currently smoke?
Patient: I'd say about three or four joints per day.
Interviewer: Have you noticed that you need more marijuana in order to feel the same effects?
Patient: Yes.
Interviewer: How much time do you spend getting and smoking marijuana?
Patient: A lot. I wake and bake in the morning, then I'll use throughout the day, I'm pretty much always high. I get hooked up from my friend who has a prescription, so it doesn't take me too long, but I definitely spend a lot of money on weed.
Interviewer: When you are not high, do you have cravings to use?
Patient: Totally. Winter break with my parents is the worst.
Interviewer: Have you ever been high in a physically dangerous situation?
Patient: I guess, but I drive slower when I'm stoned.
Interviewer: Do you feel the need to cut back on your smoking?
Patient: My girlfriend says I should.
Interviewer: Have you ever tried to cut back, and how did that work?
Patient: A few times, but I always start again.
Interviewer: When you try to stop smoking, what happens?
Patient: I have trouble sleeping, and my girl says I'm cranky.
Interviewer: Has smoking gotten in the way of work or relationships?
Patient: Well, it definitely bothers my girlfriend, and sometimes I decide to blow off work and get high. I think my boss suspects something's up. Once I failed a drug test and lost my gig at the video store. I liked working there too, I used to roll one up and watch action flicks—best job I ever had.
Interviewer: So you feel smoking has led to some negative consequences but you still smoke?
Patient: Part of me wants to stop, but I don't really see too many problems with it.

This interview highlights the key diagnostic criteria for cannabis-related disorders. Initial questions elicit necessary information regarding age at onset, volume of marijuana consumed, and tolerance (determined by inquiring about the need for more marijuana to produce the same effects over time). In individuals with chronic, heavy usage, symptoms of withdrawal are determined by inquiring about signs and symptoms when marijuana is no longer used. The interviewer also inquires about whether the individual experiences cravings for marijuana and whether he or she has made unsuccessful attempts to reduce use or stop using. In addition, the interviewer asks whether the individual has used marijuana in hazardous situations (e.g., driving under the influence). Finally, the interviewer inquires about the negative consequences of marijuana consumption and continued smoking despite awareness of these consequences.

Tips for Clarifying the Diagnosis

- Ask about symptoms of withdrawal during the evaluation of cannabis use.
- Be aware of the cultural context of use, especially reported medical uses of cannabis.
- Realize that it may be difficult for individuals to identify the social and occupational consequences of cannabis use.

- Carefully evaluate for anxiety and mood symptoms that may have been present before the onset of use or during periods of prolonged abstinence.
- Assess whether the use of cannabis is causing clinically significant impairment in the individual's ability to function, in his or her ability to perform at work or school, or in his or her interpersonal relationships.

Consider the Case

Mr. Jackson, a 23-year-old man, presents with severe features of posttraumatic stress disorder. Since returning from Iraq, he has been using 1–2 grams per day of marijuana, which he obtains through a marijuana dispensary because he has a prescription to treat his chronic pain. He says smoking helps him cope with his symptoms and relax enough to be around people. He began using intermittently as a teenager but became a daily user after returning from the war. He works as a security guard at a casino, often for late hours, coming home after 2 A.M., and he has found that smoking marijuana before going to bed "relieves the tension" in his body and allows him to sleep. If he does not use any cannabis, he reports, he generally cannot sleep at all, feels hypervigilant, and is consumed with thoughts about his time in the military. He smokes upon awakening because it helps him get out of bed: "Otherwise I'm too stiff." He reports that he has had periods of trying to stop in the past year because of the cost, but "it's the only thing that helps with my pain." He has been planning to apply to the police academy but has not filled out the applications.

The cultural acceptance of cannabis for medical purposes has made its use more acceptable and expanded its availability in certain communities. This makes teasing out symptoms that may be consequences of use more difficult for clinicians; similarly, individuals have more difficulty defining social or occupational problems resulting from use of the substance. Many individuals use cannabis in the context of the symptoms of posttraumatic stress disorder and anxiety disorders, such as generalized anxiety disorder and social anxiety disorder (social phobia). Evaluation of co-occurring psychiatric disorders is important in providing education, support, and targeted treatment to these individuals. In the case of Mr. Jackson, issues specific to his war-related disorders need to be understood and addressed in the context of his treatment.

Differential Diagnosis

The differential diagnosis of cannabis-related disorders includes consideration of the following:

- **Cannabis use disorder:** nonproblematic use of cannabis; other mental disorders (e.g., anxiety disorders, major depressive disorders)
- **Cannabis intoxication:** other substance intoxication (e.g., phencyclidine intoxication, hallucinogen intoxication); cannabis-induced mental disorders (e.g., cannabis-induced anxiety disorder, with onset during intoxication)
- **Cannabis withdrawal:** withdrawal from other substances; depressive, bipolar, anxiety, or other mental disorders; another medical condition
- **Unspecified cannabis-related disorder**

Cannabis-related disorders might be characterized by symptoms that resemble those of primary mental disorders. For example, generalized anxiety disorder needs to be distinguished from cannabis-induced anxiety disorder, with onset during intoxication. Chronic cannabis use can result in an amotivational syndrome that resembles chronic depressive disorder. Acute adverse reactions to cannabis need to be distinguished from the symptoms of panic disorder, major depressive disorder, delusional disorder, bipolar disorder, and schizophrenia. Urine screen and physical examination, which may reveal elevated pulse and red eyes, can help make the distinction. It is important to query about substance use and determine whether symptoms are present outside the context of recent use and withdrawal.

It is essential to the diagnosis to clarify that the cannabis use is problematic and creating impairments in functioning. This assessment can be tricky because social, behavioral, and psychological problems may be difficult to attribute specifically to cannabis use (especially if the individual is also using other substances). Furthermore, denial of heavy use and lack of acknowledgment that cannabis may be related to or causing substantial problems can be common in individuals presenting for treatment at the request or urging of someone else.

See DSM-5 for additional disorders to consider in the differential diagnosis. Also refer to the discussions of comorbidity and differential diagnosis in their respective sections of DSM-5.

Summary

- Cannabinoids, especially cannabis, are the most widely used illicit psychoactive substances in the United States.
- Rates of cannabis use disorder are greater among males than females.
- The abrupt cessation of daily use often results in cannabis withdrawal syndrome, which includes symptoms of irritability, anger, anxiety, depressed mood, restlessness, sleep difficulty, and decreased appetite or weight loss.
- Cannabis intoxication does not typically result in the severe behavioral and cognitive dysfunction seen in alcohol intoxication.
- It is essential to the diagnosis to clarify that the cannabis use is problematic and creating impairments in functioning.
- Cannabis-related disorders might be characterized by symptoms that resemble those of primary mental disorders.

───────────── IN-DEPTH DIAGNOSIS ─────────────
Opioid-Related Disorders

Emergency physicians treat Mr. Johnson, a 36-year-old man, at the hospital after his girlfriend found him unresponsive on the floor of his apartment and called an ambulance. They revived him by the administration of intravenous naloxone. He has a long history of drug and alcohol use, beginning in early adolescence with marijuana and alcohol. In his late teens he began using prescription opiates that he stole from family members; he initially took them orally and later intranasally. This use was followed over the course of several years by the use of intranasal heroin that he bought on the street. By his early 20s, he was using heroin intravenously. He committed petty crimes as a teenager, stealing from neighbors or stealing cars; got into multiple fights with his peers; and was frequently truant from school, ultimately dropping out of high school before obtaining his diploma. He has a history of multiple arrests, with short jail stays but no prison sentences. He was mandated to addiction treatment as a condition of probation, including three episodes of medically supervised withdrawal followed by short-term, abstinence-based residential treatment. During the year of court-mandated methadone maintenance treatment, he successfully remained abstinent from opiates, but he continued to use alcohol and benzodiazepines and left methadone maintenance treatment when his probation ended. He began using intravenous heroin again, with periods of stopping use by buying buprenorphine/naloxone or methadone on the street. When his girlfriend found him on the floor, he had taken methadone that he received illicitly.

Severe opioid-related disorders are frequently characterized by physiological dependence and intense cravings that are motivated by both positive rewards (e.g., euphoria) and negative ones (e.g., avoidance of withdrawal symptoms). Users frequently relapse, having limited response to treatment other than opioid replacement therapy such as methadone or buprenorphine/naloxone. Opioid-related disorders frequently co-occur with either antisocial personality disorder or antisocial behavior, which is understandable in that people with severe opioid use disorder need vast amounts of money to obtain their drugs and may commit crimes as a result.

Approach to the Diagnosis

Opioid-related disorders have traditionally been found primarily in users of illicit opiates, but the rise in nonmedical uses of prescription opiates is striking and of great public health concern. There has been somewhat of a shift in the use of intravenous opiates because the purity of heroin sold on the street has increased to the point that intranasal use has become a common entry point for users. There has also been a shift in the rates of opioid-related disorders from prescription opiates because the prescribing of high-potency opiates such as oxycodone and methadone has increased for non-cancer pain, chronic or otherwise. Therefore, young opiate users and older individuals who have been prescribed opiates for pain may develop opioid-related disorders without intravenous use. Unspecified opioid-related disorder can be diagnosed when an individual presents with symptoms characteristic of an opioid-related disorder that cause significant distress or functional impairment; however, the symptoms do not meet the full criteria for any specific opioid-related disorder.

The approach to different populations must consider at what point the use began (i.e., during adolescence or adulthood), whether users have other substance-related disorders, whether there are comorbid psychiatric illnesses, and whether there are co-occurring medical conditions involving pain. The hallmark of all these opioid-related disorders is the daily use of opiates, with significant periods of withdrawal and cue-conditioned use, often related to reducing symptoms of withdrawal but also related to drug craving.

Although users typically mask or hide their use, if they are not forthcoming it should not be seen as a sign of either severity or lack of willingness to engage in treatment. Questioners should pay close attention to their own responses to patients, maintaining a neutral and nonjudgmental stance. Even doing so may not allow a person to discuss freely his or her use because it is typical for individuals to expect a critical response from clinicians. Clinicians can use the principles of both Screening, Brief Intervention, and Referral to Treatment (Substance Abuse and Mental Health Services Administration 2000) and motivational interviewing (Miller and Rollnick 2013) to allow for more accurate data gathering during initial and subsequent interviews.

As stated in DSM-5, "Opioid use disorder is associated with a heightened risk for suicide attempts and completed suicides. Particularly notable are both accidental and deliberate opioid overdoses. Some suicide risk factors overlap with risk factors for an opioid use disorder. In addition, repeated opioid intoxication or withdrawal may be associated with severe depressions that, although temporary, can be intense enough to lead to suicide attempts and completed suicides. Available data suggest that nonfatal accidental opioid overdose (which is common) and attempted suicide are distinct clinically significant problems that should not be mistaken for each other" (p. 544).

Getting the History

Interviewer: When did you begin using opiates?
Patient (age 42 years): Probably when I was 20. I had some friends who got some Oxys [oxycodone tablets], and I started using them.
Interviewer: How much were you using at that time?
Patient: On the weekends with friends.
Interviewer: Were opiates the first drugs you used?
Patient: No, I used to drink in high school, mostly on weekends, and also would smoke pot.
Interviewer: How much oxycodone were you using at that time?
Patient: Just here and there. If I could get a few pills, I would. I wasn't buying them at first, but when I took them I felt like the person I was supposed to be, so I started buying them.
Interviewer: When did your drug use increase?
Patient: Kind of right away. The Oxys were so expensive, and someone I knew had heroin, so I started smoking during the day before classes.
Interviewer: When was the first time you tried to stop?
Patient: Just a few months after I started, but I would get sick—you know, like having the flu, cramps, feeling really like crap—so I would just use.
Interviewer: How much time do you spend getting and using opiates?
Patient: I pretty much plan my day around it, where I'm going to use it.
Interviewer: Have you ever tried to cut back, and how did that work?
Patient: Sometimes I used to slow down by getting some methadone or maybe Suboxone (buprenorphine/naloxone), but I always start again.
Interviewer: Have you been able to stop completely?
Patient: This is really the first time. I was taking Suboxone once but stopped going for my prescriptions, but now that I'm taking methadone I really don't feel like using.

In getting a history of opioid-related disorders, the clinician needs to obtain a history not only of the symptoms associated with use, but also of the course of treatment and attempts to stop using. Individuals who are not presenting for addiction treatment directly are likely to speak about their use in a way that minimizes the negative reaction they expect from clinicians. It is important to evaluate the symptoms and behaviors associated with use and relapse to use, paying particular attention to the cue-conditioned behaviors, whether they are hedonically driven or driven by the avoidance of negative effects common in withdrawal.

Co-occurring psychiatric conditions are common and should be evaluated concurrently. Individuals with opioid-related disorders frequently have other substance-related disorders, and these should also be evaluated concurrently in any such person.

Tips for Clarifying the Diagnosis

- Determine answers to the following questions: Is the use of opiates causing clinically significant impairment in the individual's ability to function? Has it impaired his or her ability to perform at work or school? Has it negatively affected interpersonal relationships?
- Question whether the individual has made unsuccessful attempts to cut back his or her use.
- Assess whether there is evidence of a need for increased use of opiates in order to produce the same effects (tolerance).
- Explore whether the individual has physical symptoms of withdrawal when reducing or stopping the use of opiates.
- Question whether the individual has persistent craving for opiates after use has stopped.
- Determine whether other substance-related disorders are co-occurring.

Consider the Case

A 46-year-old woman, Ms. Lark, with no past psychiatric or substance use disorder history other than a tobacco-related disorder, presents upon referral from her primary care provider after she had run out of her opiate pain medication prescription early. She had been well until 1 year prior, when she fractured her tibia and fibula and required open reduction and internal fixation. She had a difficult postoperative course and complained of ongoing pain. She was prescribed opiate pain medication through her recovery. Her doses continued to be increased after she began ambulating and her casts and splints had been discontinued. Over months Ms. Lark continued to complain of worsening pain and went on extended leave from her position in the accounting department of a manufacturing firm. Her primary care provider continued to increase her dose of opiates and prescribed a second course of physical therapy. Several months before, Ms. Lark reported taking additional opiates after physical therapy "because the pain was so bad" and because she "couldn't function without it." One month she reported that her pills spilled in the bathroom sink and she lost most of them because they got wet and went down the drain. The primary care provider told her that she could not refill any more prescriptions after that, but this month she called 2 weeks before her refill was due, stating that after a dinner party at her home her prescription bottle was empty. Therefore, the referral was made.

Most of the diversion and nonmedical use of prescription opiates is through opiate pain medication legitimately prescribed to patients, or their relatives or friends, rather than through "doctor shopping." In spite of this, many people are able to get more opiates than they were originally prescribed and for longer periods from their prescribers. It is important in the evaluation and treatment of such patients to focus on both their pain (which needs to be adequately addressed) and aspects of their use that is maladaptive. In this case, it is important to be aware of the concerns women have in seeking treatment. While in general opiate use is more prevalent in males, with a ratio of 1.5:1 in prescription opiate use disorder and 3:1 in heroin use disorder, there is evidence that female adolescents may have a higher likelihood of developing opioid use disorder.

Differential Diagnosis

The differential diagnosis of opioid-related disorders includes consideration of the following:

- **Opioid use disorder:** opioid-induced mental disorders (e.g., persistent depressive disorder [dysthymia]); other substance intoxication (e.g., alcohol intoxication; sedative, hypnotic, or anxiolytic intoxication); other withdrawal disorders (e.g., sedative-hypnotic withdrawal)
- **Opioid intoxication:** other substance intoxication (e.g., alcohol intoxication, sedative-hypnotic intoxication); other opioid-related disorders
- **Opioid withdrawal:** other withdrawal disorders (e.g., sedative-hypnotic withdrawal; anxiolytic withdrawal); other substance intoxication (e.g., hallucinogen intoxication, stimulant intoxication); opioid-induced mental disorders (e.g., opioid-induced depressive disorder, with onset during withdrawal)
- **Unspecified opioid-related disorder**

Opioid-induced mental disorders may be characterized by symptoms (e.g., depressed mood) that resemble primary mental disorders (e.g., persistent depressive disorder [dysthymia] vs. opioid-induced depressive disorder, with onset during intoxication). Opioids are less likely to produce symptoms of mental disturbance than are most other drugs of abuse. Opioid intoxication and opioid withdrawal are distinguished from the opioid-induced mental disorders (e.g., opioid-induced depressive disorder, with onset during intoxication) because the symptoms in these latter disorders are in excess of those usually associated with opioid intoxication or opioid withdrawal and are severe enough to warrant independent clinical attention.

Alcohol intoxication and sedative, hypnotic, or anxiolytic intoxication can cause a clinical picture that resembles that for opioid intoxication. A diagnosis of alcohol or sedative, hypnotic, or anxiolytic intoxication can usually be made based on absence of pupillary constriction or the lack of response to a naloxone challenge. In some cases, intoxication may be due both to opioids and to alcohol or other sedatives. In these cases, the naloxone challenge will not reverse all of the sedative effects.

The anxiety and restlessness associated with opioid withdrawal resemble symptoms seen in sedative-hypnotic withdrawal. However, opioid withdrawal is also accompanied by rhinorrhea, lacrimation, and pupillary dilation, which are not seen in sedative-type withdrawal. Dilated pupils are also seen in hallucinogen intoxication and stimulant intoxication. However, other signs or symptoms of opioid withdrawal, such as nausea, vomiting, diarrhea, abdominal cramps, rhinorrhea, or lacrimation, are not present.

See DSM-5 for additional disorders to consider in the differential diagnosis. Also refer to the discussions of comorbidity and differential diagnosis in their respective sections of DSM-5.

Summary

- Opioid-related disorders typically are associated with physiological dependence.
- Co-occurring legal problems and antisocial personality disorder are common among opioid users, especially among intravenous users.
- Opioid use disorder is often associated with other substance-related disorders, especially those involving alcohol, marijuana, stimulants, and benzodiazepines, which are often taken to reduce symptoms of opioid withdrawal or craving for opiates, or to enhance the effects of administered opiates.
- Cue-associated conditioned use is common, is associated with relapse and recurrence, and frequently persists long after cessation of use.

IN-DEPTH DIAGNOSIS

Stimulant-Related Disorders

A 36-year-old man, Mr. Wilson, comes to the clinic after getting into an accident during his job as a truck driver. Drug testing revealed he had been using methamphetamine, and his union suggested that he should get treatment. During the course of the interview, he says that he began taking stimulants in his early 20s, when he was driving a beer truck and making deliveries. He states that he was "burning the candle at both ends," trying to party and have fun but also trying to keep his job, which required long hours at times. He states that recently he has occasionally shot up, but typically he just pops pills. Mr. Wilson reports that in between truck routes (and meth use), he crashes "hard," often feeling down and irritable. He states that he has never really maintained a long-term relationship with anyone but that he likes to engage in sexual activity when using and is concerned that he may have acquired a sexually transmitted infection. He relates that he has always been anxious and describes panic attacks since childhood.

This case highlights the more prolonged course of tolerance and withdrawal associated with oral use of stimulants. Over time, tolerance occurs and use escalates. In addition, Mr. Wilson describes some of the typical patterns of withdrawal, including depressive symptoms and irritability. His use occurs in binges, coinciding with his truck driving. Engaging in unprotected sex and the transmission of infection are frequently associated with use, in particular intravenous use. Frequently, histories associated with panic attacks and anxiety symptoms are seen in individuals with stimulant-related disorders.

Approach to the Diagnosis

Stimulant-related disorders involve the use of cocaine and amphetamine-type stimulants. Both naturally derived stimulants and synthetic stimulants can produce stimulant-related disorders. This disorder group also covers amphetamine-type stimulants that are structurally different from amphetamines but have similar modes of action, such as methylphenidate and newer synthetic stimulants known as "bath salts" (e.g., mephedrone and methylone). Unspecified stimulant-related disorder can be diagnosed in cases in which symptoms characteristic of a stimulant-related disorder cause significant distress or functional impairment but do not meet the full criteria for any specific stimulant-related disorder.

Largely, the clinical presentation of amphetamine-type stimulants is very similar to that of cocaine; however, they do not contain the localized analgesic properties of cocaine and therefore may result in less risk for inducing certain medical conditions than cocaine does. The psychoactive effects of amphetamine-like substances last longer than those of cocaine, and the effects on the peripheral sympathetic nervous system may be more potent, leading to fewer incidences of use than with cocaine over a fixed period of time. Amphetamine-type stimulants may be prescribed for the treatment of attention-deficit/hyperactivity disorder, narcolepsy, and other disorders.

Stimulant-related disorders can develop over very short periods of time, even in less than a week, because of their strong euphoric effects. Tolerance occurs with repeated use, and withdrawal symptoms include hypersomnia, increased appetite, and dysphoric mood. These symptoms enhance cravings and increase the likelihood of relapse. Use may be chronic or episodic. Aggressive or violent behavior is associated with stimulant use disorder, in particular when high doses are smoked, ingested, or used intravenously. Individuals can present with intense anxiety, resembling panic disorder or generalized anxiety disorder, as well as paranoid ideation and psychotic episodes resembling schizophrenia.

Stimulants can produce rapid and potent effects on the central nervous system, producing instant feelings of well-being, confidence, and euphoria. Individuals may spend large amounts of money and engage in criminal activities to obtain stimulants. Erratic behavior, social isolation, and sexual dysfunction are often long-term sequelae of stimulant-related disorders.

Acute intoxication from high dosages of stimulants may manifest in rambling speech, headaches, transient ideas of reference, and tinnitus. Individuals may also present with paranoid ideation, auditory hallucinations, and tactile hallucinations, which they typically recognize as part of the effects of the stimulants. Individuals may present with extreme anger, threats, or acting-out behavior. Mood changes include depression, suicidal ideation, anhedonia, and emotional lability. Disturbances in attention and concentration are also common. These disturbances in mood and cognitive functioning usually resolve within hours to days after cessation of use; however, they can persist for up to a month.

Withdrawal occurs after the cessation or reduction in use of stimulants and may be characterized by fatigue, vivid/unpleasant dreams, insomnia or hypersomnia, increased appetite, and psychomotor agitation or retardation. The substance from which the person is withdrawing should be specified, be it cocaine, amphetamine, or another stimulant.

Individuals with stimulant use disorder often develop conditioned responses to drug-related stimuli (e.g., seeing a pill bottle), which often play a role in relapse and are particularly difficult to extinguish.

As stated in DSM-5, "Depressive symptoms with suicidal ideation or behavior can occur and are generally the most serious problems seen during 'crashing' or other forms of stimulant withdrawal" (p. 570).

Getting the History

Interviewer: When did you begin using stimulants?
Patient (age 38 years): I was 18.
Interviewer: How much were you using at that time?
Patient: Not much, just for tests and stuff.
Interviewer: When did your stimulant use increase?
Patient: While I was in college. At first I was using just to get my homework done, but then my buddies and I started snorting cocaine. I dropped out of school and started selling to keep up with my habit, eventually switching to shooting up because it was cheaper and easier to get my hands on.
Interviewer: How much/how often do you currently use?
Patient: Every couple of days or so.
Interviewer: Have you noticed that you need to use more in order to feel the same effects?
Patient: Yes.
Interviewer: How much time do you spend obtaining, using, and recovering from the use of stimulants?
Patient: I'm mostly always using or recovering; I'll go on a bender every couple of days and then mostly feel miserable the next couple of days.
Interviewer: Have you ever used stimulants in a physically dangerous situation?
Patient: Yes. I'll pick up women when I'm using, and I have had a lot of unprotected sex with people I don't know much about.
Interviewer: Do you feel the need to cut back on your use?
Patient: That's why I'm here.
Interviewer: Have you ever tried to cut back, and how did that work?
Patient: A few times, but I always start again.
Interviewer: When you have tried to stop using, what happened?
Patient: I get really down; I'll even get tearful sometimes. I can't focus on anything. I'm a mess.
Interviewer: Has using gotten in the way of work or relationships?
Patient: Seriously? I dropped out of school, I can't work, I'm homeless; the list goes on.
Interviewer: So you feel stimulants have led to negative consequences but you still use them?
Patient: I can't stop.

This interview highlights the key diagnostic criteria for stimulant-related disorders. Initial questions elicit necessary information regarding age at onset, volume consumed, and tolerance (determined by inquiring about the need for more stimulants to produce the same effects over time). Symptoms of withdrawal are determined by inquiring about signs and symptoms when stimulant consumption is reduced or the individual has tried to stop using. Information is also obtained about the amount of time spent consuming, obtaining, and recovering from the effects of stimulants. The interviewer also inquires about whether the individual experiences cravings for stimulants and has made unsuccessful attempts to reduce or stop use. In addition, the interviewer asks about whether the individual has used stimulants in hazardous situations. Finally, the interviewer inquires about the negative consequences of stimulant consumption and continued use despite awareness of these consequences. Ambivalence regarding stopping use is a common experience of those with stimulant-related disorders because the sequelae of tolerance and withdrawal can occur particularly rapidly in those who snort or use intravenously, and attempts to stop may have resulted in intense physiological discomfort associated with withdrawal.

Tips for Clarifying the Diagnosis

- Determine answers to the following questions: Is the use of stimulants causing clinically significant impairment in the individual's ability to function? Has it impaired his or her ability to perform at work or school? Has it negatively affected interpersonal relationships?
- Ask whether the individual has made unsuccessful attempts to cut back the volume of his or her stimulant use.
- Establish whether the individual requires increased consumption of stimulants to produce the same effects (tolerance).
- Question whether the individual has engaged in physically hazardous activities while using stimulants.
- Consider whether the individual presents with intense anxiety resembling panic disorder or generalized anxiety disorder, or with paranoid ideation and psychotic episodes resembling schizophrenia.

Consider the Case

A 31-year-old man, Mr. Rose, presents to the emergency department with paranoia and reports of hearing voices. He states that he has been walking for several days, trying to get away from the individuals who are after him. He reports that he feels safe in the hospital, although he is fearful that "they" may infiltrate the system. He calms slightly with reassurance that the hospital police force will not allow anyone to interfere with his treatment. He says that he began using drugs, including cannabis and methamphetamine, in junior high school and remembers people being out to get him over the past decade or so; he describes never staying in one place for very long in order to stay safe. He presents as tangential, appearing paranoid and internally preoccupied, telling a rambling narrative interlaced with ideas of reference concerning intricate conspiracies regarding why he was taken to this hospital and devices that are monitoring his movements. At times he becomes agitated and labile during the course of the interview. He describes his belief that thoughts and voices can be inserted into his head through computers and various appliances. His symptoms do not remit over the course of several weeks.

This case may represent stimulant-induced psychotic disorder, one of the most severe instances of stimulant toxicity, although the persistence of Mr. Rose's symptoms makes it difficult to know whether they actually result from a primary psychotic disorder. Individuals with stimulant-induced psychotic disorder may present with delusions and hallucinations that resemble schizophrenia. This man exhibits paranoia, and he describes fixed beliefs that individuals are funneling thoughts and voices into his head through household items and that others are out to get him and are monitoring him. These symptoms typically remit over time; if they do not, a psychotic disorder diagnosis is warranted. At this point, there is no definitive way to determine whether Mr. Rose's persistent psychotic symptoms are substance induced or due to a primary psychotic disorder.

Although this case may represent the typical presentation of acute intoxication, including rambling speech, emotional lability, agitation, and ideas of reference, the persistence of the psychotic symptoms lead to concerns that Mr. Rose has a psychotic disorder instead. In the case of stimulant intoxication, the severity of the intoxication symptoms exceeds those of stimulant-induced psychotic disorder and indicates separate diagnostic consideration.

Differential Diagnosis of Stimulant-Related Disorders

The differential diagnosis of stimulant-related disorders includes consideration of the following:

- **Stimulant use disorder:** primary mental disorders (e.g., schizophrenia, depressive and bipolar disorders, generalized anxiety disorder, panic disorder); phencyclidine intoxication; stimulant intoxication and withdrawal
- **Stimulant intoxication:** stimulant-induced mental disorders (e.g., stimulant-induced depressive disorder, psychotic disorder); other mental disorders
- **Stimulant withdrawal:** stimulant use disorder and stimulant-induced mental disorders (e.g., stimulant-induced intoxication delirium, stimulant-induced depressive disorder, stimulant-induced bipolar disorder, stimulant-induced anxiety disorder)
- **Unspecified stimulant-related disorder**

Individuals can present with intense anxiety resembling panic disorder or generalized anxiety disorder, which can be particularly tricky in the context of stimulant-related disorders because individuals who develop these disorders frequently also have histories of repeated panic attacks, social phobias, and generalized anxiety. Getting an accurate timeline can be particularly important, and collateral information may be essential. Urine screening in the context of acute intoxication can also be helpful because individuals may present with paranoid ideation and psychotic episodes resembling schizophrenia.

Furthermore, individuals with stimulant use disorder often have transient depressive symptoms that meet criteria for major depressive disorder. Again, it is important to establish whether these symptoms occur outside the context of use and recovery from stimulants.

In extreme cases, individuals can present with stimulant-induced psychotic disorder, with delusions and hallucinations and resembling the features of schizophrenia. When symptoms persist long after expected from intoxication, a psychotic disorder should be diagnosed.

See DSM-5 for additional disorders to consider in the differential diagnosis. Also refer to the discussions of comorbidity and differential diagnosis in their respective sections of DSM-5.

Summary

- Individuals may begin stimulant use to lose weight or to improve performance in school, work, or athletics.
- Stimulant use disorder develops rapidly when the mode of administration involves intravenous use or smoking and progresses over the course of weeks to months. Oral usage typically results in a slower trajectory (months to years).
- The large majority of individuals who present for treatment of stimulant use disorder administer via smoking (66%) rather than injecting (18%) or snorting (10%).
- Individuals tend to stop using stimulants after 8–10 years, which may be associated with the mental and physical sequelae of long-term use.
- Individuals use episodically or daily. Binges are a form of use in which high dosages are consumed over a period of hours or days. This usage pattern is typically associated with physical dependence. Binges often terminate when the supply of stimulants is depleted.
- Stimulant-related disorders can develop over very short periods of time, even in less than a week, due to their strong euphoric effects. Tolerance occurs with repeated use, and withdrawal symptoms include hypersomnia, increased appetite, and dysphoric mood. These symptoms enhance cravings and increase the likelihood of relapse.

IN-DEPTH DIAGNOSIS
Tobacco-Related Disorders

A 46-year-old man, Mr. Tam, presents with a 33-year history of smoking and is currently smoking one-and-a-half packs of cigarettes per day. He reports beginning smoking at age 13, with daily smoking by age 15. By age 18 he was smoking a pack a day. He has made four or five previous attempts to quit smoking (with abstinence for at least 1 day), with the longest period of abstinence lasting 9 months. He had tried to use a nicotine replacement patch on two of those occasions but had a local reaction to it and stopped each time after 3 or 4 days. He was once prescribed bupropion 300 mg/day, but he took it for only 2 months, stating that he "hates pills" and wanted to quit on his own.

He reports that he currently begins smoking as soon as he wakes up ("even before I go to the bathroom") and that his first cigarette of the day is the most enjoyable. He leaves his building at work to smoke outdoors, and when he cannot smoke for more than an hour or two, he becomes "really irritable—like little things can set me off." He feels that he needs to smoke to "deal with the anxiety" but remains concerned about his health and is interested in cutting down.

Most smokers begin before they are age 18, but few people who begin smoking after age 21 develop physiological dependence and have difficulty stopping. Many smokers make multiple attempts to stop, either with or without pharmacological treatment, and recurrence is common. Smokers who report smoking within 30 minutes of awakening are more likely to have a severe disorder and more difficulty stopping. It is important to distinguish between withdrawal symptoms and those of a primary anxiety or mood disorder.

Approach to the Diagnosis

Aside from the overlap of tobacco withdrawal symptoms with other substance withdrawal and psychiatric symptoms, the diagnosis of tobacco-related disorders is rather
straightforward. Contrary to general beliefs, adolescents frequently exhibit symptoms of
withdrawal, even without a history of long-term use, so withdrawal is not limited to
long-term tobacco users. Nondaily use, which accounts for 20% of cigarette smoking in
the United States, is infrequently associated with physiological dependence and usually
will not be associated with a tobacco use disorder. Unspecified tobacco-related disorder
can be diagnosed when an individual presents with symptoms characteristic of a tobacco-
related disorder that cause significant distress or functional impairment; however, the
symptoms do not meet the full criteria for any specific tobacco-related disorder.

The comorbidity of psychiatric conditions in smokers is widespread and may
mimic the symptoms of withdrawal, so any diagnostic evaluation of tobacco users
must include evaluation of past and current psychiatric conditions. Many smokers,
for instance, mistake the symptoms of withdrawal for those of anxiety or depression,
but at the same time, symptoms of anxiety and depression may make individuals less
likely to attempt to stop smoking or more likely to relapse if they do. Evaluating the
temporal relationship between symptoms and cessation of smoking (even if it was
only hours before) and the severity of withdrawal is important.

Getting the History

> Interviewer: When did you begin smoking cigarettes?
> Patient (age 54 years): When I was 14.
> Interviewer: How much were you smoking at that time?
> Patient: At first I just started taking cigarettes from my dad, but then I started hanging
> out and smoking with friends after school. Not every day, anyway.
> Interviewer: When did your smoking increase?
> Patient: By the time I was in high school, like a junior or something, I was smoking ev-
> ery day. I could buy them myself, so it wasn't a problem.
> Interviewer: How much do you currently smoke?
> Patient: Less than a pack a day, maybe 5 packs a week. Last year it was 2 packs a day,
> but I have cut down.
> Interviewer: Have you tried to completely stop?
> Patient: Yes, a few times. Once I made it a week, but the other times I started again in
> a day or two.
> Interviewer: When you try to stop smoking, what happens?
> Patient: I have trouble sleeping and am a total bear. In fact, if I have to do something
> for more than a few hours when I can't smoke, I start to get bad—like anxious and
> irritable—and my first priority is to get a smoke.
> Interviewer: So you feel that smoking has led to negative consequences, but you still
> smoke?
> Patient: Sometimes I want to stop, but at this point I can't see stopping with everything
> I have going on.

The interviewer should obtain a sense of the longitudinal history of use, including
when use started, the pattern of use over time, the involvement of symptoms of craving
and withdrawal, and attempts to stop smoking. Daily smokers are frequently unable to

stop smoking in large part because of persistent withdrawal and craving. Early use in life predicts the severity of use later, and the severity of withdrawal predicts inability to stop. Many people with tobacco-related disorders have already made multiple attempts to quit and will continue to make attempts to do so in the future; approximately half of daily smokers, for instance, ultimately attain long-term abstinence.

Tips for Clarifying the Diagnosis

- Establish when the individual first started smoking.
- Discuss whether the individual has made attempts to stop.
- Question whether the individual smokes within 30 minutes of awakening, which is often associated with significant difficulty stopping.
- Evaluate for co-occurring psychiatric conditions, which commonly occur.
- Carefully determine the severity of withdrawal.

Consider the Case

A 59-year-old woman, Ms. Schneider, reports smoking 10 cigarettes a day, although the number has been increasing over the past year since she began smoking again. She had smoked two packs per day for many years, but 2 years prior she was diagnosed with non–small cell carcinoma of the lung and had a successful resection of her right lower lobe with no mediastinal involvement. She was able to stop smoking after her surgery but eventually began smoking "a few cigarettes a day." She was prescribed varenicline, which she continued for 4 months until her insurance company denied her further treatment, and she decided not to pay for it out of pocket. Two months later she began smoking again and made several attempts to stop, being unable to do so for more than a day. She reports that she wants to smoke more than she currently is but knows that it is "bad" for her and is limiting herself to half a pack a day. She is concerned that her smoking will continue to increase in spite of her setting this limit.

Smoking affects men somewhat more than women, but in this case a woman with a severe disorder has relapsed in spite of the past health consequences of her use and her strong desire to not smoke. It is typical that smokers who stop using continue to have cravings for nicotine long after they are abstinent and may remain at risk of relapse for years.

Differential Diagnosis

The symptoms of tobacco withdrawal overlap with those of other substance withdrawal syndromes (e.g., alcohol withdrawal, caffeine withdrawal); caffeine intoxication; anxiety disorders, such as panic disorder or generalized anxiety disorder; depressive disorders; bipolar disorders; sleep disorders; and medication-induced akathisia. Voluntary smoking cessation or admission to smoke-free inpatient units can induce withdrawal symptoms that mimic, intensify, or disguise other diagnoses or adverse effects of psychiatric medications; for example, irritability thought due to alcohol withdrawal could be due to tobacco withdrawal.

See DSM-5 for additional disorders to consider in the differential diagnosis. Also refer to the discussions of comorbidity and differential diagnosis in their respective sections of DSM-5.

Summary

- Tobacco-related disorders generally begin in adolescence.
- Frequent failed attempts to stop are a hallmark of tobacco use disorder.
- An intoxication syndrome does not apply to tobacco; however, withdrawal is common, and its severity is important to assess.
- Many tobacco users have tobacco-related physical symptoms or diseases and continue to smoke.
- Tobacco withdrawal usually has an onset within 24 hours of stopping or cutting down on tobacco use, peaks at 2–3 days after abstinence, and lasts 2–3 weeks.
- Craving persists long after use has ceased and contributes to recurrences.

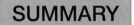

Substance-Related and Addictive Disorders

The hallmark of substance-related and addictive disorders is that they arise out of a disruption of the normal reward circuitry of the brain. The reward system is usually activated by natural rewards such as food or sex, but addictive substances and behaviors produce a more intense activation such that normal activities may be neglected.

The substance-related and addictive disorders include difficulties associated with 10 classes of drugs (alcohol; caffeine; cannabis; hallucinogens [including phencyclidine]; inhalants; opioids; sedatives, hypnotics, and anxiolytics; stimulants; tobacco; and other [or unknown] substances) and gambling. This category of disorders includes both substance use disorders and substance-induced disorders (intoxication, withdrawal, and substance/medication-induced mental disorders included elsewhere in DSM-5, such as substance-induced psychotic disorder or substance-induced depressive disorder). Many substances can cause substance-induced mental disorders that resemble other diagnoses, with the caveat that typically substance-induced symptoms only last temporarily.

Alcohol-related disorders are the most prevalent of the substance-related and addictive disorders in the United States. Individuals who present for treatment are often among those with the most severe alcohol-related problems. Most individuals have a relatively promising prognosis, with rates of abstinence 1 year following treatment varying from 45% to 65%.

Cannabinoids, typically in the form of marijuana, are the most widely used illicit psychoactive substances in the United States. The abrupt cessation of daily use often results in cannabis withdrawal syndrome, which includes symptoms of irritability, anger, anxiety, depressed mood, restlessness, sleep difficulty, and decreased appetite or weight loss.

Opioid-related disorders typically are associated with physiological dependence. Cue-associated conditioned use is common and associated with relapse and recurrence, and it frequently persists long after cessation of use.

Stimulant-related disorders develop rapidly when the mode of administration involves intravenous use or inhalation and progresses over the course of weeks to months. Oral usage typically results in a slower trajectory (months to years).

Tobacco-related disorders generally begin in adolescence, and frequent failed attempts to stop are a hallmark of tobacco use disorder. An intoxication syndrome is rare among these disorders, but withdrawal is common and its severity is important to assess. Craving persists long after use has ceased and contributes to recurrent use.

Although the term *dependence* has been removed from this diagnostic class to avoid overlap with pharmacological tolerance and withdrawal, it is important to highlight the physiological aspect of these disorders and to understand that the behavioral patterns associated with substance-related and addictive disorders develop as a result of alterations in reward pathways—both negative and positive rewards—and that individuals with substance-related and addictive disorders are typically in a cycle of relapse and recovery.

Symptoms of withdrawal and tolerance can occur during medical treatment involving prescription drugs such as opioids, benzodiazepines, and antidepressants. Tolerance and withdrawal are normal physiological responses to repeated doses of substances but do not, in and of themselves, represent a disorder of the brain's reward system. However, tolerance and withdrawal can be important physiological signs of the severity of a substance use disorder; for example, when prescription medications are used in excess of what is prescribed or for nonmedical reasons, and when other symptoms are present, substance use disorder can be diagnosed.

Diagnostic Pearls

- Tolerance and withdrawal can be important pharmacological signs of the severity of a substance use disorder.

- When tolerance and withdrawal occur during the course of medical treatment, they should not be counted toward the diagnosis of a substance-related or addictive disorder; however, when prescriptive medications are used inappropriately or in excess of what is prescribed and other symptoms are present, such a diagnosis can be made.

- Behaviors associated with substance-related and addictive disorders can often be mistakenly viewed as volitional or manipulative; however, these behavioral patterns result from alterations in reward pathways and are often tied to physiological dependence and logical sequelae of the disorders themselves.

- Symptoms associated with substance-related and addictive disorders may meet criteria for other disorders; however, these symptoms are typically transient (e.g., hallucinations associated with stimulant intoxication or anxiety associated with alcohol withdrawal).

- Many individuals use substances in various contexts; however, it is important to establish the relationship of substance use to functionally significant impairment in order to merit a diagnosis of substance use disorder.

Self-Assessment

Key Concepts: Double-Check Your Knowledge

What is the relevance of the following concepts to the various substance-related and addictive disorders?

- Factors contributing to relapse
- Nonproblematic usage
- Cue association
- Episodic versus chronic use
- Binges
- Tolerance and withdrawal
- Substance use disorders versus substance-induced disorders
- Functional consequences

Questions to Discuss With Colleagues and Mentors

1. How might an individual's cultural background affect the history obtained from him or her of a substance use disorder?
2. How do gender and cultural factors influence the recognition of symptoms in disorders of addiction?
3. How might marijuana use affect psychosocial functioning?
4. How might the co-occurrence of posttraumatic stress disorder affect making a diagnosis of substance-related and addictive disorders?
5. How do the course and associated features of substance use disorders contribute to a cyclical pattern of use and dependence?
6. When symptoms manifest in the context of acute intoxication, what is typically their course?

Case-Based Questions

PART A

Ms. Forsythe is a 43-year-old woman with bipolar I disorder, who is referred for outpatient evaluation and treatment. She was recently hospitalized for 10 days for a manic episode in the context of intermittent adherence to her complex medication regimen. During her hospitalization, she developed increasing agitation and bizarre behavior with unstable vital signs and ultimately was diagnosed with alcohol withdrawal and treated with benzodiazepines. Her mania abated as her medications were reinstituted.

Ms. Forsythe reports that since discharge she has been taking her medications as prescribed, stating, "That last time really scared me, but I still have my glass of Chardonnay every evening. It's really not something I can see giving up." She reports that her mood is "fine" and that she has no thoughts of self-harm or suicidal thoughts.

What are the diagnostic issues in this case? What are the most important principles to consider in evaluation?   Ms. Forsythe has a lifelong mood disorder and was admitted to hospital treatment for mania and was subsequently found to be in alcohol withdrawal. Consideration must be given to the role of alcohol in the development of the mood disorder and a determination made about whether the mood episode was substance induced. It is unlikely in this case, even though Ms. Forsythe's mania was temporally related to her alcohol use, because there is sufficient information to determine that she has bipolar I disorder and that her lack of medication adherence was more likely the proximate cause of her relapse. Further information needs to be gathered—even in the context of what appears to be well-documented alcohol withdrawal—to accurately diagnose the extent of her alcohol use disorder.

PART B

> Ms. Forsythe currently smokes between a half and a full pack of cigarettes a day, having started smoking in her teens. She reports making three attempts to stop smoking in the past, with the longest period of abstinence from smoking lasting 7 days. She had been diagnosed with attention-deficit/hyperactivity disorder as a child and was intermittently treated with stimulants. She began using marijuana and drinking alcohol in high school. Her first episode of depression was at age 12, she believes, and she began taking antidepressants and attending psychotherapy at that time. While in her first year of college away from home, she had an episode consistent with mania that required hospitalization, but she finished that year of schooling. She then left college, moved back to her parents' home, and finally got a bachelor's degree at a local college after 6 years.
>
> In her 20s she reports binge drinking on weekends with friends, with some cannabis use, but she began drinking regularly during the evenings after she moved out of her family home. She married at age 28 and had two children, but the marriage ended when the children were young and she shares custody of them with their father. Child protective services had been involved early in the children's lives during a period when Ms. Forsythe was severely depressed, but ultimately she was found fit to parent. She moved back to her parents' house after her divorce but lost her job working at a travel agency and found herself drinking each night, up to two bottles of wine. Because her time was unstructured and her children were at school, she would begin drinking in the late morning. "It's not as if I had the shakes or anything. I just wanted to drink." Her family has made several attempts to get her to stop drinking, including 5 years earlier when she had several days of "bad anxiety," but she went to Alcoholics Anonymous only "a few times." She began drinking again, albeit "only a few glasses a day," after 3 months. She continues to use marijuana, "three joints a week," that she states she buys at a marijuana dispensary "because of my bipolar disorder."

What additional substance use disorders can now be diagnosed? What additional information would be helpful in making these diagnoses? Bipolar disorder frequently co-occurs with substance use disorders, most commonly with tobacco use disorder but also with alcohol, cannabis, and other substance use disorders. More information is available to more precisely diagnose Ms. Forsythe's alcohol use disorder, which can be done at this time, but further information may be needed to clarify the cannabis use as a disorder. The use of marijuana as medicine is growing because more states and municipalities sanction its use.

Bipolar disorder frequently co-occurs with other psychiatric disorders, including attention-deficit/hyperactivity disorder and anxiety disorders. Further information should be gathered about those disorders because they, in and of themselves, are risk factors for the development of substance use disorders.

Short-Answer Questions

1. What are the 10 classes of drugs in the DSM-5 substance-related and addictive disorders diagnostic class?
2. Many substances can cause substance-induced mental disorders that resemble primary mental disorders. What is a distinguishing factor between them in terms of course?
3. What is the typical age at onset of first alcohol intoxication?
4. By what age do the majority of individuals develop alcohol-related disorders?
5. Alcohol withdrawal is characterized by symptoms that develop approximately how long after heavy alcohol consumption?
6. What is the most widely used illicit substance in the United States?
7. How do rates of cannabis use disorder compare in males and females?
8. What are the symptoms of withdrawal associated with cannabis use disorder?
9. How do individuals typically begin using stimulants?
10. How does the method of consumption affect the course of stimulant use disorder?
11. What is the typical method of consumption of stimulants with which individuals who have stimulant use disorder present?
12. What is episodic use of stimulants?
13. What are binges?
14. When do tobacco-related disorders typically begin?
15. What is the hallmark of tobacco use disorder?
16. How common are intoxication and withdrawal in tobacco-related disorders?
17. When does tobacco withdrawal typically begin, and how long does it last?
18. How long do tobacco cravings persist?

Answers

1. The 10 classes of drugs are alcohol; caffeine; cannabis; hallucinogens (including phencyclidine); inhalants; opioids; sedatives, hypnotics, and anxiolytics; stimulants; tobacco; and other (or unknown) substances.
2. Typically, the symptoms of substance-induced mental disorders last only temporarily, in keeping with the effects of the substance (e.g., cannabis-induced anxiety disorder, with onset during intoxication vs. generalized anxiety disorder); however, substance use and other mental disorders can be comorbid.
3. Most often first alcohol intoxication occurs during the mid-teens.
4. The majority of individuals who develop alcohol-related disorders do so by their late 30s.
5. Alcohol withdrawal is characterized by symptoms that develop approximately 4–12 hours after the reduction of prolonged heavy alcohol consumption.
6. Cannabinoids are the most widely used illicit psychoactive substance in the United States.
7. Rates of cannabis use disorder are greater among adult males (2.2%) than females (0.8%) and among 12- to 17-year-old males (3.8%) than females (3.0%).

8. The abrupt cessation of daily use often results in cannabis withdrawal syndrome, which includes symptoms of irritability, anger, anxiety, depressed mood, restlessness, sleep difficulty, and decreased appetite or weight loss.

9. Individuals may begin stimulant use in an attempt to lose weight or to improve performance in school, work, or athletics.

10. Stimulant use disorder develops rapidly when the mode of administration involves intravenous use or smoking and progresses over the course of weeks to months. Oral usage typically results in a slower trajectory (months to years).

11. The large majority of individuals who present for treatment of stimulant use disorder administer the stimulant via smoking rather than injecting or snorting.

12. Episodic use of stimulants is separated by 2 or more days of nonuse.

13. Binges are a form of use in which high dosages are consumed over a period of hours or days.

14. Tobacco-related disorders generally begin in adolescence.

15. Frequent failed attempts to stop are a hallmark of tobacco use disorder.

16. An intoxication syndrome does not apply to tobacco; however, withdrawal is common and its severity is important to assess.

17. Onset of tobacco withdrawal usually begins within 24 hours of an individual stopping or cutting down on tobacco use, peaks at 2–3 days after abstinence, and lasts 2–3 weeks.

18. Tobacco cravings persist long after use has ceased and contribute to recurrences.

References

Miller WR, Rollnick S: Motivational Interviewing: Helping People Change, Third Edition. New York, Guilford, 2013

Substance Abuse and Mental Health Services Administration, Office of Applied Studies: Substance Abuse Treatment in Adult and Juvenile Correctional Facilities: Findings from the Uniform Facility Data Set 1997 Survey of Correctional Facilities. Drug and Alcohol Services Information System Series: S-9 (DHHS Publ No SMA-00-3380). Rockville, MD, Substance Abuse and Mental Health Services Administration, 2000

20

Neurocognitive Disorders

Brian Yochim, Ph.D.

Maya Yutsis, Ph.D.

Allyson C. Rosen, Ph.D.

Jerome Yesavage, M.D.

"He keeps asking the same thing over and over."

"She left the stove on!"

The neurocognitive disorders diagnostic class includes disorders of acquired cognitive deficits. Although cognitive deficits may be present in many mental health conditions, only disorders whose *primary* and *core features* are of cognitive decline are included under the neurocognitive disorders (NCDs). People will self-report changes in their abilities, or if they lack awareness of them, a caregiver will report them to the clinician. Initial clinical presentation and referral can fall into one of two categories: 1) people who are developing cognitive deficits of unknown cause, for which the clinician must assess the nature, extent, and etiology of these changes; or 2) people who have known neurological injury (e.g., a traumatic brain injury [TBI] or stroke), for which the clinician must assess the effects of the damage. The individual's experience of the disorder can vary widely from complete awareness of the decline and associated distress to complete lack of awareness and consequent safety concerns (e.g., in regard to driving, cooking, living alone). In the encounter with the patient, the clinician must take care to express empathy related to this dramatic change in life circumstances, increase insight, and make appropriate referrals as needed.

The NCDs are unique in DSM-5 because their symptoms are almost entirely cognitive in expression and clearly connected to underlying neurobiological processes. With a thorough evaluation, including input from neurology, psychiatry, and neuropsychology, the clinician can reasonably and confidently establish a neurological etiology. The NCDs involve a decline in cognitive functioning from a previous state, as evidenced by 1) concerns from the individual, an informant, or the clinician; and 2) objective test performance. This evaluation differs from that for intellectual disabilities in that intellectual disabilities involves a baseline, impaired level of cognitive functioning.

There are three main syndromes of NCDs: delirium, major NCD, and mild NCD. Delirium can be thought of as a behavioral manifestation of an underlying metabolic disturbance that impairs central nervous system functioning to the extent that individuals show reductions in their basic ability to attend to the environment. These individuals will show impairment in at least one other cognitive ability, such as memory or language. Delirium differs from major and mild NCDs in that it develops rapidly (i.e., in hours or days) and can be linked to medical conditions, substance intoxication or withdrawal, or other causes. Delirium is also unique in that it can completely resolve if the underlying cause is treated. The DSM-5 criteria incorporate the reality that delirium can endure for long periods of time, and the clinician can specify whether the disturbance is acute (lasting hours or days) or persistent (lasting weeks or months). Indeed, in medically frail older adults, one condition causing delirium can be ameliorated while another condition surfaces, leading to the net effect of no change in the outward manifestation of delirium.

Major NCD was previously called *dementia* in prior versions of the DSM. That term has been replaced in DSM-5, in part to incorporate the reality that the NCDs lie on a continuum of severity, including major and mild. Major NCD typically involves severe impairment in *one* or more cognitive domains with accompanying impairment in activities of daily living. These criteria differ from the DSM-IV criteria for dementia, which required impairment in *two* or more domains. One exception to this difference is in major NCD due to Alzheimer's disease, which requires impairment in two or more domains. Mild NCD bears similarity to what is also called *mild cognitive impairment*. The difference between a major and mild NCD is twofold: 1) the cognitive deficits are more severe in major NCD (typically at or below the 3rd percentile) than in mild NCD (typically between the 3rd and 16th percentile); and 2) in major NCD the deficits must be severe enough to interfere with independence, whereas in mild NCD the deficits do not interfere with independence, although "greater effort, compensatory strategies, or accommodation" may be needed to remain independent. A key point about the NCDs is that the same etiologies cause the disorder, whether it is a major or a mild NCD.

Once it is established that a person has a major or mild NCD, the next step for the clinician is to determine the most likely etiologies. The etiology can be determined on the basis of a combination of symptom time course, cognitive domains involved, and associated medical or neurological condition. In some cases, a diagnosis of major or mild NCD depends on the presence of a known medical condition causing cognitive decline, as with the following etiologies: vascular disease, TBI, substance/medication use, HIV infection, prion disease, Parkinson's disease, and Huntington's disease. For other neurodegenerative etiologies, including Alzheimer's disease, frontotemporal lobar degeneration, and Lewy body disease, major or mild NCDs are diagnosed primarily on the basis of the presence of cognitive, behavioral, and functional symptoms. Many NCDs have multiple causes, and the diagnostician must undergo a process of ruling out various etiologies. The most common cause of NCD is Alzheimer's disease. This disease most typically causes memory dysfunction in its early stages, although deficits in other areas (e.g., executive functioning) can sometimes manifest as the first symptom. Other categories in this diagnostic class include major or mild NCD due to another medical condition, major or mild NCD due to multiple etiologies, and unspecified NCD.

Three substantial changes from DSM-IV to DSM-5 are as follows: 1) the inclusion of Lewy body disease and frontotemporal degeneration as etiologies and much greater detail provided for TBIs ("head trauma" in DSM-IV) as an etiology; 2) the differentiation between major or mild NCDs (DSM-IV had only the category of "dementia"); and 3) the replacement of the term *dementia* by the term *neurocognitive disorder*, which now encompasses causes such as TBI or stroke that may not be degenerative and that may even improve over time. A plethora of research has been conducted on mild cognitive impairment since DSM-IV was published, and the inclusion of mild NCDs permits the inclusion of this diagnostic entity. DSM-5 has become more specific in defining "cognitive impairment," providing increased guidance to clinicians. For major NCDs, cognitive test performance is "typically" at or below the 3rd percentile, whereas for mild NCDs, performance is typically between the 3rd and 16th percentiles. Descriptions of cognitive domains (e.g., complex attention, learning and memory, social cognition) are also provided. The diagnostic criteria for NCD have also changed in that visual perception is included as a possible area of impairment.

IN-DEPTH DIAGNOSIS

Delirium

Mr. Hancock, who is 90 years old, was brought by his daughter to the emergency department because he started to "ramble and moan" and could not answer questions or track conversations over the past 2 days. He also started yelling at her about taking his money away but quickly shifted to crying. He started to experience hallucinations of seeing strangers in his room who were "chasing" him. These symptoms worsened in the evening. He was sleeping a lot during the day and was awake much of the night. On admission, he was disoriented and did not know the date, the day of the week, or his address. He was found to have an acute urinary tract infection. Upon reviewing his medication regimen, the physicians found that he was taking a benzodiazepine for "nerves" and 10 other medications. They decided to taper him off the benzodiazepine and treat the urinary tract infection during a hospital stay. Throughout the hospital stay, Mr. Hancock was provided with a quiet environment at night to aid his sleep and frequent gentle reminders of the date and place, with this information written on a whiteboard next to his bed. His family placed family pictures around the room. After a week of hospitalization, his speech became understandable, he was no longer yelling at his loved ones, and he was able to state the date, his address, and the name of the hospital. Once the urinary tract infection cleared, Mr. Hancock was discharged home.

This case illustrates several key components of delirium. The symptoms developed abruptly and rapidly over a few days, which helped to differentiate delirium from other NCDs. Disorientation and unawareness of surroundings together with a change in sleep-wake cycle further indicated delirium. Mr. Hancock tended to become worse in the evening and had a rapid change from one emotional state to another, features that are common in delirium. Visual hallucinations are common, and people are often afraid of these experiences; when a person presents with a new onset of visual hallucinations and is older than age 45 years, it is important to consider a delirium process rather than attributing hallucinations to a psychotic disorder. As is common in delirium, Mr. Hancock was found to have more than one contributor to the symptoms: a urinary tract infection and a medication (a benzodiazepine) that is associated with delirium. Polypharmacy is another leading cause of delirium. The urinary tract infection was treated while he was tapered off the benzodiazepine. (Substance withdrawal, of course, is another cause of delirium, and benzodiazepines must be carefully tapered to prevent delirium.) The medical team made strong efforts to provide a quiet environment for him, with frequent reorientation and cues to dates and place to assist in his recovery. It is also helpful for family members or close ones to assist in reorienting the patient (e.g., with photos, as in this case).

Approach to the Diagnosis

Given the complex etiology of delirium, the first line of its assessment is gathering a comprehensive history and establishing a baseline of cognitive functioning. According to DSM-5, the key feature of delirium is a disturbance in attention and awareness that develops rapidly over a few hours to days and represents a change from a typical level of cognitive functioning for the patient. Impaired attention may include difficulty answering questions and/or repeating words and numbers; difficulty multitasking; becoming distracted by noises, other people, and objects in the room; and difficulty staying on the topic of conversation. Questions often need to be repeated because the person's attention wanders. The individual may provide the same answer to different questions (e.g., answering "35" to both "How old are you?" and "What is your address?"). Lack of awareness of the environment may result in disorientation to date, time, place, and even personal information such as age, marital status, or address. These difficulties may vary throughout the day and even hour to hour, with marked worsening in the evening and at night. The interviewer should assess whether a medical event (e.g., a fall, accident, surgery) may have triggered the aforementioned rapid changes in cognitive status. A physical examination should include a review of current medications, especially those added recently; symptoms of past or current systemic infections; blood work, urine analysis, and imaging to establish whether these changes are due to an underlying medical condition; metabolic issues such as renal or liver dysfunction, hypoxia, hypoglycemia, anemia, substance intoxication or withdrawal; medication use (e.g., benzodiazepines, anticholinergics, pain narcotics); or a combination of these factors. Because systemic infections, such as urinary tract infections or pneumonia, are a common etiology of delirium, special attention is paid in the history to any symptoms of infection, including changes in urinary symptoms, cough, shortness of breath, and fever.

Given that delirium often occurs in older adults with a preexisting major or mild NCD, which renders them more vulnerable to changes in cognitive status, a cognitive baseline must be established. Because the individual will likely have difficulty answering questions accurately due to impaired attention and disorientation to most personal information, a collateral source or review of outside medical records is needed to establish a cognitive baseline. Data from neuroimaging and other biomarkers can be used to establish whether mild or major NCD of a known etiology, such as Alzheimer's disease, is also present and further renders the person more vulnerable for delirium. In addition to the disturbance in attention and awareness, a change in at least one other cognitive area must occur, such as in recent memory; disorientation to time and place; language (e.g., rambling speech, mumbling); or perceptual disturbance, including visual hallucinations or misinterpretations. To assess for perceptual disturbances, the interviewer can ask, "Do you see things other people don't see?" If the answer is yes, the clinician can follow up with additional questions, such as, "Do you see animals (people, faces, strangers)? Do these figures appear threatening? What are they doing?" A collateral source should be asked whether the person has a previous diagnosis of mild or major NCD or variability in attention, alertness, and orientation to date and place and/or personal information. The collateral source should also be asked if the person frequently "stares into space" and appears more "confused" in the evening. A careful history of the time course of the illness is important to make a separation between delirium and other NCDs.

Getting the History

Mr. Hart, a 90-year-old man admitted to the emergency department, is unable to answer questions, appears lethargic most of the day, becomes easily distracted by nursing staff walking in and out of the room, and reports "seeing strangers in his room." The interviewer first determines the time and course of these symptoms by asking a family member who is present in the room a series of questions: "When did you first notice that he had difficulty answering questions? Were these issues triggered by a recent change in any medications? Has he fallen recently or developed a urinary tract infection? Does his alertness vary throughout the day?" If the symptoms vary and developed within the last day after he was diagnosed with a urinary tract infection, the interviewer may suspect delirium. The interviewer also assesses Mr. Hart's orientation to surroundings by asking him, "Can you tell me today's date? What is the name of this place? What is your name? How old are you?" If Mr. Hart knows his age and name but incorrectly states the date and the name of the place, he is considered disoriented to surroundings. Administering a subtest of the Montreal Cognitive Assessment, such as digit span, assesses attention. To assess digit span, the interviewer says, "I am going to say some numbers and when I am through, repeat them to me exactly as I said them," and reads a 5-number sequence at a rate of one digit per second. If the man repeats fewer than 3 numbers, his attention is impaired, further indicating delirium. Finally, the interviewer assesses perceptual disturbances by asking Mr. Hart, "Do you see things that others do not see?" If the answer is yes, the interviewer asks, "What do you see? Are these images scary? What are they doing?" The interviewer also asks the man's family member whether Mr. Hart has a history of perceptual disturbances, substance use, and other medical problems.

Given that the prevalence of delirium is highest among individuals ages 85 and older (14% prevalence rate per year), the man's age of 90 and the rapid onset of impaired attention should be the key indicators that a diagnosis of delirium should be high in the diagnostic differential. The man experiences rapid and abrupt onset of impaired attention (fewer than 3 digits repeated) and disorientation (he does not know the date and place) over 1 day, triggered by a diagnosis of urinary tract infection, thus meeting criteria for delirium. His level of alertness and inattention varied throughout the day, which further indicates delirium. The man also experienced a new onset of visual hallucinations without a previous history of psychosis or perceptual disturbances, which usually indicates a neurological problem or delirium, rather than a preexisting mood or psychotic disorder. The interviewer will want to find out the course and nature of visual hallucinations, because mild or major NCD with Lewy bodies can mimic delirium; it presents with fluctuations in alertness and attention as well as visual hallucinations. However, the short duration and rapid onset of these symptoms support the diagnosis of delirium. A full medical workup and medical chart review would be warranted to rule out other medical problems that may be contributing to the man's current difficulties.

Tips for Clarifying the Diagnosis

- Evaluate recent lab results.
- Review the person's medical record and current medications, especially ones that were added recently. Assess which over-the-counter medications the person may take that have sedating properties, such as diphenhydramine.
- Assess the time and duration of symptoms and clarify how quickly they developed.
- Explore whether deficits in attention and orientation vary throughout the day.
- Conduct a collateral interview to establish an accurate cognitive baseline for the individual and to verify the medical history and medications. Ask about previously diagnosed major NCDs.
- Evaluate for sensory misperceptions such as visual hallucinations and question whether the person is frightened by these experiences.

Consider the Case

Mr. Nelson is a 25-year-old man admitted to the hospital following a 10-foot fall from a ladder, resulting in mild TBI and a broken leg. His neighbor found him unconscious on the ground. On admission to the hospital, he was fully oriented to date, time, place, and personal information. He remembered falling off the ladder and "waking up in the ER," but he did not know who found him. Duration of posttraumatic amnesia was estimated to last less than 1 hour. On a brief mental status examination, he had difficulty counting backward from 100 in increments of 7 and recalling five newly learned words, indicative of memory impairment. His attention was intact, and he repeated up to 5 digits forward and 3 digits backward. He underwent surgery to stabilize his broken leg and was started on morphine postoperatively to aid with pain management. A catheter was also placed. One day following surgery, Mr. Nelson was unable to state the date and the name of the hospital and reported that strangers were "attacking" him. His attention declined significantly; he was unable to answer any questions or repeat 3 digits forward. A computed tomography scan of his head was negative. His brother informed the staff that Mr. Nelson was allergic to morphine. Upon discontinuation of morphine, Mr. Nelson's attention and orientation returned to his admission level within 3 days. He continued to have difficulty recalling new information, such as a list of five words and the names of new nursing staff and/or attending physicians.

Delirium can often be triggered by a new medical problem such as TBI, introduction of new medications, or surgery. When multiple risk factors are present, delirium is more likely to develop. In this case, Mr. Nelson suffered a mild TBI, resulting in memory difficulties for recently learned information, which is commonly associated with TBI. However, his attention was initially intact and he was aware of his surroundings. Following surgery, placement of a catheter, and initiation of an opiate pain narcotic, his attention and awareness of surroundings markedly declined overnight. He was unable to repeat more than 3 digits forward, to follow conversation, and to answer questions, which indicated impaired attention. (Someone his age should be able to repeat at least 5 digits forward and 3 backward.) Visual hallucinations of a frightening nature were also noted. His disorientation to date and place together with impaired attention indicated a major decline in cognitive status compared with his status at admission. Following the introduction of an opiate narcotic, he demonstrated an allergic reaction to morphine, which triggered an acute onset of delirium superimposed onto a recent mild TBI. Once the medication was discontinued, delirium appeared to clear within 3 days. He continued to have memory difficulties, as would be expected with mild TBI 1 week following the injury. Memory impairment due to mild TBI would be expected to resolve completely within 1–3 months.

Differential Diagnosis

The differential diagnosis of delirium is quite broad because the hallmark of delirium is rapid onset of impaired attention, reduced awareness or orientation to the environment, and decline in thinking abilities that includes, but is not limited to, deficits in memory, disorientation, language, visuospatial ability, and perception. These difficulties frequently occur in the context of most major NCDs, medical disorders, and substance/medication-induced side effects, especially postoperatively, with the latter two categories necessitating appropriate medical workup. Similarly, delirium may be seen in many psychiatric disorders (psychotic disorders including but not limited to schizophrenia, schizophreniform and brief psychotic disorders, bipolar and depressive disorders with psychotic features, acute stress disorder, malingering, factitious disorder, and substance use disorders). The most common differential diagnosis for delirium includes separating whether a person has major NCD or delirium, both delirium and NCD, or NCD without delirium. Memory problems are common to both delirium and major NCD, such as NCD due to Alzheimer's disease, but the person with only major NCD is typically oriented to personal information, such as his or her name, age, and children's names, and is aware of surroundings (e.g., hospital vs. home; city and state), and this awareness does not change over the course of the day. Psychotic disorders should also be considered in the differential diagnosis when perceptual changes are present, including visual hallucinations, delusions, or rambled speech. The rapid onset and fluctuation of these perceptual changes would be more consistent with delirium, whereas prolonged onset, chronicity, and stability of these symptoms would suggest presence of a psychotic disorder. Finally, in the absence of a medical condition or substance that is associated with rapid changes in thinking abilities, malingering and/or factitious disorder should be considered in the differential diagnosis.

Two associated features that help with the diagnosis of delirium include change in sleep-wake cycle and rapid changes in emotional states that can vary from hour to hour. Change in sleep-wake cycle may include increased and excessive daytime sleepiness and difficulty falling asleep and is often associated with but not required to make a diagnosis. Rarely, a complete reversal of sleep cycle occurs in which a person sleeps during the daytime and is awake during all nighttime hours. Rapid changes in emotional states include nervousness and anxiety and feeling afraid, depressed, irritable, angry, apathetic, or overly euphoric. Irritability and anger can include behaviors such as screaming, cursing, moaning, rambled speech, and unintelligible sounds. These changes occur rapidly and unpredictably, and they fluctuate hour to hour. Acute stress disorder and delirium can both be associated with intense feelings of fear, anxiety, and disorientation, but these symptoms are precipitated by an easily identifiable traumatic event in the case of acute stress disorder. Behavioral problems increase in the evening and nighttime with delirium, because the environmental cues of light and activity are absent.

See DSM-5 for additional disorders to consider in the differential diagnosis. Also refer to the discussions of comorbidity and differential diagnosis in their respective sections of DSM-5.

Summary

- A diagnosis of delirium should be considered when 1) a rapid and abrupt onset of disturbance in attention and disorientation is present, and 2) the alteration represents a change from the individual's cognitive baseline.
- Delirium may be due to substance use intoxication or withdrawal.
- A preexisting history of major NCD highly increases an individual's vulnerability to developing delirium.
- Delirium has diverse causes, including a wide range of general medical disorders (e.g., metabolic issues, hypoxia, hypoglycemia, systemic infections), polypharmacy (e.g., benzodiazepines, opiate narcotics, and anticholinergics), recent injury (e.g., TBI, stroke, hypoxia), and psychiatric disorders (e.g., substance use disorders, acute stress disorder, somatic symptom and related disorders, factitious disorder).

——————— **IN-DEPTH DIAGNOSIS** ———————

Major or Mild NCD Due to Alzheimer's Disease

Mr. Green is an 80-year-old man who reports that he is having difficulty finding the right word when speaking, but he attributes this to his age. His wife reports that he increasingly repeats stories to her and asks the same question several times a day. This has progressively worsened over the past year, with no clear precipitating event. His wife also reports that she has taken over managing the finances because he has made a few errors in bill payments in the last year. Upon interview, he is unable to describe current events in the news, other than making vague references to wars in parts of the world. On neuropsychological assessment, his performance on measures of memory, naming, and executive ability is at the 1st percentile as compared with adults his age. During the evaluation he makes several socially inappropriate comments but is friendly and cooperative. Complex attention and visuoperceptual ability are normal for his age and not suggestive of decline. He and his wife report that he has three or four alcoholic drinks per week but he has never been a heavy drinker. Each denies that he has any current symptoms of depression. He lost consciousness once for approximately 5 minutes about 20 years ago in a motor vehicle crash, with no other reported brain injuries. Magnetic resonance imaging (MRI) reveals cortical atrophy, with pronounced atrophy in the medial temporal lobes shown on a coronal scan, and age-appropriate white matter cerebrovascular changes. He is physically healthy with no acute infections and has no family history of neurological disease. No genetic testing has occurred.

This vignette highlights several important components of the assessment of major NCD due to Alzheimer's disease. Mr. Green himself does not express concern, whereas a knowledgeable informant, his wife, reports common symptoms relevant to this diagnosis. Clinicians may also see individuals who have concerns, whereas their caregivers lack concerns. Neuropsychological assessment shows impaired performance in two or more domains, with the typical finding of memory impairment associated with Alzheimer's disease. The deficits have interfered with Mr. Green's independence, as indicated by his wife's need to take over financial management. The timeline of progression over the past year and current health are not suggestive of delirium. Although Mr. Green has a past history of a brain injury, it seems unrelated to his current symptom presentation. MRI findings show atrophy in the areas typically affected by Alzheimer's disease but no evidence of strong cerebrovascular involvement. Information that would be additionally helpful would include whether or not he is experiencing hallucinations or parkinsonian symptoms or other features of Lewy body disease. The deficits in executive ability and mildly socially inappropriate behavior raise concerns about frontotemporal lobar degeneration, but his predominant memory deficits and his older age than that of typical people who have frontotemporal lobar degeneration are less consistent with that diagnosis. It is important to note that complex attention and visuoperceptual ability are normal for his age and not suggestive of decline, although "normal" performance for patients with a high baseline may be indicative of decline.

Approach to the Diagnosis

Assessing a person for the possibility of NCD due to Alzheimer's disease consists of gathering a clear history and obtaining some assessment of cognitive functioning, with an emphasis on memory. The diagnosis of Alzheimer's disease as the cause of NCD can be thought of as a process of ruling out other potential etiologies. Many, if not most, individuals will have more than one suspected etiology (e.g., Alzheimer's disease and vascular disease). These individuals should be diagnosed with major or mild NCD due to multiple etiologies.

Alzheimer's disease involves progressive decline, usually with no precipitating event; but sometimes symptoms, which may simply have not been apparent before, seem to be triggered by a discrete medical event (e.g., surgery, major illness, hospitalization) or a psychosocial event (e.g., major travel, major change in routine). In the interview, it is helpful to gather examples of memory problems, such as forgetting conversations, repeating things, or becoming unable to learn new skills that were previously easy to learn (e.g., how to use the new TV remote or the latest type of phone). Other symptoms that individuals or their caregivers may report include word-finding problems in conversation, getting lost, deficits in social functioning, difficulty handling multiple tasks, or other executive deficits described in DSM-5. It is essential to interview not only the individual but also a caregiver, because individuals can under- or overestimate their deficits.

Neuropsychological assessment, if available, is helpful in providing precise measurement of a person's cognitive abilities and comparing them with those of others of a similar age and education level. Neuropsychological testing can also detect mild deficits that screening tools miss. Data from neuroimaging and other biomarkers can be used to establish whether Alzheimer's disease is the underlying cause of deficits found through testing and/or interview.

Once a clinician suspects Alzheimer's disease as the cause, "probable" or "possible" must be specified. The criteria for probable Alzheimer's disease differ depending on whether the NCD is major or mild. For major NCD, probable Alzheimer's disease requires either 1) evidence of a causative Alzheimer's disease genetic mutation from family history or genetic testing, or 2) a combination of clear decline in memory and one other cognitive domain; progressive, gradual decline in cognition; and absence of other possible etiology. If neither of these criteria are met, possible Alzheimer's disease is diagnosed. Other biomarkers of Alzheimer's disease (e.g., neuroimaging) are not included at this time. For mild NCD, probable Alzheimer's disease is diagnosed only if there is evidence of a causative Alzheimer's genetic mutation. Possible Alzheimer's disease is diagnosed for mild NCD when there is no evidence of a causative Alzheimer's disease genetic mutation but the other clinical criteria are met.

Lastly, there are two factors to consider in differentiating major and mild NCD related to Alzheimer's disease. Although the general criteria for major NCD involve decline in *one* or more cognitive domains, the criteria for major NCD due to Alzheimer's disease require impairment of *two* domains. This is the only NCD category in which the major specification requires two domains to be impaired. The other key difference between major and mild NCD lies in the impairment in everyday activities involved in major NCD.

Getting the History

Ms. Bell reports that her 77-year-old husband's memory is getting worse. She explains that his long-term memory is normal but his short-term memory is poor. The interviewer asks, "Can you give me an example?" She reports that he repeats questions throughout the day. When asked about the effects of these memory problems on his everyday living, Ms. Bell is unable to provide a clear answer. The interviewer then asks, "Let's say you had to leave town for a few days. Would you feel comfortable leaving your husband alone at home for a few days?" Ms. Bell then exclaims, "No, I couldn't do that! He would leave on the stove burner and burn down the house! He would also become lost while driving home from the grocery store." After further discussion, the interviewer asks, "Is there some event that seemed to start these problems?" Ms. Bell cannot recall an event that seemed to trigger the problems, but she notes that she knew there was a problem when he had great difficulty learning how to operate the new television they purchased a year ago. She also mentions how their daughter from another state came for her yearly visit several months ago and was concerned about how different her father seemed.

Ms. Bell reported difficulties in her husband's "short-term memory." The terms *memory*, *short-term memory*, and *long-term memory* mean different things to different people in the lay public and require clarification when patients or caregivers use these terms. The examples they provide may lead the clinician to hypotheses about whether the person is experiencing mild or major NCD, whether the deficits are due to other causes such as a stroke or TBI, how much depression or anxiety symptoms have an impact on functioning, and so on. For instance, if a corporate executive reports difficulty remembering the names of all his or her employees, this may reflect a mild NCD, whereas if a person is reporting more serious memory problems, such as the ones in this vignette, these may be more symptomatic of major NCD due to Alzheimer's disease. Eliciting examples accomplishes another goal: assessing the effects of the deficits on everyday functioning. Individuals or their caregivers occasionally are unable to provide clear answers about everyday functioning, and the question mentioned in the vignette about leaving town for a few days can help elicit a clear answer. Lastly, this vignette illustrates how the observation of a new problem often involves the person's being placed in a new situation (e.g., learning how to operate a new appliance) or an infrequent visitor observing the change (e.g., a family member visiting after some time away).

Tips for Clarifying the Diagnosis

- Establish whether the person shows impairment in one or more cognitive domains, particularly in memory.
- Determine whether this impairment is severe enough to interfere with daily activities.
- Clarify whether the impairment has developed gradually over time or after a particular event (e.g., stroke, brain injury).
- Seek evidence to confirm whether this is a delirium or a chronic disorder.
- Verify whether the person is abusing alcohol or other substances that can cause a reversible memory impairment, or whether the person has a history of chronic alcohol abuse that may be the cause of a more permanent impairment.
- Investigate the possibility of parkinsonian motor symptoms or hallucinations related to Lewy body disease, which may suggest a different etiology than Alzheimer's disease.

Consider the Case

Ms. Sato is 85 years old and reports that her children have requested that she stop driving because she has been involved in three car accidents in the last year. She says that two of the accidents involved other vehicles that "came out of nowhere" and that she hit another car while parking. Her children also note that she sometimes calls them the wrong name when looking at them. When discussing her hobbies, she explains that she used to enjoy reading but has found it more difficult. Ms. Sato lives with her son, and his wife manages her finances and shopping needs. They are of Japanese ethnicity and attribute her symptoms to old age, stating that all older adults eventually must stop driving. Neuropsychological assessment demonstrates performance at the 1st percentile in visual perception, but intact memory, attention, language, and executive ability. She is socially appropriate, quiet, and deferential to medical professionals. She denies any hallucinations, symptoms of rapid eye movement sleep behavior disorder, or fluctuations in attention. Motor examination results are normal, and she has no parkinsonian symptoms. She denies any history of strokes or TBIs. MRI shows bilateral atrophy in the occipital and posterior parietal lobes. Ms. Sato and her children deny significant history of substance abuse. She denies feeling sad or having physical symptoms of depression, including excessive sleeping and decreased appetite.

This case illustrates atypical mild NCD due to Alzheimer's disease and important components to consider when working with older Japanese Americans. Although Alzheimer's disease typically causes predominant memory deficits early on, occasionally nonamnestic symptoms occur first. This woman is showing some symptoms of the visuospatial variant that results from posterior cortical atrophy, with difficulty perceiving other cars while driving, difficulty reading, and inability to recognize familiar faces. This diagnosis is supported by MRI findings of atrophy in the occipital and parietal lobes. Visual perception deficits can also be caused by Lewy body disease, but Ms. Sato lacks other symptoms of this disease (e.g., visual hallucinations, fluctuating attention, parkinsonian symptoms). Neuropsychological testing found impairment in one area, visual perception, but other areas were intact; thus, mild rather than major NCD would be diagnosed. Ms. Sato and her family are of Japanese ethnicity; individuals from this background are more likely to attribute their symptoms to normal aging and may not seek help when needed. When evaluating for symptoms of depression that may contribute to cognitive presentation, clinicians should keep in mind that people of Japanese ethnicity may be more likely to report physical symptoms (e.g., sleep and appetite disturbances) than depressed mood. It is also important when working with members of this ethnic group to incorporate the closeness of the family unit when planning care.

Differential Diagnosis

Major or mild NCD due to Alzheimer's disease differs from vascular NCD in that most often a discrete cerebrovascular event or a preponderance of vascular damage seen on neuroimaging can be linked with the development of vascular NCD, whereas Alzheimer's disease develops more gradually without a clear precipitant. Other diseases such as Lewy body disease or Parkinson's disease also develop gradually but have symptoms (e.g., visual hallucinations, motor symptoms) that are not characteristic of Alzheimer's disease. Symptoms of executive dysfunction and decline in social cognition can occur in both Alzheimer's disease and the behavioral variant of frontotemporal NCD, and language difficulties (e.g., poor word finding or speech production) can occur in both Alzheimer's disease and the language variant of frontotemporal

NCD. However, memory tends to be impaired as well in Alzheimer's disease, whereas it is spared in the early stages of frontotemporal degeneration. Frontotemporal NCD occurs most often in patients younger than age 65 (although 20%–25% of cases are older than 65), whereas Alzheimer's disease tends to develop later in life.

Other medical causes of cognitive dysfunction (e.g., vitamin B_{12} deficiency, thyroid disorders) should be ruled out in the assessment through lab work. Symptoms of delirium tend to develop rapidly (e.g., in hours or days), whereas symptoms of Alzheimer's disease typically manifest over the span of months.

Major depressive disorder, generalized anxiety disorder, and posttraumatic stress disorder (PTSD) in older adults can often interfere with cognitive functioning. However, these disorders typically do not lead to the cognitive profiles associated with Alzheimer's disease. For example, although individuals with these disorders may have difficulty acquiring new information on memory tasks, they are typically able to retain information over time, whereas people with Alzheimer's disease forget information over time. Likewise, language difficulties occur in Alzheimer's disease but not typically in major depressive disorder, generalized anxiety disorder, or PTSD.

Alzheimer's disease occurs later in life, when persons are more susceptible to a variety of other medical problems. Alzheimer's disease, like other conditions that compromise the brain, increases the risk of delirium, and individuals often are found to be experiencing both conditions. Vascular disease is common in older adults and increases the risk for Alzheimer's disease, in addition to directly causing NCD on its own. Comorbid vascular disease may lead to symptoms of decreased processing speed and executive dysfunction. Depressive symptoms have a strong relationship with Alzheimer's disease; some literature has found that a history of depressive symptoms may increase the risk of Alzheimer's disease, and newly diagnosed individuals with Alzheimer's disease often develop symptoms of depression in response to the diagnosis. Clinicians should be careful to assess suicidal ideation in newly diagnosed patients, particularly those who are demographically at increased risk of suicide (e.g., older white men). Comorbid depressive symptoms may also accelerate cognitive decline in individuals with Alzheimer's disease. Alcohol abuse in older adults can worsen symptoms of Alzheimer's disease, and individuals should decrease or cease their usage if a history of alcohol abuse is present.

See DSM-5 for additional disorders to consider in the differential diagnosis. Also refer to the discussions of comorbidity and differential diagnosis in their respective sections of DSM-5.

Summary

- Alzheimer's disease, the most common cause of NCD, most often involves progressive deterioration in memory and other cognitive abilities.
- Major NCD due to Alzheimer's disease involves impairment in two or more domains and interference with ability to complete everyday activities.
- Mild NCD due to Alzheimer's disease involves decline in one or more cognitive domains, but the deficits do not interfere with independence in everyday activities.

- The criteria for probable versus possible Alzheimer's disease differ depending on whether the NCD is major or mild.
- The main biomarker included in the diagnostic criteria is evidence of a causative Alzheimer's disease genetic mutation from family history or genetic testing.

IN-DEPTH DIAGNOSIS
Major or Mild NCD With Lewy Bodies

Ms. Farley, a 66-year-old woman, presents with a history of worsening anxiety and depression that began 18 months ago. According to her husband, she had the belief that there was a third person in the house, and she also saw people in the house who were not there. She often slept for several hours during the day and would have periods when she would stare into space. One night she asked her husband what he was doing in her bed, as if she did not recognize him. Her husband had taken over the laundry chores because intermittently Ms. Farley became upset and frustrated that she could not figure out how to use the washing machine, which she had used throughout their marriage. She was hospitalized briefly, during which a full evaluation was conducted with no evidence of a medical contributor to her symptoms. She was given neuroleptic medication, and at the time of her discharge from the hospital, staff noted that she had signs of a movement disorder and the medication was stopped. Neurological evaluation revealed subtle motor signs consistent with those observed in Parkinson's disease, which had previously not been noticed by the woman or her husband. Formal neuropsychological evaluation revealed that Ms. Farley has significant executive and visuospatial deficits that cannot be accounted for by a movement disorder. She has fears of falling, but her most disabling fear relates to needing to use a bathroom while away from home. Her husband says that she often turns back from leaving the house because she worries that she will need to use the bathroom but not have one available.

Formal neuropsychological assessment documented a significant deficit in executive and visuospatial functioning, so that one feature of major NCD is satisfied. Another feature of major NCD, requiring assistance in instrumental activities (i.e., laundry chores) is also met. Careful interviewing revealed that although the presenting problems are depressed mood and anxiety, they are related to a fixed delusion of a third person in the house and a core symptom, hallucinations. Ms. Farley shows examples of fluctuations in attention and alertness, notably sleeping several hours during the day and displaying episodes of staring into space. The motor signs are subtle and detected only on formal neurological evaluation, a core feature. Establishing the timing of onset is problematic with disorders that evolve gradually; however, given that there has not been a formal diagnosis of a movement disorder and the cognitive dysfunction is significant, the diagnosis of NCD with Lewy bodies (NCDLB) would be more appropriate than one of NCD due to Parkinson's disease. Associated features include difficulty with urination and potential susceptibility to falling, of which Ms. Farley appears to be aware. Urinary incontinence or difficulty with urination are not apparent early in Alzheimer's disease but are consistent with NCDLB. In summary, Ms. Farley has more than two core symptoms of functional decline and would thus receive the diagnosis of probable major NCDLB with mild behavioral disturbance.

Approach to the Diagnosis

The three core symptoms of NCDLB are fluctuations in cognition with pronounced variations in attention and alertness, visual hallucinations, and a parkinsonian movement disorder that develops after the cognitive dysfunction. A common reason for which individuals present for clinical evaluation is a late-life, new onset of visual hallucinations, which may be associated with delusions and emotional disturbance. At this point it is crucial to evaluate the other core symptoms of the disorder, because treatment with some neuroleptic medications in patients with NCDLB can lead to enduring disability and be fatal. This adverse response to these medications is described as neuroleptic sensitivity, and symptoms include worsening of movement disorder and impaired consciousness. A previous history of neuroleptic sensitivity is consistent with NCDLB and is a suggestive diagnostic feature. Fluctuations in cognition and attention can be assessed with screening measures (e.g., Ferman et al. 2004; Walker et al. 2000), and it is important to reassure families that the variability in functioning is consistent with the disorder and not intentional. Individuals also may have experienced a rapid eye movement (REM) sleep behavior disorder beginning decades before the illness. REM sleep behavior disorder is a phenomenon in which individuals do not experience the typical paralysis with sleep and may be physically violent during the dream state, which can lead to injuries. This symptom is suggestive; not all persons with REM sleep behavior disorder develop NCDLB.

The probable versus possible descriptors reflect the level of certainty of the diagnosis: probable NCDLB requires two core features or one core and one suggestive feature, whereas possible NCDLB requires one core deficit or one or more suggestive features.

Finally, the DSM-5 criteria are consistent with existing consensus statements (McKeith et al. 2005); however, it is important for clinicians working with these patients to monitor the literature for these consensus statements as more is learned about the underlying brain pathology.

Getting the History

Mr. Greene brings his 68-year-old wife for a diagnostic evaluation. She presents with fluctuations of symptoms, hallucinations, and parkinsonian features. The interviewer asks Mr. Greene about fluctuations with the following questions: "Do you find that your wife sometimes blanks out, becomes confused, does not know where she is, or can't perform something simple that she should be able to do?" An example is transient inability to perform an activity, such as brushing teeth without guidance of a caregiver. Although structured measures of fluctuation can sensitively detect NCDLB (e.g., Ferman et al. 2004; Walker et al. 2000), people using those rating scales often disagree on their ratings if they do not have significant clinical experience with patients who have NCDLB. The interviewer asks, "Is she drowsy during the day, or does she take naps for more than 2 hours?" Content items that differentiate NCDLB from NCD due to Alzheimer's disease include daytime drowsiness, daytime sleep of more than 2 hours, staring into space for long periods, and disorganized flow of ideas. The interviewer asks, "Are there times when she seems disorganized, unclear, or not logical?"

To assess hallucinations, the clinician asks Ms. Greene, "Do you see or hear people or things that others tell you are not there? Describe them." Hallucinations typically are visual, well formed, and commonly of people (less commonly of animals); however, auditory hallucinations or hallucinations of objects do occur. The interviewer asks Ms. Greene, "Does seeing these things make you upset?" It is important to assess whether there is associated emotional distress and/or delusions. For example, Capgras syndrome, the delusion that an imposter replaced a family member, can occur. The clinician can inquire into this by asking Ms. Greene's husband, "Does your wife ever treat you as if you were someone else, not her husband?" How a caregiver responds could be important for clinical management, and this information can be elicited by asking, "What do you do when she acts this way?" The interviewer assesses whether particular objects can be important triggers for Ms. Greene by asking her, "Are there places in your house/living space where you are likely to see these people?"

Parkinsonian features are evaluated by asking the patient, "Have you had any falls or difficulty getting around recently?" A neurological examination is required and typically indicates that patients are slow (bradykinesia), are stiff (rigidity), and have abnormalities in walking (gait disorder). Although tremor appears to be less common and less severe in NCDLB than in NCD due to Parkinson's disease, no motor symptoms reliably discriminate the disorders. Because there may be several contributors to falls in NCDLB (e.g., autonomic dysfunction, gait instability), falls are an early symptom and a risk for further disability. The interviewer asks if the patient has fallen repeatedly. The timing of symptom onset and monitoring of motor symptoms is important over time.

Suggestive diagnostic features include REM sleep behavior disorder and severe neuroleptic drug sensitivity. REM sleep behavior disorder can be assessed by asking Mr. Greene, "Does your wife lie still during sleep or does she behave as if she were acting out a dream, such as talking, yelling, or moving violently?" This symptom is best assessed in a formal sleep clinic. The disorder is important to identify because it is amenable to treatment. Severe neuroleptic drug sensitivity can be evaluated by asking Mr. Greene, "Has anyone ever given her medications that changed her ability to move or think clearly? Which medication was given?" Patients who have NCDLB have an extreme sensitivity to anticholinergic and antidopaminergic medications, including typical neuroleptic medications.

This case is an example of an initial interview; however, an evaluation of NCDLB should be multidisciplinary. A basic evaluation ideally includes neurological, medical, and neuropsychological assessments to characterize the motor, autonomic, and cognitive symptoms, respectively. A sleep study would be advisable if symptoms are consistent with REM sleep behavior disorder. Unless otherwise specified, questions are directed to the caregiver, particularly regarding symptoms that the patient would likely be unaware of (e.g., sleep-related behaviors). For clarity, the symptom areas are separated, but it is important to establish roughly when each symptom began to differentiate NCDLB and NCD due to Parkinson's disease.

Tips for Clarifying the Diagnosis

- If complex hallucinations first develop in an older adult or marked fluctuations in alertness develop gradually, assess for the other core symptoms of NCDLB.
- Investigate a history of neuroleptic sensitivity, which is suggestive of NCDLB.
- Arrange for a careful medical evaluation, which can assist in discriminating a delirium from NCDLB, both of which are characterized by fluctuating cognition, attention, and alertness.
- Question and warn the patient about falls, which are common among people with NCDLB and raise the risk for further disability.

- Differentiate NCDLB from NCD due to Parkinson's disease by establishing the beginning of the major NCD relative to the movement disorder symptoms: major cognitive deficits develop 1 year before symptoms of a movement disorder in NCDLB but at least 1 year after such symptoms appear in NCD due to Parkinson's disease.
- Remember that memory is relatively preserved and visuospatial and executive functions are disproportionately impaired early in NCDLB, which distinguishes the cognitive pattern from NCD due to Alzheimer's disease and normal aging.

Consider the Case

Mr. Rodriguez is a 65-year-old retired farm laborer who moved to the United States from Mexico 20 years ago. He presents at the movement disorders clinic for a presurgical evaluation for implantation of a brain stimulation device. Mr. Rodriguez and his wife do not speak English and are interviewed through an interpreter. His wife is eager for the intervention because she believes it will improve her husband's gait and stop him from having falls, symptoms that developed within the past 6 months. When interviewed alone, Mr. Rodriguez describes himself as sad and hopeless because he believes his wife is having an affair. His wife admits that a few times over the past year or two Mr. Rodriguez appeared to be talking to himself and staring off into space. When she asked him if he was hallucinating, he denied it. She is unsure how frequently this occurred because she is often away, assisting other family. Aside from the stiffness and falls, he appears to be able to care for himself. Although he has always preferred a sedentary lifestyle, he has become more sedentary over the past year and spends most of his day falling asleep in front of the television. The couple have slept separately for many years because Mr. Rodriguez has dreams in which he thrashes violently, and his wife is worried that she would be injured if she stayed in the same bed. Upon neuropsychological evaluation, the man demonstrates significant executive dysfunction. He is given a Spanish version of a word list–learning task and displays remarkably preserved memory ability.

The evaluation of non-English speakers always has limitations, even with an interpreter. Although Spanish versions of measures are available, educational and cultural differences within subgroups of Spanish speakers need to be considered. Relatively strong performance should be trusted more than dysfunction if there is reason to believe language or cultural differences could contribute to poor performance. In this case, neuropsychological testing demonstrated relatively preserved memory as evidence against a diagnosis of NCD due to Alzheimer's disease. Poor performance on measures of executive functioning would support the conclusion of a core feature of a major NCDLB, if it can be determined that this performance is not due to the English-based nature of these measures. There is no evidence that the cognitive deficit is associated with functional disability, but this conclusion should have a few caveats.

Another difficulty is the need to rely on an informant when the informant may have limited information. In this case the informant, the patient's wife, is often absent from home, and Mr. Rodriguez leads a largely sedentary life, so that his functional disability may be underrepresented given the minimal demands and his limited activities. In addition, the patient's wife is also expressing a wish that the patient undergo a deep brain stimulation surgery that they believe will improve his physical mobility, so she has an incentive to focus on motor-related symptoms and minimize other cognitive symptoms. Under this circumstance, clinicians must carefully probe for cognitive dysfunction and hallucinations and explain to patients the limitations and risks of therapeutic interventions. Mr. Rodriguez spends a large portion of his time sleeping, which would be consistent with fluctuations in alertness, a core symptom of NCDLB, and this appears to predate the onset of motor signs. Depression is an associated feature supporting the diagnosis of NCDLB.

In summary, Mr. Rodriguez has a significant cognitive deficit and at least two core features (i.e., features of parkinsonism, fluctuating alertness) and may experience hallucinations, although limited information is available. In establishing these signs and symptoms, the clinician attempted to select measures appropriate for a non-English speaker, to establish strengths and weaknesses, and to consider the entire pattern of symptoms in light of issues related to ethnic diversity and the context of the evaluation. The patient also has evidence of REM sleep behavior disorder, a feature suggestive of NCDLB. The motor symptoms are relatively more recent than the changes in alertness, thus differentiating this disorder from NCD due to Parkinson's disease. He also has other associated features, including a delusion, depressed mood, and falls, that are consistent with the diagnosis. Therefore, the diagnosis is probable major NCDLB without behavioral disturbance.

Differential Diagnosis

The pattern of symptom progression and the relative onset of cognitive and motor dysfunction are important in discriminating NCDLB from other NCDs. When fluctuations are reported, a careful medical evaluation to rule out a delirium is important. Although the patterns of cognitive deficits in NCD due to Parkinson's disease and in NCDLB are similar, major cognitive deficits develop 1 year before symptoms of a movement disorder in NCDLB. In contrast, in NCD due to Parkinson's disease, the stage of major NCD develops at least 1 year after Parkinson's disease has been diagnosed. Assessing whether the patient has suggestive features, REM sleep behavior disorder, and a history of an adverse reaction to neuroleptics further confirms the diagnosis of NCDLB. Suggestive features such as frequent falls and autonomic dysfunction such as urinary incontinence are important to describe and refer for clinical management (for an extensive review, see Ferman 2013). Once a patient develops motor symptoms and slowing, depressed scores on speeded measures of executive control will be exaggerated. A comprehensive neuropsychological assessment will thus be helpful in discriminating mild from major NCDLB and separating the contribution of cognitive dysfunction versus motor dysfunction to functional disability.

Another differential diagnosis to consider with NCDLB is NCD due to Alzheimer's disease, because the latter is the most common disorder in late life and both it and NCDLB develop gradually. The cognitive dysfunction in Alzheimer's disease typically involves memory and confrontation naming, domains that are relatively preserved in NCDLB. In contrast, executive and visuospatial dysfunctions are more typical of NCDLB. The three core features of NCDLB (visual hallucinations, motor symptoms, and fluctuating cognition and attention) are not typical of early Alzheimer's disease.

NCD due to Alzheimer's disease and NCDLB both develop gradually, unlike vascular dementia, which typically develops in a stepwise pattern and is associated on MRI with strokes and white matter hyperintensities. Fluctuations in alertness and cognition are also not consistent with Alzheimer's disease. Other disorders that lead to hallucinations are peduncular hallucinosis, a rare phenomenon that has MRI findings, and schizophrenia, which has much earlier onset.

See DSM-5 for additional disorders to consider in the differential diagnosis. Also refer to the discussions of comorbidity and differential diagnosis in their respective sections of DSM-5.

Summary

- The core diagnostic features of NCDLB are fluctuating cognition, attention, and alertness; visual hallucinations; and movement disorder symptoms.
- Neuroleptic medication can worsen functioning. This associated feature is termed neuroleptic sensitivity.
- REM sleep behavior disorder, a condition in which the normal paralysis of movement during sleep is absent, is also a suggestive feature.
- A careful description of the time course of the illness is crucial to discriminate NCDLB from NCD due to Parkinson's disease. In NCDLB, the major cognitive deficits develop before the onset of motor symptoms, but in NCD due to Parkinson's disease, the major NCD evolves long after the movement disorder is established.

——— IN-DEPTH DIAGNOSIS ———
Major or Mild Vascular NCD

Mr. Vicker, a 66 year-old man, and his partner report that he has increasing difficulty concentrating and making decisions. He takes longer to complete projects than he used to. They believe these symptoms began after a day when he experienced left leg numbness and tingling in his left hand. He denied experiencing other neurological symptoms around this time, other than a general, vague sensation of feeling "odd." Neuroimaging shows evidence of small infarctions surrounding the ventricles, predominantly on the right side of his brain. A small degree of atrophy, normal for his age, is also seen on imaging. He has a history of atrial fibrillation, diabetes, cigarette smoking, and hypertension. Neuropsychological assessment finds evidence of mild impairment (15th percentile) in speed of processing, complex attention, and executive functioning, particularly on speeded tasks. Tests of memory show mild difficulty learning new information but minimal forgetting of what he has learned. He is able to continue in his occupation, maintains his level of independence in other areas of functioning, and is aware of his weaknesses.

This case illustrates mild vascular NCD. Mr. Vicker seems to have experienced a mild ischemic event when his left side became numb and tingly. His deficits can be temporally related to this event. Neuroimaging shows evidence of cerebrovascular damage to his brain, which may be related to the event he described. He shows the typical cognitive profile of impaired information processing, complex attention, and executive functioning. Subcortical vascular damage can result in deficits in these areas. His history of atrial fibrillation, diabetes, smoking, and hypertension provides further evidence for a vascular cause. The lack of significant atrophy and his performance on memory testing help to rule out Alzheimer's disease as a cause. Although he showed impairment in three cognitive domains, the impairments are mild and do not significantly interfere with his independence. Thus, the disorder is mild in severity.

Approach to the Diagnosis

Because of the heterogeneous nature of the presentation of vascular NCD, the approach to the diagnosis also varies considerably depending on the person. Individuals may present with gradually developing cognitive symptoms that can be linked with underlying cerebrovascular disease or with severe cognitive symptoms of a recent stroke. In a general outpatient clinic, a mental health clinician is more likely to encounter individuals whose underlying cerebrovascular disease is less well established. If cognitive decline is suspected by the person, a caregiver, or the clinician, a thorough description of symptoms and medical history must be gathered. If the symptoms can be linked in time to a discrete vascular event (e.g., "that time when my right hand went numb" or a diagnosed stroke), then a vascular etiology should be suspected. Evidence of stability in symptoms without continual decline is also suggestive of vascular disease as an etiology. If the symptoms seem more reflective of poor attention, slow processing speed, or executive impairment, and less related to memory, a vascular etiology should be suspected. However, individuals occasionally have strokes in the cerebral vasculature feeding the hippocampus, which would lead to memory deficits similar to those seen in Alzheimer's disease. If possible, it is essential to obtain neuroimaging to assist in the diagnosis. If prominent vascular lesions are seen, with less evidence of atrophy, vascular disease is suspect. The clinician should also always keep in mind that many, if not most, individuals with NCD have more than one etiology and that Alzheimer's disease and vascular disease are very often comorbid, which would result in both atrophy and vascular damage being seen on neuroimaging.

Clinicians also may encounter people who were hospitalized for a stroke but whose cognitive functioning has never been formally evaluated. It is very common for family members to observe significant changes in their loved one after a stroke and to not possess a rudimentary understanding of these deficits. If clinicians uncover a history of a stroke in the recent past that seems linked in time to the onset of a person's deficits, the person should be referred to a neurologist and/or neuropsychologist for evaluation and diagnosis. Individuals and their caregivers are often very grateful for clarifying information about deficits and remaining strengths that can be used in rehabilitation.

Getting the History

Mr. Lim is 69 years old and presents to the clinic, reporting that his memory seems worse than it used to be. The interviewer asks, "Can you provide examples of what you mean?" and Mr. Lim explains that it is difficult for him to concentrate on driving if the radio is on or if a passenger is speaking to him. He also states that it is difficult for him to keep up in conversations, even though he can understand what people are saying to him. The interviewer asks, "How long have you had these symptoms?" and Mr. Lim answers that it has been almost a year. When asked, "Is there some event that seemed to start these problems?" he states that one day almost a year ago he had difficulty walking and his vision was blurry. When asked if he saw a doctor at that time, he responds that his doctor thought he may have had a "mini-stroke" and prescribed a "water pill" (diuretic). Upon interview, his wife explains that Mr. Lim seems generally slower than he used to be but that he can remember things well if she talks to him in an environment free of distraction (e.g., after turning off the television). The interviewer asks if he has difficulty making decisions (e.g., what to make for dinner or what to order at a restaurant) or if his behavior is changed (e.g., if he says inappropriate things to people), and she answers that he takes longer to make a decision but his social behavior is fine. Lastly, when asked if his problems have stayed stable or worsened since the "mini-stroke," both Mr. Lim and his wife report that they have stayed the same.

This interview highlights a few important aspects of gathering the history. First, when Mr. Lim was asked to provide examples, he did not endorse memory problems typical of Alzheimer's disease but rather difficulties with complex attention (e.g., difficulty driving with competing stimuli) and slowed processing speed. His difficulty keeping up in conversations seems more to do with slowed processing speed than with symptoms of aphasia. He connects the onset of symptoms with a vascular event described by his physician as a small stroke. His wife reports additional symptoms of executive dysfunction (difficulty making decisions) but also denies memory problems typical of Alzheimer's disease. Lastly, the stable progression of the deficits leads the interviewer toward a diagnosis of vascular NCD rather than a degenerative condition. If possible, the clinician should refer Mr. Lim for neuroimaging and neuropsychological assessment to confirm this diagnosis.

Tips for Clarifying the Diagnosis

- Suspect vascular disease as an etiology when deficits seem to be primarily in attention, processing speed, or executive functioning.
- Use neuroimaging, which is critical in establishing the presence of cerebrovascular damage.
- Take into consideration that when someone has memory deficits suggestive of Alzheimer's disease but also evidence of extensive cerebrovascular involvement, Alzheimer's disease and vascular disease may both be etiologies.
- Remember that damage to certain parts of the brain such as the thalamus or angular gyrus can lead to severe deficits that seem out of proportion to the size of the injury. Infarcts in these locations are known as "strategic" infarcts. They can result in symptoms that are more severe than larger infarcts in other parts of the brain.

Consider the Case

Ms. Garcia, a 66-year-old Puerto Rican American woman, sustained a large ischemic stroke 6 months ago; neuroimaging showed a large infarction in the territory of her left middle cerebral artery. Neuroimaging was otherwise normal, with no significant atrophy suggestive of Alzheimer's disease. She was functioning normally and proficient in

English and Spanish before the stroke, but after the stroke she had symptoms of aphasia, with halting, nonfluent speech; difficulty understanding verbal commands; and severe word-finding difficulty. She also showed severe memory impairment. After the
event, she was unable to move her right arm. Over the next 6 months, she gained back
most of her language abilities with speech therapy, but with lingering word-finding
problems and minor memory deficits, scoring at the 15th percentile in auditory memory but with normal memory for visual information. She regained use of her right arm
enough to return to work as a graphic designer. Her children are highly involved in her
care and report that she does not need assistance with her everyday activities.

Ms. Garcia's case demonstrates that a diagnosis of NCD is not necessarily permanent. With etiologies such as vascular disease (particularly in the form of an acute
stroke) and TBI, cognitive functioning may be severely impaired but improve over
time to a mild NCD or to the absence of an NCD. Ms. Garcia experienced a major vascular NCD after a large vessel infarction. Her deficits persisted for several weeks, but
with the assistance of speech therapy, she was able to regain a large part of her language functioning. It is important to assess and treat language functioning in different languages for a person who is proficient in more than one language. Ms. Garcia is
left with word-finding deficits and impaired memory for auditory information but is
intact in her other abilities and is able to return to her occupation and other activities
of daily living. Although she and her family report that she is independent in her
daily activities, family members from her culture may provide a great deal of assistance with her daily activities while reporting that she is independent in them. Her
work as a graphic designer is less likely than other occupations to require extensive
language skills, which facilitates her ability to return to work. Mild vascular NCD
thus becomes the diagnosis.

Differential Diagnosis

One key difference between vascular disease and other causes of NCD is that vascular
disease, particularly in the form of a large stroke, often can lead to a stepwise pattern
of decline, with sudden steep declines followed by periods of stability. In contrast,
Alzheimer's disease, Lewy body disease, and frontotemporal degeneration cause a
more continual, linear progression of decline. However, vascular disease in the absence of major stroke events can also cause a decline that is continual. In situations
such as this, neuroimaging can show cerebrovascular damage significant enough to
cause cognitive impairment, and can be used to assess whether there is significant atrophy suggestive of Alzheimer's disease. Notably, risk factors for vascular NCD (e.g.,
hypertension, diabetes) are also risk factors for Alzheimer's disease, and patients
with evidence of both Alzheimer's disease and cerebrovascular disease meet the criteria for NCD due to multiple etiologies. NCDLB typically involves fluctuating cognition, visual hallucinations, and parkinsonian symptoms, which do not normally
occur in vascular NCD. Lastly, frontotemporal degeneration also can cause executive
impairment, but in a more gradual fashion than what is seen in vascular NCD and
with less involvement of cerebrovascular disease.

Individuals with vascular NCD often have overlapping symptoms of depression related to damage to frontal-subcortical networks. Clinicians must take care to assess

whether a person's deficits are due to a combination of vascular disease and depression or to one factor alone. Concomitant symptoms of depression can worsen the clinical picture and unfortunately may not respond to the same treatments as a nonvascular depression.

Individuals with TBI often experience cerebrovascular damage such as hemorrhages and subdural hematomas. Although these conditions on their own cause deficits that could be considered NCD associated with vascular disease (i.e., strokes), the primary cause is the TBI, and thus the patient would be diagnosed with NCD due to TBI. Strokes in certain locations (e.g., the basal ganglia or the hippocampus) can cause deficits that mimic diseases that are highly associated with these locations (e.g., Parkinson's disease, Alzheimer's disease), but the appropriate diagnosis is vascular NCD. Individuals can also experience delirium when in the acute stages of a stroke. Lastly, other medical conditions such as brain tumors or multiple sclerosis can also result in cognitive impairment, sometimes with profiles similar to that seen in vascular NCD, and vascular NCD is not diagnosed if these conditions can account for the cognitive deficits.

See DSM-5 for additional disorders to consider in the differential diagnosis. Also refer to the discussions of comorbidity and differential diagnosis in their respective sections of DSM-5.

Summary

- Vascular NCD should be suspected if the onset of deficits is temporally linked with a cerebrovascular event or if there is decline in complex attention (including processing speed) and executive function.
- Probable vascular NCD is diagnosed if there is neuroimaging evidence of cerebrovascular disease, a temporal connection between onset of deficits and a documented cerebrovascular event, or clinical and genetic evidence of cerebrovascular disease.
- Symptoms of depression are particularly common in patients with vascular NCD.
- Many patients with vascular NCD will show a stepwise decline, whereas patients with Alzheimer's disease, Lewy body disease, and frontotemporal degeneration will show more gradual decline.

IN-DEPTH DIAGNOSIS

Major or Mild NCD Due to TBI

Ms. O'Brien is 60 years old and was involved in a car crash in which her head hit the windshield. She lost consciousness for an estimated 10–15 minutes. She recalls approaching the intersection while driving but cannot remember other details until paramedics arrived on the scene. Her Glasgow Coma Scale score was 14 at the time. She presents in an outpatient primary care clinic 2 weeks later and reports having headaches, concentration difficulties, fatigue, and increased sensitivity to light since the accident. No evidence of seizures, hemiparesis, or visual disturbances is found. A cognitive screen finds deficits in attention and working memory and on speeded tasks. Ms. O'Brien is less productive at work, and she takes twice as long to complete tasks as before the accident. She has to take frequent rest breaks every 2–3 hours and becomes easily fatigued. She left work early several times during the first week after the event but soon resumed her usual work schedule. Her medical workup is otherwise normal, and lab results are in the normal range, ruling out a delirium. An MRI does not show any damage. Three weeks after the accident, she meets diagnostic criteria for mild NCD due to TBI. Six months after the injury, she completes a neuropsychological assessment. She performs in the normal range on measures of effort, attention, working memory, processing speed, and other domains. She denies experiencing any cognitive difficulties at 6 months postinjury and feels that she is "back to normal."

This case illustrates one important aspect of mild NCD due to TBI that differs from most other NCDs: individuals can experience an NCD at one time point but recover enough that they no longer meet criteria for the NCD (this can also occur with vascular NCD). Ms. O'Brien met diagnostic criteria for mild NCD in the weeks after her injury, which is a common outcome for people who have experienced a mild TBI. It is typical for the majority of such patients to completely recover to baseline functioning within 3 months after the injury. Ms. O'Brien showed typical symptoms after the event, including headaches, fatigue, increased sensitivity to light (i.e., photosensitivity), and poor attention, working memory, and processing speed.

Approach to the Diagnosis

The first line of assessment involves a clinical interview and medical chart review to determine the nature and severity of the TBI (mild, moderate, or severe, according to DSM-5 severity ratings). Per DSM-5, TBI may include impact to the head or other mechanisms of rapid movement or displacement of the brain within the skull with one or more of the following key features: 1) loss of consciousness, 2) posttraumatic amnesia, 3) disorientation and confusion, or 4) neurological signs (e.g., neuroimaging showing injury; new onset of seizures; a marked worsening of previously diagnosed seizure disorder; visual field cuts; anosmia; hemiparesis). Finally, for an NCD to be related to TBI, the cognitive decline must manifest immediately after the TBI or present immediately after recovery of consciousness and persist past the acute postinjury period. A medical chart review should include current medications (e.g., benzodiazepines, anticholinergics, pain narcotics, sedatives, anticonvulsants), history of seizures, lab work examining blood alcohol level, metabolic issues such as renal or liver dysfunction, and substance intoxication or withdrawal.

Cognitive deficits are evaluated in a clinical interview and by a neuropsychological battery of standardized measures focused on attention; speed of processing information; memory; and executive abilities. In an interview, a clinician ascertains whether cognitive difficulties immediately follow the injury by asking about the time of onset and the nature of cognitive difficulties. Although post-TBI cognitive deficits are variable, most involve *impaired attention* (e.g., difficulty answering questions and completing tasks, multitasking, losing track in conversations, repeating questions), *executive dysfunction* (e.g., poor problem solving and planning, disinhibition, impulsivity, inability to benefit from feedback, and/or inability to create a sequence of steps for complex tasks such as cooking), *learning and memory problems* for recent information (e.g., interviewer's name and 5-word list recall), and *slowed processing speed* (longer completion time of tasks or delayed response to questions). *Personality changes* are also common and include decreased frustration tolerance, irritability, impulsivity, and inappropriate comments in social settings. In severe TBI, the following deficits are commonly seen: aphasia, visual field cuts, hemispatial neglect/inattention, and apraxia (inability to carry out purposeful movement such as brushing one's teeth).

A clinician determines whether the nature and severity of the current cognitive decline meet diagnostic criteria for mild or major NCD. There are two factors to consider when making a diagnosis. First, a diagnosis of major versus mild NCD due to TBI is determined by the extent or severity of cognitive decline from a previous level of functioning rather than the severity of TBI itself. In other words, mild TBI can result in major NCD due to TBI if there is evidence of substantial decline on cognitive testing from an estimated previous level of functioning within the first week to months following injury. Second, the course of cognitive decline can vary over time, with major NCD converting to mild NCD, if not completely resolving, because the natural course of cognitive changes involves improvement, if not complete resolution, of symptoms. Except in cases of severe TBI, the typical course of recovery is that of complete or substantial improvement in cognitive, neurological, personality, and mood changes within weeks to 3 months following mild TBI and within 1 year following moderate TBI. For individuals with moderate to severe TBI, cognitive deficits may persist long term and be further exacerbated by neurophysiological, emotional, and behavioral complications. These may include seizures, especially within 1 year after injury, developmental delays in children, PTSD, depression, anxiety, photosensitivity, hyperacusis, irritability, sleep disturbance, fatigue, apathy, and inability to return to work or school. Disruption in social and occupational functioning further negatively affects interpersonal relationships and family/marital functioning. As such, mood assessment should be routinely conducted.

Getting the History

Mr. Bates is 25 years old, had a TBI 3 months ago, and reports increased "concentration" difficulties in college. The interviewer asks, "Can you give me examples of concentration difficulties?" Mr. Bates is unable to provide examples. The interviewer asks follow-up questions: "Do you have to reread the same pages to remember them? Do you lose track of thoughts in conversations? Do you start projects and find it difficult to complete them?" Mr. Bates responds yes to all of these questions, indicating reduced attention. The interviewer then asks, "Does it take you longer to complete tasks?" and the man nods in agreement and adds that he tends to repeat himself and requires multiple repetitions to learn new information. The interviewer follows with, "When did you first notice these difficulties?" The patient responds that concentration issues started within the week of injury and have improved somewhat over the past 3 months but have not completely resolved. The duration of posttraumatic amnesia and loss of consciousness is determined by asking, "What is the last clear memory you have before your injury? What is the first clear memory following the injury? Did you lose consciousness and for how long?" The patient reports loss of consciousness of 60 minutes, feeling disoriented for 1 day following the injury, no difficulty remembering events immediately preceding the injury, and a first postinjury memory of waking up in a hospital room 2 days later. The interviewer asks, "Have you been feeling unusually blue, tearful, or nervous in the past 3 months?" and the patient denies any signs of emotional distress. Finally, the interviewer asks about difficulty in independent living and self-care (e.g., cooking, driving, managing finances and medications). Mr. Bates denies any changes in independent functioning and is diagnosed with mild NCD due to TBI.

The clinician first establishes the nature of cognitive deficits that the patient experiences. Once reduced attention and processing speed are identified, the time at onset of cognitive deficits is clarified to determine whether the patient meets criteria for mild or major NCD due to TBI, which requires the onset of cognitive difficulties immediately following the injury. Although the severity of initial TBI is not necessarily predictive of mild versus major NCD due to TBI, it is always helpful to assess for the severity of initial injury, which determines prognosis in regard to the timeline of recovery, and to assess whether persisting difficulties are due to other causes (e.g., other medical problems, substance use, anxiety, depression, pain, medication effects). For example, if the patient had suffered a mild TBI and continues to experience cognitive deficits 3 months later, other contributing factors should be explored because complete cognitive recovery should occur within weeks to 3 months after mild TBI. To rule out the presence of emotional distress that can further compound and/or contribute to ongoing cognitive deficits, the clinician rules out the presence of depression, anxiety, or emotional control issues. Finally, to differentiate between mild and major NCD, the clinician asks about changes in everyday functioning. Compared to those with mild NCD, individuals with major NCD due to TBI have difficulty completing daily activities independently and need assistance.

Tips for Clarifying the Diagnosis

- Determine severity of TBI based on characteristics at the time of injury: loss of consciousness, posttraumatic amnesia, and Glasgow Coma Scale score at the time of injury. Severity of TBI should not be determined by the severity of cognitive decline following injury.
- Establish severity (i.e., mild vs. major) of the resulting NCD due to TBI based on the severity of cognitive decline following injury and its impact on ability to perform activities of daily living.
- Clarify the history of the injury and establish the duration of posttraumatic amnesia to better describe the severity of injury:
  - Ask the patient what he or she remembers *last, before* the injury and elicit details.
  - Ask the patient what he or she remembers *first, after* the injury. Be sure to differentiate between what the patient has been informed about what happened versus what he or she remembers.
- Assess what characteristics were present before the injury in addition to what has occurred since the injury, because many characteristics associated with TBI (e.g., impulsivity, irritability, depression, anxiety, substance use, high-risk behaviors) may be present before someone experiences a TBI.

- Provide education to patients with mild TBI in regard to recovery trajectory: neurocognitive deficits will likely resolve within the first 3 months postinjury.

Consider the Case

Mr. Daimler is 24 years old and speaks English as his second language. He fell down on the sidewalk while intoxicated, and his forehead struck the concrete. He was unconscious for approximately 2 hours before paramedics awakened him. His Glasgow Coma Scale score was 10 out of 15 when paramedics arrived. Blood alcohol level was 0.12 at the hospital. He had no memory of the injury or the day before the fall. His first clear memory following the fall was of his sister visiting him at the hospital. He presents to the clinic 1 year after the fall, reporting frequent headaches, shortness of temper, and sensitivity to bright lights. He undergoes a comprehensive neuropsychological assessment and struggles with attention, multitasking, problem solving, and memory for recently learned information, with these scores ranging from the 5th to the 15th percentiles. He demonstrates adequate effort in the assessment. Since the fall, he has returned to work as a mechanic, although he takes longer to complete tasks (e.g., 90 minutes to perform a standard oil change). He remains independent in his everyday functioning, but his wife has always managed family finances. He reports increased irritability and frequent arguments with his wife. Although he was likely intoxicated at the time of the fall, he and his wife reported that he typically has no more than three to six alcoholic drinks over the course of a week. He reports some history of depressive symptoms 10 years ago and was treated with an antidepressant medication at that time. He denies feeling depressed or anxious at this time.

Mr. Daimler experienced a TBI of moderate severity, as evidenced by the Glasgow Coma Scale score of 10, loss of consciousness between 30 minutes and 24 hours, and posttraumatic amnesia between 1 and 7 days. Mr. Daimler is within the peak age range for TBI, ages 15–24 years. Because English is his second language, his neuropsychological test performance should be interpreted with caution because lower scores may underestimate his true abilities. Most cognitive measures were constructed in the English language and with Western notions of cognitive functioning. Research suggests that very few, if any, cognitive tests are immune to these influences; therefore, they may have limited validity in persons who speak English as a second language or who are from different national, ethnic, racial, linguistic, or cultural backgrounds. Although Mr. Daimler's neuropsychological test results indicate at least moderate cognitive deficits, he is independent in daily life and able to return to work, and the tests may underestimate his abilities. Based on this information, he meets diagnostic criteria for mild NCD due to moderate TBI. Alcohol was involved in the fall, which can complicate the assessment of TBI severity, because the sedating properties of severe alcohol intake can depress a Glasgow Coma Scale score and a clinician may be unable to determine whether the low score is due to the alcohol intake or the brain injury. It is also important for clinicians to determine whether cognitive impairment after a TBI is related to the TBI, or whether there is a long history of alcohol abuse that could explain the cognitive deficits, or whether the TBI and alcohol abuse history jointly contribute. Given the family's report of Mr. Daimler's infrequent alcohol use, long-term effects of alcohol on cognitive functioning can be ruled out at this time. Because he denied symptoms of depression and anxiety, it is unlikely that emotional distress is exacerbating, or can explain, his current cognitive difficulties. Lastly, it is important to assess the effort a person exerts in a cognitive evaluation after a TBI, because the possibility of compensation or relief from prior duties may lead a person to perform poorly in an evaluation despite intact cognitive functioning.

Differential Diagnosis

Although the diagnosis of major or mild NCD is not necessarily related to the initial severity of TBI, in some instances the severity of cognitive decline and/or the lack of expected improvement in symptoms over time may appear inconsistent with the nature and severity of injury. After careful medical record review and ruling out neurological complications (e.g., chronic hematoma, stroke, seizure activity), the clinician should consider the possibility of psychiatric, substance use, and somatic symptom and related disorders. PTSD can frequently co-occur with the NCD and can be the primary diagnosis explaining ongoing cognitive deficits, especially for individuals who experience cognitive deficits that are not necessarily consistent with the severity of the initial TBI. Difficulty concentrating, irritability, sensitivity to noise and light, headaches, depressed or anxious mood, and behavioral disinhibition are common to both PTSD and NCDs due to TBI, but the symptom severity usually improves, if not resolves, in NCDs due to mild to moderate TBI in 3–6 months after TBI, whereas symptoms often persist, if not worsen, when due to PTSD and other psychiatric disorders. When younger adults experience an NCD subsequent to a TBI, a clinician can be confident that the etiology is not a progressive neurodegenerative disorder such as Alzheimer's disease because of the extremely low prevalence in younger adults. TBI victims often experience vascular damage, such as hemorrhages and subdural hematomas. Although these conditions on their own cause deficits that could be considered NCD associated with vascular disease (i.e., strokes), the primary cause is the TBI; thus, the person would be diagnosed with an NCD due to TBI.

Many symptoms associated with NCDs due to TBI overlap with mood-related disorders, including depressed or anxious mood, headaches, sensitivity to light and noise, and changes in personality (e.g., behavioral disinhibition, irritability, aggressiveness). Substance use (either preexisting or following TBI) is commonly seen in those with NCDs due to TBI and can significantly compound and exacerbate cognitive deficits and functional difficulties in daily life. As noted earlier, many symptoms associated with TBI may overlap with symptoms found in cases of PTSD, and the two disorders can be comorbid, especially in military populations. Additionally, prominent neuromotor features (e.g., ataxia, loss of balance, incoordination, motor slowing) can be present in major NCD due to TBI, but medical and neurological examinations are needed to rule out other neurological causes (e.g., seizures, tumors, movement disorders).

See DSM-5 for additional disorders to consider in the differential diagnosis. Also refer to the discussions of comorbidity and differential diagnosis in their respective sections of DSM-5.

Summary

- Mild or major NCD due to TBI is determined by the severity of cognitive decline following injury and its impact on the person's ability to perform activities of daily living. Specification of mild versus major NCD due to TBI is not determined by the severity of injury.
- Severity of injury is determined by characteristics at the time of injury (i.e., loss of consciousness, posttraumatic amnesia, and Glasgow Coma Scale score), not by the severity of cognitive decline following injury.
- A high blood alcohol level at the time of injury can depress the initial Glasgow Coma Scale score and result in an inaccurate measure of injury severity.
- Unlike other NCDs, NCD due to TBI is unique in regard to recovery trajectory: the individual can experience either mild or major NCD immediately after injury, transition from major to mild NCD, and possibly recover enough that he or she no longer meets criteria for the NCD.
- For NCD due to mild TBI, the majority of patients completely recover to baseline functioning within 3 months after injury.
- The clinician should evaluate the patient's history of and current symptoms of mood and substance-related disorders. If neurocognitive deficits worsen or persist longer, it is important to consider other factors (e.g., psychiatric, substance, neurological, or somatic symptom and related disorders) that can be contributing to ongoing cognitive difficulties.

───────── SUMMARY ─────────

Neurocognitive Disorders

Table 20–1 summarizes the diagnostic guidelines covered in this chapter for NCDs due to Alzheimer's disease, NCDLB, vascular NCDs, and NCDs due to TBI. Cognitive dysfunction is a common feature of all of these NCDs. Major and mild NCDs are distinguished by the severity of cognitive dysfunction as well as functional impairment. For major NCDs, individuals must have functional impairment, defined as a need for assistance with everyday functioning. Independence in everyday functioning is characterized by the ability to complete instrumental activities of daily living without assistance, such as managing finances and medications, preparing meals, and arranging transportation. In degenerative disorders, in which there is no clear event such as a head injury, the clinician needs to specify probable versus possible, and these criteria vary across the syndromes (as described in Table 20–1). The clinician also needs to indicate whether there is behavioral disturbance. In mild or major NCDs due to TBI, it is important to identify the nature of the injury and the duration of loss of consciousness and posttraumatic amnesia, which occurs immediately after TBI and includes the coma period as well as the time after the recovery of consciousness. It can be assessed by asking a patient what the first thing is that he or she remembers after the event.

TABLE 20–1. **Summary of diagnostic guidelines for selected neurocognitive disorders (NCDs)**

Major NCD (all causes)	Mild NCD (all causes)
1. Cognitive deficits interfere with independence in everyday activities. 2. Cognition is typically ≤3rd percentile.	1. Cognitive deficits do not interfere with independence in everyday activities. 2. Cognition is typically between the 3rd and 16th percentile.

Major NCD due to Alzheimer's disease	Mild NCD due to Alzheimer's disease

Symptoms

Insidious onset and gradual progression of impairment in one or more cognitive domains. Disturbance is not better explained by another process.

Probable Alzheimer's disease
  Genetic mutation
  Or all of the following:
  1. Decline in memory and learning *and at least one other cognitive domain*
  2. Progressive and gradual decline
  3. No evidence of mixed etiology
Otherwise, possible Alzheimer's disease
	Probable Alzheimer's disease
	  Genetic mutation
	
	Possible Alzheimer's disease
	  All of the following:
	  1. Decline in memory and learning
	  2. Progressive, gradual decline
	  3. No evidence of mixed etiology

Major NCD with Lewy bodies	Mild NCD with Lewy bodies

Symptoms

Insidious onset and gradual progression of impairment in one or more cognitive domains. Disturbance is not better explained by another process.

Probable Lewy bodies
  Two core features, or at least one core and one suggestive feature
Possible Lewy bodies
  One core feature, or at least one suggestive feature

Major vascular NCD	Mild vascular NCD

Symptoms

Clinical features of vascular etiology, suggested by either
  1. Prominent decline in complex attention, processing speed, and executive function; *or*
  2. Onset of cognitive deficits is temporally related to one or more cerebrovascular events.
Evidence of cerebrovascular disease.
Disturbance is not better explained by another process.

Probable vascular NCD
  One of the following is present:
  1. Neuroimaging evidence of cerebrovascular disease *or*
  2. Cognitive deficits with onset temporally due to cerebrovascular event(s) *or*
  3. Genetic and clinical evidence
Possible vascular NCD
  Clinical criteria are met, but neuroimaging is not available and temporal relationship with one or more cerebrovascular events is not established.

TABLE 20–1. **Summary of diagnostic guidelines for selected neurocognitive disorders (NCDs)** *(continued)*

Major NCD due to TBI	Mild NCD due to TBI

Symptoms

Evidence of TBI (at least one of the following):

1. Loss of consciousness
2. Posttraumatic amnesia
3. Disorientation and confusion
4. Neurological signs

Onset is immediately after TBI or after recovering consciousness and persists past acute postinjury period.

No specification of probable or possible, because the etiology is more clearly established.

Note. TBI=traumatic brain injury.

■ ■ ■

Diagnostic Pearls

- NCDs involve a decline in cognitive functioning from a prior level. These disorders differ from intellectual disabilities, which are present from birth or from a very young age.

- Delirium occurs when a medical condition interferes with brain functioning, causing symptoms of disorientation and cognitive impairment.

- Major and mild NCDs both involve impairment in one or more cognitive domains (two or more domains are required for NCD due to Alzheimer's disease). In major NCD, significant cognitive impairments interfere with independence in everyday activities. In mild NCD, modest cognitive impairments do not interfere with independence in everyday activities.

- The best way to establish the main symptoms of the NCDs (i.e., cognitive deficits) is through cognitive testing. A patient's self-report of cognitive deficits is not sufficient for diagnosis. Moreover, the nature of some NCDs often precludes the patient's own awareness of a disorder being present.

- Unlike other psychiatric disorders, the diagnosis should be thought of as the syndrome (neurocognitive disorder) in addition to the likely neurological cause (e.g., Alzheimer's disease, TBI).

- Alzheimer's disease is the most common degenerative cause of NCD.

- NCD due to TBI can be acquired at any age, whereas the other NCDs occur most often in older adults.

- To ensure that treatable causes of cognitive dysfunction are considered, cognitive impairment in older adults should be thought of as being due to delirium, unless proven otherwise.

- Hallucinations in delirium as well as in NCDLB are most often visual, whereas hallucinations in schizophrenia are more often auditory, although each of these disorders can involve hallucinations in other modalities.

Self-Assessment

Key Concepts: Double-Check Your Knowledge

What is the relevance of the following concepts to the various NCDs?

- Posttraumatic amnesia
- Hallucinations
- Vascular disease
- Learning and memory
- Visuospatial skills
- Stroke/cerebrovascular accident
- Neuroleptic sensitivity
- Loss of consciousness
- Cerebral autosomal dominant arteriopathy with subcortical infarcts and leukoencephalopathy (CADASIL)
- Glasgow Coma Scale

Questions to Discuss With Colleagues and Mentors

1. What tools do you prefer for assessing cognition?
2. Are there certain questions you find helpful in establishing differential diagnosis?
3. How do you manage patients with NCDs who behave inappropriately with you?
4. In your practice, what do you find to be the most common triggers of delirium?
5. Which questions to significant others do you find most helpful in obtaining information in regard to establishing a cognitive baseline and decline?

Case-Based Questions

PART A

Ms. Nicolas is 75 years old and reports that her memory has been declining gradually over the past 2 years. Her partner reports that she frequently repeats questions and occasionally forgets where she set out to go on an errand. Each denies any changes in Ms. Nicolas's personality or behavior.

What disorder might be causing these symptoms?   Her symptoms sound like those of NCD due to Alzheimer's disease.

PART B

Upon clarification, these symptoms appear to have started abruptly, when Ms. Nicolas presented at the emergency department with complaints of sudden visual disturbance. She believes that the symptoms began then, but her partner believes that some memory deficits were present beforehand.

What problems can cause a sudden development or worsening of cognitive problems?   Sudden onset of memory deficits can be due to a stroke or other acute medical condition (e.g., encephalitis, expansion of a brain tumor to a critical size). Clinicians often struggle with discrepant reports; in this case, the memory deficits may have started before the event (consistent with Alzheimer's disease), may have been caused by this event (consistent with vascular disease), or may represent precipitant Alzheimer's disease worsened by a stroke.

PART C

> Ms. Nicolas undergoes an MRI, which shows evidence of a stroke in the distribution of her hippocampal memory centers and her occipital areas of visual processing. Genetic testing finds that she carries the apolipoprotein E4 gene, and she reports that both her parents had been diagnosed with Alzheimer's disease. Neuropsychological testing shows impairments in memory and visual perception but intact functioning in other areas. Review of her medications finds that she recently began taking a benzodiazepine for her "nerves."

What are all the potential etiologies of her deficits, and are any of them reversible?   The review of records uncovered three possible causes of Ms. Nicolas's memory deficits: 1) MRI evidence of a stroke in the artery that feeds the hippocampus, which would be expected to lead to memory deficits; 2) genetic testing consistent with Alzheimer's disease; and 3) recent introduction of a medication (a benzodiazepine) that often interferes with cognition. If she is experiencing symptoms of an anxiety disorder, appropriate treatment must be initiated because anxiety can also interfere with cognition. This case illustrates some of the complexities of assessing and treating cognitive deficits in older adults; many disorders are multifactorial in etiology, with some reversible causes, some stable, and some degenerative.

Short-Answer Questions

1. Which events do patients with Alzheimer's disease have the most trouble remembering: recent events or events from the distant past?
2. True or False: The diagnosis of major NCD due to Alzheimer's disease requires evidence of cognitive decline in only learning and memory.
3. Aside from cognitive test performance, what is the key distinguishing feature used to differentiate between mild and major NCD?
4. What is the essential feature of delirium?
5. Visual hallucinations can occur in NCDLB and what other NCD?
6. What are the three core diagnostic features of major or mild NCDLB?
7. Which cognitive domains are most prominently affected in major or mild vascular NCD?
8. True or False: Probable vascular NCD can be diagnosed if there is neuroimaging-supported evidence of extensive cerebrovascular disease resulting in the neurocognitive deficits.
9. Name five risk factors associated with major or mild vascular NCD.
10. True or False: The diagnosis of mild versus major NCD due to TBI is based on the initial severity of brain injury.

Answers

1. Patients with Alzheimer's disease have the most trouble remembering recent events.

2. False. One other cognitive domain must be impaired.

3. Everyday functioning is the key component used to differentiate between mild and major NCD. For mild NCD diagnosis, the patient's ability to function independently is relatively intact, whereas for major NCD diagnosis, the patient depends on others for assistance in instrumental activities of daily living.

4. The essential feature of delirium is disturbance in attention and/or awareness that is rapid in onset.

5. Visual hallucinations can occur in delirium.

6. The three core diagnostic features of major or mild NCDLB are fluctuating cognition (attention and awareness); recurrent visual hallucinations; and spontaneous features of parkinsonism, with onset after the development of cognitive decline.

7. Complex attention (including processing speed) and executive function are most prominently affected in major or mild vascular NCD.

8. True. Neuroimaging-supported evidence of extensive cerebrovascular disease resulting in the neurocognitive deficits is sufficient to be diagnosed with probable vascular NCD.

9. Risk factors associated with major or mild vascular NCD include hypertension, diabetes, smoking, obesity, high cholesterol levels, atrial fibrillation, cerebral amyloid angiopathy, and hereditary conditions such as CADASIL.

10. False. The mild versus major designation is based on the severity of cognitive deficits.

References

Ferman TJ: Dementia with Lewy bodies, in Mild Cognitive Impairment and Dementia: Definitions, Diagnosis, and Treatment (Oxford Workshop Series). Edited by GE Smith, Bondi MW. New York, Oxford University Press, 2013, pp. 255–301

Ferman TJ, Smith GE, Boeve BF, et al: DLB fluctuations: Specific features that reliably differentiate DLB from AD and normal aging. Neurology 62:181–187, 2004

McKeith IG, Dickson DW, Lowe J, et al: Diagnosis and management of dementia with Lewy bodies: third report of the DLB consortium. Neurology 65:1863–1872, 2005

Walker MP, Ballard CG, Ayre GA, et al: The Clinician Assessment of Fluctuation and the One Day Fluctuation Assessment Scale. Two methods to assess fluctuating confusion in dementia. Br J Psychiatry 177:252–256, 2000

21

Personality Disorders

Daryn Reicherter, M.D.

Laura Weiss Roberts, M.D., M.A.

"People always let me down."

"I can't do anything unless my kitchen is perfectly clean."

People with personality disorders have enduring maladaptive patterns related to their thoughts, behaviors, reactions, and internal experience that occur across social situations and lead to serious impairment in their lives. Their ability "to love and to work" is diminished, and they often suffer greatly. The disruptive, negative, or damaging behaviors of people living with personality disorders cause others around them also to suffer. By definition, personality disorders are not episodic; their enduring nature is the key to understanding this diagnostic class.

Personality disorders are not rare, and some are more prevalent in men while others are more prevalent in women. In clinical practice, co-occurring disorders, such as disorders of mood or anxiety or substance-related conditions, and significant psychosocial issues are considered the rule rather than the exception. For these reasons, the clinical care of people with personality disorders can be especially challenging, and it requires great conscientiousness, compassion, and tolerance for complexity on the part of health professionals who undertake this work.

In learning about personality disorders, it is helpful to first get a sense of the broad diagnostic class and then to become familiar with the specific criteria for the 10 individual DSM-5 personality disorders. The astute reader will note that the DSM-IV-TR criteria for personality disorders have been preserved without changes in DSM-5 Section II. Significant scientific work—for example, in the areas of temperament and personality structure—and international comparative studies suggest that future editions of DSM will have new concepts and criteria for personality disorders. The emerging thinking on this domain is detailed in DSM-5 Section III, in the chapter "Alternative DSM-5 Model for Personality Disorders." The chapter examines new approaches to consider in personality disorders and provides a more in-depth look at areas of dysfunction often seen in personalities. The chapter also includes a proposed rating scale to calibrate the level of personality functioning. The interested learner is encouraged to review this material in DSM-5.

General Personality Disorder

The criteria for the presence of a personality disorder, in general, must be met before a specific personality disorder diagnosis should be considered. Many negative personality traits may be observed in persons who never meet the general criteria for a personality disorder and who should not be classified with a specific personality disorder (e.g., borderline personality disorder, dependent personality disorder). Maladaptive personality traits may occur in isolation from other characteristics, or they may occur only in specific situations, in which case they would not constitute a personality disorder diagnosis.

In essence, to meet criteria for a personality disorder diagnosis, a person's maladaptive patterns of experience and behavior must be essentially fixed into the individual's personality. The traits must in some sense be "calcified" as an aspect of the person's way of experiencing and behaving across situations. For professionals just entering clinical work, this notion can be hard to understand when, for instance, the trait appears superficially to be dynamic (e.g., because the person is emotionally labile and engages in disruptive behavior) but is actually quite consistent across time and context. This consistency is fundamental to the diagnostic class. The enduring and pervasive nature of personality disorders is why DSM-5 specifies that these conditions be apparent across diverse situations and multiple spheres of function, be of a long duration, and be traceable to adolescence or early adulthood. Patients can meet full DSM-5 criteria for more than one personality disorder and be correctly diagnosed with each personality disorder when full criteria are met.

Personality disorder diagnoses are often deferred until after age 18 because the clinician should identify these experiences and behaviors in an adult personality as opposed to a developing personality. Personality disorders may be accurately diagnosed before the age of 18 if symptoms are clearly present for more than 1 year. The one exception is antisocial personality disorder, which cannot be diagnosed in an individual under age 18 years. It is also important to note that personality disorders are not necessarily lifelong diagnoses. Patients meeting criteria for personality disorders may develop and no longer meet the diagnostic criteria for personality disorder at another stage of life.

Personality traits are defined in DSM-5 as "enduring patterns of perceiving, relating to, and thinking about the environment and oneself that are exhibited in a wide range of social and personal contexts" (p. 647). When personality traits are maladaptive and inflexible, they constitute the patterns associated with personality disorders. Specific constellations of maladaptive personality traits constitute the 10 personality disorders as defined in DSM-5 (p. 645):

- *Paranoid personality disorder* is a pattern of distrust and suspiciousness such that others' motives are interpreted as malevolent.
- *Schizoid personality disorder* is a pattern of detachment from social relationships and a restricted range of emotional expression.
- *Schizotypal personality disorder* is a pattern of acute discomfort in close relationships, cognitive or perceptual distortions, and eccentricities of behavior.
- *Antisocial personality disorder* is a pattern of disregard for, and violation of, the rights of others.
- *Borderline personality disorder* is a pattern of instability in interpersonal relationships, self-image, and affects, and marked impulsivity.
- *Histrionic personality d*isorder is a pattern of excessive emotionality and attention seeking.
- *Narcissistic personality disorder* is a pattern of grandiosity, need for admiration, and lack of empathy.
- *Avoidant personality disorder* is a pattern of social inhibition, feelings of inadequacy, and hypersensitivity to negative evaluation.
- *Dependent personality disorder* is a pattern of submissive and clinging behavior related to an excessive need to be taken care of.
- *Obsessive-compulsive personality disorder* is a pattern of preoccupation with orderliness, perfectionism, and control.

The specific personality disorders are often thought about in three different "clusters" on the basis of similarities between the diagnoses:

- Cluster A personality disorders are those diagnoses characterized by odd beliefs and eccentric behaviors. Cluster A includes paranoid, schizoid, and schizotypal personality disorders.
- Cluster B personality disorders are those diagnoses characterized by erratic and dramatic behaviors and emotional instability. Cluster B includes antisocial, borderline, histrionic, and narcissistic personality disorders.
- Cluster C personality disorders are those diagnoses characterized by fear-based desire for control and anxiety. Cluster C includes avoidant, dependent, and obsessive-compulsive personality disorders.

It is not uncommon for personality traits to overlap within a cluster. For instance, a person who presents with the full set of signs consistent with borderline personality disorder may also have some of the traits seen in histrionic personality disorder. The clusters may help clinicians group similar clinical pictures of personality disorders.

A final subgroup, called "other personality disorders," includes personality change due to another medical condition, which is a persistent personality disturbance judged to be due to a medical condition. The "other personality disorders" subgroup also includes other specified personality disorder and unspecified personality disorder, which are used to describe a condition wherein the definition for personality disorder is met but the full criteria for a specific personality disorder diagnosis has not been met.

Distinguishing personality disorders from other mental health diagnoses, physiological effects of substances, or medical conditions can be difficult but is essential before arriving at the diagnosis of any personality disorder. Discerning whether another factor or set of factors is shaping the experiences and behaviors that appear to be "a personality disorder" can be quite difficult, given that patients often present with multiple conditions and states that must be taken into account.

People with personality disorders are often considered to represent an especially difficult patient population because they elicit strong emotional reactions from others around them—health professionals are not an exception to this pattern. People who have these disorders may not understand their traits to be pathological, even if those traits clearly compromise their well-being and effectiveness in major spheres of life. Paradoxically, people with personality disorders may be successful in some of their activities in society, and in these cases, the diagnosis may be harder to determine. Accurately identifying the presence of a personality disorder diagnosis—and then learning to respond therapeutically rather than to "react" to patients with these conditions— is the mark of a maturing and sound clinician.

This chapter focuses on these 4 of the 10 specific personality disorders found in DSM-5: borderline, obsessive-compulsive, schizotypal, and narcissistic. Each of these disorders should be considered in the greater context of the DSM-5 criteria for general personality disorder.

IN-DEPTH DIAGNOSIS

Borderline Personality Disorder

Ms. Hernandez is a 26-year-old single white woman who presents to the emergency department after consuming 20 tablets of her antidepressant medication. She says she took the pills suddenly after an intense fight and "breakup for the last time" with her boyfriend. Ms. Hernandez called her boyfriend immediately after taking the pills, and he came with her to the emergency department.

Ms. Hernandez reports that she and her boyfriend have had an "on-and-off" relationship—she says she always feels that she "needs" him but they have "lots of fights" and cannot "hold it together" for more than a couple of weeks at a time. Most of her family relationships are strained, but she says her sister is her "best friend" now that they "are on speaking terms with each other again." Ms. Hernandez says that she took the overdose because she "can't stand to be alone." She volunteers that she "sees lots of other guys" and has a pattern of risky sexual behaviors when she and her boyfriend are having problems. She engages in binge drinking ("only when I am really mad") many times each month. Ms. Hernandez reports that she has had "anger issues" and "is always suicidal" since her teenage years. She has been in therapy many times, with many different therapists because she cannot find one that "understands" her. "At first they seem to 'get me'—understand what I am going through—but then they always pull back at some point."

Throughout the interview, Ms. Hernandez is highly emotional and affectively labile, ranging from intense anger to tearfulness. The interviewer's sense is that the reactions are well out of the appropriate range for the topics discussed. Review of her medical record shows five emergency department visits for "overdose" or "suicidal thoughts" within the last year. Her overdoses have always been with small enough quantities of medication that she only required monitoring without admission to an intensive care unit.

Ms. Hernandez's thoughts, reactions, and behaviors align well with the DSM-5 description of borderline personality disorder as "a pervasive pattern of instability of interpersonal relationships, self-image, and affects, and marked impulsivity, beginning by early adulthood and present in a variety of contexts" (p. 663). Her life story fulfills at least five of the nine criteria for the diagnosis. Ms. Hernandez reports experiences that meet DSM-5 criteria for borderline personality disorder, including efforts to avoid abandonment, intense interpersonal relationships, impulsivity, suicidal gestures, affective instability, and inappropriate anger. The pattern has been pervasive across multiple social spheres and clearly has negatively affected Ms. Hernandez's ability to live a complete, happy, and healthy life.

Ms. Hernandez reports a pattern of self-damaging impulses and recurrent suicidal behaviors. Although she has not yet had a life-threatening overdose, she is at risk for premature death. The fact that she has not yet had a self-harm gesture resulting in serious health impairment or organ damage by no means should reduce the clinician's concern for grave outcomes such as completed suicide. Impulsivity and danger should be evaluated thoroughly in assessing a person with borderline personality disorder. Although she has demonstrated these symptoms in an enduring and pervasive pattern, the clinician must nevertheless make certain that there is not another mental health condition or substance abuse issue that better accounts for the pattern seen in the case.

Approach to the Diagnosis

Borderline personality disorder often manifests with dramatic flares. Intense relationships, repeated self-harm behaviors, and intense and inappropriate anger can manifest together to create a tempestuous clinical picture. Conflicted and emotionally volatile relationships are often impressive with a borderline presentation. The intense emotionality of persons with the diagnosis can sometimes be remarkable—even overwhelming—to the clinician early in assessment; however, more subtle presentations are also possible. Furthermore, the diagnosis of borderline personality disorder must be arrived at by establishing that the criteria have been present and causing dysfunction over time. Also, before this specific diagnosis of borderline personality disorder can be given, it must be clarified that the patient meets the criteria for general personality disorder (see the section "General Personality Disorder" earlier in this chapter and in DSM-5).

As with the other personality disorder diagnoses, the clinician must first clarify that the symptom cluster is not better accounted for by another mental disorder or by the use of substances. This step may be difficult, given the likelihood of comorbidity in borderline personality disorder. Discerning the diagnosis may also be challenging because the patient's stated reason for seeking care may not immediately line up with the diagnostic criteria for the disorder. A patient with borderline personality disorder may present with a stated concern of "depression" or "high and low moods," which hints of mood disorder, when in fact the underlying pathology may be the labile mood states seen in borderline personality disorder. Moreover, people living with borderline personality disorder may develop major mood, anxiety, or trauma-related disorders. Distinguishing the chronic low mood states seen in persistent depressive disorder (dysthymia) or recurrent major depressive disorder from the chronic feelings of emptiness seen in borderline personality disorder, for instance, is a challenge that requires attention to the whole clinical picture.

Another potentially confusing issue that may complicate a case is an incorrect diagnosis given in the past or a patient's identification with a different mental health diagnosis. A misdiagnosis may have become the primary issue in the thoughts of the patient. A patient with an earlier diagnosis of "bipolar disorder" or "posttraumatic stress disorder" but whose condition is more consistent with a personality disorder may focus the clinical attention on the working diagnosis from an earlier time. It is important for the clinician to be aware of these considerations and place the patient's experiences and behaviors in the greater context.

The transient presence of borderline traits under specific conditions may be another confusing clinical presentation. Some people will use coping strategies consistent with the borderline personality diagnosis but only under specific stresses or in a particular life challenge. This pattern of situational coping does not meet the criteria for a diagnosis of borderline personality disorder. The pervasive traits of borderline personality disorder will often be evidenced by a long history of psychosocial complications, such as multiple disruptive and conflicted relationships, employment problems, and/or legal problems. These impairments in function can be directly linked to behavioral manifestations of the borderline personality disorder traits.

Substance abuse is a common co-occurring phenomenon in borderline personality disorder, and patients with borderline personality disorder should be carefully evaluated for substance-related issues.

It is very useful to try to get a longitudinal history and to obtain collateral information from other people involved with the patient's life (e.g., friends, family). It is often necessary to see a patient on multiple occasions to clarify the pathology's enduring nature. The input from friends and family can clarify the pattern in multiple contexts and help to trace the pathology back to adolescence.

Getting the History

Ms. Lane, age 33 years, describes a history of a pervasive pattern of instability of interpersonal relationships and marked impulsivity beginning by early adulthood and present in a variety of contexts. But she reports that she and her family think she is "bipolar" because of her "highs and lows." She says, "I looked up *bipolarism* on the Internet, and it is a perfect description of me. I am up and down all of the time! I've been like that since I was a teenager."

To discriminate between affective instability and episodic mania, the interviewer asks, "Can you say more about your 'highs and lows'?" Ms. Lane replies, "I can be fine 1 minute, and the next minute I am so angry. I get really manic sometimes when I am angry. I will get into an argument, and the mania takes over and I start yelling." The interviewer asks, "How long does that last?" The patient replies, "It can last 20 or 30 minutes. Longer sometimes. I just feel like my emotions are out of control. Sometimes I even throw things. And then I come back down."

The interviewer asks, "When does that happen?" Ms. Lane responds, "When I fight with my boyfriend, but it can also happen out of the blue if I start thinking about all my stress."

When asked when she started noticing this, Ms. Lane responds, "I have been like that since I was little. I used to do that when I would argue with my mother. But it got worse when I started dating boys in high school." The interviewer asks, "Can you think of times when you weren't like that?" She responds, "Usually when I first start going out with a guy, everything is great, and I am fine. It's when they start turning into jerks that my bipolar gets worse." The interviewer asks, "Do you get angry like that in situations other than with boyfriends?" She says, "Yes, my boss got me all manic a few times by being an idiot, and then he tried to get me fired for it!"

Emotional dysregulation and temper outbursts exemplified in this case are consistent with the affective instability seen in borderline personality disorder. The mood lability elicited in this history is a long-standing pattern rather than distinct episodes of mania or hypomania. The clinician establishes the pattern of *reactive* mood—different from the pattern present in depression or bipolar disorder, for example. The clinician also clarifies that these mood states are transient and that emotion regulation is a pervasive problem. Ms. Lane has had anger outbursts with many boyfriends throughout her adolescence and early adulthood, as well as with her mother and her boss.

It is confusing that Ms. Lane uses technical terms such as *manic* or *mania* and that she uses the incorrect term *bipolarism*. The clinician must distinguish between DSM-5 criteria and what the patient is trying to describe about her life experience.

Tips for Clarifying the Diagnosis

- Establish that the clinical picture is consistent with the definition of general personality disorder.
- Confirm that the DSM-5 symptoms of borderline personality disorder have occurred over a long duration in multiple social settings.
- Explore other diagnoses that may better explain the observed symptoms.
- Consider episodes from mood disorder diagnoses (e.g., major depressive episode or manic/hypomanic episode) and stable mood states as defined by the time span described in DSM-5. In borderline personality disorder, mood states tend to be unstable and fluctuate rapidly.
- Remember that other mental health diagnoses are commonly associated with the diagnosis.

Consider the Case

Mr. Bush, a 29-year-old single white man, presents to a psychiatrist reporting that his girlfriend wants him to "do something for anger management." He reports a history of intense anger and "temper" problems culminating in arguments and, at times, in physical fights with his girlfriend, brothers, and neighbor.

On further interview, Mr. Bush reports that his anger has "always been out of control." He has a long history of temperamental behavior in many different social contexts that has led him to physical fights with family members and breakups with previous girlfriends. He has been hospitalized three times for suicidal thinking and self-destructive behaviors like punching himself in the face. Each hospitalization occurred after a breakup with a girlfriend. He is very impulsive, reporting uncontrolled spending and reckless driving as well as binge-drinking episodes. His unstable moods and accompanying behaviors have resulted in a criminal record, including charges for assault, appearing drunk in public, and reckless driving. His conflict-oriented interpersonal style has led to arguments with work superiors and loss of jobs.

When discussing mood, Mr. Bush reports that he has been "depressed since I was a teenager." He endorses chronic feelings of emptiness. Furthermore, he reports reactive "mood swings" that last "a few hours at a time."

On mental status examination, he is hostile and angry for much of the interview. He becomes intensely tearful when discussing his girlfriend. He has multiple piercings on his ears and nose and tattoos on his neck. He has surface cuts in different stages of healing on his forearms where he says he has cut himself with razor blades in an effort "to make the pain go away."

The case of Mr. Bush demonstrates many features of borderline personality disorder. Mr. Bush states that his intense anger is his reason for seeking help, but it is the enduring and pervasive pattern of disruptive, negative, and self-damaging feelings that has caused problems for him in multiple spheres of his life. He meets criteria for general personality disorder and exhibits at least five of the nine criteria for the diagnosis of borderline personality disorder over a wide range of experiences and in an enduring pattern.

Differential Diagnosis

Borderline personality disorder can manifest with a myriad of different behaviors or symptoms. These must be distinguished from other mental health issues that can also look similar. For example, the strong emotional content of a borderline presentation can be mistaken for mood disorder episodes. In an effort to describe their affective instability, intense anger, or impulsivity, persons with borderline personality disorder may endorse symptoms that sound consistent with major depressive episode or manic/hypomanic episode. A diagnosis of bipolar disorder might be incorrectly considered when a patient with borderline personality disorder describes frequent, intense "highs and lows," when in fact the emotional states are often unstable and more a function of mood lability. Duration of symptoms is a key element in determining episodic, pathological mood states as in depression and bipolar disorder. Borderline personality disorder tends to be characterized by chronic mood instability, whereas depression and bipolar disorder are characterized by sustained episodes of mood pathology (often with interepisode resolution of symptoms). The differential diagnosis includes, in addition to mood disorders, other personality disorders, personality change due to another medical condition, substance use disorders, and identity problems.

Borderline personality disorder may co-occur with other mental disorders or substance use disorders. Mood disorders, anxiety disorders, and eating disorders are common comorbidities that must be recognized, but each can also become a misdiagnosis when borderline personality disorder better explains the presentation. The clinician should first establish that the definition for general personality disorder has been met, and then should systematically explore the specific criteria for borderline personality disorder while also recognizing that other pathological phenomena, such as eating disorder behaviors or substance abuse, may be present. In this manner, it will be possible to determine whether a patient has additional conditions that fulfill DSM-5 diagnoses. These additional diagnoses, when present, should be noted.

Patients may also exhibit maladaptive coping strategies and behaviors that look like borderline personality disorder only in specific stressful situations, in which case the behaviors are not enduring and do not warrant the diagnosis of borderline personality disorder.

See DSM-5 for additional disorders to consider in the differential diagnosis. Also refer to the discussions of comorbidity and differential diagnosis in their respective sections of DSM-5.

Summary

Borderline personality disorder is characterized by an enduring pattern of emotional instability. Features of the disorder may include any of the following:

- Conflict-oriented, unstable relationships that are characterized by alternating extremes of devaluation and idealization.
- Disproportionate, inappropriate, and intense anger.
- Difficulty maintaining a "true sense of self"; identity disturbance.
- Impulsive and self-injurious behavior.
- Co-occurring mental and substance-related disorders are common.

IN-DEPTH DIAGNOSIS

Obsessive-Compulsive Personality Disorder

Mr. Upton, a 37-year-old man, presents with his wife to a mental health clinician for evaluation in the context of having difficulties at work. He says that he believes that he is "fine" but that his boss—and his wife, he adds reluctantly—may have a problem with his "neatness." Mr. Upton has missed opportunities for promotion at work because he has trouble completing tasks, even though he is "the most conscientious worker there." His wife reports that he is a "control freak."

He is puzzled by his boss's attitude toward him. Mr. Upton states, "I'm a real perfectionist. You would think a supervisor would like that!" Mr. Upton is inflexible about matters of morality and ethics. He points out his opinion to coworkers routinely because they are often, he says, so "woolly headed" about the basics of "right and wrong."

Interviewing the couple reveals that Mr. Upton is very devoted to work activities to the exclusion of leisure activities and family. He is very critical of his wife's inability to maintain his standard of neatness. He will come home from work and redo household cleaning tasks that his wife completed earlier the same day. He scrutinizes their financial budget and has tried to restrict his wife's spending. He says that he wants to make sure they keep some money for "future emergencies."

He reports that he has "always been a stickler for the rules, even as a kid." As a young child he recalls having fits if someone else sat in his assigned seat at the dinner table. He was socially unpopular in high school because he would report schoolmates for "tardiness." His overinvestment in rules has caused conflict in many social spheres from a very young age.

Often people with obsessive-compulsive personality disorder do not see their personality traits as maladaptive. As demonstrated in this case, these individuals see the symptoms as strengths, despite their maladaptive nature and the conflicts and dysfunction that they cause. A clinician needs to assess and interpret the patient's experiences and behaviors carefully when fitting the behavior patterns with the criteria for the disorder. Mr. Upton describes his behaviors as "conscientious," "perfectionistic," and "neat," but he also discloses the problematic nature of them and describes the disability and compromised areas of function that they cause. Mr. Upton meets criteria for general personality disorder as well as at least four of the eight criteria for obsessive-compulsive personality disorder.

Approach to the Diagnosis

DSM-5 describes obsessive-compulsive personality disorder as "a pervasive pattern of preoccupation with orderliness, perfectionism, and mental and interpersonal control, at the expense of flexibility, openness, and efficiency, beginning by early adulthood and present in a variety of contexts" (p. 678). It is important for the clinician to keep this "big picture" in mind when approaching the patient. To be certain of the diagnosis, a number of factors should be clarified—the first of which is that the patient meets criteria for a general personality disorder (see the section "General Personality Disorder" earlier in this chapter and in DSM-5)—before refining the diagnosis for a specific personality disorder. A typical presentation of obsessive-compulsive personality disorder will capture the essence of the description above, and must meet four of the eight criteria specified in DSM-5.

Persons with this disorder will have an anxious preoccupation with rules and control to the extent that it causes great interpersonal conflict and dysfunction. Their perfectionism may result in a paralysis rather than excellence. They tend to focus on the trivial details to the extent that their main goals are lost.

Patients may not be aware that their personality traits are pathological. In fact, they may be very invested in their preoccupation with rules or their perfectionism and may believe these traits to be adaptive. This creates a challenge for the clinician to uncover. A patient may present with other complaints, such as interpersonal conflicts or anxiety symptoms. The clinician may have to work to reveal the clinical picture because of the patient's lack of insight.

The transient presence of obsessive-compulsive personality disorder traits under specific conditions may create a confusing clinical presentation. Some people might exhibit these traits only under specific stresses, in a particular life challenge, or in a narrow area of their overall social function. Such a pattern does not constitute a diagnosis of obsessive-compulsive personality disorder. Moreover, in many instances rigid, rules-oriented traits and excessive attention to detail are adaptive; however, these usually happen in a context, such as in a profession that requires great attention to detail, and are not pervasive.

When establishing a diagnosis, it is very useful to try to get a longitudinal history and to obtain collateral information from other people in the patient's life (e.g., friends, family). With obsessive-compulsive personality disorder, it is not uncommon for a family member to be able to articulate the clinical picture better than the patient because of the family member's perspective. It is often necessary to see a patient on multiple occasions to clarify the pathology's enduring nature. The input from friends and family can clarify the pattern in multiple contexts and help to trace the pathology back to adolescence.

Getting the History

> Mr. Fox, age 38 years, requested assessment from a psychiatrist because he is having marital difficulties. He tells the clinician that he doesn't think he has a problem, but his wife thinks he has a "control freak personality." Inviting the patient to explain his concerns, in his own words, is an important part of getting the history needed to determine the diagnosis. In talking about his orderliness, for example, Mr. Fox mentions that he doesn't like it when his wife plays his CDs because she "doesn't put them back right." He says, "I like my CDs to be in alphabetical order and on the shelf in a certain way." The interviewer asks, "Can you tell me how you like them to be ordered?" Mr. Fox replies, "I like them to be in order by category and then alphabetically by artist's last name. And my wife doesn't even know that Miles Davis is a jazz musician, let alone how to alphabetize. She usually just leaves them out anyway. She drives me crazy." The interviewer asks, "What do you do when she leaves them out?" Mr. Fox responds, "Well, we argue. And then I put them where they go! In fact, there's no mystery when she's been playing my CDs. She leaves them all over. And out of order." The interviewer asks, "What would happen to you if you didn't put them back?" Mr. Fox answers, "I don't know. Nothing. Sometimes I don't, in fact, because I'm too busy picking up some other mess she left." The clinician asks, "Do you ever check the CDs to make sure they're in order?" Mr. Fox responds, "Not really. But that's not a bad idea to check them periodically just to make sure she hasn't messed them up." The clinician asks, "Do you find yourself thinking or worrying about the order of the CDs?" He responds, "Only if I know she was messing them up." The interviewer asks, "Do you spend a lot of time keeping things like the CDs in a particular order?" Mr. Fox replies, "Just when I see she's strewn 'em all over the place. Why do you ask? Don't you think a man's record collection should be respected?"

The interviewer, who believes that Mr. Fox has an enduring and pervasive pattern of maladaptive personality disorder traits that are consistent with DSM-5 criteria for obsessive-compulsive personality disorder, is trying to distinguish Mr. Fox's preoccupation with orderliness around the CDs from an obsessive thought or a compulsion to act, which would indicate possible obsessive-compulsive disorder (OCD). In this case, it seems that the patient is describing an example of a preoccupation with order. He has a particular system with rules that he wants for his CDs, and he shows annoyance with violations of these rules. However, he does not ruminate and worry excessively about the CD collection. He does not check the CDs spontaneously. Furthermore, he does not experience anxiety when they are out of order. He is just fixated on the orderliness of the collection to the extent that he is willing to let it cause repeated arguments with his wife.

Tips for Clarifying the Diagnosis

- Establish that the clinical picture is consistent with the definition of general personality disorder.
- Confirm that the DSM-5 symptoms of obsessive-compulsive personality disorder have occurred over a long duration in multiple social settings.
- Explore other diagnoses that may better explain the observed symptoms.
- Look for dysfunction as a result of overvalue of rules and details.
- Remember that other mental health diagnoses are commonly associated with the diagnosis.

Consider the Case

Mr. Ganeshe, a 33-year-old Indian American computer programmer, presents with symptoms of insomnia. In the interview, the psychiatrist uncovers an enduring pattern of preoccupation with orderliness and perfectionism. Further interview reveals some anxiety-based insomnia that bothers Mr. Ganeshe when he works late on projects and then cannot stop thinking about them when he tries to fall asleep.

Mr. Ganeshe goes on to describe a long history of difficulty getting his work done because of his overcommitment to making sure that "everything is perfect" before he logs out. This leads him to work late into the night on projects that colleagues would be able to finish during regular work hours. He reports frustration because his work colleagues are often praised for projects but he is not, even though his projects "have better attention to little details." He will not delegate work to others because, he says, "If you want something done right, you have to do it yourself." He does not engage in many social activities because of his devotion to work and work-related projects. In fact, he does not attend work-related social activities because he doesn't want to "waste company time."

Mr. Ganeshe lives alone and dates rarely, despite pressure from his family to get married. He says that members of his family tell him that he is "not right"—but he feels that "they are the ones who are wrong!" He reports that he cannot stay with a girlfriend because the women he meets are "never just right for me."

He does not have generalized symptoms of anxiety or panic attacks.

He believes that his behaviors make him a better programmer despite feedback that he is struggling at work. He goes on to say that his commitment to orderliness is a culturally appropriate phenomenon and that it is "very Indian." He admits that other Indian Americans in his company "have a more 'American' work ethic."

This case fits with the DSM-5 description of obsessive-compulsive personality disorder. As frequently occurs in patients with this disorder, Mr. Ganeshe does not see these behaviors as problematic and is stubborn about changing these behaviors. He views them as adaptive in the workplace despite feedback that it is not.

There can be cultural variants that will apply to evaluation of the symptoms of obsessive-compulsive personality disorder. In Mr. Ganeshe's case, the behavior pattern is enduring and pervasive and causes dysfunction in multiple spheres, and the symptoms cause significant disability. Mr. Ganeshe does not exhibit thoughts, reactions, or behaviors that align with cultural or social norms, despite the patient's insistence. A patient can normalize something pathological as a cultural nuance, when in fact, it is more of a noncultural, maladaptive trait.

Differential Diagnosis

Obsessive-compulsive personality disorder must be distinguished from other mental disorders (e.g., OCD, hoarding disorder, substance use disorders), other personality disorders and personality traits, and personality change due to another medical condition.

OCD is usually easily distinguished from obsessive-compulsive personality disorder by the presence of true obsessions and compulsions in OCD. Descriptively, very often OCD is quite uncomfortable for the individual ("ego-dystonic") on an emotional level, whereas obsessive-compulsive personality disorder is not necessarily evidently problematic for the person ("ego-syntonic"). A person with obsessive-compulsive personality disorder tends to be less aware of his or her rigidity and more aware of the conflict that arises from it. When criteria for both disorders are met, both diagnoses should be made.

Other anxiety states may bring out rigid, rules-oriented traits but should not be confused with obsessive-compulsive personality disorder.

Other personality disorders may be confused with obsessive-compulsive personality disorder because they have traits in common. Therefore, a clinician needs to distinguish among these disorders by the differences in their characteristic features. For example, narcissistic personality disorder may also describe perfectionism and a belief that others cannot do things as well; however, narcissism is usually distinguished by inflated self-importance rather than rigid adherence to rules.

Obsessive-compulsive personality traits may be adaptive in certain professional contexts or other situations that reward highly detail-oriented performance. Furthermore, for an individual, the traits may exist only in a context where the trait is adaptive, in which case the diagnosis should not be made.

See DSM-5 for additional disorders to consider in the differential diagnosis. Also refer to the discussions of comorbidity and differential diagnosis in their respective sections of DSM-5.

Summary

Individuals who have obsessive-compulsive personality disorder demonstrate an enduring pattern of preoccupation with orderliness, order, and organization. Features of the disorder may include any of the following:

- Obsessive-compulsive personality disorder includes an enduring pattern of perfectionism.
- A person with obsessive-compulsive personality disorder has an enduring pattern of reluctance to delegate tasks, believing that only he or she can do such tasks correctly.

- Obsessive-compulsive personality disorder includes an enduring pattern of rigidity and stubbornness.
- These patterns are pervasive across multiple spheres of social life and create dysfunction.
- Neither obsessions nor compulsions are present in obsessive-compulsive personality disorder, which differentiates the disorder from OCD.

IN-DEPTH DIAGNOSIS
Schizotypal Personality Disorder

Ms. Katz, a 44-year-old single woman, presents with the chief complaint "I am so afraid." She reports anxiety stemming from serious concerns about the world ending with the end of the Mayan calendar in 2012. She believes that the date was actually a miscalculation and that the "true" date is in 2018. She has been interested in the predictions of "end times" from ancient sources like the myths of the ancient Mayans and the predictions of Nostradamus. She shows the psychiatrist Web sites that describe the Mayan prediction and possible scenarios for the end of the world. She has "triangulated the data to demonstrate" that the world will end in 2018. "I don't know what is going to happen, but it will be bad," she states.

Ms. Katz says that these fears are "really serious"—she states that she has severe symptoms of anxiety to the extent that she has insomnia and worries about the end of the world. She reports that she has taken precautions for the possibility of catastrophe, like taking self-defense classes and stocking her shelves with water and canned foods. She is involved with a group that takes these predictions seriously. The members of this group are her only major social contacts. Outside this group she has very few social relationships other than first-degree relatives.

Ms. Katz is not shy about sharing her interest in other unusual topics, such as crop circles, UFOs, and her belief that "aliens have probably visited Earth."

She has a pattern of odd beliefs and fascinations with fantasy and science fiction since childhood. She was awkward socially and had a very limited social group since adolescence. She reports that she has never been married and has never had any serious romantic relationships. She is oddly dressed, wearing a pin that says, "The end is near."

Ms. Katz does not have auditory hallucinations. She does not endorse any frankly delusional ideas. She is organized in her behavior. She has never had mood episodes of mania/hypomania or depression.

Ms. Katz fulfills criteria for general personality disorder, as well as specific diagnostic criteria for schizotypal personality disorder. She has few social relationships. She has very odd beliefs that influence her behavior. These beliefs are odd and eccentric but not clearly of the delusional caliber seen in thought disorders such as schizophrenia. Furthermore, she reports that these patterns have been present for much of her adolescent and adult life. Her interest in and odd ideas around fantasy topics are consistent with the eccentric ideas seen in schizotypal personality disorder. Meanwhile, she does not exhibit the hallmark symptoms of schizophrenia (e.g., she does not have hallucinations or frank delusions, disorganized speech, disorganized behavior, or a flattened affect).

Approach to the Diagnosis

DSM-5 describes the essence of schizotypal personality disorder as "a pervasive pattern of social and interpersonal deficits marked by acute discomfort with, and reduced capacity for, close relationships as well as by cognitive or perceptual distortions and eccentricities of behavior, beginning by early adulthood and present in a variety of contexts" (p. 655). A clinician must determine first that a person fits the definition of general personality disorder (see the section "General Personality Disorder" earlier in this chapter and in DSM-5) and then that the individual meets five of the nine described criteria for the specific diagnosis. An individual with schizotypal personality disorder typically presents as odd and eccentric and has a limited social network.

Other conditions must be examined when arriving at a personality disorder diagnosis. The prodrome of schizophrenia, for instance, may look very much like schizotypal personality disorder, but the former should be distinguishable because of its timeline as well as its evolution into a primary psychotic disorder.

Individuals may not be aware of their symptoms as pathological. In fact, if they seek mental health treatment at all, they most often present for depression, anxiety, or something else other than the personality disorder traits. The clinician must therefore get at the hallmark symptoms through an interview style that uncovers these patterns.

It is very useful to try to get a longitudinal history and to obtain collateral information from other people involved in the person's life (e.g., friends, family). Given the individual's lack of insight into symptoms, it is often helpful to get background history from family members. It is often necessary to see a person on multiple occasions to clarify the pathology's enduring nature. Additional information from friends and family can clarify the pattern in multiple contexts and help to trace the pathology back to adolescence.

Getting the History

Mr. Willis, age 36 years, reports that he has a background in physical science but dropped out of his doctoral program because of conflicts with his dissertation adviser. Mr. Willis states that the adviser did not understand him, because the adviser is not a "time traveler." Mr. Willis then indicates that this is not unusual. "People who don't believe in time travel are just different from me." His language around the belief is vague and circumstantial, so the interviewer has a hard time distinguishing "odd beliefs or magical thinking" from psychotic delusion.

The clinician asks, "Can you tell me more about the time travel?" Mr. Willis replies, "There are lots of stories about it, but no one really knows if it can work or not, right? With Einstein's relativity, we know that space and time bend." The clinician asks, "But can you tell me about *your* time travel?" Mr. Willis replies, "Different objects vibrate on their own frequencies. And if you get objects from a certain era of time together, they will all vibrate on the frequencies from that time. So I think people can time travel if they have the right objects together around them." The clinician asks, "Have you ever done this time travel?" Mr. Willis replies, "I am still working on getting the right conditions. But I have read about people who have done this. And it's real!" The clinician asks, "Do you mean you've read this in fiction or in real life?" Mr. Willis responds, "It's in science fiction all the time. But I think it's based on things that really happen. And I have read real accounts of this online. The scientific community just ignores it."

The interviewer, who believes that Mr. Willis has an enduring and pervasive pattern of maladaptive personality disorder traits that are consistent with DSM-5 criteria for schizotypal personality disorder, wants to find out if there is a more bizarre idea under the stated belief of the patient. The interviewer is seeking to clarify if the unusual belief should be thought of as a psychotic delusion. The clinician asks questions to see how firm the belief is. In this case the belief is unusual, but Mr. Willis does not hold this belief as absolutely fixed, as he would if it were a psychotic delusion. Furthermore, he is not claiming to have had the experience of time travel, an elaboration that may be present in someone with psychotic symptoms; he simply believes that time travel is possible. It is more along the lines of the odd beliefs seen in schizotypal personality disorder than it is like a psychotic delusion.

Tips for Clarifying the Diagnosis

- Establish that the clinical picture is consistent with the definition of general personality disorder.
- Confirm that the DSM-5 symptoms of schizotypal personality disorder have occurred over a long duration in multiple social settings.
- Explore other diagnoses that may better explain the observed symptoms.
- Remember that although they have similarities, people with schizotypal personality disorders should be distinguished from people with primary psychotic disorders.

Consider the Case

Mr. Huffman is 42 years old. He has been referred by a physician who has performed a necessary work physical examination for evaluation of "possible" depression. The occupational health doctor refers him to a psychiatrist to "rule out a psychotic disorder" because the doctor thinks Mr. Huffman is "very odd" and seems to be "delusional."

In his visit with a psychiatrist, Mr. Huffman is dressed oddly, wearing all purple from head to toe. He reports that he likes his work as an information technology technician because he does not have to talk to anyone. He says, "I just fix computers." When asked about depressive symptoms, he says, "I'm okay, I guess. Sometimes I feel discouraged."

He has never been on a date and has never been married. He has few social contacts because he "doesn't trust anyone." He sees his mother every weekend and helps her to "get groceries and pick up the house." His main social network comes through his interaction with people through online video gaming. He is very involved in a fantasy-oriented video game that he plays late at night against other fans through the Internet. He says that the purple clothes are his "magic colors" from the video game. He wears them every day to bring good fortune and to protect him from "evil." He reports that this pattern of behavior has been present since a young age.

Mr. Huffman does not experience auditory hallucinations, and he does not describe frank delusions. He has no history of substance abuse. There is no evidence of autism spectrum disorder. He does not endorse depressive symptoms.

Mr. Huffman's case seems to be consistent with schizotypal personality disorder. The man demonstrates a pervasive pattern of odd and eccentric behaviors within the context of a solitary life with few social relationships. He meets at least five of the nine criteria listed in DSM-5 for schizotypal personality disorder. He has eccentric behaviors, odd beliefs, few social relationships, and a generally guarded and suspicious view of other people. The phenomenon described in this case with regard to the man's belief that the purple colors will protect him is an unusual belief, but it should be viewed as an instance of "magical thinking" rather than a psychotic delusion. Divergent cultural norms may make "magical thinking" a difficult phenomenon to categorize, but in this case the belief is inconsistent with any cultural or religious explanation. Cultural variations and beliefs should be considered when determining the traits of schizotypal personality disorder. For instance, a wide range of beliefs might be considered quite ordinary to one culture but as "magical thinking" in another.

Differential Diagnosis

Schizotypal personality disorder must be distinguished from other disorders with psychotic symptoms, neurodevelopmental disorders, personality change due to another medical condition, substance use disorders, and other personality disorders and personality traits.

Schizotypal personality disorder can be distinguished from delusional disorder, schizophrenia, and bipolar or depressive disorder with psychotic features because these other disorders are all characterized by a period of persistent frank psychotic symptoms. Schizotypal personality is characterized by odd and eccentric thoughts and behaviors, including ideas of reference and magical thinking, but is not characterized by frank psychotic phenomena. It may be challenging to delineate between ideas of reference and delusions and between magical thinking and psychotic delusion, particularly in the context of evaluating a person of a different cultural background. In rare cases, a transient presence of schizotypal traits under specific conditions may be a confusing clinical presentation. This transient emergence of symptoms does not warrant a diagnosis of schizotypal personality disorder.

Special care must be taken to differentiate children with schizotypal personality disorder from those who have autism spectrum disorder.

Substance use disorders can present with similar symptoms as schizotypal personality disorder and must be ruled out. Some psychoactive drugs may mimic symptoms of the disorder.

Other personality disorders may be confused with schizotypal personality disorder because they have common traits. Other Cluster A personality disorders (i.e., paranoid and schizoid personality disorders) may have similar characteristics, such as suspiciousness, lack of close personal relationships, and odd interpersonal dynamics; however, they are usually distinguishable by the broad presentation of trait cluster that defines schizotypal personality disorder. Individuals who have borderline personality disorder may also have transient, psychotic-like states, but these states tend to be related to intense emotion or dissociation.

See DSM-5 for additional disorders to consider in the differential diagnosis. Also refer to the discussions of comorbidity and differential diagnosis in their respective sections of DSM-5.

Summary

Individuals who have schizotypal personality disorder demonstrate an enduring pattern of reduced interpersonal relationships and suspicious thinking. Features of the disorder may include any of the following:

- Schizotypal personality disorder includes an enduring pattern of cognitive or perceptual distortions, including "magical thinking."
- Schizotypal personality disorder includes an enduring pattern of odd behaviors and eccentricities.
- Patterns are pervasive across multiple spheres of social interaction, and they cause dysfunction.
- Schizotypal personality disorder is not associated with auditory hallucinations or delusions.

―――――――― IN-DEPTH DIAGNOSIS ――――――――
Narcissistic Personality Disorder

Mr. Klein, a 68-year-old retired businessman, presents with concerns over interpersonal conflicts. He wants to consult with a mental health professional to learn about the pathology of his family and uncover why they are not treating him as he feels he should be treated. He feels that he has been unjustly alienated from his family. He is twice divorced, describing his ex-wives as "girls who were too simple to appreciate what they had in me." He has become estranged from his daughters and grandchildren over time because "they don't give me the respect I deserve in our visits."

Further review of his history reveals a pattern of grandiosity and excessive need for admiration. Mr. Klein describes grand stories of his business endeavors, name-dropping famous businessmen such as Donald Trump and Bill Gates as peers. He continuously focuses on his achievements in business and in social interactions. He demonstrates a lack of empathy for those "beneath" him and identifies closely with celebrity businesspeople. From the interview, it is not clear how successful he was in his career. It is clear that he ran into conflicts with superiors, limiting his ability to be promoted. He claims that his bosses "were always jealous" of his talent and never let him "get ahead."

Mr. Klein describes the current problem between him and his family as the source of conflict causing him irritability. He has refused to spend time with his daughters and grandchildren because they don't show him the "respect I deserve." He was particularly annoyed that he had to go to the daughters' houses for visits. "They should come see me on my home turf instead." He announced to them that he no longer would travel to anyone's house. For 3 years he has not seen his daughters or his grandchildren. He gets invited to holidays and to the kids' birthdays but refuses to go unless they come to his house first.

Mr. Klein says, "If they want to see me, they know what they need to do."

Mr. Klein meets DSM-5 criteria for general personality disorder, as well as specific diagnostic criteria for narcissistic personality disorder. A sense of confidence may be useful in the business world, but the pattern of grandiosity seen in this case does not generate success in business or in family life. His rigid rules around expectations for how he is to be treated and respected have been poorly adaptive to achieve his desired goals. Furthermore, there is a sense that other people involved in this man's life would have very different perspectives on the story.

Approach to the Diagnosis

Narcissistic personality disorder is described by DSM-5 as "a pervasive pattern of grandiosity (in fantasy or behavior), need for admiration, and lack of empathy, beginning by early adulthood and present in a variety of contexts" (p. 669). To make the diagnosis, the person must meet the definition of general personality disorder (see the section "General Personality Disorder" earlier in this chapter and in DSM-5) as well as at least five of the nine identified criteria for the specific disorder.

The typical presentation of narcissistic personality disorder is that of a grandiose individual with an excessive need for admiration. Individuals with this disorder believe that they are superior to others and should be recognized for their superiority. People with narcissistic personality disorder tend to lack empathy for others.

Other pathology should always be investigated. Often persons with narcissistic personality disorder will present for assessment or treatment of symptoms of major mental disorders or because of interpersonal problems. Mood disorders should be considered and ruled out. The grandiosity seen in manic or hypomanic episodes should not be mistaken for narcissistic personality disorder because of the episodic nature of grandiosity in bipolar disorders.

Substance abuse should be investigated. Cocaine intoxication, for example, can present as apparent grandiosity.

Individuals who have narcissistic personality disorder may not be aware of their symptoms. They do not often present for treatment or evaluation of their personality disorder traits. The diagnosis may be difficult to arrive at initially because of the person's lack of insight.

Adaptive variations of traits must be considered. In limited instances grandiosity and overconfidence are adaptive traits and promote success. Usually when these traits are pervasive and enduring, they cause dysfunction. To make the diagnosis of narcissistic personality disorder, the clinician must look for the pervasive pattern causing dysfunction.

It is very useful to try to get a longitudinal history and to obtain collateral information from other people involved in the person's life (e.g., friends, family). It is often necessary to see a person on multiple occasions to clarify the pathology's enduring nature. The input from friends and family can clarify the pattern in multiple contexts and help to trace the pathology back to adolescence.

Getting the History

A clinician believes that Mr. Pierce, age 37 years, may meet the DSM-5 description of narcissistic personality disorder, but the clinician is having trouble fitting the man's presentation to the specific criteria from DSM-5. The man has described his job as a manager of a paper supply store as a "waste of his talent." The clinician tries to explore this statement as an example of the DSM-5 criteria by asking more about it.

The clinician asks, "What do you mean by a 'waste of your talent'?" Mr. Pierce responds, "I mean I am way smarter than anyone in that place. I am the manager of morons. And my boss is a moron. I am the only one in that place with real brains." The clinician asks, "So do you mean you are overqualified to work there?" He responds, "No, I mean I am just way more gifted than anyone else there." The clinician asks, "Do other people see that you are gifted?" He responds, "No, and it drives me crazy." The clinician asks, "How so?" Mr. Pierce responds, "Because no one there appreciates my brains. They can't see that I am smarter. I could snap my fingers and get a better job, but the same thing will probably happen somewhere else!"

Narcissistic personality disorder may be a tricky diagnosis to make because it is unlikely that a person will answer affirmatively to questions based on the exact criteria from DSM-5. It is doubtful that someone with the disorder would have the insight to say, "Yes, I do require excessive admiration, I have a sense of entitlement, and I am interpersonally exploitative." Therefore, the diagnosis often must be made from inference on the basis of content that comes from the interview.

Tips for Clarifying the Diagnosis

- Establish that the clinical picture is consistent with the definition of general personality disorder.
- Confirm that the DSM-5 symptoms of narcissistic personality disorder have occurred over a long duration in multiple social settings.
- Explore other diagnoses that may better explain the observed symptoms.
- Remember that other mental health diagnoses are commonly associated with the diagnosis.

Consider the Case

Mr. McCoy, a 22-year-old college sophomore and football player, presents to the student mental health center with irritability after being replaced as quarterback. Despite good athletic performance, he was benched because the coach said that his "attitude stinks." Mr. McCoy says the coach "is blind if he can't see that I'm better than the other players—even the seniors." He quotes his passing and rushing statistics proudly to make the case that he should not have been demoted.

Mr. McCoy says, "They call me a prima donna but they need me. Oh yeah. They need me." He is very critical of the other players and will berate them on the field in games.

His girlfriend broke up with him recently, saying to him that she could "never love you as much as you loves yourself." He laughs at this, saying, "Oh, she'll regret leaving me—she'll never get it so good with somebody else."

Mr. McCoy reports that his "confidence" has always been a "major part of his game." He counts on his abilities to make plays and pick up yards. He says, "I have to be the best to win." He reports that part of his success relates to taking risks—"Going for it, big time!"—and that his coaches have tried to discourage this. "I say to them, 'Hey—no pain, no gain. You gotta take the risk or you won't win.' "He has had excellent performance throughout high school and early college play. He sees this trait as adaptive and productive, despite the feedback he has gotten from the coaches and other players.

This pattern has been present for Mr. McCoy throughout his adolescence and young adult life. It has caused him problems in family and intimate relationships.

Confidence can be adaptive, especially in sports, and some of the traits associated with narcissistic personality disorder can be helpful and positive in very specific contexts. However, these traits tend to be maladaptive when inflexibly applied across multiple settings and when they are unchanging over time. Mr. McCoy has applied extreme confidence and risk taking to be competitive in games, and the strategy has worked to a great enough extent that he has had success and earned the role of starting quarterback. However, his interpersonal relationships are hindered to the point that he has lost his spot on the team. Furthermore, he is failing in other areas of functioning as a result of his rigid patterns.

Differential Diagnosis

Narcissistic personality disorder must be distinguished from mania or hypomania, substance use disorders, and other personality disorders and personality traits. Grandiosity often manifests as part of manic or hypomanic episodes. The inflated sense of self that relates to bipolar disorder should be present only in the context of a mood episode, whereas it is an enduring trait of the personality disorder. Manic or hypomanic states would not necessarily mimic other traits of narcissistic personality disorder.

Narcissistic personality disorder must also be distinguished from symptoms that may develop in association with persistent or intermittent substance use.

Other personality disorders may be confused with narcissistic personality disorder because they have certain features in common. Other Cluster B personality disorders (i.e., antisocial, borderline, and histrionic personality disorders) may share the most overlap with narcissistic personality disorder traits. Antisocial personality disorder shares the characteristic lack of empathy and manipulation of others. The two disorders are usually easily distinguished by the other symptoms in the DSM-5 description. Antisocial personality disorder is usually characterized by lack of regard and violation of the rights of others as evidenced by aggressiveness, deceit, and lack of remorse, whereas the lack of empathy seen in narcissistic personality disorder is usually a result of an inflated self-ego.

Many highly successful individuals display personality traits that might be considered narcissistic. Only when these traits are inflexible, maladaptive, and persisting and cause significant functional impairment or subjective distress do they warrant a diagnosis of narcissistic personality disorder.

See DSM-5 for additional disorders to consider in the differential diagnosis. Also refer to the discussions of comorbidity and differential diagnosis in their respective sections of DSM-5.

Summary

Individuals who have narcissistic personality disorder may demonstrate an enduring pattern of grandiose sense of self-importance. Features of the disorder may include any of the following:

- People with narcissistic personality disorder may have an enduring pattern of lack of empathy.

- People with narcissistic personality disorder may have an enduring pattern of excessive need for admiration.
- These patterns are pervasive across multiple spheres of experience and they cause dysfunction.

-------------------- SUMMARY --------------------

Personality Disorders

To be diagnosed with any personality disorder, the person must first meet the threshold criteria that define the presence of a general personality disorder. Personality disorders are defined as enduring patterns of experience and behavior that are pervasive across social situations and lead to serious impairment in important areas of life function. The enduring quality is a key to understanding the concept of the diagnosis because these phenomena are related to personality traits that are generally consistent throughout adulthood and are nonepisodic.

If the clinical case meets the description of general personality disorder, a specific personality disorder diagnosis may be considered. Many maladaptive personality traits may be observed in persons who never meet general criteria for personality disorder and should not be classified with a specific personality disorder. Maladaptive personality traits may occur in isolation or only in specific situations, in which case they would not be associated with a personality disorder diagnosis.

The concept of general personality disorder suggests that the maladaptive patterns of experience and behavior are fixed into an individual's personality. This is why DSM-5 specifies that personality disorders are of long duration and must be traceable to adolescence or early adulthood. While it is possible to give a personality disorder diagnosis in a person under age 18, personality disorder diagnoses are often deferred until after age 18 because the clinician should identify these experiences and behaviors in an already firmly established personality rather than a developing personality.

Distinguishing personality disorders from other mental health diagnoses, physiological effects of substances, or medical conditions is a challenging necessity for any personality disorder diagnosis. This can be a challenging step, given that individuals often present with multiple conditions and states that must be taken into account.

---------------- ■ ■ ■ ----------------

Diagnostic Pearls

- Personality disorders are associated with maladaptive personality traits.
- In personality disorder, the maladaptive traits must be enduring over a long period of time (i.e., fixed in the personality) and pervasive across many social situations; they are not episodic.
- The enduring and pervasive pattern of maladaptive experience and behavior must lead to impaired function to be classified as a personality disorder.

- Personality disorder traits can be traced to the development of adult personality (adolescence or early adulthood).

- Specific personality disorder diagnoses can be made only if the criteria for general personality disorder are met first.

- Personality disorders may be confused with other mental disorders, substance abuse, or medical conditions. Understanding the long-lasting patterns of behavior is essential to making a correct diagnosis. This understanding usually involves knowing a person long term and/or having a very extensive and complete history.

Self-Assessment

Key Concepts: Double-Check Your Knowledge

What is the relevance of the following concepts to the various personality disorders?

- General personality disorder
- Pervasive and inflexible pattern
- Onset in adolescence or early adulthood
- Stability of pattern over time
- Ten specific personality disorder diagnoses
- Cluster A: odd or eccentric profiles
- Cluster B: dramatic, emotional, or erratic profiles
- Cluster C: anxious or fearful profiles

Questions to Discuss With Colleagues and Mentors

1. If a patient exhibits six of the nine symptoms listed in the DSM-5 criteria for borderline personality disorder only when he or she is under a particular stressor, is the diagnosis of borderline personality disorder appropriate?
2. A person develops personality disorder traits after the onset of a medical condition in the fifth decade of life. His symptom profile meets six of the seven criteria for paranoid personality disorder. What is the most appropriate way to apply DSM-5 diagnoses to this case?
3. If all of the diagnostic criteria are met for more than one personality disorder in two separate clusters, can one patient be given two diagnoses?
4. How are personality disorders different from episodic mood disorders?
5. Personality disorder traits can work to an individual's benefit in certain situations. Why is it important to examine the pervasiveness of patterns to make the diagnosis of a personality disorder?
6. How is a diagnosis of other specified personality disorder or unspecified personality disorder useful in practice?

Case-Based Questions

PART A

Ms. Bailey, a 26-year-old single white woman, presents to the clinic with a pervasive pattern of instability of interpersonal relationships, self-image, and affects, and marked impulsivity, beginning by early adulthood and present in a variety of contexts. She has a prior diagnosis of unspecified bipolar disorder. She does not report a history consistent with manic or hypomanic episodes; however, she does report a mood history consistent with having had depressive episodes. She also reports some very unusual and eccentric beliefs, but no frank delusions and no auditory hallucinations.

Ms. Bailey's presentation reveals anger outbursts and constant irritability. Identity disturbance also seems to be a serious issue. She identifies closely with a small group of friends in a club that plays a fantasy game. The few romantic relationships she has had have been with members of this group and have been unstable and intense. She claims that her identity is closely related to her character in the game (and to the fantasy club in general).

Ms. Bailey does not drink alcohol, but she does use hallucinogenic drugs fairly regularly (once every few weeks). She says she does these drugs with her friends from the fantasy club. She is odd in her dress.

What diagnosis can be made?   With the information above, it seems clear that the criteria for general personality disorder are met. Ms. Bailey seems to have traits from the DSM-5 criteria for borderline personality disorder, but the clinical picture is complicated by her odd beliefs and eccentricities. She does not seem to meet symptom criteria for bipolar disorder.

PART B

When exploring Ms. Bailey's fantasy interests more closely, the concept of schizotypal personality disorder enters the thoughts of the clinician. The woman speaks of the fantasy club in very vague terms, and she does not distinguish the members of the club from their characters in the game. In fact, she refers to herself by the name of her character about half the time. When asked about her unusual dress, she reports that this is typical dress "for an elf." When specifically asked, she reports that she does not think she is an elf, but her character in the club is. She says that like her character, she has "special gifts for reading people." When asked in more detail, she reports that her character is clairvoyant and "to some extent, so am I."

She reports that she believes that people outside of her fantasy club are untrustworthy.

When she uses hallucinogenic drugs, she reports that she "enters the real kingdom" (referring to her fantasy game). But she goes on to say, "That only happens when I trip."

Can one individual be diagnosed with more than one personality disorder?   Yes. In the second part of this case, the clinician uncovers traits consistent with schizotypal personality disorder in addition to the borderline personality disorder traits. Two specific personality disorder diagnoses can be made if the person fulfills the criteria for both. This case is complicated further by the use of hallucinogenic drugs, because they may cause odd ideas and/or magical thinking.

439

Short-Answer Questions

1. If a person meets seven of the nine criteria for borderline personality disorder, but only in the context of a hypomanic episode, is the diagnosis of borderline personality disorder appropriate?
2. A senator has an "overly inflated ego" and enjoys the admiration she gets from others. She is in a successful marriage and is high functioning without the perception of distress in her life. Should the diagnosis of narcissistic personality disorder be considered?
3. Which personality disorder is most associated with self-harm behaviors?
4. Which two symptom criteria does OCD have that obsessive-compulsive personality disorder lacks?
5. If a phenomenon that a clinician may consider to be "magical thinking" occurred in his own culture and is a widely accepted belief in the culture of a patient, how might this similarity change the way the clinician should think about the phenomenon in terms of diagnosis?
6. Can a 17-year-old be correctly given a personality disorder diagnosis?
7. Is a personality disorder necessarily a lifelong or permanent diagnosis?
8. Can personality disorders be diagnosed cross-culturally?
9. Which gender has a higher prevalence of borderline personality disorder?
10. What is in the differential diagnosis for schizotypal personality disorder?

Answers

1. No. Borderline personality disorder is not diagnosed when the criteria that are met occur in the context of a hypomanic episode.
2. No. The features of a personality disorder must cause distress or dysfunction.
3. Borderline personality disorder is the personality disorder most associated with self-harm behaviors.
4. Obsessions and compulsions occur in OCD but not in obsessive-compulsive personality disorder.
5. Cultural norms should be taken into account before using a technical term like "magical thinking." If the phenomenon is consistent with widely held systems of belief in the person's culture, it should not be considered pathological.
6. Yes. A 17-year-old can be diagnosed with a personality disorder if the features have been present for at least 1 year—with the exception of antisocial personality disorder, for which an individual must be at least age 18 to receive this diagnosis.
7. No. A personality disorder is not necessarily a lifelong or permanent condition, although when a personality disorder is present, it must have emerged early in life.
8. Yes. Personality disorders can be diagnosed cross-culturally.
9. Females have a higher prevalence of borderline personality disorder.
10. In the differential diagnosis for schizotypal personality disorder are other mental disorders with psychotic symptoms, neurodevelopmental disorders, personality change due to another medical condition, substance use disorders, and other personality disorders and personality traits.

22

Paraphilic Disorders

Richard Balon, M.D.

"I have this urge to show my genitals."

*"I have recurring sexual fantasies of being beaten
by my partner."*

The diagnostic class of paraphilic disorders includes disorders of sexual interest and behavior characterized by intense and persistent fantasies, interests, or behaviors far beyond what is considered a normative ("normophilic") sexual interest and/or behavior and that cause significant distress or impairment. The term *paraphilia* literally means love (*philia*) beyond the usual (*para*).The focus of paraphilic behavior could be either the target of sexual activity or fantasy (e.g., nonhuman objects, children or non-consenting adults, animals) or the sexual activity (e.g., various activities such as spanking or whipping a sexual partner or oneself to cause suffering or humiliation to oneself or one's sexual partner). It is important to note that this interest and/or behavior should exceed interest in what is considered regular sexual intercourse and relationship with a consenting sexual partner, because some elements of this behavior may occur during what is considered normal sexual activity.

The crucial distinction made in DSM-5 as compared to DSM-IV is between paraphilic disorder and paraphilia. *Paraphilia* is the description of specific sexual arousal and behavior (Criterion A of each paraphilic disorder, which requires a duration of at least 6 months), whereas *paraphilic disorder* is the paraphilia plus its consequences (e.g., acting on the sexual urges or fantasies with a nonconsenting person, the paraphilia causing clinically significant distress or impairment in social, occupational, or other important areas of functioning—i.e., Criterion B of each paraphilic disorder). This distinction advanced by DSM-5 avoids labeling of every non-normative sexual behavior as psychopathological and also provides more specific guidance for clinical intervention. Examples in which this distinction is important include fetishism or transvestism: if the person using a fetish or engaging in cross-dressing during sexual activity is not distressed or impaired, the diagnosis of fetishistic or transvestic disorder should not be entertained. In the absence of a disorder, clinical intervention is not indicated.

Paraphilic interest and/or behavior occurs along a spectrum from occasional nondistressing behavior during normative copulatory behavior (e.g., mildly spanking a sexual partner); to intense urges, fantasies, and behaviors that are still not distressing and not causing any impairment; to intense and/or persistent urges, fantasies, and/or behaviors that also cause distress and/or impairment in various areas of functioning; to intense and/or persistent urges, fantasies, and/or behaviors that the individual acts on with a nonconsening person or that cause distress and/or impairment in various areas of functioning. The careful use of both Criterion A and Criterion B (and also, possibly, specifiers, severity ratings, and patient self-measures) allows for clearer distinction and delineation of occasional nonconsequential behavior, paraphilia, and paraphilic disorder.

One individual may be diagnosed with more than one paraphilic disorder (e.g., pedophilic disorder and voyeuristic disorder) and/or co-occurring paraphilia and paraphilic disorder (e.g., fetishism and sexual sadism disorder). Paraphilic disorders can also be comorbid with other mental disorders (e.g., personality disorders, substance use disorders).

Interviewing individuals with suspected or diagnosed paraphilic disorder(s) or paraphilia(s) may be a challenging task. These disorders may have far-reaching medicolegal impact and consequences; thus, the individual may not be willing or eager to discuss his or her innermost fantasies, urges, and behaviors in the paraphilia realm. Thus, the interview must be conducted in an atmosphere of respect and rapport. The interviewer should be aware of his or her countertransferential feelings, which could be fairly strong in this area, especially in cases of paraphilic disorders involving children or violence. When legal issues are relevant, the limits on confidentiality should be explained. The interviewer should attempt to obtain insight into the feelings and possible suffering of the individual with paraphilic disorder. Some individuals not only recognize the problems, unacceptability, and consequences of their urges, fantasies, and behaviors to others (victims, families) and themselves, but also agonize over them despite being unable to resist them.

DSM-5 delineates eight paraphilic disorders:

- *Voyeuristic disorder:* getting sexually aroused by observing an unsuspecting person being naked, disrobing, or engaging in sexual activity.
- *Exhibitionistic disorder:* getting sexually aroused by exposing one's genitalia to nonconsenting person(s).
- *Frotteuristic disorder:* getting sexually aroused by touching or rubbing against a nonconsenting person.
- *Sexual masochism disorder:* getting sexually aroused from being humiliated, beaten, bound, or otherwise made to suffer during sexual activity.
- *Sexual sadism disorder:* getting sexually aroused by the physical or psychological suffering of another individual.

- *Pedophilic disorder:* getting sexually aroused by fantasies, urges, or behavior involving sexual activity with prepubescent children (generally those age 13 or younger).
- *Fetishistic disorder:* getting sexually aroused from using nonliving objects or highly focusing on nongenital body parts of a sexual partner.
- *Transvestic disorder:* getting sexually aroused from cross-dressing as a member of the opposite sex.

These eight paraphilic disorders do not encompass all possible paraphilias or paraphilic behaviors. Numerous paraphilias have been described, such as acrotomophilia (erotic focus: amputation in partner), necrophilia (erotic focus: corpses), telephone scatologia (erotic focus: obscene phone calls), and zoophilia (erotic focus: animals). In cases of clearly distinctive paraphilic behavior that is not included in the eight delineated disorders and that has been present for at least 6 months and is causing distress or impairment, the diagnosis of *other specified paraphilic disorder* should be used, specifying the specific reason or paraphilia. When paraphilic behavior causes significant distress or impairment in social, functional, occupational, or other areas but does not meet the full criteria for any disorder in this diagnostic class (or insufficient information is available to make a more specific diagnosis), clinicians should use the diagnosis of *unspecified paraphilic disorder*.

IN-DEPTH DIAGNOSIS
Exhibitionistic Disorder

Mr. Ward, a 25-year-old man, was referred for an evaluation by the court. He was arrested by the police after he exposed himself to a female fast-food restaurant worker. While the woman was handing him his order in his car at the drive-thru window, he exposed his genitalia. After the woman started to scream, he drove away. The woman was able to get his license plate number and contacted police immediately. He was arrested about a mile away while still masturbating in the car. During the interview he reveals that he has been exposing his genitalia to unsuspecting females for several years. Mr. Ward likes to expose himself to women with "big breasts, if possible." He has exposed himself several times to women at drive-thru restaurants or to women passing by his car in parking lots. Exposing himself to unsuspecting women and subsequently masturbating has been his preferred sexual activity, although he had a girlfriend with whom he was sexually active. Mr. Ward occasionally masturbates while imagining exposing himself to female movie stars. At times, he cannot control his urge to expose himself and drives "around to see where I can do it." He has been very nervous lately because "I have almost been caught by police several times, but I cannot stop myself. It is hopeless." He denies any other unusual sexual behavior. He works part-time and lives by himself. He occasionally has contact with his parents and rarely with coworkers.

This heterosexual man was referred for psychiatric evaluation by the criminal system. Individuals with exhibitionistic disorder do not usually seek help themselves. Mr. Ward presents a typical case of exhibitionism, in that he is a male deriving sexual arousal from exposing his genitals to unsuspecting females. The behavior has been ongoing for several years, with onset around age 20. Further, he was not seeking treatment himself, although he has been distressed by possible consequences of his behavior and the inability to stop his urges.

Approach to the Diagnosis

A substantial number of individuals who expose themselves or have a strong impulse to expose themselves may never be referred and diagnosed with exhibitionistic disorder. If these individuals are not distressed by their fantasies and urges, are not impaired by this sexual interest in other important areas of functioning, and their self-reported, psychiatric, or legal histories indicate that they do not act on their interest, they could be, according to DSM-5, ascertained as having a paraphilia (i.e., exhibitionism) but are not diagnosed with exhibitionistic disorder. Those individuals who are distressed by their behavior or are impaired in some area(s) of their functioning (e.g., relationship, occupation due to legal issues) should be diagnosed with exhibitionistic disorder. The urges, interests, fantasies, and behaviors must be intense and recurrent over at least 6 months to meet the diagnostic criteria for this disorder.

Although the paraphilic behavior or the distress/impairment is the key feature, the duration of the recurrent and intense sexual arousal is necessary for making the diagnosis. These features help to determine whether the general criteria are fulfilled for the disorder.

The intensity or severity of the disorder may vary during its course. DSM-5 provides specifiers regarding the preference of the person to whom the individual likes to expose himself or herself (i.e., prepubertal children, physically mature individuals, or both) and in what environment. The "in controlled environment" specifier was added as an acknowledgment that behavior such as exhibitionism may be difficult to assess in individuals who have limited opportunity to expose themselves because they are in a controlled environment (e.g., such exposure may not be possible in prison or during military service). The exhibitionistic disorder could also be specified as being in full remission, meaning that the individual has no distress or impairment in functioning and has not acted on exhibitionistic urges for at least 5 years while in an uncontrolled environment. DSM-5 does not specify whether the individual might have urges that he or she does not act on.

DSM-5 notes that the disorder is unusual in females and that it tends to emerge in males in adolescence or early adulthood. Little is known about its persistence over time. No specific tests are useful for making this diagnosis. Thus, the approach to this diagnosis is clinical and descriptive.

Getting the History

A 35-year-old man reports that he has been having problems being sexually aroused unless he is "in some special situations." The interviewer, even if knowing (from the referral) or suspecting that the individual exposes his genitals to unsuspecting strangers, should ask for a better description of the situation in which arousal occurs and accept the individual's description as a starting point, no matter how evasive or minimalizing the description is.

Once the occurrence of exhibitionism is established, the interviewer should ask how the individual feels during the exposure, immediately after it, and later on, and investigate whether he masturbates during or after the exposure: "Do you get really aroused when you show your genitals to some unknown woman? Do you masturbate when she is surprised or shocked?" The next questions should focus on how long, how often, and in what situations the behavior occurs: "When did you first expose yourself? How often do you expose yourself and where do you usually expose yourself?" Finally, the interviewer should ask whether the individual is disturbed by the behavior: "Does the exposing to people bother you? Do you feel upset about it? Have you had any legal or other problems related to exposing yourself?"

The interview should establish an atmosphere of trust and good rapport, without confronting the individual about his or her behavior and its legal consequences, to elicit all symptoms of exhibitionism.

The description of the behavior—exposure of genitals to unsuspecting strangers—and the fact that the behavior arouses the individual are crucial for recognizing *exhibitionistic disorder.* The questions about being distressed or impaired in some area of functioning are helpful for making the diagnosis. The individual may be evasive about his or her arousal or behavior, its frequency, and associated problems (e.g., legal trouble). The clinical interview is the cornerstone for making the diagnosis. Previous records of exhibitionistic behavior (e.g., police reports, victim statement, prior evaluations) or a corroborating interview (e.g., with parents in the case of a juvenile offender or with the individual's partner) may also be helpful. Evaluations conducted for forensic purposes have different confidentiality requirements that should be reviewed with the individual being interviewed.

Tips for Clarifying the Diagnosis

- Determine whether the exposure of genitals happens in the presence of unsuspecting strangers.
- Explore whether the individual is unable to control his or her urges to expose himself or herself.
- Establish whether the exposure is accompanied or followed by masturbation.
- Evaluate whether the individual is apprehensive about or distressed by his or her behavior.
- Investigate whether the individual has the opportunity to go out and expose himself or herself.

Consider the Case

Mr. Carson, a 50-year-old man, seeks help for "sexual deviation." "My wife caught me making calls to some pay-for-sex phone numbers and talking about sex while touching myself." Mr. Carson admits during the interview that what he calls "phone sex" is just a substitution for what he really likes: "getting out of the car in some unknown neighborhood, watching some people in their bedrooms, and then, when I get excited, finding an unknown woman to whom I show my penis. That really makes my day, when she screams and I come. But, you know, this has been a very tough winter. I cannot get out because it is really cold outside, so I tried those phone numbers." He says that he has never gotten caught over the 15 years he has been exposing himself; however, he has been a bit nervous since he read in the newspaper that police were looking for an older man who likes to expose himself. His wife, with whom he has a "regular but boring sex life," had not known about his behavior until recently. "She did not push me to seek help, but she told me I was nuts, deviant, someone with whom she does not want to have sex. That made me think."

The onset of Mr. Carson's exhibitionistic behavior developed relatively late in his life, which is unusual but possible. Although he reports himself for help and treatment, his self-referral is not totally voluntary; he has been forced by some circumstances, such as by reading about police looking for someone who is exposing himself and by his wife's comments. He is heterosexual, married, and engaged in regular sexual activity with his wife. However, he has been deriving more satisfying arousal and sexual satisfaction from paraphilic behaviors, such as watching people in their bedrooms (voyeurism), exposing himself, and talking about sex over the phone (telephone scatologia). His preferred source of paraphilic arousal is exposing himself to unsuspecting females. It is important to realize that paraphilic disorders can overlap or coexist. Exhibitionism also can occur in an individual who is involved in regular sexual activity with a partner. Organic brain changes may be considered in older individuals in which paraphilia or paraphilic disorder develops totally de novo. However, Mr. Carson has shown no signs of cognitive impairment and has no history of brain injury. A further neurological workup may be needed to anchor the diagnosis.

Differential Diagnosis

The differential diagnosis of exhibitionistic disorder is relatively narrow because the description of the paraphilic behavior is specific—exposing one's genitalia to unsuspecting strangers. This behavior may occur strictly within exhibitionistic behavior or within the frame of several co-occurring paraphilic disorders (e.g., voyeuristic disorder, fetishistic disorder). The exposure of genitals may also occur in psychosis (where the exposure would probably be more nondiscriminatory), conduct disorder, antisocial personality disorder, and substance use disorders (especially during intoxication). The exhibitionistic disorder should also be distinguished from nudism—individuals with exhibitionistic disorder usually do not expose themselves at nudist places.

The course of the disorder likely varies with age and little is known about persistence over time when it emerges in adolescence or early adulthood. Advancing age may be associated with decreasing exhibitionistic sexual preferences and behavior. Depression and substance use may develop as a consequence of exhibitionistic disorder and then affect the clinical presentation. Denial or minimization of the behavior could hinder the differential diagnosis.

See DSM-5 for additional disorders to consider in the differential diagnosis. Also refer to the discussions of comorbidity and differential diagnosis in their respective sections of DSM-5.

Summary

- Exhibitionistic disorder involves recurrent and intense sexual arousal from the fantasies, urges, or behavior of exposing one's genitalia to nonconsenting, unsuspecting strangers.

- In the context of an intense exhibitionistic sexual interest, the diagnosis of exhibitionistic disorder can be made if the individual has exposed his or her genitalia to a nonconsenting person, or when the individual has distress or impairment in various areas of functioning because of the exhibitionistic urges or fantasies.
- Careful history should help to rule out other mental disorders (e.g., psychotic disorder, substance use disorder, personality disorder) and other paraphilic disorders.

IN-DEPTH DIAGNOSIS

Pedophilic Disorder

Mr. Flynn, a 50-year-old businessman, reports being attracted to "little girls, when they barely have any breasts and have no body hair. Their bodies enormously arouse me." He says that he has always been sexually attracted to female children. His first sexual encounter around age 16 was with a "neighbor's girl. She was about 9. She excited me, unlike my classmates." He started to touch her and then undressed them both and fondled her genitalia, although "she was pushing me away." He then masturbated in front of her. He adds that when both their parents found out, his parents punished him, but the "whole thing was swept under the rug. Everybody said that kids are curious and like to play." He states that although he has had sexual intercourse with adult women and is married, he has always been much more excited by "those little girls." He regularly masturbates while viewing child pornography. He has had sex with female children around the country. "You know, in some cities, you can get a little girl easily." He has also traveled to other countries to have sex with girls because "it is quite easy to get girls in some countries. Their families offer them for almost nothing." He has spent all his money on travel to "get girls" and on child pornography. His wife divorced him when she found him masturbating using child pornography. He has no friends because "nobody would understand me." He has the urge to look at "pictures" at work and is afraid that he will be fired, should he follow the impulse and be discovered.

Mr. Flynn has always been aroused by prepubescent girls. His parents and others considered his first sexual encounter with a girl child's play or an act of curiosity. It is difficult to establish a firm sexual interest during adolescence because many children and young adolescents are curious about seeing other children naked, but they lose their curiosity during puberty. This man has remained sexually aroused by prepubescent girls as an adult and clearly prefers sex with prepubescent girls over sex with adult females. He has acted on his fantasies and urges, either masturbating while watching child pornography or having sex with prepubescent girls. He does not seem to be distressed by his attraction (some individuals with pedophilic disorder are not distressed by and do not feel guilty about what they consider to be a sexual "preference"). Mr. Flynn's pedophilia (sexual attraction to prepubescent girls, acting out on his fantasies and preferences) has caused a significant impairment in his social functioning (divorce, no friends), in his work setting, and probably in personal finances (spending substantial money on child pornography and travel for sex). As sexual arousal decreases with age, it is possible that his pedophilic activities and their frequency may decrease.

Approach to the Diagnosis

Most individuals with pedophilic disorder are evaluated after being caught or reported for having sex with children (prepubescent or pubescent), soliciting sex with children, trading child pornography, or being caught watching child pornography. Individuals with pedophilia or pedophilic disorder frequently deny sexual attraction to children because they are aware of the legal ramifications of their sexual attraction. It is important to note that pedophilia is not synonymous with sexual offending against children. Some individuals may report sexual attraction to children (prepubescent males or females), yet they do not feel guilty, ashamed, or distressed about it, and they have never acted on their fantasies or urges. Thus, the interviewer may ascertain that these individuals have pedophilia but not pedophilic disorder.

Pedophilic disorder occurs mostly in males, although it also occurs in females. Pedophilia or pedophilic disorder develops around the time of puberty and is usually stable across the lifespan. Pedophilic disorder should be suspected in any adult individual whose behavior suggests sexual interest in or preference for children.

Some individuals with pedophilic disorder are not distressed and do not feel guilty or ashamed about their sexual attraction and behavior. However, they should be diagnosed with pedophilic disorder if they have acted on their fantasies or urges with a prepubescent child or children or if they have been socially, economically, or otherwise impaired because of their sexual preferences (e.g., divorce, job loss).

The age difference of 5 years between the individual acting on pedophilic urges and fantasies and the child is an important issue and an area where medicine and law may differ. An 18-year-old male who has been having sex with a fully sexually developed 14- to 15-year-old girl is not considered to have pedophilia or pedophilic disorder in medical terms; however, he may be labeled as a sexual offender in many jurisdictions, which may have lifelong consequences.

The diagnosis of pedophilic disorder should specify whether it is *exclusive type* (attracted only to children) or *nonexclusive type* (attracted to children as well as sexually mature adults), as well as whether the individual is sexually attracted to males, females, or both (gender specifier). Finally, it should be specified whether the pedophilic disorder is limited to incest.

Assessment tools that may help in diagnosing pedophilic disorder in special settings include penile plethysmography (sensitivity and specificity may vary from place to place), viewing time (using photographs of nude children may be difficult because owning such photographs may violate American law regarding possessing child pornography), and self-report measures.

Getting the History

The individual evaluated for possible pedophilic disorder has usually been suspected of, if not clearly "caught," being involved in pedophilic behavior. To the extent possible, the interviewer should establish an atmosphere of trust, because many individuals deny their pedophilic urges, fantasies, and behavior. The interviewer should ask first about the individual's understanding of the reasons for the evaluation and clarify what happened. Then the interviewer should move to more specific questions, such as determining the sexual attraction: "Do you get sexually aroused by fantasizing about sex with adults, young adults, kids? Have you ever masturbated while thinking about sex with younger persons? How old were they? Does watching pornography arouse you sexually? What kind of pornography? How frequently do you do this?" Then the interviewer should determine whether the individual acted on his or her urges, which may be difficult information to obtain. The interviewer may start asking about touching children, spending time with them, and the activities the individual did with children.

Once the existence and nature of the pedophilic disorder is established, the individual should be asked about the distress and/or possible consequences: "How have you been feeling about being sexually aroused by children? Have you ever had any problems because of watching child pornography? What about your relationships with others—have they said anything about your sexual interests? Have you been in any legal troubles because of your sexual urges and acting on them?" It may be useful to watch the reactions to such questions, such as hesitation to answer, pauses, vehement denial, and refusal to answer, and then modify subsequent questions due to these reactions.

Tips for Clarifying the Diagnosis

- Investigate whether the individual becomes sexually aroused by fantasizing about having sex with children.
- Explore whether the individual has acted on these fantasies or urges.
- Verify whether the individual is at least age 16.
- Confirm that the individual is at least 5 years older than the child or children of interest.
- Clarify whether the individual is attracted only to children.
- Assess the sexual preferences in terms of gender (males, females, both).
- Determine whether the individual's urges, fantasies, and/or sexual behaviors are limited to children in his or her nuclear family only (i.e., biological or stepchildren).

Consider the Case

Ms. Dixon, a 25-year-old nanny, and a 12-year-old boy were found naked by his parents when they came home unexpectedly. She admitted that she has been "playing with him for a few months." She says that she has been sexually aroused by looking at him since she started to work for his family a year ago. She used to bathe him and his sister and enjoyed playing with his genitals when drying him off. She fantasized about having oral sex with him. When he started to get erections while she was playing with his genitals, she finally performed fellatio on him. They have been engaged in regular sexual activities since then, whenever his parents were not at home. Ms. Dixon usually performs oral sex on him and masturbates during it. She admits feeling guilty and anxious and worried about being caught all the time. She says, "I know it's illegal, but I could not help it. I love him and love his young body." She had an older boyfriend when she was 18 but did not like having sex with him. "He had too much body hair and was a bit rough." She has not had a boyfriend since she ended that relationship and has not been sexually attracted to adult males. However, she has been fantasizing about sex with young boys, "just as they stop being little." She was dismissed from her previous job as a nanny because her employers became suspicious when she was rubbing their son for a long time after he took a bath.

Pedophilic disorder occurs mostly in males, but rare cases of female pedophilia or pedophilic disorder have been reported. Ms. Dixon started to fantasize about having sex with pubescent boys shortly after ending an adult sexual relationship with an older male, when she realized that she was not sexually attracted to adult males. She gradually started to act on her fantasies, fondling the boy's genitals and finally performing oral sex and masturbating while having sex with him. She clearly prefers sex with pubescent boys, has been intensely aroused by pubescent boys, and has acted on her fantasies and urges. At 25 years old, she is more than 5 years older than pubescent boys. She has been feeling guilty, knows it is illegal, and is worried about her behavior. She has been dismissed from one job. She clearly meets the criteria for pedophilic disorder in that she has pedophilic fantasies and urges, acts on them, and is distressed about her behavior and losing her job because of it.

Differential Diagnosis

The differential diagnosis of pedophilic disorder includes other paraphilic disorders (e.g., sexual sadism disorder, voyeuristic disorder), antisocial personality disorder, substance use disorders, neurocognitive disorders, obsessive-compulsive disorder, intellectual disability (intellectual developmental disorder), and brain injury. The distinction between pedophilic disorder and other paraphilic disorders should focus on the object of arousal (children) and character of sexual behavior (sexual intercourse, masturbation). Individuals with pedophilic disorder may also be diagnosed with antisocial personality disorder; however, personality disorder does not explain pedophilic disorder and should not supplant it. Individuals with substance use disorders may get involved in sex with children while intoxicated, but their pedophilic activity usually occurs during intoxication only and does not have chronic character. Individuals with neurocognitive disorders may fondle children, but this behavior develops uncharacteristically in older age and within the context of neurocognitive impairment. Obsessive-compulsive disorder may include obsessions involving sex with children, but individuals with obsessive-compulsive disorder do not act on those urges. Individuals with intellectual disability may get sexually involved with children, and the evaluation of the adaptive functioning and determination of IQ will be helpful in the differential diagnosis in such cases. The time frame should be considered in pedophilic behavior that developed after a brain injury.

Individuals with pedophilic disorder may have comorbid anxiety, depression, substance use disorder, or personality disorder. These disorders may affect the presentation of pedophilic disorder—for example, depression may be associated with profound feelings of guilt not necessarily about the pedophilic disorder. The pedophilic behavior may get more disinhibited in individuals with substance use disorders, especially during intoxication. The comorbid antisocial personality disorder psychopathology may also affect the presentation of pedophilic disorder, in terms of a lack of distress or impairment in various areas of functioning.

See DSM-5 for additional disorders to consider in the differential diagnosis. Also refer to the discussions of comorbidity and differential diagnosis in their respective sections of DSM-5.

Summary

- The defining feature of pedophilic disorder is intense sexual arousal from fantasies, urges, and behaviors involving sexual activity with prepubescent children.
- To meet the criteria of pedophilic disorder, the individual must act on these sexual urges; or the urges or fantasies cause marked distress or interpersonal difficulty.
- The individual with pedophilic disorder should be at least age 16 and at least 5 years older than the child or children for whom he or she feels sexually aroused.
- Pedophilic disorder occurs predominantly in males, but the disorder has been reported in females.
- Pedophilic preference, age difference between the individual and child, and acting on the preference—or experiencing distress or interpersonal difficulty resulting from the sexual urges and fantasies—all must be present to make the diagnosis of pedophilic disorder.
- Careful history should help to differentiate pedophilic disorder from other mental disorders and other paraphilic disorders.

IN-DEPTH DIAGNOSIS

Fetishistic Disorder

Mr. Griffith, a 30-year-old man, reports being ashamed and stressed out about "my sexual practices." Since he became sexually active over 10 years ago, he has been extremely aroused by holding his partners' "used panties and smelling them while having sex or while masturbating." He also asks his partners to cut a substantial piece of their hair, which he uses to play with while masturbating or puts over his partner's face during sex. Mr. Griffith says that he has had sex or masturbated without these objects, but "it is not the same and I am not even able to come without them at times." He adds that alternatively, when he has everything "together," "the sex could be pretty amazing, I get very aroused." He was not originally distressed by using fetishes. However, because several of his girlfriends were turned off by his practices and called him "a pervert," he started to wonder whether he "was normal." He began to feel more guilty that "I am not able to have sex without bothering my girlfriend with those panties and hair." His current girlfriend has flatly refused to let him cut her hair and use her panties during sex. She has threatened to leave him unless he stops this behavior.

Mr. Griffith's use of fetishes during sexual intercourse and masturbation developed in his late teens and was not originally associated with distress, so at first he had a fetishism. However, over the years, his sexual partners have been complaining about his use of fetishes, and he has gradually become distressed. He has started to doubt himself and feels a lot of shame. His relationships with several girlfriends have been impaired due to his adamant requirement for fetishes during intercourse. Thus, he now meets the criteria for fetishistic disorder. He has been using more than one fetish, and his behaviors have included holding and smelling underwear and requiring his partner to have pieces of her hair on her face during intercourse. Interestingly, he reports lesser arousal during intercourse when not using any fetish—impaired sexual functioning may occur when a preferred fetish is not available during intercourse or masturbation.

Approach to the Diagnosis

Most individuals with fetishism (use of fetishes during sexual intercourse or masturbation or fantasizing about using them) do not seek help or get diagnosed. Their sexual
partners may tolerate their behavior. The diagnosis of fetishistic disorder is made only
when the individual has significant distress or impairment in important areas of functioning due to his or her fetishism. Individuals with either distress or impairment due
to using fetishes—thus meeting the diagnostic criteria for fetishistic disorder—are
more likely to be diagnosed because their distress or impairment may bring them to
clinicians. Fetishistic disorder is usually considered harmless unless it leads to criminal
activity, such as stealing to have a specific fetish or collection of fetishes (some could
be quite special or expensive). Fetishes involve not only nonliving objects but also may
include very specific nongenital parts of the body, such as feet, toes, and hair.

Individuals (mostly male) with fetishistic disorder may use one specific fetish,
more than one fetish, or a specific combination of fetishes. Behaviors involving fetishes may include holding them, rubbing them, smelling them, touching them, in-
serting them, asking a sexual partner to wear them, and kissing or sucking them (e.g.,
nongenital body parts), all during sexual intercourse with a partner, masturbation, or
intense sexual fantasies. The fetishistic behavior should not be limited to cross-dressing or to use of devices designed to increase sexual stimulation, such as vibrators. It
is important to note that the diagnosis of fetishistic disorder does not require the use
of fetishes during sexual intercourse. The condition could involve using fetishes during masturbation or fantasies only.

Impairment of sexual functioning may occur when a preferred fetish is not available during sexual intercourse. The sexual dysfunction due to the lack of fetish should
be distinguished from sexual dysfunction due to other reasons, such as physical illness, depression (even due to fetishistic disorder), or medication use.

The diagnosis should specify whether nonliving objects or specific body parts are
the focus of fantasies, urges, or behaviors. The diagnosis should also specify whether
the behavior is in full remission and whether it occurs in a controlled environment.

Fetishes can develop before adolescence or, more commonly, during puberty. Fetishistic disorder tends to be a chronic condition that fluctuates in intensity and frequency of urges or behavior. In clinical samples, it is nearly exclusively reported in
males. No specific tests are useful for making this diagnosis. Thus, the approach to
this diagnosis is clinical and descriptive and relies on clinician judgment.

Getting the History

The individual will usually present to the clinician his or her focus on a fetish in sexual
fantasies, urges, and behaviors (e.g., intercourse, masturbation). The interviewer
should further explore whether the individual derives intense arousal from using fetishes and what kind of fetishes by asking, "Do you get aroused using some objects—
for instance, panties, bras, or your girlfriend's shoes? Does kissing or sucking your girlfriend's feet or toes excite you during sex? Does any other part of her body, besides her
breasts and private parts, arouse you sexually?" Once the interviewer establishes that
the individual becomes aroused by using a fetish or fetishes, further clarification
should focus on duration and intensity: "How long have you been using these (e.g.,

panties, bras, socks, toes) to get aroused during intercourse/masturbation/fantasizing about sex? Are you able to have sex (or masturbate) without using them?" The interviewer should also rule out other paraphilic disorders by asking, for example, "Do you wear women's clothes during sex? Does it excite you? Do you use your fetish to slap or beat your partner during sex?"

Finally, the interviewer should establish whether the use of a fetish is causing any distress or impairment by asking, "What does your partner think about using your fetish during sex? How do you feel about using the fetish or fetishes? Do you feel guilty or ashamed that you have to use it? Have you had any problems related to your use of fetishes, such as being chastised or being apprehended getting a fetish that did not belong to you?"

The description of the behavior—using various fetishes such as undergarments or a partner's foot or toe—and the fact that the behavior arouses the individual are crucial for recognizing *fetishistic behavior* or *fetishism*. The questions about being distressed or impaired in some area of functioning are crucial for making the diagnosis of *fetishistic disorder*. Obtaining a detailed description of the objects, behaviors involved (e.g., touching, smelling), and their frequency may be straightforward; however, the individual may be evasive about some associated problems, such as a partner's tolerance, associated sexual dysfunction when a fetish is not used, or associated criminal activity. It is important to establish a trusting atmosphere to elicit all symptoms of fetishism. The clinical interview is the cornerstone for making the diagnosis.

Tips for Clarifying the Diagnosis

- Explore whether the individual becomes sexually aroused by use of nonliving objects or a focus on nongenital body parts.
- Question whether the individual uses fetishes during sexual intercourse or masturbation or whether he or she fantasizes about using them during sexual activities.
- Determine whether this behavior has been ongoing or is an occasional experimentation.
- Consider whether this behavior is limited to use of a vibrator.
- Investigate whether the individual derives his or her sexual arousal from cross-dressing.
- Evaluate whether the individual is apprehensive or distressed by his or her behavior.

Consider the Case

Mr. Owen, a 45-year-old man, was arrested for breaking a fashion clothing store window and stealing a couple of female mannequins but no clothing. This was his third arrest for the same offense. During the interrogation by police, he admitted, "I needed them for sex. I cannot help it." He was referred for an evaluation by the court. He reports, "These slender mannequins really excite me when I hold them while I masturbate or when I look at them while having sex with my wife." He prefers mannequins without any clothing. He says he does not know why he likes to use them, but "I really like them." He has not tried to have sex with mannequins; he just touches them or looks

at them during intercourse or masturbation. He describes that his attraction to mannequins developed over the past 5 years, after he and his wife moved from a small town
to a big city where he started frequenting shopping malls with stores that have mannequins in their windows. Mr. Owen says that his wife tolerates him having the mannequins at home but threw the previous ones out "when the kids started to ask why we
have them in our bedroom. She tolerated me having them because our sex has become
better since I got my first mannequin and I do not chase other women."

Mr. Owen developed the attraction and use of a fetish—slender female mannequins—at a relatively late age of 40. Most paraphilic disorders, including fetishistic
disorder, develop during puberty or adolescence. He has been touching and/or looking at the fetish (mannequin) during sexual intercourse or masturbation. The presence of the mannequin enhances his sexual arousal. The use of fetishes is frequently
accepted or tolerated by sexual partners. This man's wife tolerates his attraction to
mannequins because their sex life has improved since he has been using them. He has
not used mannequins as sexual surrogates. He could not explain his attraction to
mannequins, and most individuals with fetishistic behavior are unable to explain
their attraction to fetishes. He has displayed serious functional impairment because
he has been arrested for burglary and destroying property several times. He has not
been able to control his illegal behavior.

Differential Diagnosis

The differential diagnosis of fetishistic disorder is relatively narrow. Fetishistic disorder
should be distinguished from other paraphilias, namely transvestic disorder (sexual
arousal derived from using a fetish vs. sexual arousal derived from cross-dressing—
in both cases, female undergarments may be used) and sexual masochism disorder
(sexual arousal derived from using fetishes to touch, smell, or hold oneself vs. sexual
arousal derived from the sexual partner using various objects to slap, hit, or bind the
individual). Fetishistic disorder may co-occur with other paraphilic disorders. The distinction between fetishistic and transvestic disorder could be difficult at times because
their phenomenology is similar; however, this differential diagnosis is fairly straightforward—in transvestic disorder, the articles of clothing are worn exclusively during
cross-dressing. Fetishistic disorder is not diagnosed when the object used is genitally
stimulating because it was designed for that purpose (e.g., a vibrator).

Some individuals may use fetishes (e.g., licking partner's toes; wearing leather
boots) during foreplay or sexual activity and not be distressed about it—this behavior
should be categorized as fetishistic behavior without fetishistic disorder. Fetishistic
disorder may also occur in individuals with other mental disorders, such as personality disorders, mood disorders, and impulse-control disorders.

Fetishistic disorder occurs mostly in males and the course of the disorder is
chronic. Depression and substance use may develop as a consequence of fetishistic
disorder and then affect the clinical presentation. Sexual dysfunction may develop
during the times when fetishes are not available. Denial or minimization of the behavior could hinder the differential diagnosis. Occasionally, an injury may occur when a
fetish is inserted or when fetishistic behavior such as sucking gets extreme or switches
to more harmful behavior such as biting.

See DSM-5 for additional disorders to consider in the differential diagnosis. Also refer to the discussions of comorbidity and differential diagnosis in their respective sections of DSM-5.

Summary

- The hallmark of fetishistic disorder is the use of nonliving objects (e.g., undergarments) or nongenital body parts (e.g., partner's feet, toe, hair) to get sexually aroused.
- Establishing the use of fetishes for sexual arousal allows confirmation of the presence of fetishism, not fetishistic disorder.
- Distress over the fantasies, urges, or behavior—or impairment in various areas of functioning—is necessary for establishing the diagnosis of fetishistic disorder.
- Careful history should help to rule out other mental disorders (e.g., psychotic disorder, substance use disorder, personality disorder, impulse-control disorder) and other paraphilic disorders, such as transvestic disorder and sexual masochism disorder.

--------- **SUMMARY** ---------

Paraphilic Disorders

Paraphilic disorders are rare in routine practice. The diagnostic class includes disorders with sexual interest and behavior characterized by intense and persistent fantasies, interests, or behaviors beyond what is considered a normophilic sexual interest and/or behavior. Examples of paraphilic behaviors include being sexually aroused by any of the following: watching a nonconsenting person who is naked, disrobing, or having sex; exposing one's genitals to nonconsenting strangers; rubbing or touching a nonconsenting person; being humiliated, beaten, or otherwise made to suffer; causing the physical or psychological suffering of another person; having sexual activity with prepubescent or pubescent children; using a nonliving object or nongenital body part during sexual intercourse or masturbation; and cross-dressing. Some sexual interests and behaviors may be relatively harmless (e.g., fetishism, transvestism) and at times they do not distress individuals; in those cases, only paraphilia is identified and paraphilic disorder is not diagnosed. The origin or basis of paraphilic behavior or disorder is unknown.

Paraphilic disorders occur almost exclusively in males (with the exception of sexual masochism disorder), for unclear reasons. Paraphilic disorders usually develop during late childhood or puberty/adolescence and have a chronic, lifelong course.

■-■-■

Diagnostic Pearls

- The diagnostic class of paraphilic disorders includes intense or persistent sexual interest or behavior that is not conventionally considered normal sexual interest or behavior.

- The diagnosis of paraphilic disorder is made if the individual with the non-normative sexual behavior (e.g., fetishism, cross-dressing) describes being distressed by his or her behavior or having impairment in various areas of functioning due to the behavior.

- In the absence of distress or impairment regarding the paraphilia, if the individual has acted on the sexual urges with children (pedophilic disorder) or nonconsenting persons (exhibitionistic disorder, frotteuristic disorder, or sexual sadism disorder), diagnosis of the paraphilic disorder applies.

- The delineation of the paraphilic urges, fantasies, and behaviors as "intense" and "persistent" may be difficult in some cases and should then be defined as paraphilic only if greater or equal to normophilic sexual interest and behavior.

- The urges, fantasies, and/or behaviors should occur over a period of at least 6 months.

- Most paraphilic disorders occur almost exclusively in males, with sexual masochism disorder being an exception.

- Although paraphilic preferences may persist to the end of an individual's life, it is believed that paraphilic expressions or performances of paraphilic behavior decrease with age.

- Paraphilic disorders may overlap with other disorders within the diagnostic class (e.g., fetishistic disorder and sexual masochism disorder) or may be comorbid with other mental disorders (e.g., depressive disorders, substance use disorders, personality disorders).

Self-Assessment

Key Concepts: Double-Check Your Knowledge

What is the relevance of the following concepts to the various paraphilic disorders?

- Normophilic behavior
- Sexual fantasies, urges, and behaviors
- Sexual preferences for object of behavior (fetish, nonconsenting stranger)
- Marked distress over sexual preferences or behavior
- Recurrence of fantasies, urges, and behaviors
- Exposure of genitals
- Fetish—nonliving object, nongenital body part
- Age difference between perpetrator and child in pedophilic disorder
- Role of a controlled environment

Questions to Discuss With Colleagues and Mentors

1. Do you routinely discuss sexual functioning, preferences, and behaviors with your patients?
2. If you suspect paraphilic behavior or preferences, what specific questions do you ask?
3. Do you have difficulties asking your patients about their sexual practices? Do you avoid certain questions about their preferences and practices? Why?

Case-Based Questions

PART A

Mr. Foster, a 20-year-old man, reports that he is a bit uneasy about being fixated on his need to have his sexual partners (of both sexes) wear a special tight leather garter belt, "otherwise I don't really get excited. But some of my previous partners got really upset with me and refused to wear it."

What diagnosis would you consider for Mr. Foster's behavior at this point? He seems to have fetishism because he gets really aroused only when his partner wears a specific piece of clothing. He requires both males and females to wear it, but because he does not wear it, it is not related to cross-dressing. He seems to be uneasy about his demand. The existence of distress and the duration of 6 months need to be explored to establish the diagnosis of fetishistic disorder.

PART B

Upon further questioning, Mr. Foster also states that he is sexually attracted to boys and girls and he does not get excited thinking about having sex with adults. He says that he prefers sex with both boys and girls "a few years younger than I am, when they have some pubic hair, but no body hair, their skin is soft, girls' breasts are just budding." He has had sex with several boys and girls looking like that. "They really arouse me."

Does the additional information change your diagnostic consideration? Would you change Mr. Foster's diagnosis or add another one? In addition to his fetishism, Mr. Foster has pedophilic disorder and is sexually attracted to both males and females. It would be important to establish how old his sexual partners are and what the age difference is, but he clearly prefers early pubescent males and females, has acted on this interest by having sex with several boys and girls, and thus meets the diagnostic criteria for pedophilic disorder. Various paraphilic disorders may co-occur.

Short-Answer Questions

1. How long must any paraphilic fantasies, urges, or behaviors last to meet the diagnostic criteria for paraphilic disorder?
2. What is the difference between paraphilia and paraphilic disorder?
3. What is the usual age/time period of onset of paraphilic disorders?

4. What are the usual fetishes?
5. In which gender does paraphilia almost exclusively occur?
6. What are some examples of paraphilias/other specified paraphilic disorders?
7. What personality disorder must be considered in the differential diagnosis of pedophilic disorder?
8. What is the minimal age difference between the individual with pedophilic disorder and his or her victim?
9. Why was the specifier "in a controlled environment" included in the diagnostic criteria of most paraphilic disorders?
10. Can substance use modify paraphilic behavior? Can paraphilic behavior appear during substance use and during intoxication?

Answers

1. Any paraphilic fantasies, urges, or behaviors must last 6 months to meet the diagnostic criteria for paraphilic disorder.
2. The diagnosis of paraphilic disorder includes the paraphilia and the distress or impairment caused by the paraphilia. In the absence of distress or impairment regarding the paraphilia, if the individual has acted on the sexual urges with children (pedophilic disorder) or nonconsenting persons (exhibitionistic disorder, frotteuristic disorder, or sexual sadism disorder), diagnosis of the paraphilic disorder applies.
3. Childhood through puberty or adolescence is the usual age/time period of onset of paraphilic disorders.
4. The usual fetishes are nonliving objects (e.g., undergarments) and nongenital body parts (e.g., feet).
5. Paraphilia almost exclusively occurs in males.
6. Some examples of paraphilias/other specified paraphilic disorders include acrotomophilia/acrotomophilic disorder, necrophilia/necrophilic disorder, telephone scatologia/telephone scatophilic disorder, and zoophilia/zoophilic disorder.
7. Antisocial personality disorder must be considered in the differential diagnosis of pedophilic disorder.
8. Five years is the minimal age difference between the individual with pedophilic disorder and his or her victim.
9. It may be more difficult to objectively assess an individual's propensity to act on paraphilic urges when the individual has no opportunity to act on those urges (e.g., because of being in a controlled environment, such as prison).
10. Yes. Substance use can modify paraphilic behavior, and paraphilic behavior can appear during substance use and during intoxication.

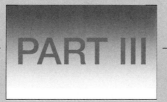

PART III

Test Yourself

In this section, we provide a series of questions to help learners apply and consolidate their knowledge of the concepts presented in the *Study Guide to DSM-5.* Many of the questions are embedded in a series of fictional cases that exemplify "classic" diagnoses from DSM-5 or that highlight phenomena that relate to key diagnostic features. Other questions test terms that are important for accurate understanding and communication of diagnoses in DSM-5.

23

Questions and Answers

Laura Weiss Roberts, M.D., M.A.

Sepideh N. Bajestan, M.D., Ph.D.

Richard Balon, M.D.

M. Rameen Ghorieshi, M.D., M.P.H.

Honor Hsin, M.D., Ph.D.

Alan K. Louie, M.D.

Daniel Mason, M.D.

Yasmin Owusu, M.D.

Daryn Reicherter, M.D.

Margaret Reynolds-May, M.D.

Yelizaveta I. Sher, M.D.

QUESTIONS

1. A 10-year-old boy who has severe developmental delay exhibits immediate and involuntary repetition of ambient sounds and vocalizations made by other people. What is the term for this phenomenon?

    A. Dysarthria.
    B. Echolalia.
    C. Echopraxia.
    D. Word salad.

2. A 19-year-old college freshman wears a wizard hat every day around campus. When asked why, he tells people it is because "the hat helps me think better." He has had few friends but enjoys participating in medieval role-playing games. He earns excellent grades in class and grooms himself appropriately every day. His speech is fluent. His thought process is linear, although he perseverates on various wizard spells he has learned online. His affect is restricted. He denies any hallucinations or any changes in sleep, mood, appetite, or energy. His unusual "style" has interfered with his getting a job, which he needs to remain in school. What is the likely diagnosis?

    A. Bipolar I disorder.
    B. Schizoaffective disorder.
    C. Schizophrenia.
    D. Schizotypal personality disorder.

3. Theravada Buddhist monks living at a temple bring a 27-year-old Laotian man to the hospital. The man apparently has fasted for 17 days. The man is acutely dehydrated and emaciated. The patient is admitted to the medicine service. He is delirious at first, but when he improves, the psychiatric consult service is called because of his "odd manner." The patient is unkempt and unshaven, which is in sharp contrast to the two other members of his order. The patient does not speak English and one of the monks translates to help the psychiatrist with the evaluation. The patient appears withdrawn and responds very briefly to the other monks, at times laughing inappropriately. The monks say that the man's family, who had recently emigrated from Laos, brought him to the order nearly 1 year ago. Although he has been withdrawn since they have known him, the monks say that this is the first time he has embarked on such a fast. He told them that he was instructed to do so by "spirits," who watch his daily activities and comment on whether he is being appropriately observant. The members of his order are familiar with the names of the spirits from Lao folk traditions, but they are not familiar with this particular tradition of fasting. They acknowledge that the man is from a remote part of Laos, of which they are unfamiliar with the customs. What is the likely diagnosis?

    A. Culturally appropriate behavior.
    B. Major depressive disorder.

    C. Psychotic disorder due to another medical condition.

    D. Schizophrenia.

4. Match each description with the personality disorder for which it is most highly characteristic (each disorder may be used once, more than once, or not at all):

    A. Antisocial personality disorder.

    B. Borderline personality disorder.

    C. Histrionic personality disorder.

    D. Narcissistic personality disorder.

    _____ Consistently uses physical appearance to draw attention to oneself.

    _____ Failure to conform to social norms and without remorse.

    _____ Frantic efforts to avoid real or imagined abandonment.

    _____ Grandiose sense of self-importance.

    _____ Self-dramatization, theatricality, and exaggerated expression of emotion.

5. Match each mental disorder with the most accurate statement regarding prevalence by gender (each item may be used once, more than once, or not at all):

    A. More prevalent among men.

    B. More prevalent among women.

    C. Equally prevalent among men and women.

    _____ Restless legs syndrome.

    _____ Major depressive disorder.

    _____ Generalized anxiety disorder.

6. A 45-year-old man presents to his primary care doctor, complaining of chronic chest pain for the past year. He has seen multiple specialists, who tell him the pain is from uncomplicated acid reflux; however, he thinks he must have serious heart disease. He continues to worry about his heart despite reassurance from multiple cardiologists; he acknowledges that it is possible the cardiologists are correct. He denies hallucinations, and there is no evidence of delusional content. His concern about his heart has prevented him from vacationing with his family. He denies feeling depressed or anxious or having any problems with sleep or appetite, and he continues to enjoy hobbies at home. What is the likely diagnosis?

    A. Generalized anxiety disorder.

    B. Illness anxiety disorder.

    C. Major depressive disorder.

    D. Panic disorder.

7. A 22-year-old college student presents to a mental health clinic for an initial visit. She has not turned in any of her papers on time this term because she worries about getting poor grades, and this worry has affected her ability to

concentrate. She is also very concerned about getting a job after she graduates, despite multiple meetings with a career counselor. She says that she is concerned with the sanitation at the local gym and prefers not to play recreational sports because she might be injured. She does not have any rituals or checking behaviors. She describes her mood as "irritable" and says that she feels "tense all the time." Her appetite has not changed, and she continues to enjoy watching movies. She denies low energy and has not had any thoughts of harming herself. She tried cocaine last year but has not used any illicit substances or alcohol recently. What is the likely diagnosis?

A. Adjustment disorder.
B. Generalized anxiety disorder.
C. Major depressive disorder.
D. Obsessive-compulsive disorder.

8.   To meet criteria for premenstrual dysphoric disorder, how long must symptoms be present?

A. 1 week.
B. 1 month.
C. 6 months.
D. 1 year.

9.   A 16-year-old boy presents to his high school counselor after running out of his programming class because he was asked to explain a piece of code. He had trouble answering and had felt this sort of difficulty in the past, but today it was worse. He is not able to explain clearly to the counselor what happened because he is still having the same speaking problems that he had in class. He speaks in broken words and keeps getting stuck on sounds like "aye" and "ah." He seems to spit out words. He writes down on a piece of paper that he has been thinking about dropping out of school because of his difficulty speaking; his older brother dropped out of school for similar problems. The counselor later observes him working in the computer lab and notices no abnormal behavior. What is the likely diagnosis?

A. Autism spectrum disorder.
B. Childhood-onset fluency disorder (stuttering).
C. Social anxiety disorder (social phobia).
D. Tourette's disorder.

10.   Police bring a 30-year-old homeless man to the psychiatric emergency department after he called 911 because he thought people were controlling his mind through "microwaves." He has no previous psychiatric or medical history, and his urine toxicology screen is negative for illicit substances. On interview, he appears very guarded, with limited cooperation, because he feels that he does not belong on a psychiatric unit. "I am not the problem," he says. "These microwaves are all around us, even if you cannot feel them." He denies any mood symptoms. Until a few years ago he was working full time, but he refuses to

divulge his occupation "because I do not trust anyone." On examination, his speech is fluent with normal volume and rate, but his thought process is occasionally disorganized. His affect is blunted, and no psychomotor abnormalities are noted. He denies any hallucinations, but during the interview he occasionally stares behind the interviewer very intently, without responding to any questions. Which term best describes the man's experience of "microwaves"?

A. Delusion.
B. Hallucination.
C. Ideas of reference.
D. Illusion.

11.   A 22-year-old woman is brought to the hospital after being found wandering on a school playground. She is not able to read or fill out basic paperwork. On exam, she is noted to be perusing the picture books in the pediatric waiting area and laughing in a childlike manner. She is wearing a T-shirt, sweatpants, and shoes with hook-and-loop fasteners and has a wristband with her identification and her mother's contact information. The woman can say her name and address and answer simple yes/no questions but cannot answer compound or complicated questions. She begins to cry after not being able to answer many questions. A review of her records indicates that she has no psychiatric history but still sees her pediatrician, accompanied by her mother. Recent testing places her at an IQ of 50. She has no basic laboratory abnormalities and a negative urine toxicology screen. What is the likely diagnosis?

A. Conduct disorder.
B. Dissociative identity disorder.
C. Intellectual disability (intellectual developmental disorder).
D. Selective mutism.

12.   A 40-year-old woman sees a psychiatrist for the first time. She complains of having had low energy and fatigue for the past year and endorses additional symptoms of depressed mood, poor sleep, and decreased concentration. She exhibits significant psychomotor retardation on exam. She denies any suicidal ideation or hallucinations. She takes medication for hypothyroidism but has not seen a primary care doctor in over 10 years. Her thyroid-stimulating hormone level is 7.6, and her urine toxicology screen is negative. What is the likely diagnosis?

A. Bipolar II disorder.
B. Depressive disorder due to another medical condition.
C. Insomnia disorder.
D. Major depressive disorder.

13.   A 41-year-old man reports to the psychiatrist that he is afraid of dentists. He has a history of extreme anxiety upon entering a dental office, to the point that he feels dizzy and nauseated. He becomes excessively anxious in the waiting room and has a very difficult time completing visits. He is so fearful about den-

tists that he reports he cannot take his own children to their dentist because he has "anxiety attacks" in the office. Rather, he insists that his wife take the children. His aversion to dentists has led to his missing regular appointments for more than 6 years. He plans to go soon, only because he has severe tooth pain and believes he may need a root canal. He does not have anxiety in other contexts. What is the likely diagnosis?

A. Adjustment disorder with anxiety.
B. Generalized anxiety disorder.
C. Posttraumatic stress disorder.
D. Specific phobia.

14. Match each mental disorder with the age at onset noted in the diagnostic criteria:

A. Age at onset under 5 years.
B. Age at onset under 18 years.
C. Age at onset not specified.

_____ Tourette's disorder.
_____ Separation anxiety disorder.
_____ Global developmental delay.

15. A 25-year-old man with no medical or psychiatric history other than anemia travels frequently for his job. He has trouble on long flights because he feels the need to move his legs about and unfasten his seat belt to do so. When he is not permitted to get up, especially on "red eye" flights, he feels symmetrical burning and tingling in his legs. He is also very exhausted and notes that his sleep is not restful. He takes no medications except a daily multivitamin. What is the likely diagnosis?

A. Adjustment disorder.
B. Akathisia.
C. Parkinson's disease.
D. Restless legs syndrome.

16. A 26-year-old man seen in the emergency department acknowledges persistent substance use until about the last 2 days, when he was evicted from his apartment. Which cluster of symptoms is typical of stimulant withdrawal?

A. Depression, fatigue, insomnia.
B. Diarrhea, nausea, anxiety.
C. Hypertension, tachycardia, seizures.
D. Vivid dreaming, nightmares, confusion.

17. A 33-year-old man presents to a psychiatrist with concern about his excessive hand washing. He reports that he has a ritualistic washing routine that takes at least 20 minutes, which he performs multiple times per day for fear of contam-

ination with infectious disease. When further interviewed, he states that he has recurrent and persistent thoughts about hand washing and risk of contamination, which he tries unsuccessfully to suppress. He reports an overwhelming sense of anxiety if he does not wash his hands or if he does not complete the "ritual." He says the behavior is "out of control." He recognizes these thoughts as functions of his own mind. He has no other symptoms. What is the likely diagnosis?

A. Obsessive-compulsive disorder.

B. Obsessive-compulsive personality disorder.

C. Schizophrenia.

D. Specific phobia.

18. A 28-year-old woman seeks psychiatric consultation. She explains that 10 years ago, she had a panic attack while presenting her project at the high school science fair. Since then she has developed an intense fear of being embarrassed or humiliated in a public venue. She is constantly worried that others are scrutinizing her. She is very self-conscious and afraid that she will have heart palpitations, trembling, or stuttering or that her mind will go blank. She refuses to go on dates and is not being considered for a new job because she declined the interview. She is tired of living such an isolated life. What is the likely diagnosis?

A. Avoidant personality disorder.

B. Obsessive-compulsive disorder.

C. Panic disorder.

D. Social anxiety disorder (social phobia).

19. A woman brings her 32-year-old husband to a psychiatrist for "unusual behavior." She says that for the past 5 days he has been cleaning the house extensively, often late into the night. He wakes up 2 hours earlier than usual the next morning but does not appear tired. He says he feels "very happy and productive—the best I have ever been!" His wife denies any dangerous behaviors at home and reports he is able to continue working at his current job, albeit more productively than before. She recalls that 6 months ago, he seemed very depressed, with loss of interest, poor sleep, low energy, and impaired concentration that lasted 1 month. The patient has not been hospitalized previously. On interview, he is pleasant and cooperative. His speech is pressured but redirectable. His thought process is linear, and he denies any hallucinations. His urine toxicology screen is negative. What is the likely diagnosis?

A. Bipolar I disorder.

B. Bipolar II disorder.

C. Schizophrenia.

D. Substance/medication-induced bipolar and related disorder.

20. The emergency department calls a psychiatrist to evaluate a 35-year-old homeless, English-speaking man, identifying him as Native American. The police brought in the man after bizarre posturing in a park while talking to himself.

The man describes having special relationships with animals. He believes that he can communicate with them through telepathy. He reports that this communication with nature is a common belief in his culture and that he has this special "gift." He says that he receives "special signals" from birds that influence his behavior and he can "hear them talk to him." Upon further exploration, he reports that he has mental powers that influence animals and nature. He insists that he is "not crazy." His hygiene is poor and he is malodorous. He has very odd habits around eating based on his auditory hallucinations, resulting in poor nutrition and weight loss. He looks emaciated. He does not have a reasonable plan for shelter and sleeps in a field. His clothes are soiled. He has odd mannerisms throughout the interview, including laughing inappropriately. His urine drug toxicology is negative for substances of abuse. He has a history of multiple hospitalizations and involuntary commitments for grave disability starting around age 22 years. What is the likely diagnosis?

A. Alcohol use disorder.
B. Culturally appropriate behavior.
C. Major depressive disorder.
D. Schizophrenia.

21.   A 29-year-old woman and her new boyfriend had an unplanned pregnancy culminating in a first-trimester miscarriage last year. She has always considered herself an anxious person but has felt even more anxious after the miscarriage. She became pregnant a second time, again unplanned, and she gave birth to a healthy baby boy after an emergent C-section delivery. Their son is now 4 months old. Her boyfriend has become emotionally distant. He moved out of their apartment a couple of weeks after the birth, stating, "I am not ready for this life." For the past several weeks, she has experienced escalating low mood, irritability, tearfulness, poor sleep, and constant fatigue. The patient reports that she is frightened by what she is thinking. She states, "Sometimes I feel I could not care less about taking care of my son or, even worse, that I want to just physically push him away. It is really scary. How can I ever be a good mother to him? I am miserable. I do not know if I can take it anymore." Her first psychiatric contact was at age 22, when she was treated with citalopram for a depressive episode precipitated by being laid off from her first job after college. She says, "I have never quite been happy again since then. Life has been hard." What is the likely diagnosis?

A. Bipolar II disorder, current episode depressed, with peripartum onset.
B. Brief psychotic disorder, with peripartum onset.
C. Major depressive disorder, with peripartum onset.
D. Persistent depressive disorder.

22.   Which statement is correct regarding the domains DSM-5 evaluates in the Clinician-Rated Dimensions of Psychosis Symptom Severity?

   A. The scale assesses only the three most important domains of hallucinations, delusions, and disorganized speech.
   B. The scale is based on symptoms experienced by the patient in the previous 7 days.
   C. The scale is most accurate if patients, rather than clinicians, provide the responses.
   D. The scale should only be completed if the clinician is certain of the symptom severity.

23.   For which DSM-5 diagnosis is there a greater prevalence in women than men?

   A. Alcohol use disorder.
   B. Bipolar I disorder.
   C. Major depressive disorder.
   D. Schizophrenia.

24.   A 12-year-old girl persistently misbehaves at home. Recently she called 911, reporting that her parents were forcing her to go to school and threatening to run away. She also locked her younger siblings out of the house in cold weather. Although her parents attempt to set limits, she frequently responds with prolonged tantrums—crying and shouting, flailing her arms, and breaking objects in her home. Once she "gets her way" she settles down immediately. After one serious tantrum, her parents took her to the emergency department and the girl was admitted to the psychiatric unit. The patient was viewed as quite charming by several members of the staff, whereas others thought she was "a very, very difficult patient." What is the likely diagnosis?

   A. Attention-deficit/hyperactivity disorder.
   B. Conduct disorder.
   C. Intermittent explosive disorder.
   D. Oppositional defiant disorder.

25.   A 47-year-old police officer presents in an outpatient clinic for evaluation of a "weird experience." He says he was "out of my mind, really paranoid" for a full 2 weeks, but then completely recovered. His symptoms began shortly after one of his colleagues was inexplicably shot during a routine traffic stop. Although everyone in the department had been upset by the event, the patient found himself increasingly preoccupied with what he called "mysterious signs and circumstances" around the time of the tragedy and what he felt was the police chief's desire to "sweep it all under the carpet." Two days after the event, he began to hear voices on his car radio warning him about surveillance by "corrupt" members of the police department, who were "trying to bring him over" to their side with "brainwashing KGB techniques." Soon after, he began to hear a "whine" from his earpiece, which he recognized as the brain-

washing. Unable to bear it any longer, he crushed the earpiece. Although he was able to pass this off as an accident at the time, he remains terrified that he might "lose it" again. Subsequently, he returned to his usual state and did not experience further psychotic symptoms. What is the likely diagnosis?

A. Brief psychotic disorder.
B. Delusional disorder, persecutory type.
C. Schizophrenia.
D. Schizophreniform disorder.

26.   A 21-year-old college student complains that he has developed "an uncomfortable relationship with food." His current symptoms seem to be consistent with an eating disorder. Which of the following pieces of information would help distinguish between anorexia nervosa and bulimia nervosa?

A. He has lost significant weight and appears emaciated.
B. He is highly critical of his body.
C. He regularly binges on high-calorie, high-fat foods.
D. He uses large quantities of laxative tablets each day.

27.   A 32-year-old woman presents to the emergency department, requesting help for back pain. She says that she has wrestled with this pain for 2 years, after a minor skiing accident, and no medications or interventions have helped. No physical evidence explains the degree of pain she reports. The pain prevents her from working as a ballerina. She loves her job but says that for the past few years, budget cuts have stressed the entire ballet company. She denies any problems with sleep, anxiety, or mood. Her body weight is 90% of expected, and she denies any problems with her weight or diet. She is cooperative, and her thought process is linear. What is the likely diagnosis?

A. Adjustment disorder.
B. Anorexia nervosa.
C. Major depressive disorder.
D. Somatic symptom disorder, with predominant pain.

28.   A 3-year-old girl in a park attempts to sit on the lap of a homeless person. She is pulled away by her mother who recently had been out of town. While the mother was away, the girl had been under the care of a grandmother who spent little time with the girl. The girl does not respond to the affection shown to her by her mother or grandmother. The girl is indiscriminately affectionate with strangers. She has no evidence of motor abnormalities and has met all developmental milestones appropriately. What is the likely diagnosis?

A. Autism spectrum disorder.
B. Mental retardation.
C. Reactive attachment disorder.
D. Rett syndrome.

29. A 30-year-old retail manager at a cosmetics store with no previous psychiatric history finds herself experiencing distinct periods of intense anxiety two to three times per day. She is concerned because she has never experienced anything like this in the past. During the episodes she feels tremulous, hot, and faint, with palpitations and fear of loss of control. She denies any drug use and any recent stressors. This problem has been getting worse over the past few months and has affected her ability to function at work. She also has been losing weight and eating more. She is worried that her health has affected her appearance because her skin looks different, her hair is thinning, and she has swelling in her neck. What is the likely diagnosis?

    A. Agoraphobia.
    B. Anxiety disorder due to another medical condition.
    C. Generalized anxiety disorder.
    D. Social anxiety disorder (social phobia).

30. A 20-year-old college freshman is brought to the attention of the dormitory resident assistant because she is not attending meals in the dining hall. The student says she feels anxious about being in the crowded kitchen and dining hall. Similarly, she has ordered all of her schoolbooks online to avoid being in the bookstore because "it is too overwhelming." She also has not attended some of her crowded lectures. The student is able to have a good conversation in the hall of the dormitory with the resident assistant. The student denies fearing scrutiny by others. She explains that she avoids some places because she found that in malls or other crowded areas, she feels very worried, faint, sweaty, and dizzy. She is afraid of losing control and in being in situations where she cannot escape. What is the likely diagnosis?

    A. Acute stress disorder.
    B. Agoraphobia.
    C. Posttraumatic stress disorder.
    D. Social anxiety disorder.

31. A 24-year-old woman experiences severe dysphoria and anhedonia affecting her ability to perform well at her job. Which of the following additional pieces of information would be more consistent with a diagnosis of major depressive disorder than a diagnosis of premenstrual dysphoric disorder?

    A. The patient has been feeling cognitively hazy, confused, and forgetful.
    B. The patient has had suicidal thoughts every day for the past 3 weeks, and yesterday she searched "how to kill yourself" on the Internet.
    C. The patient was very irritable and rejection sensitive for 4 days last week, followed by rapid resolution.
    D. The patient's symptoms have caused strain in her relationship with her boyfriend.

32.   Match each description with the sexual dysfunction diagnosis for which it is
       most highly characteristic (each disorder may be used once, more than once, or
       not at all):

       A. Erectile disorder.
       B. Female orgasmic disorder.
       C. Genito-pelvic pain/penetration disorder.
       D. Premature (early) ejaculation.

       _____ Involves inability to attain and maintain arousal.
       _____ Involves inability to have vaginal intercourse or penetration.
       _____ Involves inorgasmia or delayed orgasm.
       _____ Involves orgasm before the person desires.

33.   A man brings his 34-year-old girlfriend to the emergency department for wors-
       ening depression and suicidal thoughts. She reports feeling more depressed
       and isolated from her friends and family during the past month. She worries
       about being watched by her neighbors and thus has been avoiding going out-
       side. She has difficulty falling asleep at night and has poor energy during the
       day. She has not showered in 5 days. She admits that she has been hearing
       voices that make derogatory statements about her. She had several previous
       depressive episodes and two psychiatric hospitalizations with similar presen-
       tations. Which piece of information would help diagnose schizoaffective disor-
       der in this woman?

       A. She has auditory hallucinations that are present only in the context of her
          mood symptoms.
       B. She has had one manic episode.
       C. She has been hearing voices for weeks without depressed or elevated
          mood.
       D. She has heard similar voices before when she was depressed.

34.   A 56-year-old biologist has had a very successful career, publishing extensive
       research on the aging process. Now he believes he has found the key to eternal
       life. For the past several months, he has been quite secretive and refuses to
       come to work group meetings regarding upcoming projects. He has installed a
       dead bolt on his office at home and insists that extra security personnel be
       hired to guard his research lab. He refuses to present his material or discuss it
       with his colleagues or family, claiming the knowledge is too powerful to be
       made public. He is not having any visual or auditory hallucinations, and he is
       able to support his statements with logical arguments. He has a history of de-
       pression. What is the likely diagnosis?

       A. Cocaine intoxication, without perceptual disturbances.
       B. Delusional disorder, grandiose type.
       C. Major depressive disorder with psychotic features.
       D. Schizophrenia.

35. A 33-year-old man arrives at the hospital by ambulance after his girlfriend called the police during a dispute. While arguing with his girlfriend, the patient had locked himself in a bathroom and swallowed a dozen tablets from the medicine cabinet. On evaluation, the patient is drowsy but responsive to voice. He has thin, linear, parallel scars on the extensor surface of his left wrist. He states that he wanted to show his girlfriend how much she was hurting him and then says, "She is probably going to leave me, just like everyone else has." What is the likely diagnosis?

   A. Adjustment disorder.
   B. Borderline personality disorder.
   C. Dependent personality disorder.
   D. Histrionic personality disorder.

36. Which statement is correct regarding how DSM-5 diagnoses and documents personality disorders?

   A. DSM-5 has eliminated personality disorder diagnoses.
   B. DSM-5 has introduced new personality disorder subtypes.
   C. DSM-5 has maintained the use of the Axis II system for documenting personality disorders.
   D. DSM-5 has preserved the same diagnostic criteria as in DSM-IV-TR for personality disorders.

37. A 50-year-old Iranian woman being treated for an ankle sprain casually reports having had a conversation with a deceased relative. The emergency department physician is concerned that she has had both auditory and visual hallucinations and asks the psychiatrist to rule out psychotic disorder. At the interview, the woman endorses having had, on multiple occasions, visits from her deceased mother, in which she has conversations with her and gets advice concerning psychosocial matters. She is not distressed by the incidents and, in fact, finds these experiences to be spiritual blessings. She does not exhibit any other symptoms of psychotic disorder. Her mental status examination is remarkable for a pleasant and cooperative demeanor, normal mood, and full range of affect. Her thought process is linear. During the interview, her husband corroborates her attitude that these are real spiritual experiences and wonders why a psychiatrist has been called to interview his wife. The Farsi-speaking interpreter says that the woman's story is common among Iranian immigrants. What is the likely diagnosis?

   A. Brief psychotic disorder.
   B. Culturally appropriate behavior.
   C. Schizophrenia.
   D. Shared psychotic disorder (*folie à deux*).

38.   A 35-year-old man tells his therapist that he is having marital problems be-
       cause the object of his sexual arousal is his wife's underwear. He reports that
       he and his wife have sexual intercourse in a limited fashion, much less often
       than he prefers. He does not wear women's clothing, but he fulfills his sexual
       desires through masturbation while holding his wife's underwear or other
       women's undergarments that he has purchased. This activity is his long-stand-
       ing pattern of sexual behavior and has been problematic in the relationship
       with his wife from early on. He reports that his wife has "caught" him mastur-
       bating with women's undergarments on multiple occasions and she thinks he
       is "weird." What is the likely diagnosis?

       A. Erectile disorder.
       B. Fetishistic disorder.
       C. Gender dysphoria in adolescents and adults.
       D. Transvestic disorder.

39.   A 27-year-old man presents to a psychiatrist for evaluation of anxiety. He ex-
       plains that he recently got a promotion at his job, which requires frequent trav-
       eling. Although he is excited about his new role, he is terrified about the
       prospect of flying. He describes that the last time he flew, 5 years ago, he felt
       extremely anxious, with rapid heart rate, rapid breathing, nausea, and tingling
       in his hands. He was terrified that the plane would crash and he would die. He
       has avoided flying ever since, but he can also feel extremely anxious to the
       point of hyperventilating when even a discussion of flying comes up. Now he
       has a business trip in 3 weeks and he is "mortified." He is considering whether
       to ask for a demotion. He denies feeling anxious in any other situations. What
       is the likely diagnosis?

       A. Generalized anxiety disorder.
       B. Panic disorder.
       C. Simple phobia.
       D. Social anxiety disorder.

40.   A mother brings her 3-year-old daughter to the pediatrician because she "does
       not talk very much." Her vocabulary consists of only 10 words, and she speaks
       only one word at a time. Her past medical history is notable for delays in de-
       velopmental milestones: she walked independently at age 2, developed a pin-
       cer grasp at 15 months, and continues to have stranger anxiety. A hearing test
       completed in the clinic was normal. What is the likely diagnosis?

       A. Autism spectrum disorder.
       B. Global developmental delay.
       C. Selective mutism.
       D. Tic disorder.

41. Match each term with the correct definition (each term may be used once, more than once, or not at all):

    A. Compulsion.
    B. Obsession.
    C. Phobia.
    D. Somatization.

    _____ Repeated behavior that a person feels driven to perform.
    _____ Repeated expression of psychological issues through physical symptoms, concerns, or complaints.
    _____ Repeated, irrational, and enduring fear of an object or situation.
    _____ Repeated thought or image that provokes anxiety.

42. A primary care doctor refers a 46-year-old woman with many physical complaints for psychological assessment after extensive medical testing reveals no evidence of physical issues. The psychologist learns that the patient has an extensive history of bodily complaints without medical basis. Her physical symptoms have been multisystemic and do not resemble the constellation of symptoms associated with specific medical illnesses. The referring doctor also reports that the patient has frustrated many primary care doctors in the past and has transitioned from one to another. The patient expresses her distress to the psychologist. She says, "None of this is in my head. It is real. I have talked to so many doctors and those doctors just can't figure it out. I have no answers, and I feel worse and worse." What is the likely diagnosis?

    A. Body dysmorphic disorder.
    B. Conversion disorder (functional neurological symptom disorder).
    C. Factitious disorder.
    D. Somatic symptom disorder.

43. A 40-year-old woman says she is "very anxious about public speaking," to the point of having episodes that resemble panic attacks when she faces speaking before even small groups of familiar coworkers. Her division chief expects that employees will present at conferences before he will promote them. She is not only unable to give presentations to large audiences but also avoids most social events related to her work. She feels as if she is "acting like an idiot" when she is with colleagues, especially her work superiors. The anticipation of a meeting with her boss can cause her to worry and lose sleep for days. She does not have anxiety in other contexts. What is the likely diagnosis?

    A. Generalized anxiety disorder.
    B. Major depressive disorder.
    C. Obsessive-compulsive personality disorder.
    D. Social anxiety disorder.

44.   Which statement is correct regarding the bipolar disorders diagnostic class of DSM-5 in comparison with earlier versions of DSM?

    A. Anxious distress has been eliminated as a feature of bipolar disorder.
    B. Bipolar disorders have been consolidated under the diagnostic class of depressive disorders.
    C. Cyclothymia has been eliminated.
    D. Increased activity or energy has been added as a new core mood elevation symptom.

45.   A woman brings her 26-year-old boyfriend, an army veteran, to a psychiatric clinic after his primary care physician refers him for evaluation of "stress." She says that after her boyfriend's return from Iraq, they moved in together, but they already need to sleep in separate beds after two episodes in which he punched her while she was sleeping. The events both occurred in the early morning and were so violent that she has bruises on her neck and arms. The man looks extremely distraught. He says he frequently dreams that he is back in the Middle East, in hand-to-hand combat, and is afraid that these dreams will cause his girlfriend to leave him. Her friends already say that he is a "crazy vet" who will "end up killing her." The thought of this is deeply painful to him, because they have a supportive, caring relationship and have spoken about getting married and starting a family. A review of systems is negative, except for increasing insomnia (delayed sleep onset). A thorough history and collateral information indicate that he does not meet criteria for posttraumatic stress disorder. He works as a vendor at the local baseball stadium, a job that he says he enjoys, but he is afraid that his poor sleep is beginning to affect his performance at work. What is the likely diagnosis?

    A. Bipolar I disorder, current episode manic.
    B. Generalized anxiety disorder.
    C. REM sleep behavior disorder.
    D. Schizophrenia.

46.   A gynecologist refers a 32-year-old hospital employee to a psychiatry clinic, noting that the patient requested testosterone shots and also a surgical referral. From the past medical records, the psychiatrist learns that the patient has normal female development and anatomy with no known abnormalities. The patient wears bland-colored baggy clothing, has very short hair, and goes by the name "Jo." She is initially brief with her answers but, after some time, is tearful, explaining that she has never been comfortable as a woman and is positive she is "supposed" to be a man. She feels ostracized at work and isolated socially. She has feelings of low self-worth and some depressed mood. What is the likely diagnosis?

    A. Adjustment disorder.
    B. Anorexia nervosa.
    C. Depersonalization/derealization disorder.
    D. Gender dysphoria in adolescents and adults.

47.   A 55-year-old woman is referred for psychiatric consultation. She has a history of HIV, contracted from a former sexual partner. She has been prescribed highly active antiretroviral therapy but for years has been only intermittently adherent. Currently, her CD4 count is 200 and her HIV viral load has been escalating. She complains that over the past several months she has been less mentally agile than in the past. She says it takes her significantly longer to read the newspaper each morning. When she wants to communicate with her daughter, concentrating on writing a text message is difficult and she even finds "my fingers do not cooperate with me when I try to type." Her fine motor skills appear to be worsening. The woman denies any other physical symptoms, such as fever or headache. There are no focal findings on neurological exam. Head computed tomography (CT), magnetic resonance imaging (MRI), electroencephalography, lumbar puncture, non-HIV viral polymerase chain reaction testing, antibody screens, metabolic parameters including hepatic and renal function, and urine toxicology are all negative. Neuropsychological testing shows impairment in information processing speeds, motor skills, and attention. What is the likely diagnosis?

   A. Cryptococcal meningitis.
   B. Major depressive disorder.
   C. Mild neurocognitive disorder due to HIV infection.
   D. Vitamin B_{12} deficiency.

48.   A 5-year-old child believes that his thoughts, words, and actions cause specific outcomes in nature, and these outcomes defy what are the commonly understood laws of cause and effect. What is this phenomenon called?

   A. Grandiosity.
   B. Hallucination.
   C. Illusion.
   D. Magical thinking.

49.   A man brings his 36-year-old wife to a new primary care doctor because she has lost patches of her hair recently. He notes that her last doctor sent her to a dermatologist, who felt that an underlying skin condition was unlikely. In a private exam room without her husband present, she says that she secretly pulls out her hair in clumps to relieve tension. The act of pulling her hair brings her relief. She denies changes in mood, sleep, concentration, or energy level. What is the likely diagnosis?

   A. Generalized anxiety disorder.
   B. Major depressive disorder.
   C. Tic disorder.
   D. Trichotillomania.

50. A 50-year-old woman presents to the local hospital complaining of "a drug problem." She says that for the past 3 years her use of cocaine has been uncontrollable, to the point that she has lost her housing and her job. She reports using increasing amounts of cocaine over the past year to "reach the same high." When she stops using cocaine, she experiences intense symptoms of anxiety, depression, fatigue, and nausea. She has tried multiple times to quit using cocaine altogether, but her efforts have been unsuccessful. She suffered a transient stroke once during a cocaine binge. She denies any mood problems or hallucinations prior to using substances. What is the likely diagnosis?

     A. Bipolar I disorder.
     B. Cocaine intoxication, without perceptual disturbances.
     C. Cocaine withdrawal.
     D. Moderate cocaine use disorder.

51. Match each description with the appropriate phrase (each item may be used once, more than once, or not at all):

     A. False negative diagnosis.
     B. False positive diagnosis.
     C. True negative diagnosis.
     D. True positive diagnosis.

     _____ A woman receives the diagnosis of bipolar disorder, manic phase, when her clinical presentation was actually due to amphetamine intoxication.
     _____ An elderly man receives no psychiatric diagnosis 2 months after the death of his wife; he sometimes is tearful and sad and once each week has difficulty sleeping when he thinks of her.

52. A 53-year-old woman presents for a psychiatric evaluation for her long-standing depression. She has had several depressive episodes and was once hospitalized after a serious suicide attempt. She describes sexual abuse by her father and neglect by her mother during her teenage years. During the interview, while talking about her childhood, she suddenly switches to talking in a childlike, high-pitched voice, while pulling her legs under her in a chair and starting to rock backward and forward. While rocking, she says, "Don't hurt me, don't hurt me." Later during the interview, when she is talking and behaving in her original manner, she endorses not being able to recount her activities during several hours per day on a number of occasions in the past year. What is the likely diagnosis?

     A. Major depressive disorder and dissociative identity disorder.
     B. Major depressive disorder and schizoaffective disorder.
     C. Major depressive disorder and schizophrenia.
     D. Major depressive disorder and somatic symptom disorder.

53. Match each term with the correct definition (each term may be used once, more than once, or not at all):

    A. Anhedonia.
    B. Anorexia.
    C. Cataplexy.
    D. Catatonia.

    ____ Loss of appetite.
    ____ Loss of interest or pleasure.
    ____ Loss of muscle tone, with weakness.
    ____ Loss of response to outside stimuli and muscular rigidity.

54. A 55-year-old woman presents to the hospital for treatment of acute myeloid leukemia, which was diagnosed 1 month ago. Her husband passed away 1 year ago from a cancer that he had battled for 3 years. She reports seeing a therapist for the "past couple of years" while dealing with her husband's illness and death. Her primary care team noted that she is frequently tearful in the hospital and looked relieved when a psychiatric evaluation was suggested. On interview, she reports feeling sad much of the day but that she is trying to stay upbeat about her treatment. She also reports feelings of hopelessness. Her appetite and sleep have been poor, and she has lost 50 pounds since the death of her husband. She feels guilty—"I wish I had taken better care of my husband in the end." She reports feeling isolated from friends and family as well. She makes a vague complaint of anxiety, which "comes and goes" throughout the day and is being treated with a round-the-clock schedule of benzodiazepines. She says that she "does not care if cancer kills her too." What is the likely diagnosis?

    A. Adjustment disorder.
    B. Generalized anxiety disorder.
    C. Major depressive disorder.
    D. Uncomplicated bereavement.

55. A 12-year-old girl is getting along poorly with her parents and teachers. She is highly argumentative and defiant at home. She has attempted to embarrass her teacher in front of the other students and uses profane language. She never seems to take responsibility for the hostility that appears to be present in many of her social interactions. Due to her constant "negativity" with her teachers, other students have begun to keep their distance from her. In the past 5 years, the girl's parents have gotten divorced. Her mother then remarried, but that marriage ended in a rapid divorce. The girl is cooperative in responding to questions during the psychiatric interview. What is the likely diagnosis?

    A. Antisocial personality disorder.
    B. Conduct disorder.
    C. Major depressive disorder.
    D. Oppositional defiant disorder.

56. Which of the following has been eliminated from the criteria for the diagnosis of schizophrenia in DSM-5 in comparison with earlier versions of DSM?

    A. The duration criteria.
    B. The negative symptom criteria.
    C. The paranoid subtype.
    D. The requirement for a delusion, hallucination, or disorganized speech.

57. A primary care physician refers a 60-year-old Cambodian man to a psychiatrist to rule out a psychotic disorder. The man was previously given a diagnosis of schizophrenia because he "hears voices." He has been prescribed a large dose of an antipsychotic medication, which he takes daily, with very little symptom relief. He states that the medicine helps him sleep. The psychiatrist learns that the man is a survivor of the Cambodian genocide of the 1970s who survived torture under the Khmer Rouge regime, witnessed executions, and endured forced labor in Communist Cambodia. The man reports that subsequent to the extremes of traumatic experience he sustained, he has had chronic symptoms of anxiety with panic attacks. He also reports a concern of "thinking too much." When asked to clarify what he means, he describes ruminating, worried thoughts about his past traumas. He reports severe insomnia and nightmares about Cambodia at night. He describes hearing voices other people do not hear. Further questioning reveals that the voices he hears are of Khmer Rouge officers, and he "hears" them when he is remembering his experiences of violence. When the psychiatrist asks him to clarify this, he says the "voices" are more like memories than hallucinations. What is the likely diagnosis?

    A. Bipolar I disorder, current episode manic.
    B. Panic disorder.
    C. Posttraumatic stress disorder.
    D. Schizophrenia.

58. On which of the following diagnostic frameworks are the DSM-5 and ICD classification systems based?

    A. Binary.
    B. Categorical.
    C. Fuzzy.
    D. Probabilistic.

59. A 62-year-old veteran underwent lung transplantation for idiopathic pulmonary fibrosis 6 months ago. His postoperative course has been complicated by a prolonged stay in the intensive care unit, renal insufficiency dependent on dialysis, atrial fibrillation, pneumonia, and severe deconditioning. He has difficulty working on his strengthening with physical therapy because he becomes anxious and worries about his perceived shortness of breath. He frequently asks to avoid or postpone these sessions and has been described as noncooperative with his treatment. This behavior, in turn, impedes his recovery. On

evaluation by psychiatry, the patient denies depressed mood, reports enjoying visits from his family and watching the news, and is hopeful about his recovery. What is the likely diagnosis?

A. Adjustment disorder.
B. Generalized anxiety disorder.
C. Posttraumatic stress disorder.
D. Psychological factors affecting other medical condition.

60. A 67-year-old man has been living by himself for decades in an apartment, but his daughter is concerned about his safety there. His rooms are stacked to the ceilings with items such as books and souvenirs, to the point that he cannot move around without shifting items. She worries that he may trip and fall in the apartment and has offered to help discard items; however, he finds it distressing to remove anything because he thinks everything will be of use to him someday. He denies any anxiety with his current living situation and prefers that it remain this way. What is the likely diagnosis?

A. Delusional disorder.
B. Generalized anxiety disorder.
C. Hoarding disorder.
D. Obsessive-compulsive personality disorder.

61. A 76-year-old widowed, retired history professor comes to the clinic with his daughter to seek help for his memory difficulties, which started about 3 years ago and have progressed gradually. He stopped driving 6 months ago after being involved in a car accident. He recently moved in with his daughter, and she has been taking him to appointments, managing his finances, and attending to his care. A recent brain CT scan shows cortical atrophy and ventricular enlargement. His thyroid-stimulating hormone and B_{12} levels are within normal limits. His daughter starts crying while reporting that he has had many verbal disagreements with her. Lately he has been accusing her of controlling him and becomes very agitated. What is the likely diagnosis?

A. Delirium.
B. Intermittent explosive disorder.
C. Major neurocognitive disorder due to Alzheimer's disease.
D. Major neurocognitive disorder with Lewy bodies.

62. A diagnosis of conduct disorder, childhood-onset type, has been associated with preceding which of the following disorders?

A. Antisocial personality disorder.
B. Attention-deficit/hyperactivity disorder.
C. Narcissistic personality disorder.
D. Oppositional defiant disorder.

63.   A doctor sees a middle-aged homeless man who was admitted to the medical
        unit 24 hours earlier for a workup of heart failure. The man has received ap-
        propriate medication for his heart but reports puzzling symptoms unrelated to
        his cardiac condition, such as feeling very dysphoric, with nausea and vomit-
        ing, muscle aches, and insomnia overnight. On physical exam, the man is
        sweating profusely, and his pupils are dilated. He keeps asking the nurse for
        "morphine for pain." At admission he was positive for opioids. What is the
        likely diagnosis?

        A. Alcohol withdrawal.
        B. Factitious disorder.
        C. Opioid intoxication.
        D. Opioid withdrawal.

64.   A husband brings his 35-year-old wife to a psychiatrist because he thinks she
        has been buying a lot of jewelry over the past few years. In private, she admits
        that she stole all her jewelry from department stores. She describes feeling ex-
        cited by the prospect of stealing and then gratified after each theft. She denies
        hallucinations or mood disturbances or any other motives for acquiring the
        jewelry. She denies any distress associated with the desire to steal or the act of
        theft. On exam, her thought process is linear with fluent, normal speech, and
        no evidence of psychomotor agitation. She denies any problems with sleep.
        What is the likely diagnosis?

        A. Bipolar I disorder.
        B. Delusional disorder.
        C. Kleptomania.
        D. Obsessive-compulsive disorder.

65.   A man brings his 35-year-old wife, who has a history of previous psychiatric
        hospitalizations, to the emergency department because of her unusual behav-
        ior. He states that she just spent $3,000 on a shopping spree. She speaks anima-
        tedly and loudly: "I just remembered all these things I wanted to buy!" She
        looks down at her hand and says, "I need *this* ring on my finger for good luck."
        She has been sleeping 5 hours per night, and her days are "packed with events,
        booked from morning to evening!" She describes her mood as "stressed" and
        her affect is labile. Her mental status examination is notable for a slender,
        well-groomed woman with meticulous makeup and good eye contact. She is
        cooperative on interview, but is difficult to interrupt. Her thought process is
        occasionally tangential, and her speech is fluent, with rapid rate. She denies
        any hallucinations. There is no evidence of psychomotor abnormalities or neu-
        rological deficits. Her urine toxicology screen is negative for illicit substances.
        What is the likely diagnosis?

        A. Bipolar I disorder.
        B. Borderline personality disorder.
        C. Obsessive-compulsive disorder.
        D. Schizophrenia.

66. A man with schizophrenia manifests a failure to express feelings either verbally or nonverbally, even when talking about issues that would be expected to engage the emotions. His expressive gestures are very limited, and there is little animation in his facial expression or vocal inflections. Which term best describes the man's affect?

    A. Blunt.
    B. Depressed.
    C. Inappropriate.
    D. Labile.

67. A mother brings her 6-year-old son to the pediatrician because of difficulty at school. His mathematical abilities are below his grade level, but he is otherwise an average student in all his other classes. His mother denies any problems with hyperactivity or impulsivity, and he is social with peers at school. He does not have behavioral problems at school, and his teachers say he is a pleasant and attentive student. He met all his developmental milestones appropriately. What is the likely diagnosis?

    A. Attention-deficit/hyperactivity disorder.
    B. Autism spectrum disorder.
    C. Global developmental delay.
    D. Specific learning disorder.

68. Which developmental stage represents the usual time of onset of pedophilic disorder in males?

    A. Childhood.
    B. Late life.
    C. Middle age.
    D. Puberty.

69. A mother who recently moved to a new area brings her 6-year-old son for evaluation by a pediatrician. She worries that he is having diarrhea because she finds stool stains on his underwear. She is not sure how often he goes to the bathroom or the nature of his stools because for many years she has worked two to three jobs and has had to leave him in day care centers. On exam, he is shy and avoidant of social interaction but appears to have no developmental delay with respect to cognition and language. The pediatrician notes a hard golf ball–sized structure on the patient's left abdomen on deep palpation. What is the likely diagnosis?

    A. Conduct disorder.
    B. Encopresis.
    C. Enuresis.
    D. Mental retardation.

70.   A woman brings her 45-year-old husband to a neurologist for "memory and behavior" problems. She states that for the past several years, he has been alternately dependent or hostile toward her, as if he were two distinct individuals. When he is dependent, he follows her around everywhere, like a child. When he is hostile, he ignores her and will curse at her if she asks him to do household chores. He also tells her to call him by a different name. Each phase lasts for months at a time. He has forgotten important details of his childhood, such as the names of his parents and the town where he grew up. His wife denies that he uses any alcohol or other substances and denies that he has a history of seizures or sleep disturbances. She has not noticed any impulsive or unsafe behaviors. On exam, the man is silent and stares blankly at the wall, without evidence of psychomotor abnormalities. He responds very briefly to questions but denies any hallucinations, changes in mood, or elevated anxiety. A thorough workup including CT and electroencephalography testing fails to reveal any clear neurological abnormalities. What is the likely diagnosis?

       A. Bipolar I disorder.
       B. Dissociative identity disorder.
       C. Major depressive disorder with psychotic features.
       D. Schizophrenia.

71.   A mother brings her 15-year-old daughter to a psychiatrist's office. The mother says that for the past year, her daughter has not said a word to her teachers. With her family members or friends, however, she is very talkative and engaging, without any speech impairments or language abnormalities. The mother notes that her daughter met all developmental milestones appropriately and reached puberty at age 14. She never had to repeat a grade in school, although her grades this year are faltering because she does not speak in class. She is otherwise attentive and does well on homework. The mother denies any impulsive behavior. The patient does not speak to the psychiatrist when addressed, but shakes her head no when asked if she has experienced any hallucinations, mood disturbances, or traumatic episodes in her past. She sits patiently in her chair, smiling, without any fidgeting or unusual movements. What is the likely diagnosis?

       A. Attention-deficit/hyperactivity disorder.
       B. Autism spectrum disorder.
       C. Schizophrenia.
       D. Selective mutism.

72.   A plastic surgeon refers a 22-year-old hairdresser with no known history of mental illness to a psychiatrist. She underwent facial reconstruction and other surgeries after a disfiguring fire at her salon. When she was seen at a 1-year follow-up appointment, the exam room mirror alarmed her. She said that she "felt apart from" her body and was markedly distressed. She described the sensation as disabling because it occurs often at work. However, she is not able to

clearly characterize her symptoms, aside from feeling "outside" herself. Aside from emotional distress from her symptoms, she has intact reality testing ability. What is the likely diagnosis?

A. Acute stress disorder.
B. Conversion disorder (functional neurological symptom disorder).
C. Depersonalization/derealization disorder.
D. Dissociative amnesia with dissociative fugue.

73. A young man comes to the clinic. He is a 26-year-old veteran who previously was involved in combat in the Middle East, where he was exposed to a few explosions. Since he returned about 4 months ago, he has had difficulty sleeping and has experienced frequent nightmares. He has avoided going out, because any loud noise startles him, disturbs him significantly, and brings back memories of the explosions. He sees himself as a failure and believes that he was not strong enough to tolerate combat. When his friends have approached him, their comments and jokes irritate him, and he isolates himself more. He has not been able to concentrate well and failed to pass the online courses he had been taking for his college degree. His mother has become increasingly concerned and encouraged him to come to the clinic. What is the likely diagnosis?

A. Acute stress disorder.
B. Adjustment disorder.
C. Posttraumatic stress disorder.
D. Social anxiety disorder.

74. A primary care physician refers a 45-year-old married man to a psychiatrist for evaluation of his anxiety. The patient explains that he worries that there is something seriously wrong within his abdomen but that his primary care doctor has not been able to identify it. He shares that he has had intermittent pain in his abdominal area. Although physical exam, laboratory work, endoscopy, imaging, and expert consultation have not revealed abnormalities, he is worried that his pain is a sign of cancer that is being missed. He relays lifelong concerns about his health. His wife shares that he is always hypervigilant about any signs of illness, and she embarrassingly chuckles that their primary care doctor "must be a very patient man" because her husband constantly e-mails and calls him with various concerns. She describes her husband as an overall healthy man. The patient denies feeling depressed but again states how anxious he is that something serious is being missed. What is the likely diagnosis?

A. Body dysmorphic disorder.
B. Generalized anxiety disorder.
C. Illness anxiety disorder.
D. Somatic symptom disorder.

75. A wife brings her husband, a 55-year-old man who has chronic conditions of diabetes, obesity, and hypercholesterolemia, to his primary care doctor. She is upset that her husband has no energy to go on outings with her and that he is

always tired; she says that even though he would like to do things with the family, he consistently declines to do so. She gave him her own prescription for sleeping medication ("I know I should not do that! I was just hoping it would help us!"), but all that she noticed afterwards is that he snored "more than usual." She is worried about the well-being of their marriage, given her husband's changes. The man notes that he is interested in life, their marriage, going out to dinner, and so on, but he does not know why he feels so exhausted. What is the likely diagnosis?

A. Adjustment disorder.
B. Anorexia.
C. Major depressive disorder.
D. Obstructive sleep apnea hypopnea.

76. A woman brings her 73-year-old father to the hospital because she is extremely concerned that he has virtually no memory of the day's events. He cannot recall where he has been or what he has done. Which additional piece of information would be more consistent with a diagnosis of dissociative amnesia than neurocognitive disorders?

A. He cannot name the current president.
B. He has a hand tremor and slowing on rapid-alternating-movements testing.
C. He has extensive history of chronic alcohol use.
D. He was the victim of a mugging that morning.

77. What term best describes a person's mental status when he or she is responsive to external stimuli but is unable to stay awake?

A. Agitated.
B. Comatose.
C. Delirious.
D. Lethargic.

78. A woman takes her 32-year-old roommate, who has a history of migraines, to the hospital after the roommate experienced sudden-onset blindness in both eyes. Her last migraine was 1 month ago, and she was not experiencing any headache symptoms at the time of exam. The preliminary visual exam revealed no blink to visual threat in either eye. The woman was unable to describe colors or identify people standing near her bed. Her CT and MRI were normal, and a cerebral vascular accident was ruled out. Ophthalmological exam revealed no abnormal findings. The blindness persisted for 3 days, during which time she was hospitalized. Further discussion with medical providers revealed that her boyfriend broke up with her the night before admission. What is the likely diagnosis?

A. Conversion disorder (functional neurological symptom disorder).
B. Dissociative identity disorder.

C. Major depressive disorder.

D. Somatic symptom disorder.

79. An 18-year-old single mother presents to the clinic after 6 weeks of low mood and trouble sleeping. At first, she attributed her poor sleep to getting up every 2 hours to feed her 8-week-old daughter, but more recently her mother has been caring for the baby at night. Despite this, the patient reports continuing poor sleep, with low energy and poor concentration. She is less interested in leaving the house and seeing others and less excited about playing with her daughter. She is not very interested in eating but pushes herself to eat, "because I want to make good milk for the baby." She denies wanting to harm herself or others and feels that, with her mother's help, she is able to care for the baby well. What is the likely diagnosis?

    A. Bipolar I disorder, current episode depressed, with peripartum onset.

    B. Major depressive disorder, unspecified.

    C. Major depressive disorder, with peripartum onset.

    D. Persistent depressive disorder.

80. Police arrest a 21-year-old man for arson, and a psychiatrist evaluates him in jail. On interview, the man describes having had an intense fascination with fire since his teenage years. He feels excited whenever he lights matches and enjoys watching the flames "dance" before him. He denies a history of unstable relationships, getting into fights, or deceiving others. He denies any suicidal or homicidal ideation, attempts, or gestures. His record shows no other legal charges besides arson. He denies hallucinations or unstable mood, and his thought process is linear. What is the likely diagnosis?

    A. Borderline personality disorder.

    B. Conduct disorder.

    C. Delusional disorder.

    D. Pyromania.

81. For which of the following DSM-5 diagnoses is there a far greater prevalence in men than women?

    A. Depersonalization/derealization disorder.

    B. Exhibitionistic disorder.

    C. Major depressive disorder.

    D. Narcolepsy.

82. A young woman, age 21, is a talented sophomore at a prestigious college, where she lives in a dormitory. She describes herself as "shy" and "slow to warm up" in social situations. She used to drink one or two cans of beer on social occasions. She found that drinking alcohol reduced her anxiety, so she started taking her "social lubricant" before most social events. After a difficult breakup with her boyfriend about 15 months ago, she began drinking larger

amounts of alcohol to "forget him." She has become irritable and impatient with friends and lost many of them. Her mother found empty bottles of hard liquor in her room during a visit and confronted her. The daughter exploded and yelled at her mother but finally admitted that alcohol was contributing to her erratic behavior and promised to cut back. Despite her efforts, she has found it difficult to reduce her drinking. Every night, she decides to drink only one beer but craves more and eventually ends up drinking a few shots as well and fails to do her schoolwork. She has been skipping her morning classes because she feels sick and has to have a drink to prevent shaking, sweating, and anxiety. She has also stopped hiking with friends on the weekends, because she worries that she may start shaking in the middle of a hike. Once, she fell off her bike while she was drunk and broke her wrist. Her grades have started to deteriorate. An instructor asked her to see a doctor after he became aware of her drinking behavior. What is the likely diagnosis?

A. Adjustment disorder.
B. Alcohol intoxication.
C. Alcohol use disorder.
D. Alcohol withdrawal.

83.   A mother brought her 12-year-old son to the clinic. He is a pleasant student who has developed difficulty staying awake in class for the past 6 months. He is very upset that no matter how much he tries, he suddenly becomes very sleepy, even during his favorite classes, and then falls asleep and naps. He feels refreshed after these naps but feels embarrassed when other students laugh at him or when teachers notice these episodes, which happen at least three times per week. His parents ensure that he goes to sleep at a regular time and sleeps for at least 8 hours, but this regularity has not helped with his lapses into sleep during the day. Recently, he started having episodes where he suddenly loses muscle tone and falls but remains conscious. These falls usually happen when he is excited or laughs. He has had a few such falls over the past month. Last time, it happened when he got very excited because his school's basketball team won the state championship, and he felt very embarrassed in front of his classmates. He has begun avoiding social events at school because he is worried he may have one of these falls. The extensive neurological and cardiac workups were unrevealing. The nocturnal sleep polysomnography shows rapid eye movement (REM) sleep latency of less than 15 minutes. What is the likely diagnosis?

A. Circadian rhythm sleep-wake disorder.
B. Narcolepsy.
C. Non–rapid eye movement sleep arousal disorder.
D. Rapid eye movement sleep behavior disorder.

84.   Concerned parents bring a 33-year-old man to the psychiatrist. He appears to be his stated age, with erythematous face and holding his reddened and chapped hands away from his body. He takes a few minutes to adjust into the seat. He appears very embarrassed during the evaluation as he shares his story.

He describes being very concerned about getting sick from the germs in the environment. This concern translates into frequent hand washing and showering. He explains that he has a particular ritual for these grooming procedures and that if he feels that he made a mistake, he has to repeat the whole procedure from the start. He spends approximately 5 hours per day on his grooming rituals. He also shares that things in his room have to be in a particular order; otherwise, he feels very uncomfortable and thus spends significant time readjusting these items. Moreover, when driving, he frequently worries that he ran over someone, and he has to go back to make sure that no body is lying on the ground. This worry has led him to avoid driving. He realizes that his concerns are irrational but cannot stop his rituals because they help with the significant anxiety that accompanies his troubling thoughts. He has not worked for the past 5 years because his rituals and worries caused him to be late and inefficient at his job. He currently lives with and is supported by his parents. He finally agreed to come in for an evaluation at their urging. What is the likely diagnosis?

A. Generalized anxiety disorder.
B. Obsessive-compulsive disorder.
C. Obsessive-compulsive personality disorder.
D. Panic disorder.

85.   Women account for more than 90% of the diagnoses for which of the following disorders?

A. Bulimia nervosa.
B. Major depressive disorder.
C. Obsessive-compulsive disorder.
D. Schizophrenia.

86.   A mother brings her 11-year-old daughter for assessment. The girl's teachers are uncertain whether she should advance to the next grade level. She enjoys doing math problems and is always enthusiastic when doing experiments in the science lab. However, in English and history class, she seems like a very different student. She sits in the back of the classroom, looking distracted, and avoids reading out loud when asked. When she does read aloud, her reading lacks fluidity and is often peppered with inaccuracies. Her reading comprehension test results show that she is well below grade-level expectation. She does not make spelling mistakes in her homework assignments. What is the likely diagnosis?

A. Specific learning disorder.
B. Specific learning disorder, with impairment in mathematics.
C. Specific learning disorder, with impairment in reading.
D. Specific learning disorder, with impairment in written expression.

87.   DSM-5 assigned to new diagnostic classes some diagnoses that DSM-IV in-
       cluded in disorders usually first diagnosed in infancy, childhood, or adoles-
       cence. Which of the following statements is correct regarding these changes?

       A. Selective mutism was added to anxiety disorders.
       B. Selective mutism was added to depressive disorders.
       C. Separation anxiety disorder was added to dissociative disorders.
       D. Separation anxiety disorder was added to schizophrenia spectrum and
          other psychotic disorders.

88.   Each week a 52-year-old woman bakes bread using the recipe and techniques
       taught to her by her grandmother. She describes this behavior as an important
       "ritual" in her life. When does this behavior become a symptom that would ap-
       propriately be considered a part of a diagnostic assessment?

       A. At all times this behavior should be considered a symptom.
       B. At no time should this behavior be considered a symptom.
       C. When engaging in this behavior is no longer of interest or is distressing to her.
       D. When engaging in this behavior is very time consuming for her.

89.   A 21-year-old college student is preoccupied with the appearance of her nose.
       She has a small, 0.2-cm soft tissue nodule from a biking accident many years
       ago, but the area is well healed. She feels it is a serious flaw on her face, how-
       ever, and is thinking about plastic surgery to correct the defect. She is con-
       cerned about dating anyone as long as she has this nodule on her nose,
       although she continues to enjoy spending time with friends. She denies any
       pain or discomfort, and she has no concerns about her body weight, which is
       average for her height. She continues to bike the same route daily at school.
       What is the likely diagnosis?

       A. Anorexia.
       B. Body dysmorphic disorder.
       C. Posttraumatic stress disorder.
       D. Somatic symptom disorder.

90.   Which statement is correct regarding the World Health Organization Disability
       Assessment Schedule 2.0 included in DSM-5?

       A. The scale assesses only the three most important domains of hallucinations,
          delusions, and disorganized speech.
       B. The scale is based on symptoms experienced by the patient in the previous
          30 days.
       C. The scale is most accurate if patients, rather than clinicians, provide the re-
          sponses.
       D. The scale should only be completed if the clinician is certain of the symp-
          tom severity.

91.   A mother reports that her son, who is now in first grade, has not seemed to fit in with his classmates since he was in kindergarten. He has a difficult time fully engaging in conversations with them. Instead, he seems to talk "at" them. For example, in a monotone voice he persistently shares elaborate and detailed information about his favorite subject, classic cars, even when the other children are very disinterested. Although this child met all motor milestones appropriately, he often exhibits a repetitive behavior of stacking his cars in a line. He does not have auditory problems. What is the likely diagnosis?

   A. Autism spectrum disorder.
   B. Global developmental delay.
   C. Language disorder.
   D. Social anxiety disorder (social phobia).

92.   An 8-year-old boy wets the bed approximately 2 nights a week. He has been invited to a weeklong summer sleep-away camp but feels afraid to go because of his bed-wetting. He is particularly upset because he did not have this problem last year. He feels a little less embarrassed when he finds out that his dad had the same problem when he was a boy. His father moved out of the home last year after marital separation. The boy does not take any medications and has no known medical problems. What is the likely diagnosis?

   A. Encopresis.
   B. Enuresis, diurnal only.
   C. Enuresis, nocturnal and diurnal.
   D. Enuresis, nocturnal only.

93.   Police arrest a 26-year-old man for smashing the windows of a coworker's car after an argument at work. The man's wife says that he has a history of destroying property or items of value when provoked, in a manner that is "extreme" as compared to the magnitude of the inciting trigger or event. He denies any history of head trauma, difficulty with attention, depressed or labile mood, restlessness, or any problems with sleep or appetite. When he is not provoked, he is calm and pleasant. He denies any alcohol or substance use, and his wife corroborates this information. There is no evidence of fidgeting or psychomotor agitation on exam. What is the likely diagnosis?

   A. Attention-deficit/hyperactivity disorder.
   B. Bipolar I disorder.
   C. Intermittent explosive disorder.
   D. Panic disorder.

94.   A 66-year-old moderately obese man has a long history of hypertension. He is seen by his primary care physician for a follow-up appointment after his second stroke, which happened about 2 months ago. He reports that the weakness in his right leg is improving with physical therapy, but he has had difficulty finding his way back from the rehabilitation center, which is only a few blocks from his home. His wife reports that after her husband's first stroke, which

happened about 2 years ago, he started having memory difficulties. The man used to enjoy playing chess with his grandchildren, but his memory deteriorated so significantly after his second stroke that he is unable to play and even forgets their names frequently. The man is pleasant, articulates words well, but shows significant difficulty finding words. He is not oriented to time, performs poorly in calculation, and is unable to name familiar objects, such as a pen or watch. While the clinician reviews the man's medications, the man shows significant difficulty remembering the medications' names and instructions. He appears frustrated and asks for a pen to write down the instructions. What is the likely diagnosis?

A. Delirium.
B. Major neurocognitive disorder due to Alzheimer's disease.
C. Major neurocognitive disorder due to another medical condition.
D. Major vascular neurocognitive disorder.

95.   Match each description with the paraphilic disorder for which it is most highly characteristic (each disorder may be used once, more than once, or not at all):

A. Exhibitionistic disorder.
B. Fetishistic disorder.
C. Pedophilic disorder.
D. Sexual sadism disorder.
E. Voyeuristic disorder.

_____ Involves exposing one's genitalia to unsuspecting people.
_____ Involves intense sexual arousal from observing an unsuspecting person disrobing or being naked.
_____ Involves intense sexual arousal from prepubescent children.
_____ Involves intense sexual arousal from the significant physical or psychological suffering of another person.

96.   A 34-month-old boy rarely initiates eye contact with his mother and does not seem to engage in play with other children in his peer group at day care. At times, he behaves aggressively toward the other children. He is only minimally communicative with speech but, when vocal, is prone to repetitively use only single words. He gets very upset when his mother varies his morning clothing routine, always insisting, for example, that she put on his right sock first, before any other piece of clothing. What is the likely diagnosis?

A. Autism spectrum disorder.
B. Global developmental delay.
C. Intellectual disability (intellectual developmental disorder).
D. Major depressive disorder.

97. Using the DSM-5 criteria to "diagnose" celebrities on the basis of media reports is not considered ethically acceptable in the profession for many reasons, but especially for which reason?

    A. Celebrities do not like to be diagnosed.
    B. DSM-5 diagnostic criteria do not apply to celebrities.
    C. DSM-5 diagnostic criteria rely on information gathered through a comprehensive evaluation.
    D. Media do not accurately portray celebrities.

98. A mother has learned during a conference with her 6-year-old son's teacher that her son tends to blurt out answers when students are asked to raise their hands. Also, he often intrudes on other children's activities during playtime, which has caused some disputes with his classmates. The mother notes that he often forgets to bring home his schoolwork. In addition, he often willingly starts a chore around the house, such as cleaning his room, but often switches to another activity and fails to finish the original task. What is the likely diagnosis?

    A. Attention-deficit/hyperactivity disorder.
    B. Obsessive-compulsive disorder.
    C. Oppositional defiant disorder.
    D. Tourette's disorder.

99. Match each description with the personality disorder for which it is most highly characteristic (each disorder may be used once, more than once, or not at all):

    A. Avoidant personality disorder.
    B. Paranoid personality disorder.
    C. Schizoid personality disorder.
    D. Schizotypal personality disorder.

    _____ Behavior that is odd, eccentric, or peculiar, with odd beliefs or magical thinking that influence behavior and are inconsistent with cultural norms.
    _____ Neither desires nor enjoys close relationships, with emotional coldness, detachment, or flattened affective responses to others.
    _____ Suspects that others are exploiting or deceiving him or her, and persistently bears a grudge against others for perceived insults or slights.

100.   Match each term with the correct definition (each term may be used once, more
       than once, or not at all):

       A. Agnosia.
       B. Anhedonia.
       C. Aphasia.
       D. Apraxia.

       ____ Problems in comprehending language despite intact sensory function.
       ____ Problems in performing purposeful motor activities despite intact motor
            function.
       ____ Problems in producing language despite intact motor function.
       ____ Problems in recognizing objects despite intact sensory function.

101.   A 29-year-old graduate student is accompanied by her parents for an initial ap-
       pointment with a psychiatrist. The student reports that her boyfriend broke up
       with her 2 months ago, and she continues to feel devastated. She immediately
       moved back into her parents' home for support. Her parents are used to this,
       she says, because "this happens all the time." Her parents help her with every-
       thing, including choosing her clothes each morning, washing her laundry, and
       making all of her meals. They recall, "Her boyfriends would always pay her
       bills and even choose her friends for her. She has never made it on her own."
       Despite their concerns, in many ways her parents like having her at home be-
       cause she is always agreeable and respectful. She even volunteers to scrub all
       the bathrooms from top to bottom; she says, "Whatever I have to do so they will
       let me stay there until I find a new boyfriend." What is the likely diagnosis?

       A. Avoidant personality disorder.
       B. Borderline personality disorder.
       C. Dependent personality disorder.
       D. Generalized anxiety disorder.

102.   A young girl is in second grade. Last year her paternal grandfather died from
       cancer. Since then her parents have become increasingly concerned about her.
       Last week a babysitter said that the girl sat staring at the front door almost the
       entire night, waiting for her parents to return from their date night. Their
       daughter keeps asking to stay home from school. She pleads for her mother to
       stay home with her, stating, "I do not want you to drive to work. What if you
       get in an accident? Just stay home with me." Before she goes to bed at night,
       she complains of headaches, which only seem to subside if she sleeps in her
       parents' room. They have stopped allowing her to sleep in their room, but
       some mornings they find her sleeping in the hallway right outside their bed-
       room door. She refuses to attend sleepovers with friends because she always
       feels "sick" while she is there. What is the likely diagnosis?

       A. Major depressive disorder.
       B. Panic disorder and agoraphobia.
       C. Separation anxiety disorder.
       D. Social anxiety disorder.

103. Partners in a long-term affectionate and intimate relationship have recently begun to "experiment" with wearing costumes with especially soft fabrics and engaging in role-play during their sexual encounters. They are enjoying this practice and find that it enriches their sexual life together. Does this pattern meet criteria for fetishistic disorder?

    A. No, because neither partner is experiencing distress.
    B. No, because soft fabrics do not represent a fetishistic object.
    C. Yes, because role-playing represents a fetish.
    D. Yes, because this "experimentation" is new.

104. For a diagnosis of bipolar I disorder, an individual must have experienced in the past which of the following events, even if the event was not formally documented or diagnosed and did not lead to an episode of clinical care?

    A. Depressive episode.
    B. Head injury.
    C. Manic episode.
    D. Psychological trauma.

105. Police bring a woman to the hospital after they find her in an alley behind a restaurant. She appears to be in her late 20s. She cannot say who she is or where she lives. When asked what she was doing earlier, she recounts a reasonable story about having dinner at a restaurant and then having a few drinks. However, she looks worn, as though she has been living on the streets and exposed to the elements for hours or days. She is negative for alcohol and drugs on laboratory testing. Aside from mild dehydration, she is medically stable. Physical exam shows no neurological abnormalities. Finally, staff members find in her belongings an employee identification card from a mall where a shooting occurred 2 days earlier. When asked about that event, she has no recollection of it and seems unbothered. Her speech is clear and fluent, and she denies any perceptual changes. Police match her to a missing person report that her mother placed the previous day. What is the likely diagnosis?

    A. Bipolar I disorder.
    B. Depersonalization/derealization disorder.
    C. Dissociative amnesia with dissociative fugue.
    D. Schizophrenia.

106. Police arrest a 26-year-old man who got into a fight in a bar after he was discovered in the act of stealing the wallet of another customer. He defended his behavior to the police, stating that the other man had provoked him earlier in the evening by calling him a profane name. Review of his criminal record reveals charges, including some as a minor, for credit card fraud and selling cocaine. He lives alone and is currently unemployed. He has no psychiatric history. He does not report any recent hallucinations or changes in his mood or sleep. What is the likely diagnosis?

A. Antisocial personality disorder.
B. Conduct disorder.
C. Moderate cocaine use disorder.
D. Narcissistic personality disorder.

107. A 37-year-old single mother divorced her husband about 8 months ago and has custody of their two daughters. She went back to work full-time "to make ends meet." About 2 months ago, while at work, she began to feel extremely anxious. Within a few minutes, she had heart palpitations and difficulty breathing and almost fainted. Her coworkers rushed her to the hospital. A thorough medical workup was performed and no underlying medical cause was identified. Within 1 week, she had another attack at the local grocery store and felt embarrassed because she had to lie down on the floor for about 10 minutes while she was surrounded by the store's concerned customers until the symptoms subsided. She has had two other "freak outs" in different situations. She has constant concern that the problem will "happen again." She has been skipping meetings at work to avoid embarrassment in front of her coworkers in case she "goes crazy" again. What is the likely diagnosis?

A. Generalized anxiety disorder.
B. Panic disorder.
C. Social anxiety disorder (social phobia).
D. Specific phobia.

108. A child is struggling in second grade. Her teacher called her parents for a conference due to concerns that she has become forgetful in class, is often seen to be daydreaming, and has serious difficulty following multistep directions. Her mother noted that "in second grade there is some real homework and she cannot sit down and focus on doing it. Half the time she even forgets it at home in the morning." Her teacher recalls careless errors on simple mathematics assignments. The child's father reminds them, "She has been this way for years. You cannot get her to focus, even if it is on making her bed or brushing her teeth." What is the likely diagnosis?

A. Attention-deficit/hyperactivity disorder, predominantly hyperactive-impulsive presentation.
B. Attention-deficit/hyperactivity disorder, predominantly inattentive presentation.
C. Conduct disorder.
D. Major depressive disorder.

109. Which statement is correct regarding the depressive disorders diagnostic class of DSM-5 in comparison with earlier versions of DSM?

A. Brief depressive disorder has been added as a new diagnosis.
B. Disruptive mood dysregulation disorder has been eliminated as a diagnosis.
C. Persistent depressive disorder has been eliminated as a diagnosis.
D. Premenstrual dysphoric disorder has been added as a new diagnosis.

110. The hematology service requests a psychiatric consult for a 45-year-old woman with generalized bruising. The hematology team cannot find a cause for her physical findings, which have led to three hospital admissions in the past 5 months. The patient is a nurse at the hospital. On interview she is very tearful. Bruising is predominantly circumferential on her arms and legs, with none on her face or torso. She does have some venipuncture marks on her abdomen, however, as well as a wristband from another hospital. She appreciates the consult but asks the psychiatrist to leave when her ex-husband comes for his daily visit to watch videos of their daughter. She explains that they lost their daughter to a chronic illness at age 8. What is the likely diagnosis?

    A. Conversion disorder (functional neurological symptom disorder).
    B. Factitious disorder.
    C. Malingering.
    D. Somatic symptom disorder.

111. The neurology department refers a 39-year-old woman to psychiatry because she has been experiencing tonic-clonic movements of extremities without loss of consciousness for the past 2 months. An extensive neurological workup has been performed and no abnormalities are evident. The patient is cooperative throughout the session but shows restricted range of affect. Her husband says that she has been under treatment for infertility for many years and miscarried during a much desired pregnancy about 3 months ago. She does not show significant changes in her affect in reaction to this information from her husband. What is the likely diagnosis?

    A. Conversion disorder (functional neurological symptom disorder).
    B. Depressive disorder due to another medical condition.
    C. Factitious disorder.
    D. Somatic symptom disorder.

112. Match each description with the most appropriate diagnosis (each disorder may be used once, more than once, or not at all):

    A. Bipolar I.
    B. Bipolar II.
    C. Cyclothymia.

    ____ Meets criteria for mania.
    ____ Meets criteria for hypomania but not mania.
    ____ Does not meet criteria for hypomania or mania.

113.   A 12-year-old boy feels tired of "standing out so much" at school. Several times a day he feels an uncomfortable sensation in his throat and then feels he "has to" cough or grunt, which temporarily makes the uncomfortable sensation go away. He also repeatedly shrugs his shoulders and stomps his feet at what appear to be random moments throughout the day. The other students no longer make fun of him the way they did when they were younger, but he still feels demoralized because he just wants to fit in with them. What is the likely diagnosis?

   A. Obsessive-compulsive disorder.
   B. Obsessive-compulsive personality disorder.
   C. Persistent motor or vocal tic disorder.
   D. Tourette's disorder.

114.   Match each time criterion with the most appropriate diagnoses (each time criterion may be used once, more than once, or not at all):

   A. Symptoms persist less than 1 month.
   B. Symptoms persist more than 1 month.

   _____ Acute stress disorder.
   _____ Delusional disorder.
   _____ Posttraumatic stress disorder.
   _____ Brief psychotic disorder.

115.   A 19-year-old college student is brought to the psychiatric emergency department by his friends because he had not slept for 4 days, was speaking loudly, felt "exuberant" and "on top of the world," and because he had attempted to lift a car with his "bare hands." He was an avid weight lifter and recently had started taking steroids (purchased "on the streets") to help him "bulk up." What is the most appropriate diagnosis?

   A. Bipolar I.
   B. Bipolar II.
   C. Substance/medication-induced bipolar and related disorder.
   D. Substance/medication-induced psychotic disorder.

———————— ANSWERS ————————

1. B. Echolalia.

2. D. Schizotypal personality disorder.

3. D. Schizophrenia.

4. C. Histrionic personality disorder—Consistently uses physical appearance to draw attention to oneself.

    A. Antisocial personality disorder—Failure to conform to social norms and without remorse.

    B. Borderline personality disorder—Frantic efforts to avoid real or imagined abandonment.

    D. Narcissistic personality disorder—Grandiose sense of self-importance.

    C. Histrionic personality disorder—Self-dramatization, theatricality, and exaggerated expression of emotion.

5. B. More prevalent among women—Restless legs syndrome.

    B. More prevalent among women—Major depressive disorder.

    B. More prevalent among women—Generalized anxiety disorder.

6. B. Illness anxiety disorder.

7. B. Generalized anxiety disorder.

8. D. 1 year.

9. B. Childhood-onset fluency disorder (stuttering).

10. A. Delusion.

11. C. Intellectual disability (intellectual developmental disorder).

12. B. Depressive disorder due to another medical condition.

13. D. Specific phobia.

14. B. Age at onset under 18 years—Tourette's disorder.

    C. Age at onset not specified—Separation anxiety disorder.

    A. Age at onset under 5 years—Global developmental delay.

15. D. Restless legs syndrome.

16.   A.   Depression, fatigue, insomnia.

17.   A.   Obsessive-compulsive disorder.

18.   D.   Social anxiety disorder (social phobia).

19.   B.   Bipolar II disorder.

20.   D.   Schizophrenia.

21.   C.   Major depressive disorder, with peripartum onset.

22.   B.   The scale is based on symptoms experienced by the patient in the previous 7 days.

23.   C.   Major depressive disorder.

24.   D.   Oppositional defiant disorder.

25.   A.   Brief psychotic disorder.

26.   A.   He has lost significant weight and appears emaciated.

27.   D.   Somatic symptom disorder, with predominant pain.

28.   C.   Reactive attachment disorder.

29.   B.   Anxiety disorder due to another medical condition.

30.   B.   Agoraphobia.

31.   B.   The patient has had suicidal thoughts every day for the past 3 weeks, and yesterday she searched "how to kill yourself" on the Internet.

32.   A.   Erectile disorder—Involves inability to attain and maintain arousal.
      C.   Genito-pelvic pain/penetration disorder—Involves inability to have vaginal intercourse or penetration.
      B.   Female orgasmic disorder—Involves inorgasmia or delayed orgasm.
      D.   Premature (early) ejaculation—Involves orgasm before the person desires.

33.   C.   She has been hearing voices for weeks without depressed or elevated mood.

34.   B.   Delusional disorder, grandiose type.

35.   B.   Borderline personality disorder.

36. D. DSM-5 has preserved the same diagnostic criteria as in DSM-IV-TR for personality disorders.

37. B. Culturally appropriate behavior.

38. B. Fetishistic disorder.

39. C. Simple phobia.

40. B. Global developmental delay.

41. A. Compulsion—Repeated behavior that a person feels driven to perform.
    D. Somatization—Repeated expression of psychological issues through physical symptoms, concerns, or complaints.
    C. Phobia—Repeated, irrational, and enduring fear of an object or situation.
    B. Obsession—Repeated thought or image that provokes anxiety.

42. D. Somatic symptom disorder.

43. D. Social anxiety disorder.

44. D. Increased activity or energy has been added as a new core mood elevation symptom.

45. C. REM sleep behavior disorder.

46. D. Gender dysphoria in adolescents and adults.

47. C. Mild neurocognitive disorder due to HIV infection.

48. D. Magical thinking.

49. D. Trichotillomania.

50. D. Moderate cocaine use disorder.

51. B. False positive diagnosis—A woman receives the diagnosis of bipolar disorder, manic phase, when her clinical presentation was actually due to amphetamine intoxication.
    C. True negative diagnosis—An elderly man receives no psychiatric diagnosis 2 months after the death of his wife; he sometimes is tearful and sad and once each week has difficulty sleeping when he thinks of her.

52. A. Major depressive disorder and dissociative identity disorder.

53.   B.   Anorexia—Loss of appetite.
      A.   Anhedonia—Loss of interest or pleasure.
      C.   Cataplexy—Loss of muscle tone, with weakness.
      D.   Catatonia—Loss of response to outside stimuli and muscular rigidity.

54.   C.   Major depressive disorder.

55.   D.   Oppositional defiant disorder.

56.   C.   The paranoid subtype.

57.   C.   Posttraumatic stress disorder.

58.   B.   Categorical.

59.   D.   Psychological factors affecting other medical condition.

60.   C.   Hoarding disorder.

61.   C.   Major neurocognitive disorder due to Alzheimer's disease.

62.   A.   Antisocial personality disorder.

63.   D.   Opioid withdrawal.

64.   C.   Kleptomania.

65.   A.   Bipolar I disorder.

66.   A.   Blunt.

67.   D.   Specific learning disorder.

68.   D.   Puberty.

69.   B.   Encopresis.

70.   B.   Dissociative identity disorder.

71.   D.   Selective mutism.

72.   C.   Depersonalization/derealization disorder.

73.   C.   Posttraumatic stress disorder.

74.   C.   Illness anxiety disorder.

75.   D.   Obstructive sleep apnea hypopnea.

76. D. He was the victim of a mugging that morning.

77. D. Lethargic.

78. A. Conversion disorder (functional neurological symptom disorder).

79. C. Major depressive disorder, with peripartum onset.

80. D. Pyromania.

81. B. Exhibitionistic disorder.

82. C. Alcohol use disorder.

83. B. Narcolepsy.

84. B. Obsessive-compulsive disorder.

85. A. Bulimia nervosa.

86. C. Specific learning disorder, with impairment in reading.

87. A. Selective mutism was added to anxiety disorders.

88. C. When engaging in this behavior is no longer of interest or is distressing to her.

89. B. Body dysmorphic disorder.

90. B. The scale is based on symptoms experienced by the patient in the previous 30 days.

91. A. Autism spectrum disorder.

92. D. Enuresis, nocturnal only.

93. C. Intermittent explosive disorder.

94. D. Major vascular neurocognitive disorder.

95. A. Exhibitionistic disorder—Involves exposing one's genitalia to unsuspecting people.
     E. Voyeuristic disorder—Involves intense sexual arousal from observing an unsuspecting person disrobing or being naked.
     C. Pedophilic disorder—Involves intense sexual arousal from prepubescent children.
     D. Sexual sadism disorder—Involves intense sexual arousal from the significant physical or psychological suffering of another person.

96. A. Autism spectrum disorder.

97. C. DSM-5 diagnostic criteria rely on information gathered through a comprehensive evaluation.

98. A. Attention-deficit/hyperactivity disorder.

99. D. Schizotypal personality disorder—Behavior that is odd, eccentric, or peculiar, with odd beliefs or magical thinking that influence behavior and are inconsistent with cultural norms.

    C. Schizoid personality disorder—Neither desires nor enjoys close relationships, with emotional coldness, detachment, or flattened affective responses to others.

    B. Paranoid personality disorder—Suspects that others are exploiting or deceiving him or her, and persistently bears a grudge against others for perceived insults or slights.

100. C. Aphasia—Problems in comprehending language despite intact sensory function.

    D. Apraxia—Problems in performing purposeful motor activities despite intact motor function.

    C. Aphasia—Problems in producing language despite intact motor function.

    A. Agnosia—Problems in recognizing objects despite intact sensory function.

101. C. Dependent personality disorder.

102. C. Separation anxiety disorder.

103. A. No, because neither partner is experiencing distress.

104. C. Manic episode.

105. C. Dissociative amnesia with dissociative fugue.

106. A. Antisocial personality disorder.

107. B. Panic disorder.

108. B. Attention-deficit/hyperactivity disorder, predominantly inattentive presentation.

109. D. Premenstrual dysphoric disorder has been added as a new diagnosis.

110. B. Factitious disorder.

111. A. Conversion disorder (functional neurological symptom disorder).

112. A. Bipolar I—Meets criteria for mania.

     B. Bipolar II—Meets criteria for hypomania but not mania.

     C. Cyclothymia—Does not meet criteria for hypomania or mania.

113. D. Tourette's disorder.

114. A. Acute stress disorder—Symptoms persist less than 1 month.

     B. Delusional disorder—Symptoms persist more than 1 month.

     B. Posttraumatic stress disorder—Symptoms persist more than 1 month.

     A. Brief psychotic disorder—Symptoms persist less than 1 month.

115. C. Substance/medication-induced bipolar and related disorder.

Index

Page numbers printed in **boldface** *type refer to tables or figures.*